THE DEVELOPING HEART

THE DEVELOPING HEART

Editors

Bohuslav Ošťádal, M.D., C.Sc.
Professor
Institute of Physiology
Academy of Sciences of the Czech Republic
Prague, Czech Republic

Makoto Nagano, M.D., Ph.D.
Professor Emeritus
Jikei University School of Medicine
Tokyo, Japan

Nobuakira Takeda, M.D., Ph.D.
Associate Professor
Department of Internal Medicine
Aoto Hospital
Jikei University School of Medicine
Tokyo, Japan

Naranjan S. Dhalla, Ph.D., M.D. (Hon.)
Distinguished Professor and Director
MRC Group in Experimental Cardiology
Institute of Cardiovascular Sciences
St. Boniface General Hospital Research Centre
Faculty of Medicine, University of Manitoba
Winnipeg, Canada

Lippincott - Raven
PUBLISHERS
Philadelphia • New York

Acquisitions Editor: Ruth W. Weinberg
Developmental Editor: Renee A. Gagliardi
Manufacturing Manager: Dennis Teston
Production Manager: Lawrence Bernstein
Production Editor: Dee Josephson
Cover Designer: Patty Gast
Indexer: Kathy Unger
Compositor: Compset, Inc.
Printer: Maple Press

Printed in the United States of America

9 8 7 6 5 4 3 2 1

Library of Congress Cataloging-in-Publication Data

The developing heart / editors, Bohuslav Ostádal ... [et al.].
p. cm.
Includes bibliographical references and index.
ISBN 0-397-58779-1
1. Heart—Growth—Congresses. I. Ostádal, Bohuslav.
DNLM: 1. Heart—embryology. WG 201 D4884 1997]
QP111.4.D476 1997
612.1'7—dc21
DNLM/DLC
for Library of Congress 96-50463
CIP

Care has been taken to confirm the accuracy of the information presented and to describe generally accepted practices. However, the authors, editors, and publisher are not responsible for errors or omissions or for any consequences from application of the information in this book and make no warranty, express or implied, with respect to the contents of the publication.

The authors, editors, and publisher have exerted every effort to ensure that drug selection and dosage set forth in this text are in accordance with current recommendations and practice at the time of publication. However, in view of ongoing research, changes in government regulations, and the constant flow of information relating to drug therapy and drug reactions, the reader is urged to check the package insert for each drug for any change in indications and dosage and for added warnings and precautions. This is particularly important when the recommended agent is a new or infrequently employed drug.

Some drugs and medical devices presented in this publication have Food and Drug Administration (FDA) clearance for limited use in restricted research settings. It is the responsibility of the health care provider to ascertain the FDA status of each drug or device planned for use in their clinical practice.

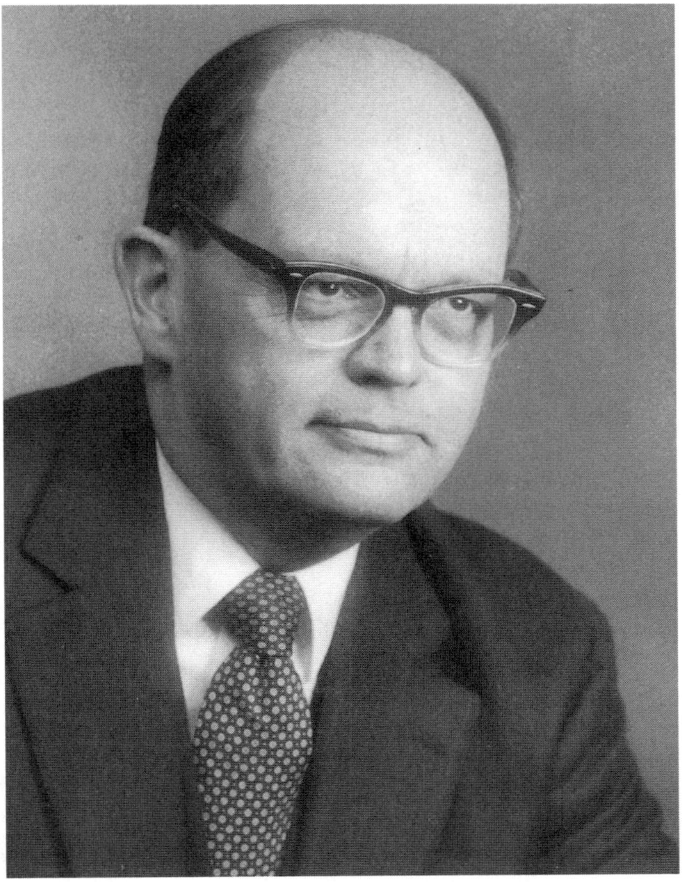

This book is dedicated to Dr. Howard E. Morgan, Senior Vice-President for Research of the Sigfried and Janet Weis Center for Research with the Geisinger Clinic, Danville, Pennsylvania for his superior leadership in the field of molecular and cellular cardiology, his strong commitment to excellence in heart research, his clear vision for blending basic sciences with clinical cardiology, and his deep devotion in helping young cardiovascular scientists to reach their potential.

A TRIBUTE TO HOWARD E. MORGAN, M.D.

Howard E. Morgan, M.D. is Senior Vice-President for Research of the Sigfried and Janet Weis Center for Research with the Geisinger Clinic and is Adjunct Professor of Physiology at Jefferson Medical College. At Geisinger, Dr. Morgan directs a strong program of basic investigation in cardiovascular disease and developmental biology. He has drawn together forty researchers who occupy laboratories in the Sigfried and Janet Weis Center for Research. The research program at Geisinger is named in honor of Henry Hood, M.D., Past President and CEO of Geisinger, who was instrumental in founding the program. Prior to coming to Geisinger, Dr. Morgan was Associate Dean for Research, as well as Evan Pugh and J. Lloyd Huck Professor and Chairman of Physiology at the Milton S. Hershey Medical Center of the Pennsylvania State University. These appointments illustrate his high profile leadership and outstanding ability in creative organization of medical research.

He was educated at the Johns Hopkins School of Medicine from which he received an M.D. in 1949. He completed his internship and residency at Vanderbilt University and held faculty appointments in Vanderbilt's Department of Physiology from 1954 to 1967. While on the faculty of Vanderbilt University, Dr. Morgan became interested in the regulation of heart metabolism. His early studies focus on the metabolism of glucose and glycogen. In association with James R. Neely, Dr. Morgan developed the isolated perfused working heart preparation from adult rats that is used extensively in metabolic studies. In 1967, Dr. Morgan founded the new Department of Physiology at the Milton S. Hershey Medical Center of Penn State University. While at Penn State, he embarked on a program to investigate the regulation of protein turnover in heart muscle. His studies have collectively provided much of the current information on the regulation of protein turnover by hormones, by increased work of the heart, and by metabolic factors. His current research efforts center around unraveling the intracellular signaling systems that are responsible for accelerated growth and hypertrophy of cardiac muscle cells. He has more than 250 scientific publications. His work has been named three times as a "Citation Classic" by Current Contents. That designation acknowledges more than 500 citations in published research for each article. Clearly, the excellence and significance of his research work place him among the greatest experimental cardiologists of this century.

Dr. Morgan served as President of the American Heart Association from 1987–1988 and as President of the International Society for Heart Research from 1983–1986. He served as President of the American Physiological Society from 1985–1986. He was Coordinator of the U.S./U.S.S.R. Exchange Program dealing with cardiovascular biology and medicine for 20 years. He has been serving as Chairman of the Council of Molecular and Cellular Cardiology of the International Society and Federation of Cardiology for the past 5 years.

In addition to serving as editor of *Physiological Reviews* (1973–1978) and *American Journal of Physiology* (Cell Physiology Section: 1981–1984), he has been and/or is on the editorial boards of more than 10 journals in the field of cardiovascular sciences. His commitment to promote the scientific basis of cardiology and young talents in heart research is unparalleled.

Due to excellence in research and strong leadership, Dr. Morgan has received the Award of Merit, the Distinguished Achievement Award, and the Gold Heart Award from the American Heart Association, and Carl J. Wiggers Award and Ray G. Daggs Award from the American Physiological Society. He was given the Peter Harris Award for outstanding contributions to Cardiovascular Research by the International Society for Heart Research. He has been cited for distinguished service by the American Society of Biological Chemists and has been named a Hughes Scholar by the Howard Hughes Medical Institute. He is a fellow of the American Association for the Advancement of Sciences and a member of the Institute of Medicine of the National Academy of Sciences. This global recognition demonstrates the wide-spread admiration and affection in which he is regarded worldwide.

Bohuslav Ošťádal, Prague
Makoto Nagano, Tokyo
Nobuakira Takeda, Tokyo
Naranjan S. Dhalla, Winnipeg

Contents

Development of Excitation-Contraction Coupling

Contributors

Michael Artman, M.D.
Professor of Pediatrics and Physiology
Department of Pediatric Cardiology
Molecular and Cellular Research Laboratories (Tisch 501)
New York University Medical Center
560 First Avenue
New York, New York 10016

Durisamy Balaguru, M.D.
Department of Pediatric Cardiology
Molecular and Cellular Research Laboratories (Tisch 501)
New York University Medical Center
560 First Avenue
New York, New York 10016

Cathy J. Beinlich, Ph.D.
Research Scientist
Sigfried and Janet Weis Center for Research
Geisinger Clinic
100 North Academy Avenue
Danville, Pennsylvania 17822-2601

Sanford P. Bishop, D.V.M., Ph.D.
Professor of Pathology
University of Alabama at Birmingham
1670 University Boulevard
Birmingham, Alabama 35294-0019

Samuel Y. Boateng, B.Sc.
Cardiothoracic Surgery
Imperial College School of Medicine
National Heart and Lung Institute
Dovehouse St.
London SW3 6LY
United Kingdom

Scott R. Boerth, M.D., Ph.D.
Research Associate
Department of Pharmacology
University of South Alabama College of Medicine
2120 Medical Sciences Building
Mobile, Alabama 36688

Kenneth R. Boheler, Ph.D.
Lecturer
Division of Cardiothoracic Surgery
Imperial College School of Medicine
National Heart and Lung Institute
Dovehouse Street
London SW3 6LY
United Kingdom

Nancy T. Brissie
Department of Pathology
University of Alabama at Birmingham
1670 University Boulevard
Birmingham, Alabama 35294-0019

Marco A. de Paula Brotto, C.T. (chemistry technologist), BSN/RN, M.S.
Research Scientist
Institute for Molecular Medicine and Genetics
Department of Cellular Biology and Anatomy and
Heart Development Group
Medical College of Georgia
Augusta, Georgia 30912-2000

Jarrett L. Burch, B.S.
Research Assistant III
Developmental Biology Program
Institute for Molecular Medicine and Genetics
Medical College of Georgia, CA4041B
Augusta, Georgia 30912-2640

Jan Černohorský, Mgr.
Institute of Physiology
Academy of Sciences of the Czech Republic
Videňská 1083
1402 20 Prague 4
Czech Republic

Jane C. Chu, B.A.
Research Assistant IV
Department of Physiology and Endocrinology
Medical College of Georgia
Augusta, Georgia 30912-3000

William A. Coetzee, D.Sc.
Associate Professor
Department of Pediatric Cardiology
Molecular and Cellular Research Laboratories (Tisch 501)
New York University Medical Center
560 First Avenue
New York, New York 10016

Tony L. Creazzo, Ph.D.
Associate Professor
Developmental Biology Program
Institute for Molecular Medicine and Genetics
Medical College of Georgia, CA4004
Augusta, Georgia 30912-2640

Annica Dahlström, M.D.
Professor of Medicine
Department of Anatomy and Cell Biology
Göteborg University
Medicinaregatan 3-5
Göteborg S-41390
Sweden

Naranjan S. Dhalla, M.D., (Hon) Ph.D.
Distinguished Professor and Director
Institute of Cardiovascular Sciences
St. Boniface General Hospital Research Centre
351 Tache Avenue
Winnipeg, Manitoba R2H 2A6
Canada

Ian M. C. Dixon, Ph.D.
Assistant Professor of Physiology
Institute of Cardiovascular Sciences
St. Boniface General Hospital Research Centre
351 Tache Avenue
Winnipeg, Manitoba R2H 2A6
Canada

Zdenka Dobešová, Ph.D.
Institute of Physiology
Academy of Sciences of the Czech Republic
Videnšká 1083
142 20 Prague 4
Czech Republic

Masao Endoh, M.D., Ph.D.
Professor of Pharmacology
Department of Pharmacology
Yamagata University School of Medicine
2-2-2 Iida-Nishi
Yamagata 990-23
Japan

Gary L. Engelmann, Ph.D.
Professor of Medicine and Cell Biology
Cardiovascular Institute
Department of Medicine
Loyola University Chicago Medical Center
Stritch School of Medicine
2160 South First Avenue
Maywood, Illinois 60153

Diego Franco, Ph.D.
Doctor in Biological Sciences
Department of Anatomy and Embryology
Academic Medical Center
University of Amsterdam
Meibergdreef, 15
1105 AZ Amsterdam
The Netherlands

Susan Y. Fu, M.D., Ph.D.
Post-Doctoral Fellow
Department of Biochemistry
University of Alberta
424 Heritage Medical Research Centre
Edmonton, Alberta T6G 2S2
Canada

Robert E. Godt, Ph.D.
Professor
Department of Physiology and Endocrinology
Medical College of Georgia
Augusta, Georgia 30912-3000

Shyamal K. Goswami, Ph.D.
Research Assistant Professor
Department of Anatomy and Cell Biology
State University of New York
Health Science Center at Brooklyn
Brooklyn, New York 11203

Patricia S. Grutkoski, B.A.
Graduate Student
Cardiovascular Institute
Department of Medicine
Loyola University Chicago Medical Center
2160 South First Avenue
Maywood, Illinois 60153

Peter S. Haddock, Ph.D.
Research Assistant Professor
Department of Pediatric Cardiology
New York University Medical Center
560 First Avenue
New York, New York 10016

Jacqueline E. Hance
Graduate Student
Department of Biochemistry
University of Alberta
424 Heritage Medical Research Centre
Edmonton, Alberta T6G 2S2
Canada

Marcia I. Heron, Ph.D.
Post-Doctoral Fellow
Cardiovascular Institute
Department of Medicine
Loyola University Chicago Medical Center
2160 South First Avenue
Maywood, Illinois 60153-5589

Robert J. Hoeschen, M.D., FRCP(C)
Professor of Medicine
Faculty of Medicine
University of Manitoba
St. Boniface General Hospital
409 Tache Avenue
Winnipeg, Manitoba R2H 2A6
Canada

Charlene M. Hohl, Ph.D.
Department of Medical Biochemistry
Ohio State University
333 Hamilton Hall
1645 Neil Avenue
Columbus, Ohio 43210-1218

Bohumil Hučín, M.D., D.Sc.
Professor of Surgery
Department of Pediatric Kardiocentrum
University Hospital Motol
V Uvalu 84
Prague 5CZ-150 00
Czech Republic

Sixtus Hynie, MUDr., Dr.Sc.
Professor of Pharmacology
Institute of Pharmacology
1st Faculty of Medicine
Charles University
Prague
Czech Republic

Akira Ishihata, M.D., Ph.D.
Assistant Professor
Department of Pharmacology
Yamagata University School of Medicine
2-2-2 Iida-Nishi
Yamagata 990-23
Japan

Haisong Ju, M.D., M.Sc.
Ph.D. Student
Institute of Cardiovascular Sciences
St. Boniface General Hospital Research Centre
University of Manitoba
351 Tache Avenue
Winnipeg, Manitoba R2H 2A6
Canada

Yumi Katano, Ph.D.
Professor of Medicine
Division of Theoretical Nursing
Department of Nursing
Yamagata University School of Medicine
2-2-2 Iida-Nishi
Yamagata 990-23
Japan

Yasuhiro Katsube, M.D., Ph.D.
Visiting Scientist
Department of Molecular and Cellular Physiology
PO Box 670576
University of Cincinnati
Cincinnati, Ohio 45267-0576

Frank J. Kelly, B.Sc., Ph.D.
Senior Lecturer in Biochemistry
Department of Cardiovascular Research
St. Thomas' Hospital
The Rayne Institute
London SE1 7EH
United Kingdom

Jagdish C. Khatter, M.Sc., Ph.D.
Associate Professor of Medicine and Pharmacology and Therapeutics
Departments of Medicine and Pharmacology and Therapeutics
University of Manitoba
Health Sciences Centre
GF328-700, William Avenue
Winnipeg, Manitoba R3E 0Z3
Canada

Lorrie A. Kirshenbaum, Ph.D.
Assistant Professor
Department of Physiology and Institute of Cardiovascular Sciences
University of Manitoba
St. Boniface General Hospital Research Centre
351 Tache Avenue
Winnipeg, Manitoba R2H 2A6
Canada

Věra Klenerová, MUDr., Dr.Sc.
Associate Professor
Institute of Pharmacology
1st Faculty of Medicine
Charles University
128 00 Prague 2
Czech Republic

Maren U. Koban, B.Sc.
Imperial College School of Medicine
National Heart and Lung Institute
Department of Cardiothoracic Surgery
Dovehouse Street
London SW3 6LY
United Kingdom

Frantisek Kolář, Ph.D.
Institute of Physiology
Academy of Sciences of the Czech Republic
Videňská 1083
142 20 Prague 4
Czech Republic

Jaroslav Kuneš, Ph.D.
Institute of Physiology
Academy of Sciences of the Czech Republic
Videňská 1083
142 20 Prague 4
Czech Republic

Wouter H. Lamers
Department of Anatomy and Embryology
Academic Medical Center
University of Amsterdam
Meibergdreef, 15
1105 AZ Amsterdam
The Netherlands

Anton Lukas, Ph.D.
Associate Professor of Medicine
Department of Physiology
Institute of Cardiovascular Sciences
St. Boniface General Hospital Research Centre
351 Tache Avenue
Winnipeg, Manitoba R2H 2A6
Canada

William A. Lutin, M.D., Ph.D.
Associate Professor of Medicine
Department of Pediatrics
Medical College of Georgia
Augusta, Georgia 30912

Noboru Machida, D.V.M., Ph.D.
Faculty of Agriculture
Tokyo University of Agriculture and Technology
3-5-8 Saiwai-cho, Fuchi-shi
Tokyo 183
Japan

Hiroshi Masuda, M.D., Ph.D.
Assistant Professor of Pediatrics
Department of Pediatrics
Hiroshima University School of Medicine
Hiroshima 734
Japan

Marvin J. McBroom, Ph.D.
Professor of Physiology
Department of Physiology and Neuroscience
St. George's University School of Medicine
St. George's, Grenada
West Indies

E. Howard Merry
Department of Pediatrics
Medical College of Georgia
Augusta, Georgia 30912

Marek Michalak, Ph.D.
Professor
Department of Biochemistry
University of Alberta
423 Heritage Medical Research Centre
Edmonton, Alberta T6G 2S2
Canada

Marie Milerová
Institute of Physiology
Academy of Sciences of the Czech Republic
Videňská 1083
142 20 Prague 4
Czech Republic

Antoon F. M. Moorman
Academic Medical Center
University of Amsterdam
Meibergdreef, 15
1105 AZ Amsterdam
The Netherlands

Howard E. Morgan, M.D.
Senior Vice-President for Research
Henry Hood MD Research Program
Geisinger Clinic
Sigfried and Janet Weis Center for Research
100 North Academy Avenue
Danville, Pennsylvania 17822-2601

Tomoe Y. Nakamura, Ph.D.
Research Fellow
Department of Pediatric Cardiology
Molecular and Cellular Research Laboratories (Tisch 501)
New York University Medical Center
560 First Avenue
New York, New York 10016

Njanoor Narayanan, Ph.D.
Professor of Physiology
Department of Physiology
University of Western Ontario
Medical Sciences Building
London, Ontario N6A 5C1
Canada

Thomas J. Netticadan, Ph.D.
Post-Doctoral Fellow
Institute of Cardiovascular Sciences
St. Boniface General Hospital Research Centre
351 Tache Avenue
Winnipeg, Manitoba R2H 2A6
Canada

Mohinder S. Nijjar, B.Sc., M.Sc., Ph.D.
Visiting Professor of Physiology
Institute of Cardiovascular Sciences
University of Manitoba
Faculty of Medicine
St. Boniface General Hospital Research Centre
351 Tache Avenue
Winnipeg, Manitoba R2H 2A6
Canada

L'udmila Okruhlicová, Ph.D.
Doctor of Natural Sciences
Department of Morphology
Institute for Heart Research
Slovak Academy of Sciences
Dúbravaská cesta 9
842 33 Bratislava
Slovak Republic

Bohuslav Ošťádal, M.D., Dr.Sc.
Professor of Medicine
Institute of Physiology
Academy of Sciences of the Czech Republic
Videňská 1083
142 20 Prague 4
Czech Republic

Ivana Ošťádalová, M.D.
Institute of Physiology
Academy of Sciences of the Czech Republic
Videňská 1083
142 20 Prague 4
Czech Republic

Václav Pelouch, Ph.D.
Associate Professor
Institute of Physiology
Academy of Sciences of the Czech Republic
Videňská 1083
142 20 Prague 4
Czech Republic

Tomas Pexieder, M.D.
Professor of Medicine
Institute of Histology and Embryology
Faculty of Medicine
University of Lausanne
1005 Lausanne
Switzerland

Karel J. Rakusan, M.D., Ph.D.
Professor of Physiology
Department of Physiology
Faculty of Medicine
University of Ottawa
451 Smyth Road
Ottawa, Ontario K1H 8M5
Canada

Lydie Rappaport, Ph.D.
Director of Research CNRS
INSERM U127
Hopital Lariboisière
41 Bd de la Chapelle
75010 Paris
France

Anna Ratajska, Ph.D.
Adjunct Professor
Department of Pathological Anatomy
Medical University of Warsaw
Chablulinskiesyo 5, 02-004, Warsaw
Poland

Hideaki Sada, M.D., Ph.D.
Associate Professor of Pharmacology
Department of Pharmacology
Yamaguchi University School of Medicine
2-2-2 Ida Nishi
Yamaguchi 990-23
Japan

Milan Šamánek, M.D.
Professor
Kardiocentrum University Hospital Motol
University Hospital Motol
V úvalu 84
Prague 5-Motol, 150 06
Czech Republic

Jane-Lyse Samuel, M.D., Ph.D.
Director of Research
INSERM U127
Hopital Lariboisière
41 Bd de la Chapelle
75010 Paris
France

Michael J. Shattock, B.Sc, Ph.D.
British Heart Foundation Senior Lecturer
Cardiovascular Research
The Rayne Institute
St. Thomas' Hospital
London SE1 7EH
United Kingdom

M. A. Q. Siddiqui, Ph.D.
Professor and Chairman
Department of Anatomy and Cell Biology
State University of New York
Health Science Center at Brooklyn
Brooklyn, New York 11203

Jana Slaviková, M.D., C.Sc.
Associate Professor of Physiology
Department of Physiology
Medical Faculty
Charles University
Lidická 1
301 66 Plezň
Czech Republic

Ján Slezák, M.D., D.Sc.
Professor of Medicine
Department of Morphology
Institute for Heart Research
Slovak Academy of Sciences
Dúbravaská cesta 9
842 33 Bratislava
Slovak Republic

Richard Southworth, B.Sc.
Post-Graduate Student
Cardiovascular Research
The Rayne Institute
St. Thomas' Hospital
London SE1 7EH
United Kingdom

Nicholas Sperelakis, Ph.D.
The Joseph Eichberg Professor Emeritus of Physiology and Biophysics
Department of Molecular and Cellular Physiology
College of Medicine
P.O. Box 670576
University of Cincinnati
Cincinnati, Ohio 45267

Catherine Sreenan
Department of Pathology
University of Alabama at Birmingham
1670 University Boulevard
Birmingham, Alabama 35294-0019

Rana M. Temsah
Institute of Cardiovascular Sciences
St. Boniface General Hospital Research Centre
351 Tache Avenue
Winnipeg, Manitoba R2H 2A6
Canada

Robert J. Tomanek, Ph.D.
Professor of Anatomy and Cell Biology
Department of Anatomy and Cell Biology
University of Iowa
Bowen Science Building
Iowa City, Iowa 52242

Narcisa Tribulová, Ph.D.
Doctor of Natural Sciences
Department of Morphology
Institute for Heart Research
Slovak Academy of Sciences
Dúbravaská cesta 9
842 33 Bratislava
Slovak Republic

Matti Vornanen, Ph.D.
Senior Research Associate
Department of Biology
University of Joensuu
P.O. Box 111
80101 Joensuu
Finland

Gerry T. M. Wagenaar, Ph.D.
Doctor in Biology
Department of Anatomy and Embryology
Academic Medical Center
University of Amsterdam
Meibergdreef, 15
1105 AZ Amsterdam
The Netherlands

Carin Wittnich, D.V.M., M.Sc. (Experimental Surgery)
Associate Professor of Surgery and Physiology
Department of Surgery and Physiology
Division of Cardiovascular Surgery
Hospital for Sick Children
University of Toronto
Medical Sciences Building
Toronto, Ontario M5S 1A8
Canada

Ande Xu, B.Sc.
Research Assistant
Department of Physiology
University of Western Ontario
London, Ontario N6A 5C1
Canada

Jing Ya, Ph.D. Student
Graduate in Biology
Department of Anatomy and Embryology
Academic Medical Center
University of Amsterdam
Meibergdreef, 15
1105 AZ Amsterdam
The Netherlands

Josef Zicha, M.D., Ph.D.
Institute of Physiology
Academy of Sciences of the Czech Republic
Videňská 1083
142 20 Prague 4
Czech Republic

Barbara Ziegelhöffer Mihalovičová
Ph.D. Student
Magister of Biology
Institute for Heart Research
Slovak Academy of Sciences
Dúbravaská cesta 9
842 33 Bratislava
Slovak Republic

Preface

The importance of the developmental approach for experimental and clinical cardiology is indisputable. Clinical-epidemiological studies have clearly shown that the risk factors of serious cardiovascular diseases, such as arteriosclerosis and ischemic heart disease, are already present during the early phases of ontogenetic development. Thus, experimental studies of the pathogenetic mechanisms of these disturbances must shift to the early developmental periods. Furthermore, congenital cardiovascular malformations remain the single largest cause of infant mortality from congenital defects in industrial countries. In spite of dramatic progress in surgical prevention, heart defects in many patients are not cured. The primary goal of medical progress must be prevention, not more and better treatment alone. It is therefore not surprising that the interest of theoretical and clinical cardiologists in the developmental approach keeps increasing. Advances in molecular biology accelerated this trend substantially.

This book is based on the symposia on developmental cardiology presented at the XV World Congress of the International Society for Heart Research (ISHR) in Prague in July 1995. The International Advisory Board in cooperation with the Organizing Committee provided for the first time in the history of ISHR congresses an excellent scientific forum for a meeting of developmental cardiologists to discuss problems related to this topic from the molecule up to the patient's bed. The book contains selected papers for the benefit of those who were unable to attend the symposia. It is organized into sections: on the molecular biology of the developing heart, cardiac growth and development, development of excitation-contraction coupling, effect of increased workload, and effect of hypoxia and ischemia. It is our contention that the biological, electrophysiological, morphological, functional, biochemical, and pharmacological approaches employed by distinguished scientists worldwide will provide the reader with a global picture for changes characterizing the developing heart. It should stimulate the curiosity of cardiovascular scientists in gaining insight into the mechanisms of normal and pathological development.

Bohuslav Ošt'ádal, Prague
Makoto Nagano, Tokyo
Nobuakira Takeda, Tokyo
Naranjan S. Dhalla, Winnipeg

Acknowledgments

The organization of the XV World Congress of the International Society for Heart Research with the five symposia devoted to the developing heart and publication of this book would not have been possible without the support of several scientific societies and pharmaceutical companies. The editors wish to thank the Council of the International Society for Heart Research (ISHR) and its American, Japanese, and European Sections, International Society and Federation of Cardiology, Knoll Ltd. BASF Pharma, Hoechst AG, Lachema a.s., Léčiva a.s., Merck Darmstadt, Merck Frosst Canada, Pfizer Inc., Pfizer Czech Republic Ltd., Pulsus Group Inc., and Philips Medizin Systeme.

The help of Susan Zettler for the preparation of this book is highly appreciated. Special thanks to Ruth Weinberg and the editorial staff at Lippincott-Raven Publishers for their patience, interest, and hard work in assembling this volume.

PART I

Introduction

The Developing Heart,
edited by Bohuslav Ošťádal et al.
Lippincott-Raven Publishers,
Philadelphia © 1997.

1

Developmental Cardiology

Bohuslav Ošťádal

Institute of Physiology, Academy of Sciences of the Czech Republic, Prague

DEVELOPMENTAL MEDICINE

Historical Remarks

The origin of developmental biology and medicine as a scientific discipline dates back to the discoveries of Darwin and Mendel in the second half of the nineteenth century. When Darwin brought forward the theory of the origin of species by natural selection, there were no other evolutionary theories to compete with it. Its rapid acceptance was due to the fact that evolution was "in the air" at the time. Darwin realized that an understanding of heredity was essential for evolutionary studies, but he apparently never came across Mendel's paper, and he stated in the last edition of the *Origin of Species* that the fundamental principles of heredity were still unknown (1). Only six years after the publication of Darwin's famous book, Mendel described the laws of heredity. His words were unfortunately long forgotten and were only rediscovered 16 years after his death; today the tenets of Mendel's principles are at the basis of most studies in evolution. It is only through an irony of fate that at the beginning of its existence Mendelism was often interpreted as the opposite of Darwinism.

It took, however, a long time before both of these basic theories became an integral part of modern physiology and medicine. In the second half of the nineteenth century these disciplines profited from the work of another scientific genius—Claude Bernard. This French physiologist formulated for the first time the concept of stability of the internal environment (homeostasis), which for a long time formed the basis of most physiological investigations. Bernard himself during his work on the theory of homeostasis had no clear view on evolution, and his originally vitalistic ideas changed only before the end of his life. So it happened that the two most important theories of life sciences, the idea of the internal milieu and the idea of evolution, were for a long time studied separately. In this connection it is interesting to mention that the lack of logic of this situation was first recognized by scientists studying evolution: it took a substantially longer time before physiologists started with an investigation of the previous history of their experimental models (2). This is also the reason that classical physiology, as is obvious from many textbooks, is predominantly the physiology of adults: the developmental approach is lacking.

At any rate, the beginning of the twentieth century provided new stimuli. An example can be found in the nutritional experiments connected with the name of F. G. Hopkins. Hopkins introduced into physiology the time factor, because prolonged studies taught researchers to wait for results for weeks or months. Simultaneously, a new, important term appeared—*adaptation*—describing the transformation of functions and, later, the structures induced by the chronic influence of altered environmental conditions on the organism. Adaptation is one of the starting points of physiology toward evolution (2).

DEVELOPMENTAL APPROACH TO CARDIOLOGY

The importance of the developmental approach for experimental and clinical cardiology is indisputable. Clinical-epidemiologic studies have shown that the risk factors of serious cardiovascular diseases, such as atherosclerosis and ischemic heart disease, are present already during the early phases of ontogenetic development (3). Some of them, such as excessive food intake and an increased level of cholesterol, operate just after birth. They are followed by smoking, where the connection with ischemic heart disease is beyond any doubt, stress, and decreased physical activity. Last but not least, genetic factors are present even before birth. Atherosclerosis and ischemic heart disease are thus no longer diseases of the fifth and higher decades of life, rather, their origins and consequences may be influenced by risk factors acting during development. It follows that experimental studies of the pathogenetic mechanisms of these disturbances must shift to the early ontogenetic periods. Furthermore, congenital cardiovascular malformations remain the single largest cause of infant mortality from congenital defects in industrialized countries. In spite of dramatic advances in surgical therapy, many patients' heart defects are not cured. There is a lingering morbidity and mortality that increases with age after surgery. The primary goal of medical progress must be prevention, rather than more or better treatment alone (4). It is therefore unsurprising that the interest of theoretical and clinical cardiologists in the developmental approach keeps increasing. Recent advances of molecular biology and the developing possibilities of prenatal cardiology (5) accelerated this trend substantially.

Developmental cardiology is an integral part of the so-called adult cardiology, but it has some of its own specificities. Research in this field can generally be divided into four closely related areas:

1. study of normal structural, functional, and biochemical development of the cardiovascular system;
2. study of the sensitivity of the developing cardiovascular system to different pathogenetic factors;

3. possibilities of protective influences; and
4. late effects of early disturbances of the cardiovascular system.

There are, however, many controversies concerning the mechanisms of developmental variations in cardiovascular responsiveness; the obvious discrepancies may be partly due to different experimental procedures used for studying different animal species (6,7). Nevertheless, it is worth noting that ontogenetic conclusions are often based on observations from two or three developmental stages, such as fetal, newborn, and adult. It is, therefore, necessary to point out that the possible developmental changes between selected (and not exactly defined) points remain undetermined. The precise knowledge of individual ontogenetic periods critical for cardiac ontogeny (prenatal, neonatal, suckling, weaning, adolescence, adulthood) is thus crucial for the prediction and explanation of cardiac reactions to various pathogenetic stimuli (8,9). Furthermore, experimental data on ontogenetic differences in cardiac responsiveness were obtained almost exclusively from healthy individuals. However, such an approach is far from clinical situations, where interventions applied in the critical developmental periods may have serious consequences for further maturation. The complications observed after the use of inotropic drugs during early development (10,11) may serve as warning examples.

MOLECULAR VERSUS INTEGRATIVE VIEW

The advances in molecular and cell biology over the last few decades amount to a very major revolution in our knowledge of the development of living systems. Twenty years ago we knew very little about the structure, organization, and expression of genes in eukaryotic cells, although we knew quite a bit about the bulk fractions of nuclear DNA. The advent of cloning methods provided molecular biologists with the tools to study genes at the molecular level, leading to detailed knowledge of gene structure (12). The recent development of in vitro systems has advanced our understanding of the ways in which gene expression is controlled in a cell-specific way. The field of developmental cardiology is now on the threshold of a molecular era, and our understanding of cardiogenesis will expand exponentially. By using in vivo molecular analysis of cardiovascular embryology and physiology, recent advances in mouse genetics are beginning to merge the fields of cardiac molecular biology and pediatric cardiology. Elucidation of the precise molecular switches that control various steps of cardiac growth and development continues to be one of the central questions in cardiovascular biology and medicine (13).

It is, however, necessary to mention that the integrative, synthetic view of different developmental problems is still indispensable. The multicellular or whole-organ problems with which cardiology was concerned before the massive switch to the cell and molecular level were often unresolved or inadequately worked out or even not yet defined. Furthermore, the systems, whose overall behavior we are trying to predict from mechanisms involving cells and molecules, are highly nonlinear (14). To meet the challenge of comprehending the process of developmental biology as a whole, we must then combine these two approaches. Such an understanding would place the descriptive facts and approximate mechanisms of molecular and cell biology into an integrative context (15,16).

SUMMARY

Developmental biology and medicine form a rational combination of an individual medical science, describing functional adaptation of a particular system, and evolution, which is the science of how biological systems came to exist. The developmental approach in medical sciences and particularly in cardiology offers new possibilities in the experimental studies of pathogeny, prevention, and therapy of cardiovascular diseases. Recent advances of new methodology, particularly molecular biology and genetics, may substantially help in the laborious search for a better understanding of the underlying mechanisms. Nevertheless, molecular analysis in developmental cardiology is unthinkable without a comprehensive and well-integrated view of the field.

REFERENCES

1. Dodson EO. *Evolution: process and product.* New York: Reinhold, 1960.
2. Poupa O. Homeostasis, evolution and adaptation. In: *The development of homeostasis, with special reference to factors of the environment.* Proceedings of a symposium. Prague: Czech Academy of Science, 1962.
3. Fejfar Z. Prevention against ischemic heart disease: a critical review. In: Oliver MF, ed. *Modern trends in cardiology.* Boston: Butterworth-Heinemann, 1975.
4. Clark EB, Markwald RR, Takao A. Developmental cardiology comes of age. In: Clark EB, Markwald RR, Takao A, eds. *Developmental mechanisms of heart disease.* Armonk, NY: Futura, 1995.
5. Šamánek M, Škovránek J, Trubačová D, Dunovská V. Nation wide project of prenatal detection of heart diseases and its results in high risk population. *Pediatr Cardiol* 1988;9:188–189.
6. Ošt'ádal B, Beamish RE, Barwinsky J, Dhalla NS. Ontogenetic development of cardiac sensitivity to catecholamines. *J Appl Cardiol* 1989;4:467–486.
7. Artman M. Developmental changes in myocardial contractile responses to inotropic agents. *Cardiovasc Res* 1992;26:3–13.
8. Ošťádal B, Kolář F, Škovránek J, Ošťádalová I. Ontogenetic development of cardiac inotropic responsiveness. In: Ošťádal B, Dhalla NS, eds. *Heart function in health and disease.* Boston: Kluwer, 1993.
9. Ošťádalová I, Kolář F, Ošťádal B, Rohlíček V, Rohlíček J, Procházka J. Early postnatal development of contractile performance and responsiveness to Ca, verapamil and ryanodine in the isolated rat heart. *J Mol Cell Cardiol* 1993;25:733–740.
10. Benedetti TJ. Life threatening complications of beta mimetic therapy for pre-term labor inhibition. *Clin Perinatol* 1986;13:843–852.
11. Škovránek J, Ošťádal B, Pelouch V, Procházka J. Ontogenetic differences in cardiac sensitivity to verapamil in rats. *Pediatr Cardiol* 1986;7:25–29.
12. Southern EM. Physiology and genes. In: Boyd CAR, Noble D, eds. *The logic of life.* Oxford: Oxford University Press, 1993.
13. Chien KR. Overview: molecular analysis of cardiac developmental phenotypes: problems, progress and perspectives. In: Clark EB, Markwald RR, Takao A, eds. *Developmental mechanisms of heart disease.* Armonk, NY: Futura, 1995.
14. Noble D, Boyd CAR. The challenge of integrative physiology. In: Boyd CAR, Noble D, eds. *The logic of life.* Oxford: Oxford University Press, 1993.
15. Diamond JR. Evolutionary physiology. In: Boyd CAR, Noble D, eds. *The logic of life.* Oxford: Oxford University Press, 1993.
16. Ošťádal B. Developmental cardiology. *Cor Vasa* 1994;36:65–67.

PART II

Molecular Biology of the Developing Heart

The Developing Heart,
edited by Bohuslav Ošťádal et al.
Lippincott-Raven Publishers,
Philadelphia © 1997.

2

Molecular Basis of Cardiogenesis

Regulatory Factors Involved in Cardiomyocyte Specification

M. A. Q. Siddiqui and Shyamal K. Goswami

The Center for Cardiovascular and Muscle Research and the Department of Anatomy and Cell Biology, State University of New York Health Science Center, Brooklyn, NY 11203

Despite the significant progress in our understanding of the molecular basis of skeletal muscle development (see ref. 1 for review), relatively little is known about the regulatory events that initiate and propagate the presumptive cardiac muscle cells to terminally differentiated cardiac myocytes. The lack of progress can, in part, be attributed to the nonavailability of a true cardiac muscle cell line amenable to differentiation in vitro. However, this limitation has been compensated to some extent by the volume of information that has accumulated over the past decade on the development of cardiovasculature (2–4) and on the role of peptide growth factors in heart development (5–7). Recent progress on understanding the development of cardiovasculature came from three distinct approaches: (a) mapping analysis of the myocardial cell lineage (2,3), (b) genetic analysis of the development of the cardiovasculature (4), and (c) identification of regulatory factors that ultimately lead the progenitor cells to differentiated cardiocytes (8). This review focuses mainly on recent progress, on understanding of the cardiac and skeletal myogenic process, and identification and characterization of key regulatory/transcription factors with the potential to play a role in cardiomyocyte specification.

ROLE OF PEPTIDE GROWTH FACTORS IN CARDIAC MUSCLE DIFFERENTIATION

In skeletal muscle differentiation, cell proliferation and differentiation are mutually exclusive; in cardiac muscle they are not (9–11). In the early developing heart, differentiated cardiac myocytes retain the ability to proliferate and are characterized by the presence of embryonic gene expression program (12) (Fig. 2–1). Neonatal cardiocytes lose their ability to proliferate and, if necessary, adapt to subsequent pressure/volume overload, resulting in an increase in size (hypertrophy) (13). On the other hand, cycling skeletal myoblasts do not express differentiated phenotype, and following differentiation the mature myocytes permanently withdraw from the cell cycle (9,10). The mechanism by which cardiac myocytes retain their ability to proliferate while maintaining their differentiated state is not known. Although there has been significant progress in understanding the role of polypeptide growth factors in the establishment of the body plan and the recruitment of the skeletal muscle precursor cells into the myogenic pathways (14,15), their role in cardiac organogenesis is largely unknown (5–7). There are fundamental differences in the effects of growth factors on cardiac and skeletal muscle differentiation programs. In skeletal muscle, peptide growth factors inhibit muscle-specific transcription by targeting the myogenic bHLH proteins (9–10). Two of the most potent inhibitors of skeletal myoblast differentiation in vitro are fibroblast growth factor

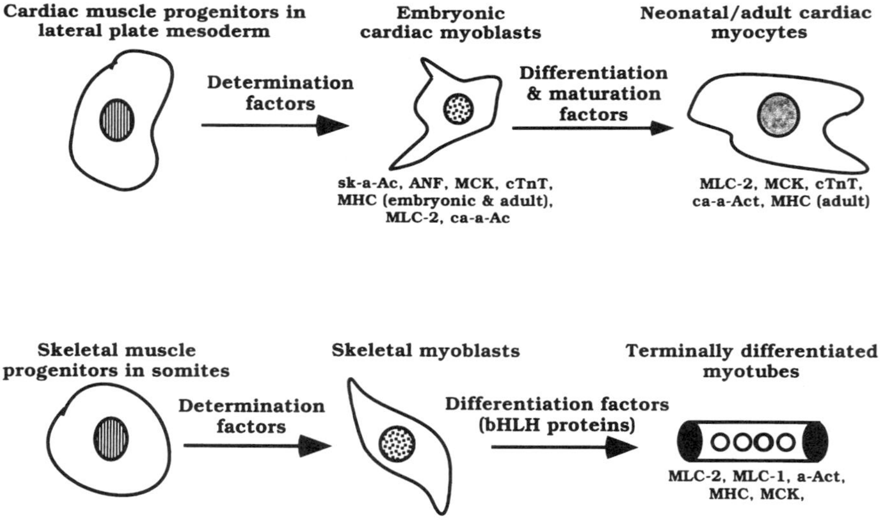

FIG. 2–1. Schematic presentation of cardiac and skeletal muscle differention program during embryonic development. *Top panel:* Cardiac muscle development starts from the splanchnic mesenchyme of the anterior lateral plate mesoderm. Commitment of mesodermal cells to the cardiogenic lineage occurs when the cells migrate to form the cardiogenic area during 18–20 h in chicken embryogenesis. The embryonic cardiac muscle cells can proliferate and are characterized by a distinct transcriptional program expressing a set of genes such as shown above. The neonatal cardiac myocytes lose their ability to proliferate and express a different set of genes. *Bottom panel:* Skeletal muscle development starts from the somites of the dorsal (paraxial) mesoderm. Under the influence of the myogenic determination factors, these cells are determined to proliferating myoblasts that subsequently lose proliferative capacity and become terminally differentiated multinucleated myotubes. Unlike the cardiac myocytes, skeletal muscle cells do not express the muscle specific markers until terminally differentiated.

(FGF) and transforming growth factor type-β (TGF-β) (9). In the developing heart, however, the proliferative cardiac myocytes themselves produce aFGF and bFGF, which stimulate cardiac growth (5). TGF-β is also involved in cardiac muscle growth and differentiation (6,7) and has been shown to induce differentiation of the presumptive cardiac mesoderm explanted from axolotl (16). An array of sarcomeric proteins is induced in QCE-6 cells (derived from splanchnic mesoderm of the Japanese Quail) by TGF-β_2 and -β_3 (17). Thus, the signaling cascades activated by these growth factors are divergent in cardiac and skeletal muscle cells. In this context, the role of AP-1 in cardiac and skeletal muscle specific gene expression is quite intriguing. AP-1 is a dimeric complex of c-*fos* and c-*jun* gene products that binds to the sequence TGACTCA. The oncogenes c-*fos* and c-*jun* are considered as the immediate early genes that are at the receiving end of a plethora of signaling pathways (18). During skeletal muscle differentiation, the peptide growth factors induce AP-1 activities, which in turn inhibit differentiation by attenuation of the myogenic bHLH factors (19). On the other hand, in cardiac muscle a variety of stimuli that elicit hypertrophic response induce AP-1; therefore, AP-1 is implicated as a positive regulator of gene expression in cardiac muscle (13). We have recently observed that, unlike in skeletal muscle cells, where it acts as global inhibitor of differentiation, AP-1 plays a more complex role as a modulator of gene expression in cardiac muscle (Goswami et al., in preparation). c-*Jun,* a component of AP1, has an inhibitory effect on cardiac muscle gene transcription. The inhibition is independent of its DNA binding property, and its ability to heterodimerize, presumably with different partner proteins, can account for its potential to repress or activate transcription. Treatment of quiescent cardiac myocytes with TPA and Ang II, both of which induce AP1/Jun activity, causes a differential effect on the expression of endogenous MLC-2 gene. Whereas TPA is an inhibitor of MLC-2 gene expression, Ang II has a stimulatory effect (Goswami et al., unpublished data). We postulate that the precise biological effect of induction of AP-1 in cardiac muscle cells depends upon the composition of the AP-1 complexes, their relative levels of expression, and their interaction with other, yet unknown, regulatory factors.

ROLE OF HOMEODOMAIN AND GATA-4 PROTEINS IN CARDIAC DEVELOPMENT

As with other organs, the development of cardiovasculature involves coordinated development of various cell types, their differentiation, morphogenesis, innervation, and attachment with other body structures. In the developing embryo, homeobox genes are involved in the specification of the body plan, pattern formation, and determination of cell fate (20,21). Based on transcript localization and gene inactivation, a number of these genes have been implicated in heart development (22–24). For example, in mice, inactivation of Hoxa-3 has caused atrial and left ventricular hypertrophy, as well as aortic and pulmonic valve defects in addition to other noncardiac abnormalities (22). Studies with NK class of homeo-

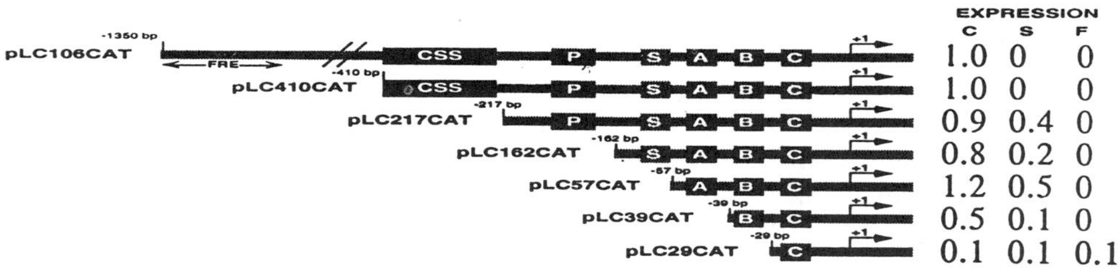

FIG. 2–2. Role of various regulatory domains of cardiac MLC-2 promoter in its tissue specific expression. The 1.3-kb promoter fragment fused to the CAT reporter sequence (pLC106CAT) was sequentially deleted from the 5′ end and the deletion mutants were tested for expression in cardiac muscle (C), skeletal muscle (S), and fibroblast (F) cells. The relative level of expression of each mutant is shown on the right. The CSS element is involved in the cardiac tissue–specific expression (75). Element P is a positive element and element S is a negative element in both cardiac and skeletal muscle (74). Element A is a CArG-like sequence, and its deletion results in down-regulation of the promoter in both cardiac and skeletal muscle (45). Element B is a MEF-2-like sequence that binds to both MEF-2 and a cardiac-specific factor BBF-1 and acts as cardiac-specific activator (45).

domain proteins (25) in both invertebrates and vertebrates have established a critical role for NK in the establishment of myogenic lineage during embryonic development. In *Drosophila,* homeodomain protein encoded by the *tinman* gene was shown to be essential for heart and visceral muscle formation (23). A murine NK gene, Nkx-2.5, is expressed in early cardiac progenitor cells prior to activation of the myogenic program (24). Nkx-2.5 transcripts are subsequently found in the myocardial layer of the embryonic and adult heart and other noncardiac tissues (24). The homology between Nkx-2.5, XNkx-2.5 (amphibian homolog of Nkx-2.5) and *tinman* and similarities in their expression pattern suggest a conserved role of these proteins in heart development (26). Targeted inactivation of Nkx-2.5 resulted in heart morphogenic defects at embryonic day 8.5. A beating linear heart tube developed, but subsequent looping was impaired (27). In addition, there was a selective inactivation of MLC-2 gene expression even though the DNA element CTNNAGTG targeted by Nkx-2.5 is absent in the MLC-2 promoter (27,28; see Fig. 2–2). One possibility is that Nkx-2.5 regulates one chain of events during the heart development and affects the expression of MLC-2 via regulation of other transcription factors located further downstream in that cascade. Support for this notion comes from the recent studies on the role of the GATA family of factors in heart formation. A member of the GATA family, GATA-4, is involved in cardiac-specific transcription of polypeptide hormones ANP and BNP (29). Antisense inactivation of GATA-4 transcripts in embryonal carcinoma P19 cells blocked its differentiation to beating cardiocytes (30). Therefore, it appears that both Nkx-2.5 and GATA-4 are involved in differentiation pathways in early cardiogenesis; it remains to be seen how they interact to dictate the pattern of gene expression in the developing heart.

CONTROL OF SARCOMERIC GENE EXPRESSION IN THE DEVELOPING HEART

Although differentiated cardiac muscle cells do not form multinucleated myotubes like skeletal myocytes, they contain the sarcomeric arrays with structural organization and function similar to those in skeletal muscle. Many contractile protein genes are members of the multigene families that express differentially in cardiac chambers and in different skeletal muscle types (31), whereas other muscle genes, such as muscle creatine kinase (MCK), are encoded by a single gene expressing in both cardiac and skeletal muscle (32). As such, it was expected that the molecular mechanisms that drive the expression of common genes in cardiac and skeletal muscles share common features (33). This notion was further enforced by the observations that several muscle-specific genes contain regulatory elements essential for their expression in both cardiac and skeletal muscles (33) and that in hypertrophied cardiac myocytes, a genetic reprogramming occurs that allows the expression of genes that are otherwise expressed in skeletal muscles only (13). However, it is now becoming clear (see later) that cardiac muscle cells have a transcriptional strategy distinct from that of skeletal muscle cells for regulation of gene expression.

During embryonic development, establishment of various cell lineages are the reflection of a regulated transcriptional program. The ultimate spectrum of genes that are expressed in a differentiated cell type depends upon the response of the genomic apparatus to a variety of intrinsic and extrinsic stimuli. It is generally believed that each facet of differentiation depends upon a unique combination of tissue-specific and ubiquitous regulatory factors that interact with a distinct set of sequence elements (*cis*- elements) present in the regulatory regions of the genes (34). Regulation of sarcomeric gene expression has long been investigated as the paradigm of muscle development. The muscle genes characterized so far can be divided into four categories: (a) genes that are tissue restricted, (b) genes that express in both cardiac and skeletal muscle cells, (c) genes whose expression is developmentally regulated, and (d) genes that are normally expressed in skeletal muscle but that are activated in cardiac muscle following the hypertrophic stimuli. Intriguingly, the regulatory regions of these genes share a number of *cis*-elements, indicating the presence of a common transcriptional mechanism in the two muscle types (33). Yet it appears now that the mechanisms by which these regulatory sequences contribute to the cardiac- and skeletal-muscle-specific transcription are distinct.

Common *Cis*-Elements and Cognate Binding Proteins Exhibit Divergent Regulatory Activity

The CArG (CCA/T_{rich}GG) sequence is one of the several well-characterized *cis*-elements present in the regulatory regions of the muscle genes that was assigned a role as muscle-specific activator of transcription (35–37). Subsequently, it was shown that the core sequence of the serum response element (SRE) of c-*fos* gene also contains the CArG box, and the proteins binding to this element in muscle (CArG binding protein) and nonmuscle cells (serum response factor) are indistinguishable (38,39). The distal enhancer of MCK gene, expressed in both cardiac and skeletal muscle cells, contains a CArG box that plays little regulatory role in skeletal muscle but is the prime determinant of the promoter activity in cardiac cells (32). Studies with the rabbit MCK promoter-enhancer, on the other hand, showed that whereas the cardiac-muscle-specific expression is determined by a single CArG element present in the proximal promoter region, the skeletal-muscle genes are regulated by an upstream enhancer (40). Another intriguing aspect of the CArG box function in cardiac- and skeletal-muscle-specific transcription is that other transcription factors, distinct from the CArG/SRE binding proteins, are involved in the negative regulation that is mediated by the CArG sequence (41). Therefore, it appears that the ubiquitous CArG-binding factor can differentially contribute to muscle-tissue-specific transcription of various genes via cooperative interactions with other factors and cofactors (42).

Another notable example is the A/T-rich sequence, TTATTTTTA, identified as MEF-2 (myocyte enhancer factor-2) binding site and extensively characterized by its role in muscle-specific transcription. MEF-2 was originally identified as a *cis* regulatory element in the MCK enhancer (43) and, subsequently, in the promoter/enhancer regions of several cardiac- and skeletal-muscle-specific genes, including the gene for cardiac MLC-2 (32,37,44,45). MEF-2, present in both cardiac and skeletal muscle cells, belongs to the MADS-box (*M*CM1, *a*gamous and *d*eficiens and *s*erum response factor) family of transcription factors. It is characterized by (a) its specificity for its target sequence TTATTTTTA; (b) the presence of the conserved MADS domain at the amino-terminus; (c) the presence of an additional domain, MEF-2 domain, which is located at the carboxyl terminal side of the MADS box and is conserved only among the members of the MEF-2 family; and (d) the existence of multiple isoforms generated from different genes and/or by alternative splicing of the primary transcripts (see ref. 44). Four MEF-2 genes have so far been identified in vertebrates (46–48). Recent data from our laboratory and others have implicated MEF-2 in cell lineage determination (49,50). It appears that the MEF-2-mediated effects are caused by a group of MEF-2 proteins rather than by a single polypeptide (44, 46–48). Some members of MEF-2 proteins are tissue restricted, whereas others are ubiquitous (46–48, 51). The fact that multiple isoforms of MEF-2 proteins, generated by alternative splicing, bind to the TTATTTTTA sequence as dimmers considerably increases their potential in performing diverse regulatory functions. At least one member of the MEF-2 family, BBF-1, appears preferentially early in the cardiogenic mesodermal cells (49, Ghatpande et al. unpublished results). Taken together, these observations strongly suggest that the MEF-2 proteins play a pivotal role in control of myogenesis and point to their potential as regulators of cell commitment (44,49,50). However, the precise mechanism of their tissue-specific activity remain unclear. As in the case of the CArG sequence, the MEF-2 sequence present in the MCK enhancer also contributes differentially to its expression in cardiac and skeletal muscle (32). Interestingly, a number of other transcription factors, which lack the preceding features but bind the MEF-2 sequence with specificity, have also been reported (52,53).

Following the discovery of MyoD (54), a member of the myogenic basic-helix-loop-helix (bHLH) family of transcription factors that acts as the determinant of skeletal muscle development, a substantial effort was made to assign a role to the E-box sequence, the binding site for bHLH proteins, in cardiac-muscle-specific genes (55). In spite of the fact that the E-box sequence is present in the regulatory regions of a number of genes in cardiac muscle cells (56,57), no bHLH family of factors, other than the ubiquitously expressed E2 gene products, was detected in cardiac myocytes (54). Targeted inactivation of genes encoding MyoD family of factors in transgenic mice demonstrated normal heart development (58). However, for human cardiac α-actin gene expression in neonatal rat cardiomyocytes, a regulatory domain containing the E-box was found to be necessary (56), but the regulatory protein that occupies this sequence in cardiac myocytes is not known. Our laboratory has recently shown that the cardiac-tissue-specific MLC2 promoter, which lacks a functional E-box, can be transactivated by the ectopic expression of MyoD in fibroblast cells (59), suggesting that a common regulatory factor(s) that can mediate activation of both skeletal and cardiac genes might be the target of MyoD in cardiac muscle cells. Recent reviews (54,55,58) have dealt extensively with the role of bHLH family of transcription factors in muscle-specific transcription; therefore, further discussion of these proteins in muscle-specific gene expression is unwarranted here.

Divergent Regulation of Genes Common to Cardiac and Skeletal Muscles

A number of sarcomeric genes, such as cardiac α-actin and cardiac troponin T (cTnT), are expressed in both cardiac and skeletal muscle cells during early embryonic development but are subsequently turned off in one or the other muscle types (12,60). Skeletal α-actin gene is induced, for example, in cardiac myocytes under the influence of several pathophysiological stimuli, which requires a 700-bp-long regulatory promoter region shown to be nonessential for its expression in skeletal muscle cells (61). Similarly, the regulatory elements involved in the cardiac-tissue-restricted expression of cTnT gene has also been dissociated from those required for its expression in skeletal muscle. During early chicken embryonic development, the cTnT gene is expressed at a low level in both skeletal and cardiac muscles, but after 12 days, its expression goes up dramatically in cardiac muscle and is repressed concomitantly in skeletal muscle (60). Although the proximal region up to –129 bp in the cTnT promoter is sufficient for its expression in skeletal muscle, the cardiac-tissue-specific expression requires an additional sequence located at –247 to –201. This region contains two distinct *cis*-acting elements, an A/T-rich sequence that is indistinguishable from the MEF-2 site and a unique sequence that recognizes a novel cardiac factor, CEBF (62,63). These two elements work in conjunction with two M-CAT sequences located in the proximal cTnT promoter (62,63). Similar studies with mouse cardiac troponin C (cTnC) gene also identified divergent regulatory pathways for its expression in cardiac and slow skeletal muscle (64,65).

Mammalian cardiac muscle cells contain two isozymes of myosin heavy chain (MHC), namely α and β, of which the β-isoform is expressed in slow skeletal muscle, whereas α-MHC is expressed exclusively in cardiac muscle (66). In small mammals, such as the rat and mouse, the expression of both isoforms is developmentally and hormonally (thyroid hormone) regulated (66). During fetal development, the β-isoform is predominant and its expression is down-regulated after birth, whereas that of α-MHC goes up (66). Functional analysis of rat β-MHC promoter in transient transfection assay suggests that the same muscle-specific enhancer—conserved among rat, rabbit, mouse, and humans (67)—activates β-MHC expression in both cardiac and skeletal muscle (68,69). This enhancer consists of three subregions, known as βe2, C-rich, and βe3, of which the βe2 domain is necessary and sufficient for conferring cardiac- and skeletal-muscle specificity to heterologous promoters (68). The βe-2 region of the human β-MHC enhancer binds a nuclear factor, βF1, present only in cardiac myocytes and related to the M-CAT binding factor (69).

Transgenic animal studies, however, revealed notable differences in sequence requirements for optimal promoter activity. Although the relatively small 600-bp promoter region was sufficient for muscle-specific expression of the recombinant gene in transient transfection, a 5600-bp upstream region was needed for its optimal expression in vivo (70). Likewise, in transgenic mice harboring the human cardiac α-actin promoter, the elements identified by in vitro analysis as necessary for optimum regulation in cardiac and skeletal muscle were enough only for basal-level promoter activity (71). Surprising results were observed during analysis of the α-MHC promoter in transgenic mice. The inactivation of the CArG element in the proximal promoter had no effect on its level of expression and tissue specificity, but that of the MEF-2 site showed an unexpected upregulation of its expression in cardiac and other nonmuscle tissues (72,73). Therefore, it appears that the mechanism of cardiac-tissue-restricted gene expression is far from resolved and requires an extensive analysis in vivo.

IDENTIFICATION OF A CARDIAC LINEAGE–ASSOCIATED PROTEIN (CLAP)

We have established in our laboratory that expression of cardiac MLC-2 gene is regulated by a number of *cis*-elements, including the MEF-2 sequence (element B) (45,49), a CArG sequence (element A) (74), a distinct negative regulatory element CSS (cardiac-specific sequence) that accounts for its repression in skeletal muscle (75) in addition to other elements P and S (45,74). Sequential deletion analysis of the regulatory region of the MLC2 promoter demonstrated that whereas CSS accounts for its repression in skeletal muscle cells, elements A and B are required for its activation in cardiac muscle (Fig. 2–2). The functional domain of CSS consists of three distinct protein binding sites with a common motif (GAAG) essential for repression of MLC-2 gene transcription. CSS-mediated transcriptional inhibition is contingent upon the presence of a downstream modulatory sequence that also contains the GAAG motif. Several element-B and CSS-specific DNA binding protein factors have also been isolated and their cDNAs cloned.

The MyoD family proteins, which are considered the hallmark of skeletal myogenesis, are absent in cardiac muscle, and there is no known marker for cardiac muscle differentiation during early embryonic development. It appears that tissue-specific regulatory factors divergent from the myogenic bHLH proteins are involved in activation of cardiogenic program. Recent evidence suggests that a common myogenic program that includes the key members of MEF-2 family proteins must be involved in specification of both cardiac and skeletal muscle lineages (49,50). We have recently identified and characterized a new transcription factor, BBF-1, in chicken embryonic cardiac muscle that recognizes the MEF-2 binding site. BBF-1 is distinguishable from MEF-2 since it is not immunoprecipitated by the MEF-2-specific antibodies (45,49). Also, unlike MEF-2, which is present in both cardiac and skeletal muscle cells, and possibly in other tissues, expression of BBF-1 is restricted to cardiac tissue only (45). Since MEF-2 has been implicated in myogenic lineage determination and BBF-1 appears to be a cardiac-specific transcription factor that binds to MEF-2 sequence, we examined the potential of BBF-1 as an early regulator of cardiac muscle differentiation. In avian embryo, the mesodermal precursors of the cardiac muscle have been mapped and the location, movement, and differentiative transition of these cells have been delineated, beginning with the assignment of cardiogenic fate at stage 4 (~20 hours) in gastrulating embryo (76–78). The molecular aspects of these early embryonic changes, especially during the period beginning from the assignment of the cardiogenic fate to the onset of morphogenetic differentiation, have not been studied, and it is not clear what developmental and spatial signals responsible for cardiac tissue specification emanate during early embryogenesis. The genes appearing during this critical period, especially those appearing at or immediately before the cardiac fate assignment at stage 4 (76), are the candidates for cardiac-lineage-specific regulatory factors. We therefore analyzed the onset of cardiac myogenesis by monitoring the appearance of cardiac-muscle-specific MLC2 and cardiac α-actin mRNAs in single embryos followed by that of BBF-1 and MEF-2 binding activities at defined stages of early blastodermal development. We also examined the same single embryos for the appearance of mRNA for CMD1, the chicken homolog of MyoD. We observed that the first discernible signals for cardiac and skeletal MLC2 mRNAs appear at stages 5 and 8, respectively. Consistent with the onset of MLC2, cardiac α-actin mRNA was also detected at stage 5 and skeletal α-actin at stage 7 (Fig. 2–3 and see ref. 49 for details). It is well established that the first heart-forming precursor cells can be located in the bilateral regions around Henson's node at the

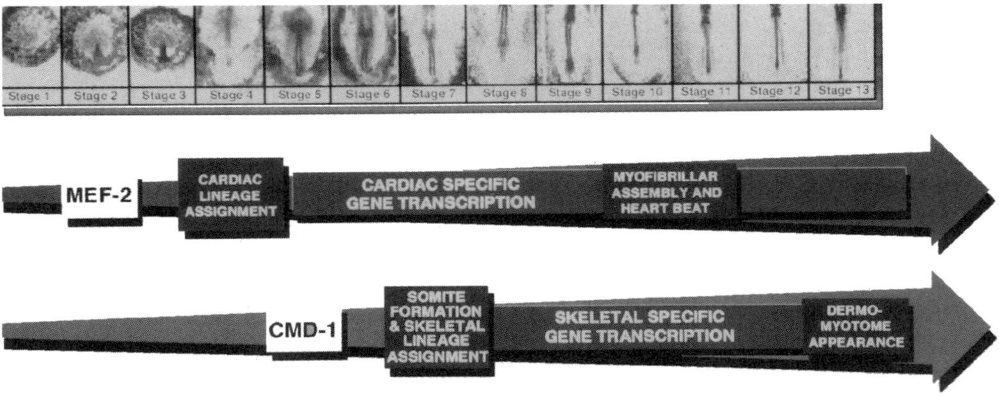

FIG. 2–3. Expression of different marker genes during myogenic lineage determination in developing embryo. *Top panel:* Different stages (76) of chicken embryonic development are shown. *Bottom panel:* Temporal expression of different marker genes is identified. The myogenic regulatory factor MEF-2 appears at stage 2. The cardiac myocyte–specific factor BBF-1 appears at stage 4, when the transcripts for cardiac MLC-2 and cardiac α-actin appear. The skeletal muscle specification factor CMD1 appears at stage 5, prior to the appearance of the first somite and the skeletal MLC-2 transcripts.

full primitive streak stage, stage 4, of chicken development (76,78), whereas the first progenitors of somite cells can be located in stage 7 blastoderms. Therefore, it appears that the cardiac and skeletal muscle differentiation begins at or immediately after the assignment of the respective cell lineage at stages 4 and 7 in developing embryo, which is well before the onset of morphological differentiation at stages 10 and 13, respectively. The temporal separation of the two transcriptional events (stages 5 and 7) is consistent with the established separation in appearance of the two tissue-specific morphological characteristics (stages 10 and 13). We also observed that the first signal of CMD1 can be detected as early as stage 5, that is, prior to the appearance of first somite and the onset of transcription of skeletal MLC2 gene at stage 8. This is consistent with the expected role of HLH proteins in programming only the skeletal, but not the cardiac, myogenesis.

The BBF-1 DNA binding activity appears first at stage 5, whereas the MEF-2-like activity begins to appear only at stage 8 and becomes defined at stage 12 (49). Subsequent analysis of protein extracts from isolated heart tubes of embryos at stage 12 of development and that from the remaining embryos further confirmed that the origins of BBF-1 and MEF-2 activities were predominantly located in the heart tube (49). Because the functional appearance of BBF-1 is temporally linked to the appearance of cardiac-muscle-specific transcripts, we propose that BBF-1 is the earliest marker of the onset of cardiogenic differentiation. To delineate the precise regulatory role BBF-1 plays in development of the cardiac muscle lineage, we recently isolated a recombinant plasmid (pCLP-1) as a candidate for BBF-1 from a cDNA library constructed from mRNA isolated from the heart-forming region of stage 6 chick embryo. Characterization of this cDNA following its expression in *Escherichia coli* shows its binding to the MEF-2 sequence (unpublished results). In situ hybridization analysis demonstrated its expression in the precardiac mesodermal region during early stages of development. The nucleotide sequence analysis of the cDNA clone and DNA binding properties of the bacterially expressed recombinant protein revealed that BBF-1 is novel transcription factor, with no homology to known MEF-2 proteins. Antisense oligonucleotide, when administered in vivo, caused specific inhibition of the heart tube formation with impairment of early somatogenesis as well. Taken together, these data suggest that CLP-1 is an important regulator of the cardiogenic lineage in avian development. Further confirmation of the role of this putative cardiac lineage–associated protein will depend upon its successful expression in noncardiogenic cells and its capacity to transform them to the cardiogenic lineage.

SUMMARY

Despite the extensive analysis and identification of the skeletal muscle–specific regulatory factors that led to dramatic insights into activation of myogenic cell lineage, the molecular basis of cardiac muscle gene specification remains enigmatic. In view of the complexity of the cardiovascular system, it might be that a hierarchical and transitional appearance of several regulators occurs during the progression of cells entering the cardiogenic fate. Recent observations led to speculations that key members of the MEF-2 family proteins, which appear sequentially, but preferentially earlier than the assignment of cardiogenic fate, are candidate regulators of cardiac cell determination. While they are in skeletal muscle cells, it is believed that MEF-2 proteins are involved in regulatory interactions with myogenic bHLH factors; it is likely that such interactions with other factors are also obligatory in cardiac progenitors. Whether such factors appear in these cells remains to be seen. One member of the MEF-2 family, CLP, recently identified in our laboratory, appears in early chicken embryonic development in a pattern that is consistent with the movement of presumptive cardiac mesodermal cells. In ovo administration of antisense oligonucleotide to arrest CLP mRNA resulted in interference with heart development. Further support of the involvement of CLP in cardiogenic commitment must come from selective inactivation of the CLP gene, currently in progress in our laboratory. Judicious application of the various tools of molecular biology will thus facilitate dissection of events responsible for cell commitment to heart development.

REFERENCES

1. Buckingham M. Molecular biology of muscle development. *Cell* 1994;78:15–21.
2. Yutzey KE, Bader D. Diversification of cardiomyogenic cell lineages during early heart development. *Circ Res* 1995;77:216–219.

3. Kirby ML, Waldo KL. Neural crest and cardiovascular patterning. *Circ Res* 1995;77:211–215.
4. Fishman MC, Stainie DY. Cardiovascular development: prospects for a genetic approach. *Circ Res* 1994;74:757–763.
5. Engelmann GL, Dionne CA, Jaye MC. Acidic fibroblast growth factor and heart development: role in myocyte proliferation and capillary angiogenesis. *Circ Res* 1993;72:7–19.
6. Brand T, Schneider MD. The TGF beta superfamily in myocardium: ligands, receptors, transduction, and function. *J Mol Cell Cardiol* 1995;2785:5–18.
7. Schneider MD, Kirshenbaum LA, Brand T, MacLellan WR. Control of cardiac gene transcription by fibroblast growth factors. *Mol Reprod Dev* 1994;39:112–117.
8. Chien KR, Zhu H, Knowlton KU, Miller-Hance W, van-Bilsen M, O'Brien TX, Evans SM. Transcriptional regulation during cardiac growth and development. *Annu Rev Physiol* 1993;55:77–95.
9. Olson EN. Interplay between proliferation and differentiation within the myogenic lineage. *Dev Biol* 1992;154:261–272.
10. Olson EN, Brennan TJ, Chakraborty T, Cheng TC, Cserjesi P, et al. Molecular control of myogenesis: antagonism between growth and differentiation. *Mol Cell Biochem* 1991;104:7–13.
11. Mima T, Ueno H, Fischman DA, Williams LT, Mikawa T. Fibroblast growth factor receptor is required for in vivo cardiac myocyte proliferation at early embryonic stages of heart development. *Proc Natl Acad Sci USA* 1995;92:467–491.
12. Buckingham M, Houzelstein D, Lyons G, Ontell M, Ott MO, Sassoon D. Expression of muscle genes in the mouse embryo. *Symp Soc Exp Biol* 1992;46:203–217.
13. Chien KR, Knowlton KU, Zhu H, Chien S. Regulation of cardiac gene expression during myocardial growth and hypertrophy: molecular studies of an adaptive physiologic response. *FASEB J* 1991;5:3037–3046.
14. Gurdon JB, Lemaire P, Kato K. Community effects and related phenomena in development. *Cell* 1993;75:831–834.
15. Melton DA. Pattern formation during animal development. *Science* 1001;252:234–241.
16. Muslin AJ, Williams LT. Well-defined growth factors promote cardiac development in axolotl mesodermal explants. *Development* 1991;112:1095–1101.
17. MacLellan WR, Brand T, Schneider MD. Transforming growth factor-beta in cardiac ontogeny and adaptation. *Circ Res* 1993;73:783–791.
18. Karin M. The regulation of AP-1 activity by mitogen-activated protein kinases. *J Biol Chem* 1995;270:16483–16486.
19. Olson EN. Proto-oncogenes in the regulatory circuit for myogenesis. *Semin Cell Biol* 1992;3:127–136.
20. Lawrence PA, Morata G. Homeobox genes: their function in *Drosophila* segmentation and pattern formation. *Cell* 1994;78:181–189.
21. Olson EN, Rosenthal N. Homeobox genes and muscle patterning. *Cell* 1994;79:9–12.
22. Chisaka O, Capecchi MR. Regionally restricted developmental defects resulting from targeted disruption of the mouse homeobox gene hox-1.5. *Nature* 1991;350:473–479.
23. Azpiazu N, Frasch M. Tinman and bagpipe: two homeo box genes that determine cell fates in the dorsal mesoderm of *Drosophila. Genes Dev* 1993;7:1325–1340.
24. Lints TJ, Parsons LM, Hartley, L, Lyons I et al. Nkx-2.5: a novel murine homeobox gene expressed in early heart progenitor cells and their myogenic descendants. *Development* 1993;119:419–431.
25. Kim Y, Nirenberg M. *Drosophila* NK-homeobox genes. *Proc Natl Acad Sci USA* 1989;86:7716–7720.
26. Tonissen KF, Drysdale TA, Lints TJ, Harvey RP, Krieg PA. Xnkx-2.5, a *Xenopus* gene related to Nkx-2.5 and tinman: evidence for a conserved role in cardiac development. *Dev Biol* 1994;162:325–328.
27. Lyons I, Parsons LM, Hartley L, Li R, Andrews JE, Robb L, Harvey RP. Myogenic and morphogenetic defects in the heart tubes of murine embryos lacking the homeo box gene Nkx2-5. *Genes Dev* 1995;9:1654–1666.
28. Chen CY, Schwartz RJ. Identification of novel DNA binding targets and regulatory domains of a murine tinman homeodomain factor, nkx-2.5. *J Biol Chem* 1995;270:15628–15633.
29. Grepin C, Dagnino L, Robitaille L, Haberstroh L, Antakly T, Nemer M. A hormone-encoding gene identifies a pathway for cardiac but not skeletal muscle gene transcription. *Mol Cell Biol* 1994;14:3115–3129.
30. Grepin C, Robitaille L, Antakly T, Nemer M. Inhibition of transcription factor GATA-4 expression blocks in vitro cardiac muscle differentiation. *Mol Cell Biol* 1995;15:4095–4102.
31. Wade R, Kedes L. Developmental regulation of contractile protein genes. *Annu Rev Physiol* 1989;51:179–188.

32. Amacher SL, Buskin JN, Hauschka SD. Multiple regulatory elements contribute differentially to muscle creatine kinase enhancer activity in skeletal and cardiac muscle. *Mol Cell Biol* 1993;13: 2753–2764.
33. Sartorelli V, Kurabayashi M, Kedes L. Muscle-specific gene expression. A comparison of cardiac and skeletal muscle transcription strategies. *Circ Res* 1993;72:925–931.
34. Nothias JY, Majumder S, Kaneko KJ, DePamphilis ML. Regulation of gene expression at the beginning of mammalian development. *J Biol Chem* 1995;270:22077–22080.
35. Minty A, Kedes L. Upstream regions of the human cardiac actin gene that modulate its transcription in muscle cells: presence of an evolutionarily conserved repeated motif. *Mol Cell Biol* 1986;6:2125–2136.
36. Jaynes JB, Johnson JE, Buskin JN, Gartside CL, Hauschka SD. The muscle creatine kinase gene is regulated by multiple upstream elements, including a muscle-specific enhancer. *Mol Cell Biol* 1988;8:62–70.
37. Ernst H, Walsh K, Harrison CA, Rosenthal N. The myosin light chain enhancer and the skeletal actin promoter share a binding site for factors involved in muscle-specific gene expression. *Mol Cell Biol* 1991;11:3735–3744.
38. Tuil D, Clergue N, Montarras D, Pinset C, Kahn A, Phan-Dinh-Tuy F. CC Ar GG boxes, cis-acting elements with a dual specificity: muscle-specific transcriptional activation and serum responsiveness. *J Mol Biol* 1990;213:677–686.
39. Taylor M, Treisman R, Garrett N, Mohun T. Muscle-specific (CarG) and serum-responsive (SRE) promoter elements are functionally interchangeable in *Xenopus* embryos and mouse fibroblasts. *Development* 1989;106:67–78.
40. Vincent CK, Gualberto A, Patel CV, Walsh K. Different regulatory sequences control creatine kinase-M gene expression in directly injected skeletal and cardiac muscle. *Mol Cell Biol* 1993;13:1264–1272.
41. Lee TC, Shi Y, Schwartz RJ. Displacement of BrdUrd-induced YY1 by serum response factor activates skeletal alpha-actin transcription in embryonic myoblasts. *Proc Natl Acad Sci USA* 1992;89:9814–9818.
42. Sartorelli V, Webster KA, Ledes L. Muscle-specific expression of the cardiac alpha-actin gene requires MyoD1, CarG-box binding factor, and Sp1. *Genes Dev* 1990;4:1811–1822.
43. Gossett LA, Kelvin D, Sternberg E, Olson EN. A new myocyte specific enhancer binding factor that recognizes a conserved element associated with multiple muscle specific genes. *Mol Cell Biol* 1989;9:5022–5033.
44. Olson EN, Perry M, Schulz RA. Regulation of muscle differentiation by the MEF-2 family of MADS box transcription factors. *Dev Biol* 1995;172:2–14.
45. Zhou MD, Goswami SK, Martin ME, Siddiqui MA. A new serum-responsive, cardiac tissue–specific transcription factor that recognizes the MEF-2 site in the myosin light chain-2 promoter. *Mol Cell Biol* 1993;13:1222–1231.
46. Breitbart RE, Liang CS, Smoot LB, Laheru DA, Mahdavi V, Nadal-Ginard B. A fourth human MEF-2 transcription factor, hMEF2D, is an early marker of the myogenic lineage. *Development* 1993;118:1095–1106.
47. McDermott JC, Cardoso MC, Yu YT, Andres V, Leifer D, Krainc D, Lipton SA, Nadal-Ginard B. hMEF2C gene encodes skeletal muscle- and brain-specific transcription factors. *Mol Cell Biol* 1993;13:2564–2577.
48. Leifer D, Krainc D, Yu YT, McDermott J. Breitbart RE, Heng J, Neve RL, Kosofsky B, Nadal-Ginard B, Lipton SA. MEF2C, a MADS/MEF2-family transcription factor expressed in a laminar distribution in cerebral cortex. *Proc Natl Acad Sci USA* 1993;90:1546–1550.
49. Goswami S, Qasba P, Ghatpande S, Carleton S, Deshpande AK, Baig M, Siddiqui MA. Differential expression of the myocyte enhancer factor 2 family of transcription factors in development: the cardiac factor BBF-1 is an early marker for cardiogenesis. *Mol Cell Biol* 1994;14:5130–5138.
50. Edmondson DG, Lyons GE, Martin JF, Olson En. Mef2 gene expression marks the cardiac and skeletal muscle lineages during mouse embryogenesis. *Development* 1994;120:1251–1263.
51. Han TH, Prywes R. Regulatory role of MEF-2D in serum induction of the c-jun promoter. *Mol Cell Biol* 1995;15:2907–2915.
52. Zhu H, Nguyen VT, Brown AB, Pourhosseini A, Garcia AV, Van Bilson M, Chien KR. A novel, tissue restricted zinc finger protein (HF-1n) binds to the cardiac regulatory element (HF-1b/MEF-2) in the rat myosin light chain-2 gene. *Mol Cell Biol* 1993;13:4432–4444.
53. Cserjesi P, Lilly P, Hincley C, Perry M, Olson EN. Homeodomain protein Mhox and MADS protein myocyte enhancer-binding factor-2 converge on a common element in the muscle creatine kinase enhancer. *J Biol Chem* 1994;269:16740–16745.

54. Olson EN, Klein WH. BHLH factors in muscle development: dead lines and commitments, what to leave in and what to leave out. *Genes Dev* 1994;8:1–8.
55. Olson EN. Regulation of muscle transcription by the MyoD family. The heart of the matter. *Circ Res* 1993;72:1–6.
56. Sartorelli V, Hong NA, Bishopric NA, Kedes L. Myocardial activation of the human cardiac alpha actin promoter by helix-loop-helix proteins. *Proc Natl Acad Sci USA* 1990;89:4047–4051.
57. Molkentin JD, Brogan RS, Jobe SM, Markham BE. Expression of the alpha-myosin heavy chain gene in the heart is regulated in part by an E-box-dependent mechanism. *J Biol Chem* 1993;268:2602–2609.
58. Weintraub H. The MyoD family and myogenesis: redundancy, networks, and thresholds. *Cell* 1993;75:1241–1244.
59. Goswami S, Siddiqui MAQ. Transactivation of cardiac MLC-2 promoter by MyoD in 10T1/2 fibroblast cells is independent of E-Box requirement but depends upon new proteins that recognize MEF-2 site. *Cell Mol Biol Res* 1995;41:199–205.
60. Ordahl CP. Developmental regulation of sarcomeric gene expression. *Curr Top Dev Biol* 1992;26: 145–168.
61. Bishopric NH, Kedes L. Adrenergic regulation of the skeletal alpha-actin gene promoter during myocardial cell hypertrophy. *Proc Natl Acad Sci USA* 1991;88:2132–2136.
62. Iannello RC, Mar JH, Ordahl CP. Characterization of a promoter element required for transcription in myocardial cells. *J Biol Chem* 1991;266:3309–3316.
63. Mar JH, Ordahl CP. M-CAT binding factor, a novel trans-acting factor governing muscle-specific transcription. *Mol Cell Biol* 1990;10:4271–4283.
64. Schreier T, Kedes L, Gahlmann R. Cloning, structural analysis, and expression of the human slow twitch skeletal muscle/cardiac troponin C gene. *J Biol Chem* 1990;265:21247–21253.
65. Parmacek MS, Vora AJ, Shen T, Brar E, Jung F, Leiden JM. A novel myogenic regulatory circuit controls slow/cardiac troponin C gene transcription in skeletal muscle. *Mol Cell Biol* 1994;14: 1870–1885.
66. Mahdavi V, Izumo S, Nadal-Ginard B. Developmental and hormonal regulation of sarcomeric myosin heavy chain gene family. *Circ Res* 1987;60:804–814.
67. Knotts S, Rindt H, Neumann J, Robbins J. In vivo regulation of the mouse beta myosin heavy chain gene. *J Biol Chem* 1994;269:31275–31282.
68. Thompson WR, Nadal-Ginard B, Mahdavi V. A MyoD1-independent muscle-specific enhancer controls the expression of the beta-myosin heavy chain gene in skeletal and cardiac muscle cells. *J Biol Chem* 1991;266:22678–22688.
69. Flink IL, Edwards JG, Bahl JJ, Liew CC, Sole M, Morkin E. Characterization of a strong positive *cis*-acting element of the human beta-myosin heavy chain gene in fetal rat heart cells. *J Biol Chem* 1992;267:9917–9924.
70. Rindt H, Subramaniam A, Robbins J. An in vivo analysis of transcriptional elements in the mouse alpha-myosin heavy chain gene promoter. *Transgenic Res* 1995;4:397–405.
71. Dunwoodie SL, Joya JE, Arkell RM, Hardeman EC. Multiple regions of the human cardiac actin gene are necessary for maturation-based expression in striated muscle. *J Biol Chem* 1994;269:12212–12219.
72. Adolph EA, Subramaniam A, Cserjesi P, Olson EN, Robbins J. Role of myocyte-specific enhancer-binding factor.
73. Subramaniam A, Jones WK, Gulick J, Wert S, Neumann J, Robbins J. Tissue-specific regulation of the alpha-myosin heavy chain gene promoter in transgenic mice. *J Biol Chem* 1991; 266:24613–24620.
74. Qasba P, Lin E, Zhou MD, Kumar, A, Siddiqui MA. A single transcription factor binds to two divergent sequence elements with a common function in cardiac myosin light chain 2-promoter. *Mol Cell Biol* 1992;12:1107–1116.
75. Shen RA, Goswami SK, Mascareno E, Kumar A, Siddiqui MA. Tissue-specific transcription of the cardiac myosin light-chain 2 gene is regulated by an upstream repressor element. *Mol Cell Biol* 1991;11:1676–1685.
76. Hamburger V, Hamilton HL. A series of normal stages in the development of the chick embryo. *J Morphol* 1951;88:49–92.
77. Manasek FJ, Monroe RG. Early cardiac morphogenesis is independent of function. *Dev Biol* 1972;27:584–588.
78. Gonzalez-Sanchez A, Bader D. In vitro analysis of cardiac progenitor cell differentiation. *Dev Biol* 1990;139:197–209.

The Developing Heart,
edited by Bohuslav Ošťádal et al.
Lippincott-Raven Publishers,
Philadelphia © 1997.

3

TGF-β Ligands and Receptors

Expression and Function in Heart Development

Patricia S. Grutkoski and Gary L. Engelmann

Molecular Biology Program, Cardiovascular Institute,
Loyola University Medical Center, Maywood, IL 60153

Development of the heart, like that of many other organs and systems, appears to be under partial control by several growth factors that work in an autocrine or paracrine manner. The presence of growth factors in the developing embryonic and fetal hearts appears to be differentially regulated in that they are expressed in both temporally and spatially discrete times and sites; and many are produced by the ventricular myocytes (cardiomyocytes) themselves. In the postnatal and mature myocardium, growth factors are produced by both cardiomyocytes and the surrounding nonmyocyte populations of fibroblast, smooth muscle, and endothelial cells. In the developing ventricle, cardiomyocyte-derived growth factors are believed to be involved in several separate yet interrelated processes: (a) cardiomyocyte proliferation and differentiation; (b) the formation of biomechanical structures such as the valves; (c) vasculogenesis, capillary angiogenesis, and neovascularization; and (d) nonmuscle cell-produced extracellular matrix (ECM) formation.

Among the growing list of growth factors that appear to have an active part in heart development are members of the transforming growth factor-beta (TGF-β) family. TGF-β is the prototypic member of a large peptide growth factor family that includes the TGF-βs, activins, inhibins, bone morphogenetic proteins, mullerian inhibiting substance, and products of the *decapentaplegic* (*Drosophila*) and *Vgl* (*Xenopus*) genes. The members of this family and their structures, general biological actions, receptors, and mechanisms of action have been extensively reviewed (1–5) and thus will not be covered in great detail here.

The general biological functions of TGF-β can be broadly grouped into three major, albeit overlapping, categories: (a) those that affect cellular proliferation and migration; (b) those involved in cell adhesion and ECM formation; and (c) those that affect a cell's phenotype (1,6). In general, all these actions can be mediated by any of the five TGF-β isoforms presently known: TGF-β_{1-3} (mammalian), TGF-β_4 (avian), and TGF-β_5 (amphibian). Each of these TGF-β isoforms has been highly conserved throughout evolution, suggesting specific roles for each. In addition, each TGF-β isoform shares a high degree of amino acid sequence homology in its mature, bioactive domain. These isoforms are often co-expressed and co-localized, and they generally elicit similar mechanisms of action on cells in culture.

To date, nine distinct protein bands have been found, by TGF-β_1 cross-linking studies, on cell surfaces of a diverse array of cell types that bind TGF-βs (2). Three of these proteins in mammalian cells are classified as functional TGF-β receptors: type I (βRI), type II (βRII), and type III (βRIII). It appears that all three mammalian isoforms of TGF-β ligands mediate their responses through the dynamics of their interactions with βRI and βRII. These two receptors belong to the serine/threonine kinase receptor family and are thought to act by forming heterodimers (or heterotetramers) upon ligand binding and initiate "downstream" signal transduction pathways that remain poorly defined at this time. The exact function of each member of the heterodimer remains to be fully elucidated; yet the evidence to date suggests that βRII is critical for TGF-β ligand binding, whereas βRI is essential for initiating the signal transduction pathways. In contrast, βRIII has been postulated to be involved in TGF-β ligand presentation (particularly for TGF-β_2) or ligand sequestration yet is devoid of any signal transduction capabilities on its own.

EXPRESSION PATTERNS

TGF-β Ligands in the Heart

Although most of what is known about the TGF-β ligands has been ascertained from their genetic organization derived from their cloning, biosynthesis and pleotrophic actions in vitro, determination of their expression patterns in vivo provides critical data needed to begin to elucidate their functions in development. Expression patterns for the TGF-β ligands during heart development have been best studied in the murine, rat, and chicken systems. These expression patterns, in general, are similar, but some significant species-related differences have been found. The expression patterns of the three TGF-β ligands are very distinct, both temporally and spatially, suggesting that although they have similar effects in vitro, they may play very specific roles in vivo.

TGF-β_1 expression was undetected in the chicken embryonic heart or cultured myocytes obtained from embryonic hearts (7,8), which may be explained by the fact that TGF-β_4 is the chicken isoform of TGF-β_1 (9). However, TGF-β_1 is expressed during rodent heart development. The earliest detectable expression of TGF-β_1 mRNA is in cardiac precursor cells within the splanchnic mesoderm (10). However, expression later in heart development, which is more defined, has also been documented (6,10,11). At 9 days post coitum (dpc), TGF-β_1 is strongly localized to those tissues that are undergoing epithelial to mesenchymal (e–m) transformation, a phenomenon that occurs during the formation of the heart valves (6,10). At 11–12 dpc, TGF-β_1 can be detected in the ventricular myocardium in a uniform manner with TGF-β_1 being localized to the myocytes themselves (6,10,11). The expression levels of β_1 increase significantly in the late fetal (18 dpc), early neonate, and in the mature heart (11). Similarly, TGF-β_4 can be localized to myocytes within the atria and ventricles of the developing avian heart from as early as stage 22 (day 4) through adulthood, with ligand expression increasing as the chick matures (8,12).

TGF-β_2 expression patterns suggest that it may play an important role in heart development in chickens as well as rodents. However, these expression patterns deviate markedly from one another. In the murine heart, TGF-β_2 is expressed at 9.5–10.5 dpc in both the atrioventricular (AV) region and in the prevalvular myocardium (10,13). However, by 12.5 dpc, TGF-β_2 expression cannot be detected in the myocardium; yet it is still highly expressed in the AV region, particularly in the valves (10,13). In contrast to the distinct temporal and regional changes in TGF-β_2 expression in the mouse, TGF-β_2 expression in the developing chicken heart appears to be in both heart regions at Hamilton-Hamburger stages 15–20 (this corresponds to the time in which differences were seen in mice) (7,8) and decreases with age after stage 29 (14).

TGF-β_3 expression appears to be the most limited of the three primary TGF-β isoforms. In the chicken, TGF-β_3 has a distinct localization to the AV canal and has been implicated to be critical in the epithelial–mesenchymal (e–m) transition associated with valve formation (see later) (7). Interestingly, TGF-β_3 cannot be detected in the early mouse heart at similar stages (7,13), suggesting that a different isoform or family member may be involved in the e–m transition/valve formation. TGF-β_1 and TGF-β_2 expression patterns suggest they may "substitute" or compensate for TGF-β_3 in the mouse. Later in heart development (11.5–16.5 dpc) TGF-β_3 can be detected in the ECM and mesenchyme of the valves as well as in the atrial and ventricular myocardium (10,15) and continues to be expressed at relatively high levels in the ventricular myocardium in the immediate postnatal period and through weaning, when the expression levels drop off markedly (16).

TGF-β Receptors in the Heart

Although expression patterns of the TGF-β ligands indicate where they may be important for various developmental processes, an understanding of the expression patterns of the TGF-β receptors is also necessary to fully appreciate the role(s) TGF-β plays in development. The expression of the three primary TGF-β receptors has been studied to varying degrees in chicken (17), murine (18,19), and rat (20) systems. In general, the expression patterns observed in these three systems are similar within the heart. Although data are limited on early heart development, neither βRI nor βRII could be detected by PCR analysis at 6.5–7.5 dpc in the three mouse embryo germ layers, but they could be detected by 14 dpc through adulthood (18,19). Similarly, expression of βRII and βRIII can be detected in the chicken heart at low levels in the stage 26 embryo in atrial and ventricular cells (17). This expression significantly increases between stage 26, day 6, and day 10, and greatly increases upon hatching. It is interesting to note that in the fetal avian heart, the protein levels of all three receptors (determined by receptor cross-linking) are approximately 10 times higher in the atria than in the ventricles (17). Expression of the three receptors was extensively studied in the rat from the late fetal stage through adulthood, and these results support and extend those obtained in the mouse and chicken (20). βRI and βRIII mRNA levels were readily detected in total RNA from ventricular tissue of 18 dpc through 9-week postnatal animals; with only a modest increase in transcript abundance. However, βRII expression was more restricted with low to undetectable levels in the late fetal periods, but expression increased markedly at or around birth and increased through the postnatal to mature stages of development (20). Immunolocalization of βRII within the ventricle was primarily in the cardiomyocytes, but surrounding nonmyocytes also expressed the receptor (20). There were no significant differences in steady-state transcript abundance between the different regions of the mature heart (right ventricle, left ventricle, and septum) (20). These studies in the rat did not address the expression of the receptors in the atria; however, it is expected that mRNA patterns would resemble those seen in other rodents, such as the mouse.

CONTROL OF EXPRESSION

The distinct temporal and spatial expression patterns observed for both TGF-β ligands and receptors suggest that each is regulated in separate ways that may occasionally overlap. Regulation of both ligands and receptors may occur at both the transcriptional and posttranscriptional levels through the use of different promoters, regulatory transcription factors, and untranslated regions (UTRs), as well as posttranslational processing and protein turnover, or "latency." These regulatory mechanisms may respond to humoral, neurohumoral, and mechanical stimuli differently, supporting the hypothesis that each TGF-β ligand and receptor may have distinct physiological and development functions.

Promoters/UTRs

The promoter and 5′ UTR from both the mouse and human TGF-β_1 gene have been cloned and well characterized (21,22). The 2.7 kilobases (kb) of DNA upstream of the translational start site in the TGF-β_1 gene are highly conserved, having 66% nucleotide identity between the murine and human sequences. The promoter is unique among TGF-β ligands in that it does not contain a CAAT or TATA box near the transcription start site. However, several Sp1- and AP-2-like, but not AP-1-like, sequences are found in the TGF-β_1 promoter. Through mutational studies, it has been shown that not all Sp1 sites contribute to TGF-β_1 transcriptional regulation (23). Rather, there are Sp1 sites distal to the transcriptional start site that appear to have no inducing capability as ascertained by cotransfection experiments of Sp1 with numerous TGF-β_1 promoter-cat constructs (23). Additionally, within the first 113 basepairs (bp) upstream of the transcriptional start site, a *ras*-responsive element was found that greatly increased transcription (21).

It appears that both the 5′ and 3′ UTRs control the production of the TGF-β_1 peptide, with the 5′ UTR of the TGF-β_1 mRNA as the best-characterized regulatory UTR among this family of ligands. It has been shown that retinoic acid (RA) can increase TGF-β_1 mRNA without an increase in peptide secretion and that progestin can increase peptide production without affecting mRNA levels (24). Therefore, both positive and negative regulatory regions must exist in the UTRs that mediate these effects. The 5′ UTR of TGF-β_1 is a GC-rich segment 840 bp long that contains two putative sequences that are capable of forming stem-loop structures (24). These stem-loop sequences are highly conserved in porcine, murine, and human TGF-β_1 genes and have been found to suppress translation in their native location or when inserted into another gene as a hybrid 5′ UTR (24,25). The 5′-loop has been found to inhibit translational initiation and to bind a 25-kDa cytosolic factor that has yet to be identified and may play a role in the inhibitory process (25). In contrast to the inhibitory activity of the 5′ UTR, the 3′ UTR appears to increase translation and decrease the stability of the mRNA (26). These effects are mediated by a region within the 3′ UTR of the TGF-β_1 mRNA that is also GC-rich, conserved among several mammalian species, and not seen in any of the other TGF-β isoforms. Interestingly, this 3′ UTR GC-rich domain can stimulate protein production only in the sense orientation, while decreasing mRNA levels and protein production in the antisense orientation (26).

The TGF-β_2 promoter and 5′ UTR are the least well characterized of the three mammalian TGF-β isoforms. The identified GC-rich promoter and 5′ UTR cover approximately 1350 bp upstream of the translational start site and contain a TATA box, cAMP responsive element (CRE)/ATF-like element, and AP-2 sequence motifs (27,28). Upstream of these elements, a negative element that suppresses transcription in a cell type–specific manner has been identified (27). Additionally, the identified ATF-1 and ATF-2 recognition sites have different binding affinities and activating potentials that are operative in a tissue-specific manner, thereby suggesting interactions with other co-regulators (27). Unlike TGF-β_1, the 5′ UTR for TGF-β_2 is not conserved across all species with the avian 5′ UTR displaying no homology with the mouse, human, and *Xenopus* 5′ UTRs, which are highly homologous (28–30).

Finally, the TGF-β_3 promoter and 5′ UTR are well characterized. Like the TGF-β_2 promoter, the human TGF-β_3 promoter is GC-rich, located within a CpG island, and contains a TATA box, CRE sites, and AP-1 and AP-2 sites (28,31). Although AP-2 sites are found in the promoter, purified AP-2 does not bind to or activate this promoter (32). In contrast, no consensus sites for Sp1 were found; yet this promoter is greatly activated by purified Sp1. In fact, the TGF-β_3 promoter is more sensitive to Sp1 than the TGF-β_1 promoter which has consensus Sp1 sites (23). Just upstream of the AP-2 sites, a sequence was found that is likely to regulate the developmental and tissue-specific expression of TGF-β_3 (32). This segment, referred to as 3xTCCC, contains three consecutive repeats of TCCC and binds a novel protein that activates the promoter approximately 63% above the "basal" levels obtained from the sequences just upstream of the transcriptional start site. Mutations within the 3xTCCC element result in the loss of binding of the novel protein as well as activation of gene transcription. Like the human promoter, the chicken TGF-β_3 promoter has a TATA box, CRE, AP-1, and AP-2 consensus binding sites; however, unlike its human counterpart, this promoter also has 10 Sp1 binding sites (33).

Like the UTRs of the other isoforms, the TGF-β_3 5′ UTR has also been found to inhibit translation/production of the TGF-β_3 peptide. The human 5′ UTR is a 1.1-kb region that contains 12 ATG codons (11 open reading frames), polypurine stretches, and uridine-rich regions (28,34). Although the exact function of these regions is unclear, deletion of any of them increases translational efficiency. The role of the ATG codons has been hypothesized to produce short, nonfunctional peptides, resulting in lower translation from the downstream, proper ATG start codon. In contrast, the chicken 5′ UTR is only 132 bp and contains no open reading frames (33).

Only one promoter has been well characterized for the TGF-β receptors, the human βRII promoter (35,36). Examination of a total of 1.9 kb upstream of the transcriptional start sites revealed that most, if not all, regulatory regions lie within the first 1.2 kb (36). This region lacks both TATA and CAAT boxes near the transcription start sites but contains two positive regulatory regions—the first, which contains two Sp1 and two AP-1 binding sites, and two negative regulatory regions, which have yet to be fully characterized (35,36).

Regulation of TGF-β Ligand and Receptor Expression

The production of mRNAs and proteins for TGF-β_{1-3} and their receptors is influenced by many diverse factors. One of these factors may be the TGF-β ligand itself. In cardiac myocytes isolated from 10-day chicken embryos, addition of TGF-β_{1-3} results in an increase in steady-state expression levels of TGF-β_{3-4}, but not of TGF-β_2 (37). Autoinduction of TGF-β_1 is also seen in rat neonatal ventricular myocytes after treatment with exogenous TGF-β_1 (38,39). Although this appears to be a direct feedback loop on TGF-β expression, another positive feedback loop can be demonstrated with ECM proteins. Mammary epithelial cells plated on ECM express a much lower level of TGF-β_1 than those plated on plastic, whereas TGF-β_2 expression appears unaffected (40). These data suggest a mechanistic, positive feedback loop wherein low ECM stimuli stimulate TGF-β_1 expression, which in return may stimulate ECM production. Once ECM concentrations reach a critical level, they may down-regulate TGF-β_1 gene expression, thereby down-regulating ECM production and completing the loop.

It should be noted that teratogenic doses of retinoic acid (RA) cause cardiac defects. Although none on the TGF-β promoters have classic retinoid response elements, RA induces TGF-β_{2-3} gene expression and peptide secretion (28,41). Other factors that have been found to regulate TGF-β gene expression in myocytes are calcium, estradiol, phorbol esters, cAMP, and steroids (28,41). The role of these inducers, whether direct or indirect, and the signaling pathways relevant to cardiomyocytes and heart development are still under investigation.

EFFECTS ON HEART DEVELOPMENT

The roles that the TGF-βs are thought to play in the development of the heart, as mentioned earlier, involve three important aspects: (a) cellular differentiation, (b) ECM deposition and tissue remodeling, and (c) cellular proliferation. Although it has been determined that TGF-β_1 may regulate cardiomyocyte gene expression through a signaling pathway that involves the activation of *ras* and immediate early genes such as c-*fos* and c-*jun* (38), other pathways are also involved, and their regulatory role, if any, remains to be fully elucidated. However, regardless of the pathway or mechanism of action, TGF-βs are known to mediate changes in gene expression, mRNA translation, and protein production.

Differentiation and ECM Deposition

For many of the muscle-specific, contractile proteins, isoform switching occurs between the fetal-to-neonatal and the neonatal-to-adult stages. Regulation of contractile protein isoform switching is still under investigation, but it has been shown that TGF-βs can influence the expression of several of these genes in cardiomyocyte cultures. In cultured neonatal rat cardiomyocytes, TGF-β_1 treatment decreases the expression of alpha-myosin heavy chain (α-MHC) and sarcoplasmic reticulum ATPase (SR Ca^{2+}-ATPase), increases β-MHC and α-skeletal actin, while having no effect on α-cardiac actin (38,42). Whether TGF-β_1 has these same effects on fetal myocytes has yet to be completely determined.

One of the classic effects of TGF-β stimulation is the regulation of ECM deposition. This regulation involves the stimulation of ECM protein production and secretion, inhibition of protease synthesis and increasing synthesis of protease inhibitors, and stimulation of integrin receptor production, which enhances the cell's ability to interact with the ECM and each other (6). Although many examples can be cited, the regulation of type I collagen demonstrates the ability of TGF-β_1 to regulate both its transcription and translation (43). Type I collagen is made up of two subunits, α1(I) and α2(I). Upon TGF-β_1 treatment, α1(I) mRNA levels increase, resulting in increased collagen protein production. However, α2(I) mRNA levels are unchanged; yet by an unknown mechanism, TGF-β_1 induces and/or increases translation from the "basal level" of this specific mRNA, resulting in an equal increase in both type I collagen protein subunits.

Cellular Proliferation

TGF-βs have significant antiproliferative activities on most cell types in culture, including cardiomyocytes (1,2,11,44,45). These antiproliferative activities can be divided into two groups: (a) those that interrupt the stimulation of proliferation by other growth-promoting stimuli and (b) those that regulate the production or activities of proteins involved in the normal progression through the cell cycle.

Epidermal growth factor (EGF), acidic and basic fibroblast growth factor (a-/b-FGF), and the insulin-like growth factors (IGF) -I and -II are five "mitogenic" growth factors that are found within the heart at various developmental stages, particularly during embryonic and fetal development, when most of the proliferative expansion of the cardiomyocyte population occurs. Co-stimulation of embryonic chicken cardiomyocytes with TGF-β_1 and b-FGF or IGF-II decreased or canceled out, respectively, their stimulatory effects on subsequent DNA synthesis and cell division (44). Downregulation of the expression of the receptors for b-FGF by TGF-β_1 has been hypothesized to play a role in this inhibition. Similar results were seen in rat cardiomyocytes, both fetal and neonatal, treated with IGF-I or IGF-II with TGF-β_1 (11). These results demonstrate that one of the antiproliferative activities of TGF-β_1 involves interfering with other proliferative stimuli commonly found in the developing heart. Another example of TGF-βs modulating the activity of another growth factor is that seen in co-treatment of neonatal rat cardiomyocytes with TGF-β_1 and EGF (45). TGF-β_1 has the ability to decrease the cAMP elevation resulting from EGF stimulation in a time- and dose-dependent manner. This decrease is bifunctional, with TGF-β_1 decreasing the EGF receptor's kinase function as well as altering the activity of the catalytic subunit of adenylyl cyclase (45).

In addition to interfering with other proliferative signals, TGF-βs have been found to influence the activities and/or production of several key components of the cell cycle (46–54). The retinoblastoma (Rb) gene is a critical cell cycle regulatory protein that becomes phosphorylated in late G_1, and its activity is necessary for entry into S phase and DNA replication. TGF-β_1 has been found to maintain Rb in its unphosphorylated state, leading to G_1 arrest (46). TGF-β_1 added at the mid to late G_1 stage of the cell cycle did not have any effect on the Rb that was already phosphorylated, but it inhibited further phosphorylation, thus regulating the phosphorylation and not the dephosphorylation of Rb (46). To date, no studies of cardiomyocyte proliferation have investigated TGF-β's effects on cell cycle–related events.

Of growing importance to our understanding of the regulatory role TGF-βs play on cell proliferation is that TGF-β_1 has been found to regulate the cyclin/cdk activities needed during G_1 to S-phase transitions. Although cyclin synthesis appears not to be directly affected by TGF-βs, synthesis of one of the cyclin co-activators, cyclin-dependent kinase (cdk) 4, is suppressed by TGF-β_1 in a posttranscriptional manner (47,48). This suppression appears to be critical in preventing the formation of active cyclin E/cdk4 complexes in cells treated with TGF-β_1. An inhibitor (p27,Kip1,Cip1) of cdk2 and cdk4 was identified as a protein that was in excess in contact-inhibited or TGF-β_1-treated cells (49–51). However, excess Kip1 was caused not by increased production of the protein itself, but by decreased competition for binding from cyclin D/cdk4 complexes that resulted from downregulated cdk4 synthesis in response to TGF-β_1. Additionally, another inhibitor of cdk4, p15^{INK4B}, was identified that inhibits cdk4 and cdk6 (52). p15^{INK4B} is induced approximately 30-fold in response to TGF-β_1, and although it may not result in the release of Kip1 from cyclin D/cdk4 complexes, it inhibits cyclin activity needed for progression through G_1. Additionally, it has been shown that TGF-β induction of Cip1 and p15^{INK4B} relies on Sp1 consensus binding sites within their respective promoters, indicating that the activity of the Sp family of transcription factors is also regulated by TGF-β (53,54). It is important to note that these studies have not been done in cardiomyocytes. Therefore, the role that TGF-βs may play in the regulation of cardiomyocyte proliferation at the level of specific cell cycle–related proteins is speculative but provides a basis on which hypotheses can be drawn.

Epithelial–Mesenchymal (e–m) Transitions

The formation of mesenchymal tissue from an epithelial sheet is a developmentally significant event and often is mediated by ECM proteins (55). This phenomenon is especially important since the valves and membranous portions of the atrial and ventricular septum are derived from cells that are endothelial in origin. Transformation is regionally specific within the heart and occurs only in the atrioventricular (AV) canal. This process of e–m transformation in the heart, as well as similar transformations earlier in embryonic development, has been recently reviewed (55). To study this phenomenon in the heart, a collagen gel culture system is employed in which explants (AV canal explants that contain myocardium and endothelium) from the embryonic heart can be cultured and allowed to grow/differentiate in a 3-D system (7). In these cultures, the myocardium aggregates into a beating myoball, the endothelium expands across the gel surface, and the mesenchymal cells can migrate into the matrix of collagen. It is these migrating cells that are the products of e–m transformation.

As mentioned earlier, TGF-β_1 is expressed in the AV canal in the chicken embryo at the time of the e–m transformation. A series of experiments has been performed in which it has been determined that TGF-β_1 plays a role in this transformation. In the first set of experiments, stage 14 AV canal explants were cultured in the presence of TGF-β_1 and TGF-β_2 $\pm$ either b-FGF or EGF (56). However, when the "AV myoball" was replaced with ventricular myocardium, e–m transitions occurred, while the myocardium itself could not induce the transformation. To support this, an antibody against all three forms of TGF-β was added to the cultures and was able to block the transformation (56). This suggested that a TGF-β along with a ventricularly produced co-factor could induce the e–m transformation.

Because exogenous TGF-βs are able to elicit similar functions when added to cells *in vitro,* an alternative method was used to determine which TGF-β isoform(s) is important for the e–m transformation. In this approach, oligonucleotides complementary to the nonconserved 5′-ends of the TGF-β mRNA transcripts were used to block production of endogenous TGF-βs (57). These oligonucleotides were topically applied to the explants 12 hours after cultures were started, and then the explants were allowed to "grow" for 12–18 hours in which e–m transformations occur. It was demonstrated that only the oligonucleotides specific for TGF-β_3 were able to inhibit transformation by 80%, whereas oligonucleotides to β_1 and β_2 mRNA had no effect. These data suggested that "only" TGF-β_3 is essential for the e–m transformation as judged by the appearance/migration of mesenchymal cells into the collagen matrix and further shows that even though an added substance can elicit a certain function *in vitro,* it may not truly reflect what actually occurs *in vivo.*

TGF-β1 Knockouts and Developing Hearts

Because the expression pattern for each TGF-β isoform is distinct, each ligand appears to have its own role in the development of the heart that may be independent of the other isoforms present in the heart. Because of the ability of each TGF-β isoform to mediate similar effects *in vitro,* such models can give an unrealistic picture of what may actually occur during *in vivo* heart development. Therefore, *in vivo* studies are necessary to elucidate the distinct role each TGF-β isoform may have on heart development, as well as those that may overlap with other isoforms or TGF-β family members. These *in vivo* models, which make use of gene ablation, transgenic mouse technologies, have been reported for the "parent" isoform TGF-β_1.

Using embryonic stem cells, TGF-β_1-deficient mice were created by knocking out a TGF-β_1 allele by homologous recombination (58–60). Crosses were performed between the resulting heterozygous animals that were phenotypically normal and fertile. Although not all the homozygous mutant (−/−) mice were born (only 40–50%), those that made it to term were indistinguishable from littermates and had no gross developmental abnormalities upon external anatomic examination. However, these animals developed a wasting syndrome and ultimately died within the first 3 weeks because of cardiopulmonary failure. Upon more detailed histologic examination, it was noted that the primary cause of death was a dysfunctional immune/inflammatory response system that is normally held in check, at least in part, by TGF-βs. Between 7 and 20 days after birth, mononuclear inflammatory cells infiltrated the lungs and heart, both the myocardium and pericardium, resulting in lesions and myocyte lysis as well as tissue necrosis.

Although it appeared that TGF-β_1 was not essential for embryonic or fetal heart development, one observation was made in the myocytes of the −/−pups that reflected one of the characteristic effects of TGF-β: inhibition of proliferation. Several myocytes from a 5-day-old TGF-β_1 null mouse were found to have mitochondrial changes that were characterized as being enlarged and having a decreased number of cristae, suggesting extended proliferation in the absence of TGF-β_1 (61). Additionally, in animals in which the inflammatory response was suppressed, nuclear labeling (by Bromodeoxyuridine) indicated hyperplasia in cardiac tissue isolated from 5-week-old animals (62). However, in TGF-β_1 null mice devoid of lymphocytes (backcrossed onto a SCID background), evidence of myocyte proliferation was not seen. This suggests that it is not the absence of TGF-β_1 but the absence of lymphocytes, by a yet unknown mechanism, that has an effect on the extended proliferation of cardiac cells (62). Additionally, TGF-β_3-null mice have also been created (63). Like the TGF-β_1 null mice, no gross abnormalities in the heart were seen in the TGF-β_3-null animals. Nevertheless, these animals died within 24 hours after birth because of their inability to breathe properly as a result of cleft palate, so possible roles of TGF-β_3 in early neonatal and adult development could not be analyzed.

Although the importance of either TGF-β isoform in heart development appears to be minimal in data from these transgenic murine models, we cannot rule out the apparent "rescue" effect other TGF-β isoforms or TGF-β family members may have in compensating for the missing isoform. Because of ligand abundance and overlap in ligand specificity for the TGF-β receptors, TGF-β receptor knockout studies may better address the role TGF-β plays in heart development as well as in cardiac structure–function relationships.

Conclusions and Discussion

Although cardiomyocytes express many of the peptide growth factors that are familiar with many cell lineages, developmental aspects of the heart are quite atypical and cannot be readily compared to other organs or be predicted from other systems. The simplest example can be drawn from the comparison of skeletal muscle development to that of cardiac muscle. In skeletal muscle development, the cells proliferate as nondifferentiated myoblasts that do not express muscle-specific genes and have no or limited contractile ability. Upon withdrawing from the cell cycle, these cells terminally differentiate and fuse to form contractile myofibers. This process is influenced by many extracellular factors, including TGF-βs, which appears to be necessary for differentiation (64). In contrast, embryonic and fetal cardiomyocytes are fully differentiated, contractile cells functioning before TGF-β ligands or type II TGF-β receptors are avidly detected in the heart. In addition to performing their contractile functions, cardiomyocytes maintain their ability to proliferate throughout fetal development, yet permanently withdraw from the cell cycle in the early neonatal period. Again, these processes of cardiomyocyte growth and heart development are influenced by many extracellular factors, such as TGF-β, but obviously not in the same regulatory scheme as that for skeletal myocyctes.

Although the TGF-β knockout studies indicate no gross developmental abnormalities in the hearts of these mice, the distinct expression patterns for the TGF-β ligands and receptors suggest a definitive role for each in development. Although compensation for missing ligands in the knockout mice is possible, it is also possible that the roles the TGF-βs play in the heart are more subtle than those associated with skeletal muscle development. The patterns of TGF-β ligand and receptor expression in ventricular tissue have been associated with documented changes in myocyte proliferation, ECM biogenesis, capillary angiogenesis, and possible contractile protein isoform switches. Therefore, studies that address the direct effects TGF-β have on cardiomyocytes are needed at the cellular and molecular level. To begin to address some of these questions, ventricular myocyte cell lines (65) and primary cultures of fetal and neonatal cardiomyocytes are being used to better characterize, at the molecular and biochemical levels, the effects TGF-βs may have on cardiomyocyte growth and maturation within a growth factor–influenced paradigm of heart development (16).

In our myocyte cell lines, the role of TGF-β is being addressed by manipulating these cells' ability to respond to TGF-β ligands by TGF-β receptor manipulations. Kinase-deficient βRII (dominant negative) mutant primary myocyte cultures and several cell lines have been used to address TGF-β's effects (66–69). These studies indicate that TGF-β may be directly involved in several of the processes (proliferation, muscle protein isoform expression, ECM biogenesis) that occur in the cardiomyocyte during heart development. However, because of the inconsistencies seen in responses between different cell types, only assumptions can be made from these studies (only one of which was performed in primary cultures of cardiomyocytes) as to the role(s) TGF-βs may have on cardiomyocytes; but they give a firm base on which to form and test such hypotheses.

SUMMARY

As this review shows, significant progress has been made in our understanding of the role TGF-β plays in heart development in both chicken and rodent systems. Numerous studies have been performed to establish the expression patterns of the ligands and receptors during multiple phases of embryonic and fetal development. In the heart, it has been demonstrated that each of the ligands and receptors have distinct temporal, spatial, and, in some cases, species-specific expression patterns. This is reflected by the differences seen in the promoters and UTRs that are unique for each gene. These data suggest that a distinct role exists for the different TGF-β ligand isoforms and/or their receptors in the numerous processes involved in normal heart development.

As noted in the last sections of this review, experimental designs are being implemented to address the roles for each ligand in heart development. For example, gene ablation studies indicate that the absence of TGF-β_1 and TGF-β_3 does not cause gross anatomic heart defects in the mouse. This may be explained by a possible "rescue" by other TGF-β or TGF-β-related isoforms. However, no studies have yet addressed the more subtle, cellular events that may be occurring in these hearts. Additionally, these studies highlight species differences in the role TGF-β may play in heart development. Although TGF-β_3 null mice have no gross defects in their hearts, similar studies in the chicken would be expected to be strikingly different, since e–m transformation, and thus valve formation, has been suggested to require TGF-β_3. Therefore, only the tip of the iceberg has been uncovered, and further studies, both on the anatomic and on the cellular level, are needed to better understand the effects, either direct or indirect, TGF-β may have on heart development among different species, including man.

ACKNOWLEDGMENTS

Partial support for these studies were provided by the American Heart Association of Metropolitan Chicago, NHLBI HL-42218, and the Bane Estate to GLE, NIAAA AA-05404 to PSG.

REFERENCES

1. Massague J. The transforming growth factor-β family. *Annu Rev Cell Biol* 1990;6:597–641.
2. Sporn MB, Roberts AB. Transforming growth factor-β: recent progress and new challenges. *J Cell Biol* 1992;119(5):1017–1021.
3. Attisano L, Wrana JL, Lopez-Casillas F, Massague J. TGF-β receptors and actions. *Biochimica Biophys Acta* 1994;1222:71–80.
4. Kingsley DM. The TGF-β superfamily: new members, new receptors, and new genetic tests of function in different organisms. *Genes Dev* 1994;8:133–146.
5. Bassing CH, Yingling JM, Wang XF. Receptors for the TGF-β ligand family. *Vit Horm* 1994;48: 111–156.
6. Roberts AB, Sporn MB. Differential expression of the TGF-β isoforms in embryogenesis suggests specific roles in developing and adult tissues. *Mol Reprod Dev* 1992;32:91–98.
7. Runyan RB, Potts JD, Weeks DL. TGF-β3-mediated tissues interaction during embryonic heart development. *Mol Reprod Dev* 1992;32:152–159.
8. Jakowlew SB, Dillard PJ, Winokur TS, Flanders KC, Sporn MB, Roberts AB. Expression of transforming growth factor-βs 1–4 in chicken embryo chondrocytes and myocytes. *Dev Biol* 1991;143: 135–148.
9. Burt DW, Paton IR. Evolutionary origins of the transforming growth factor-β gene family. *DNA Cell Biol* 1992;11(7):497–510.
10. Schneider MD, Parker TG. Cardiac growth factors. *Prog Growth Factor Res* 1991;3:1–26.
11. Engelmann GL, Boehm KD, Birchenall-Roberts MC, Ruscetti FW. Transforming growth factor-beta1 in heart development. *Mech Dev* 1992;38:85–98.
12. Jakowlew SB, Ciment G, Tuan RS, Sporn MB, Roberts AB. Pattern of expression of transforming growth factor-β4 mRNA and protein in the developing chicken embryo. *Dev Dyn* 1992;195:276–289.
13. Akhurst RJ, Fitzpatrick DR, Fowlis DJ, Gatherer D, Millan FA, Slager H. The role of TGF-βs in mammalian development and neoplasia. *Mol Reprod Dev* 1992;32:127–135.
14. Jakowlew SB, Ciment G, Tuan RS, Sporn MB, Roberts AB. Expression of transforming growth factor-β2 and β3 mRNAs and proteins in the developing chicken embryo. *Differentiation* 1994;55:105–118.
15. Burton PBJ, Quirke P, Sorensen CM, Nehlsen-Cannarella SL, Bailey LL, Knight DE. Growth factor expression during rat heart development: a comparison of TGF-β3, TGF-α, bFGF, PDGF, and PDGF-R. *Int J Exp Pathol* 1993;74:87–96.
16. Engelmann GL. Coordinate gene expression during neonatal rat heart development. A possible role for the myocyte in extracellular matrix biogenesis and capillary angiogenesis. *Cardiovasc Res* 1993;27:1598–1605.
17. Barnett JV, Moustakas A, Lin W, et al. Cloning and developmental expression of the chick type II and type III TGFβ receptors. *Dev Dyn* 1994;199:12–27.
18. Lawler S, Candia AF, Ebner R, et al. The murine type II TGF-β receptor has a coincident embryonic expression and binding preference for TGF-β1. *Development* 1994;120:165–175.
19. Roelen BAJ, Lin HY, Knezevic V, Freund E, Mummery CL. Expression of TGF-βs and their receptors during implantation and organogenesis of the mouse embryo. *Dev Biol* 1994;166:716–728.

20. Engelmann GL, Grutkoski PS. Coordinate TGF-β receptor gene expression during rat heart development. *Cell Mol Biol Res* 1994;40(2):93–104.
21. Geiser AG, Kim SJ, Roberts AB, Sporn MB. Characterization of the mouse transforming growth factor-β1 promoter and activation by the Ha-*ras* oncogene. *Mol Cell Biol* 1991;11(1):84–92.
22. Kim, S-J, Glick A, Sporn MB, Roberts AB. Characterization of the promoter region of the human transforming growth factor-β1 gene. *J Biol Chem* 1989;264:402–408.
23. Geiser AG, Busam KJ, Kim SJ, et al. Regulation of the transforming growth factor-β1 and -β3 promoters by transcription factor Sp1. *Gene* 1993;129(2):223–228.
24. Kim SJ, Park K, Koeller D, Kim KY, Wakefield LM, Sporn MB, Roberts AB. Post-transcriptional regulation of the human transforming growth factor-β1 gene. *J Biol Chem* 1992;267(19):13702–13707.
25. Romeo DS, Park K, Roberts AB, Sporn MB, Kim SJ. An element of the transforming growth factor-β1 5′-untranslated region represses translation and specifically binds a cytosolic factor. *Mol Endocrinol* 1993;7:759–766.
26. Scotto L, Assoian RK. A GC-rich domain with bifunctional effects on mRNA and protein levels: implications for control of transforming growth factor β1 expression. *Mol Cell Biol* 1993;13(6):3588–3597.
27. O'Reilly MA, Geiser AG, Kim SJ, Bruggeman LA, Luu AX, Roberts AB, Sporn MB. Identification of an activating transcription factor (ATF) binding site in the human transforming growth factor-β2 promoter. *J Biol Chem* 1992;267(28):19938–19943.
28. Burt DW, Paton R, Dey BR. Comparative analysis of human and chicken transforming growth factor-β2 and -β3 promoters. *J Mol Endocrinol* 1991;7:175–183.
29. Miller DA, Lee A, Pelton RW, Chen EY, Moses HL, Derynck R. Murine transforming growth factor-β2 cDNA sequence and expression in adult tissues and embryos. *Mol Endocrinol* 1989;3(7):1108–1114.
30. Rebbert ML, Bhatia-Dey N, Dawid IB. The sequence of TGF-β2 from *Xenopus laevis. Nucleic Acids Res* 1990;18(8):2185.
31. Lafyatis R, Lechleider R, Kim SJ, Jakowlew S, Roberts AB, Sporn MB. Structural and functional characterization of the transforming growth factor β3 promoter. *J Biol Chem* 1990;265(31):19128–19136.
32. Lafyatis R, Denhez F, Williams T, Sporn M, Roberts A. Sequence specific protein binding to and activation of the TGF-β3 promoter through a repeated TCCC motif. *Nucleic Acids Res* 1991;19(23):6419–6425.
33. Jakowlew SB, Lechleider R, Geiser AG, et al. Identification and characterization of the chicken transforming growth factor-β3 promoter. *Mol Endocrinol* 1992;6:1285–1298.
34. Arrick BA, Lee AL, Grendell RL, Derynck R. Inhibition of translation of transforming growth factor-β3 mRNA by its 5′ untranslated region. *Mol Cell Biol* 1991;11(9):4306–4313.
35. Humphries DE, Bloom BB, Fine A, Goldstein RH. Structure and expression of the promoter for the human type II transforming growth factor-β receptor. *Biochem Biophys Res Comm* 1994;203(2):1020–1027.
36. Bae HW, Geiser AG, Kim DH, et al. Characterization of the promoter region of the human transforming growth factor-β type II receptor gene. *J Biol Chem* 1995;270(49):29460–29468.
37. Jakowlew SB, Cubert J, Danielpour D, Sporn MB, Roberts AB. Differential regulation of the expression of transforming growth factor-β mRNAs by growth factors and retinoic acid in chicken embryo chondrocytes, myocytes, and fibroblasts. *J Cell Physiol* 1992;150:377–385.
38. MacLellan WR, Brand T, Schneider MD. Transforming growth factor-β in cardiac ontogeny and adaptation. *Circ Res* 1993;73(5):783–791.
39. Flanders KC, Holder MG, Winokur TS. Autoinduction of mRNA and protein expression for transforming growth factor-βs in cultured cardiac cells. *J Mol Cell Cardiol* 1995;27:805–812.
40. Streuli CH, Schmidhauser C, Kobrin M, Bissell M, Derynck R. Extracellular matrix regulates expression of the TGF-β1 gene. *J Cell Biol* 1993;120(1):253–260.
41. Roberts AB, Sporn MB. Mechanistic interrelationships between two superfamilies: the steroid/retinoid receptors and transforming growth factor-β. *Cancer Surv* 1992;14:205–220.
42. Parker TG, Packer SE, Schneider MD. Peptide growth factors can provoke "fetal" contractile protein gene expression in rat cardiac myocytes. *J Clin Invest* 1990;85:507–514.
43. Fine A, Goldstein RH. Regulation of type I collagen mRNA translation by TGF-β. *Reg Immunol* 1993;5:218–224.
44. Kardami E. Stimulation and inhibition of cardiac myocyte proliferation in vitro. *Mol Cell Biochem* 1990;92:129–135.

45. Nair BG, Yu Y, Rashed HM, Sun H, Patel TB. Transforming growth factor-β1 modulate adenylyl cyclase signaling elements and epidermal growth factor signaling in cardiomyocytes. *J Cell Physiol* 1995;165:232–239.
46. Laiho M, DeCaprio JA, Ludlow JW, Livingston DM, Massague J. Growth inhibition by TGF-β linked to suppression of retinoblastoma protein phosphorylation. *Cell* 1990;62:175–185.
47. Ewen ME, Sluss HK, Whitehouse LL, Livingston DM. TGFβ inhibition of Cdk4 synthesis is linked to cell cycle arrest. *Cell* 1993;74:1009–1020.
48. Ravitz MJ, Yan S, Herr KD, Wenner CE. Transforming growth factor β-induced activation of cyclin E-cdk2 kinase and down-regulation of p27Kip1 in C3H 10T1/2 mouse fibroblasts. *Cancer Res* 1995;55:1413–1416.
49. Polyak K, Kato J, Solomon MJ, Sherr CJ, Massague J, Roberts JM, Koff A. p27Kip1, a cyclin-Cdk inhibitor, links transforming growth factor-β and contact inhibition to cell cycle arrest. *Genes Dev* 1994;8:9–22.
50. Polyak K, Lee MH, Erdjument-Bromage H, Koff A, Roberts JM, Tempst P, Massague J. Cloning of p27Kip1, a cyclin-dependent kinase inhibitor and a potential mediator of extracellular antimitogenic signals. *Cell* 1994;78:59–66.
51. Toyoshima H, Hunter T. p27, a novel inhibitor of G1 cyclin-Cdk protein kinase activity, is related to p21. *Cell* 1994;78:67–74.
52. Hannon GJ, Beach D. $p15^{INK4B}$ is a potential effector of TGF-β-induced cell cycle arrest. *Nature* 1994;371:257–261.
53. Li J-M, Nichols MA, Chandrasekharan S, Xiong Y, Wang X-F. Transforming growth factor β activates the promoter of cyclin-dependent kinase inhibitor $p15^{INK4B}$ through an Sp1 consensus site. *J Biol Chem* 1995;270(45):26750–26753.
54. Datto MB, Yu Y, Wang X-F. Functional analysis of the transforming growth factor β responsive elements in the WAF1/Cip1/p21 promoter. *J Biol Chem* 1995;270(48):28623–28628.
55. Huang JX, Potts JD, Vincent EB, Weeks DL, Runyan RB. Mechanisms of cell transformation in the embryonic heart. *Ann NY Acad Sci* 1995;752:317–330.
56. Potts JD, Runyan RB. Epithelial-mesenchymal cell transformation in the embryonic heart can be mediated, in part, by transforming growth factor β. *Dev Biol* 1989;134:392–401.
57. Potts JD, Dagle JM, Walder JA, Weeks DL, Runyan RB. Epithelial-mesenchymal transformation of embryonic cardiac endothelial cells is inhibited by a modified antisense oligodeoxynucleotide to transforming growth factor β3. *Proc Natl Acad Sci USA* 1991;88:1516–1520.
58. Kulkarni AB, Huh CC, Becker D, et al. Transforming growth factor β1 null mutation in mice causes excessive inflammatory response and early death. *Proc Natl Acad Sci USA* 1993;90:770–774.
59. Kulkarni AB, Ward JM, Yaswen L, et al. Transforming growth factor-β1 null mice: *an animal model for inflammatory disorders. Am J Pathol* 1995;146(1):264–275.
60. Shull MM, Ormsby I, Kier AB, et al. Targeted disruption of the mouse transforming growth factor-β1 gene results in multifocal inflammatory disease. *Nature* 1992;359:693–699.
61. Boivin GP, O'Toole BA, Orsmby IE, Diebold RJ, Eis MJ, Doetschman T, Kier AB. Onset and progression of pathological lesions in transforming growth factor-β1-deficient mice. *Am J Pathol* 1995;146(1):276–288.
62. Diebold RJ, Eis MJ, Yin M, et al. Early-onset multifocal inflammation in the transforming growth factor β1-null mouse is lymphocyte mediated. *Proc Natl Acad Sci USA* 1995;92(26):12215–12219.
63. Proetzel G, Pawlowski SA, Wiles MV, et al. Transforming growth factor-β3 is required for secondary palate fusion. *Nat Genet* 1995;11(4):409–414.
64. Filvaroff EH, Ebner R, Derynck R. Inhibition of myogenic differentiation in myoblasts expressing a truncated type II TGF-β receptor. *Development* 1994;120:1085–1095.
65. Engelmann GL, Birchenall-Roberts MC, Ruscetti FW, Samarel AM. Formation of fetal rat cardiac cell clones by retroviral transformation: retention of select myocyte characteristics. *J Mol Cell Cardiol* 1993;25:197–213.
66. Zhao Y, Young SL. Requirement of transforming growth factor-β (TGF-β) type II receptor for TGF-β-induced proliferation and growth inhibition. *J Biol Chem* 1996;271(5):2369–2372.
67. Chen R-H, Ebner R, Derynck R. Inactivation of the type II receptor reveals two receptor pathways for the diverse TGF-β activities. *Science* 1993;260:1335–1338.
68. Brand T, MacLellan WR, Schneider MD. A dominant-negative receptor for type β transforming growth factors created by deletion of the kinase domain. *J Biol Chem* 1993;268(16):11500–11503.
69. Brand T, Schneider MD. Inactive type II and type I receptors for TGFβ are dominant inhibitors of TGFβ-dependent transcription. *J Biol Chem* 1995;270(14):8274–8284.

The Developing Heart,
edited by Bohuslav Ošťádal et al.
Lippincott-Raven Publishers,
Philadelphia © 1997.

4

Reactivation of DNA Synthesis and Cell Cycle Progression in Ventricular Myocytes by Adenovirus Early Region 1 Proteins

Lorrie A. Kirshenbaum

Institute of Cardiovascular Sciences, St. Boniface General Hospital Research Centre, Department of Physiology, Faculty of Medicine, University of Manitoba, Winnipeg, Manitoba R2H 2A6, Canada

Shortly after birth, cardiac muscle cells lose their ability to replicate and exit from the cell cycle (1,2). As a result, subsequent growth of the myocardium occurs by cellular hypertrophy, as manifested by an increase in cell volume and myofibrillar protein content (2–4) rather than by cellular hyperplasia. Terminally differentiated adult ventricular myocytes have long been viewed as postmitotic with a limited capacity for DNA synthesis and replication (4–6). Loss of proliferative capacity of normal ventricular muscle has profound clinical and physiologic implications, most obviously in the context of the meager adaptive growth that follows myocardial ischemia or infarction. Though of considerable scientific and clinical interest, little is known regarding the molecular events that govern cell cycle exit and terminal differentiation in cardiac muscle cells. The ability to reactivate cardiomyocyte proliferation and/or differentiation could be of significant therapeutic value following myocardial injury.

Recently, increasing awareness from studies in skeletal muscle and other model systems suggest that the so-called tumor suppressor "pocket proteins," which include the retinoblastoma gene product Rb, may be involved in this process. Rb, the prototypic member of a family of cellular tumor suppressor proteins (which also include p107 and p130), was first identified as a putative negative regulator of cell growth by the observation that functional loss or inactivation of Rb correlated with the development of a variety of human malignancies (7,8). These include childhood retinoblastoma (9); breast, bladder, and prostate carcinomas; and glioblastoma and leukemias (9–11). The biochemical mechanisms by which Rb suppresses tumor growth have largely been attributed to its ability to negatively regulate the cell cycle in G0/G1. In this regard, Rb has been postulated to be a downstream target for cyclins (D and E) and cyclin-dependent protein kinases (cdk2, cdk4) that functionally regulate Rb by phosphorylation in a cell cycle–dependent manner in response to growth or mitogenic signals. Cells in G0/G1 express an (active) unphosphorylated form of Rb (8,12,13), whereas cells in S and/or M phases of the cell cycle display a hyperphosphorylated (inactive) form of Rb. A key to the mechanism of Rb function with respect to cell cycle control and growth more generally involves the formation of protein complexes via its pocket domain and the cellular transcription factor E2F. Of note, E2F was first characterized as a cellular sequence–specific DNA binding factor, necessary for the transactivation of the early adenoviral promoter region E2A. Several cellular genes that participate in DNA synthesis and cell growth also contain E2F consensus binding sites within their promoters, supporting a role for E2F in transactivation of S phase–dependent genes (14,15).

Concurrently, a role for pocket proteins has recently been proposed for differentiation of striated muscle (16). This model suggests that pocket proteins serve as a necessary platform for the action of myogenic transcription factors, for cell cycle exit, and for transactivation of muscle-specific genes required for terminal differention. Displacement or dissociation of myogenic factors from pocket proteins would abrogate their function, repress muscle gene transcription, and impair muscle differentiation (16,17). Despite the fact that Rb and p107 are distinct proteins, they share similar properties with respect to cell cycle regulation and growth control more generally. Studies by Zhu and colleagues (1993) (15) have recently demonstrated that p107 can functionally substitute for Rb to induce growth arrest and cell cycle exit in Rb-deficient cells. However, functional similarity and biochemical similarity may not necessarily be equivalent, because in Rb-/- null mice p107 was sufficient to substitute for Rb for cell cycle exit and differentiation of skeletal muscle myoblasts but could not maintain the differentiated muscle phenotype in Rb-/- myotubes when challenged with serum growth factors (17). Although cardiac-specific determination factors such as those found in skeletal muscle have not been identified, potential candidates such as the MADS box family of transcription factors that include the MEF2 family of transcription factors (17,18) may serve as putative targets for pocket proteins during cardiogenesis and differentiation. These in turn may operate in a fashion analogous to myogenic bHLH proteins in skeletal muscle differentiation.

Importantly, certain proteins of DNA tumor viruses—including the advenovirus early region 1A protein (E1A), SV40 large T antigen, and human papilloma virus E7—have been shown to physically interact with pocket proteins and disrupt their function. Thus, viral oncoproteins with distinct cellular targets can be used to study the molecular mechanisms by which pocket proteins influence the cell's ultimate growth and/or differentiation. Evidence for the existence and operation of a pocket protein–dependent pathway in cardiac muscle is largely provided by studies in transgenic mice that demonstrated augmented atrial and ventricular muscle growth in the presence of the SV40 large T antigen (an analog of adenovirus E1A); these studies provide a conceptual rationale for the current investigations (19).

As a first step toward identifying positive and negative regulators of cardiac muscle cell growth and to verify the postulated role of pocket proteins as the "lock" for cell cycle exit in cardiac muscle, we studied the impact of adenovirus E1A oncoproteins on cardiac gene expression and DNA synthesis in neonatal ventricular myocytes, which retain a limited ability to respond to exogenous growth signals (20,21). The rationale for using adenovirus E1A proteins in our studies was based on the following: (a) precedent of E1A's impact on skeletal muscle gene transcription (22,23): (b) well-characterized domains of E1A and delineation of interactions with specific cellular targets (24,25); (c) unlike the SV40-large T antigen, which interacts with both pocket proteins and the tumor suppressor protein p53, E1A protein segregates binding to p53, permitting pocket protein disruption to be addressed more directly in cardiac muscle (26); (d) we previously demonstrated that we can deliver foreign genes into cardiac muscle cells with uniformity and high efficiency using recombinant adenovirus (27).

ADENOVIRUS EARLY REGION 1 PROTEINS (E1A)

The E1A gene is a complex transcription unit that gives rise to two major alternatively spliced gene products that yield 13S and 12S mRNA transcripts. These two transcripts give rise to 289 a.a. and 243 a.a. proteins, respectively. The amino terminus and conserved regions (CR) 1, CR2, and CR3 are shared among adenovirus serotypes and are essential for protein binding and biological activity. CR3 encodes a domain required for the transactivation of late viral genes and hence is required for virus replication but is absent from all 12SE1A proteins. Several different active sites within the E1A protein for binding cellular targets have been identified. In this regard, CR1 and CR2 together are sufficient to bind to pocket proteins (25,28); whereas a second active site comprises the amino terminus along with CR1 that binds to p300 a recently cloned bromodomain transcription factor with CREB-like properties (29). A double missence mutation of E1A in the amino terminus together with CR2, R2GC124G abrogates binding not only to pocket proteins but also to p300. This mutation is sufficient to disrupt all known functions of E1A and is inert in all cell types studied previously (25). More selective mutations of E1A that abrogate binding to either pocket proteins alone (Y47HC124G) or p300 (R2G) alone can be used to test the involvement of these pathways specifically (25,30).

METHODS AND EXPERIMENTAL DESIGN

Cell Culture—Ventricular

Ventricular myocytes were isolated from 2-day-old Sprague Dawley rats, and subjected to Percoll gradient centrifugation, for purification and submitted to primary culture as previously reported (21,31). After overnight incubation in Dulbecco's modified Eagle's medium/Ham's nutrient mixture F-12, 1:1, 17 mM HEPES, 3 mM (milli Molar) $NaHCO_3$, 2 mM L-glutamine, 50 μg/ml gentamicin, and 5% horse serum, cells were transferred to serum-free medium (21,31).

Recombinant Adenoviruses

Adenoviruses were propagated and titered using human 293 cells as previously described (28,31). The "12S. E1A + E1B" denotes virus 12S.WT (25), containing the "R2G + E1B," "Y47H,C124G + E1B," and "R2G,C124G + E1B" designate the exact amino acid substitutions of viruses 12S.RG2, 12S.YH47/928, and 12S.RG2/928 (25). Each of the four viruses indicated earlier also confers E1B. "12S E1A-E1B" indicates virus 12S.E1B—containing a deletion in the E1B gene (25). The CR3 domain of E1A protein is required for transactivation of early promoters and viral replication, and is absent from all 12S E1A proteins described. Neonatal ventricular myocytes were incubated in serum-free medium for 24 hours, and then in serum-free medium containing virus for 6 hours, and were analyzed after another 24–72 hours under serum free conditions.

Assays of Apoptosis and DNA Synthesis

Live and dead cells were distinguished using 2 μM calcein acetoxymethyl ester and 2 mM ethidium homodimer-1, respectively (molecular probes). To visualize nuclear morphology, cardiac myocytes were identified using indirect immunofluorescence microscopy for sarcomeric myosin heavy chain (MHC) and were counterstained with Hoechst dye 33258 and MF20 hybridoma supernatant (32). Nucleosomal DNA laddering was analyzed by 1% agarose gel electrophoresis. DNA synthesis was monitored using a 4-hour pulse of 10 μM 5′-bromodeoxyuridine (BrdU), from 44 through 48 hours after infection, and was detected using mouse monoclonal antibody against BrdU. For immunofluorescence microscopy, fluorescein-conjugated mouse IgG, against BrdU was used at 10 μg/ml; sarcomeric MHC was visualized using MF20 and rhodamine-conjugated second antibody.

Transfection

Cells were infected with recombinant adenovirus 18–24 hours after plating and were transfected immediately after removal of the viral stocks. Cells were incubated with the DNA–DEAE–dextran complex, containing 2.5 μg of a cytomegalovirus promotor-driven *E. coli* β-galactosidase plasmid, luciferase reporter gene, and 2.5% calf serum, (21,31,32). Cells were maintained in the serum-free medium described earlier and were harvested 48 hours after transfection. Luciferase and lacZ activity were monitored as described (31). Results were compared by Scheffe's multiple comparison test for analysis of variance and the unpaired two-tailed t test, using a significance level of $p < 0.05$.

Immunoprecipitation and Western Blot Analysis

Cardiac myocytes were harvested 48 hours post infection in NP-40 lysis buffer (1.0% NP-40, 0.5% sodium dodecyl sulfate, 150 mM Tris HCl, pH 7.4). Cell lysates were incubated overnight at 4°C with mouse monoclonal antibody (M73) directed toward E1A, followed by immunoprecipitation with protein A-G beads (Santa Cruz) for 1 hour at 4°C. After washing protein A-G complexes were mixed with 2X SDS sample buffer and boiled for 5 min. Immunoprecipitates were resolved on a 12% polyacrylamide gel and electrophoretically transferred to nitrocellulose membrane. The nitrocellulose filter was subsequently incubated with the M73, anti-E1A antibody for 4 hours at room temperature. For detection of E1A proteins the filter was washed three times and incubated with an antimouse conjugated peroxidase antibody followed by chemiluminescence reaction with ECL reagents (Amersham).

DNA Content and Analysis

To determine DNA content in cardiac nuclei, neonatal ventricular myocytes were harvested 48 hours post infection in 150 mM NaCl, 10 mM Na_2HPO_4, 10 mM EDTA pH 7.4. Cells were centrifuged at 13,000 × g for 10 min and resuspended in the same buffer and streaked onto glass slides and allowed to dry for 5 min. Cells were subsequently fixed in 150 mM NaCl, 10 mM Na_2HPO_4 pH 7.4, and 10% formaldehyde for 30 min at room temperature. For Feulgen staining of cardiac nuclei, fixed cells were incubated in 5 *N* HCl for 60 min followed by 0.1% Feulgen stain in 0.1 *N* HCl for 60 min. Slides were washed and dehydrated in 100% ethanol with two consecutive changes for 3 min each, cleared with xylene and mounted with glass cover slips. Detailed image analysis of Feulgen-stained nuclei was performed using a CAS 200 instrumentation system (Cell Analysis Systems). Normal diploid rat liver was used as an internal control for calibration of the instrument. At least 300 cardiac nuclei were examined, in two or three replicate cultures for each determination.

RESULTS AND DISCUSSION

Though little attention was given to the occurrence of "programmed cell death" or apoptosis with E1A in skeletal muscle, it has become increasingly apparent that adenovirus E1A proteins in the absence of another adenovirus protein, E1B has been reported to cause apoptosis in a variety of different cell types (26,33). To formally test for this possibility in cardiac muscle cells, we infected our neonatal cardiac ventricular myocytes with recombinant adenoviruses that express either the 12SE1A+E1B (wild type), or 12SE1A-E1B. Cells were then analyzed for the number of live and dead cells, respectively, at 24 and 72 hours. In the presence of E1B, cells infected with the wild-type 12SE1A+E1B versus the inactive form of E1A,

R2GC124G were indistinguishable from uninfected control cells (Fig. 4–1). In contrast, myocytes infected with the 12SE1A-E1B showed a significant seven-fold increase in cell death at both 24 hours and 72 hours post infection (Fig. 4–1). To confirm our inference that apoptosis was the mechanism of myocyte death induced by adenovirus E1A proteins in the absence of E1B, neonatal myocytes were infected with respective adenoviruses and analyzed for the presence of apoptotic nuclei by Hoechst 32258 staining and nucleosomal DNA laddering, another hallmark and indicator of apoptosis. Uninfected control myocytes or those infected with 12SE1A + E1B were not significantly different from each other with respect to nuclear morphology and showed no evidence of nucleosomal DNA fragmentation and thus displayed no apparent evidence of apoptosis. However, cells infected with the 12SE1A-E1B displayed nuclei that were rounded in appearance that showed evidence of nuclear fragmentation and nucleosomal DNA laddering on gel electrophoresis (data not shown). Thus, to circumvent this possibility in our subsequent experiments we utilized recombinant adenoviruses that express the wild-type 12SE1A, mutations of 12SE1A in tandem with E1B.

To examine the effects of E1A proteins on cardiac gene expression, cardiac myocytes were infected with recombinant adenoviruses and subjected to conventional plasmid transfection with luciferase reporter plasmids driven by either the α-skeletal actin, α-cardiac actin, HSVTk, or cytoplasmic β-actin promoter. The CMV-driven β-galactosidase gene from *Escherichia coli* was also transfected into cardiac myocytes to control differences in transfection efficiency. As seen in Figure 4–2, transcription of the α-skeletal actin promoter was repressed to 80% of baseline activity by wild-type 12SE1A + E1B and was not significantly affected by the inactive mutation of E1A, R2GC124G. Similar effects were also observed for the α-cardiac actin promoter. Notably, mutations that abrogate binding to p300 alone or pocket protein binding alone both retained their ability to repress transcription of the α-skeletal and α-cardiac actin promoter. In contrast, transcription of the HSVTk pro-

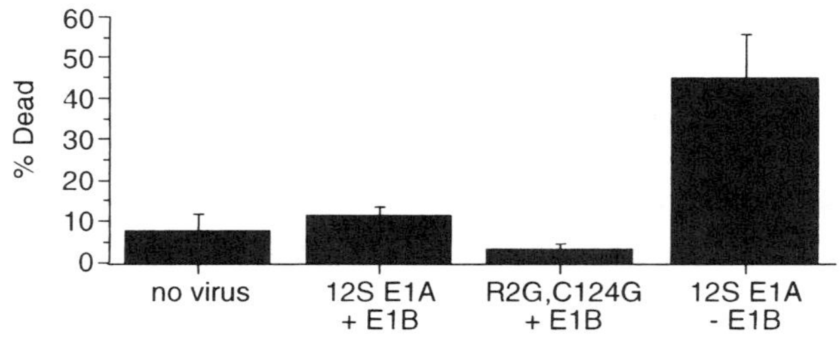

FIG. 4–1. Adenovirus E1A proteins in the absence of E1B provokes cell death in neonatal ventricular myocytes. Following 24 hours of adenovirus infection, cardiac myocytes were stained with calcein-AM and ethidium homodimer-1 to mark the number of live and dead cells, respectively. Histogram denotes a sevenfold increase in cell death of cardiac myocytes induced by E1A, in the absence of E1B. (Data represent ≥ 200 cells for each condition illustrated. Reprinted with permission from ref. 30.)

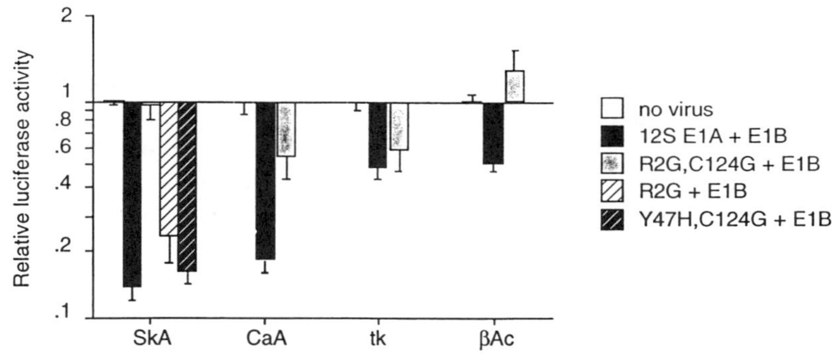

FIG. 4–2. Adenovirus E1A proteins preferentially repress muscle specific gene transcription in cardiac myocytes. Data represent relative luciferase activity as a measure of transcriptional activity of *SkA,* α-skeletal actin; *CaA,* α-cardiac actin; *tk,* herpes simplex thymidine kinase; β*Ac,* cytoplasmic β-actin normalized to β-galactosidase for transfection efficiency (mean ± S.D.). (Reprinted with permission from ref. 30.)

moter or cytoplasmic β-actin promoter was much less sensitive to the effects of E1A proteins than either the skeletal or cardiac actin genes. Moreover, the preferential repression of lineage restricted genes by E1A observed was not limited to the α-skeletal or α-cardiac actin promoters since both the αMHC and βMHC promoters were also repressed to a similar extent by E1A proteins (data not shown).

To confirm that all four E1A proteins were expressed to comparable levels and efficiently expressed in cardiac myocytes, cardiac cell lysate was immunoprecipi-

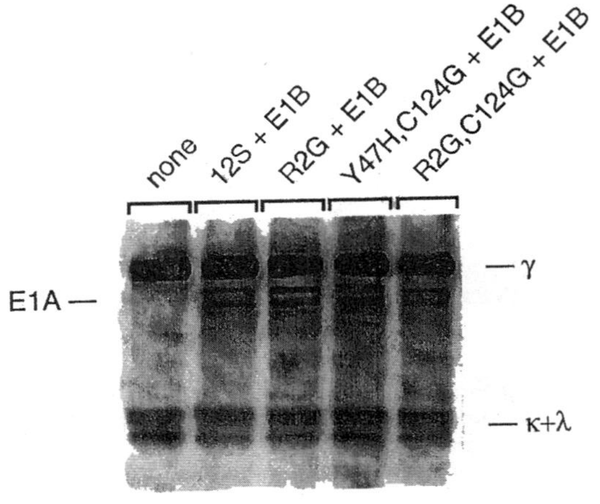

FIG. 4–3. Expression of adenovirus E1A proteins in cardiac myocyte. Cell lysate was immunoprecipated with an antibody directed against E1A and visualized by Western blot analyzed by chemiluminescence with an antimouse conjugated peroxidase antibody.

tated with an antibody directed toward E1A followed by Western blot analysis. As shown in Fig. 4–3, after adenoviral gene delivery, all four E1A proteins were expressed to comparable levels in cardiac myocytes, compared to uninfected control cells that do not express E1A proteins. In addition, indirect immunocytochemistry staining of myocytes for E1A revealed that all four E1A proteins were uniformly expressed and appropriately targeted to the nucleus (data not shown). Taken together, these results indicated that the effects of adenovirus E1A proteins on cardiac gene transcription were not due to relative differences in E1A protein delivery, protein expression, or targeting of E1A proteins to the nucleus.

To determine whether E1A proteins could reactive DNA in cardiac muscle cells, DNA synthesis was measured by immunoperoxidase staining for the incorporation of bromodeoxyuridine (BrdU). The 12SE1A + E1B provoked DNA synthesis in up to 80% of neonatal myocytes between 44 and 48 hours (Fig. 4–4) and did not differ significantly with higher multiplicities of infection. Moreover, mutations of E1A that abrogate binding to p300 binding alone or pocket protein binding alone were also sufficient to induce DNA synthesis in cardiac muscle cells. In contrast, however, the inactive form of E1A, R2GC124 + E1B, had no apparent effect on DNA synthesis. No increase in cell number was observed at this time point as expected from the fact that the majority of the cell population was in the S phase of the cell cycle. However, even up to 72 hours post infection none of the E1A proteins studied was sufficient alone to induce cell proliferation under the serum-free conditions employed for our studies (34).

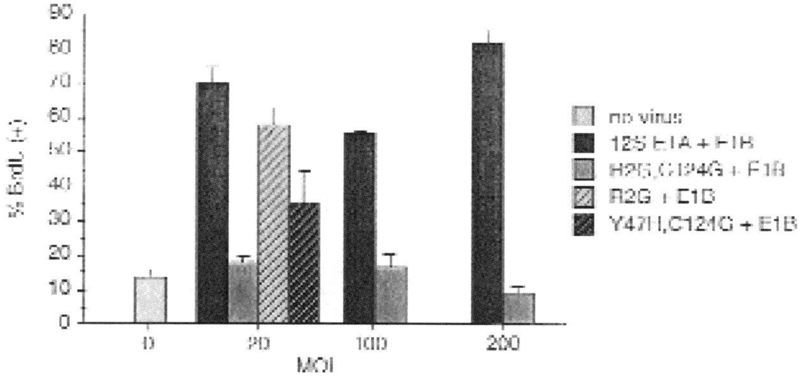

FIG. 4–4. Adenovirus E1A proteins induce DNA synthesis in neonatal ventricular myocytes. Cardiac myocytes were pulsed with bromodeoxyuridine (BrdU) at 44–48 hour post infection. The number of BrdU-positive nuclei was quantitated for each condition and shown below. To ensure DNA was occurring predominantly in cardiac myocytes, myocytes were double-immuno-stained with antibodies directed toward sarcomeric myosin and BrdU to simultaneously detect the number of BrdU myocytes. *MOI* represents the multiplicity of infection and represents the number of viral particles per cardiac cell. (Reprinted with permission from ref. 30.)

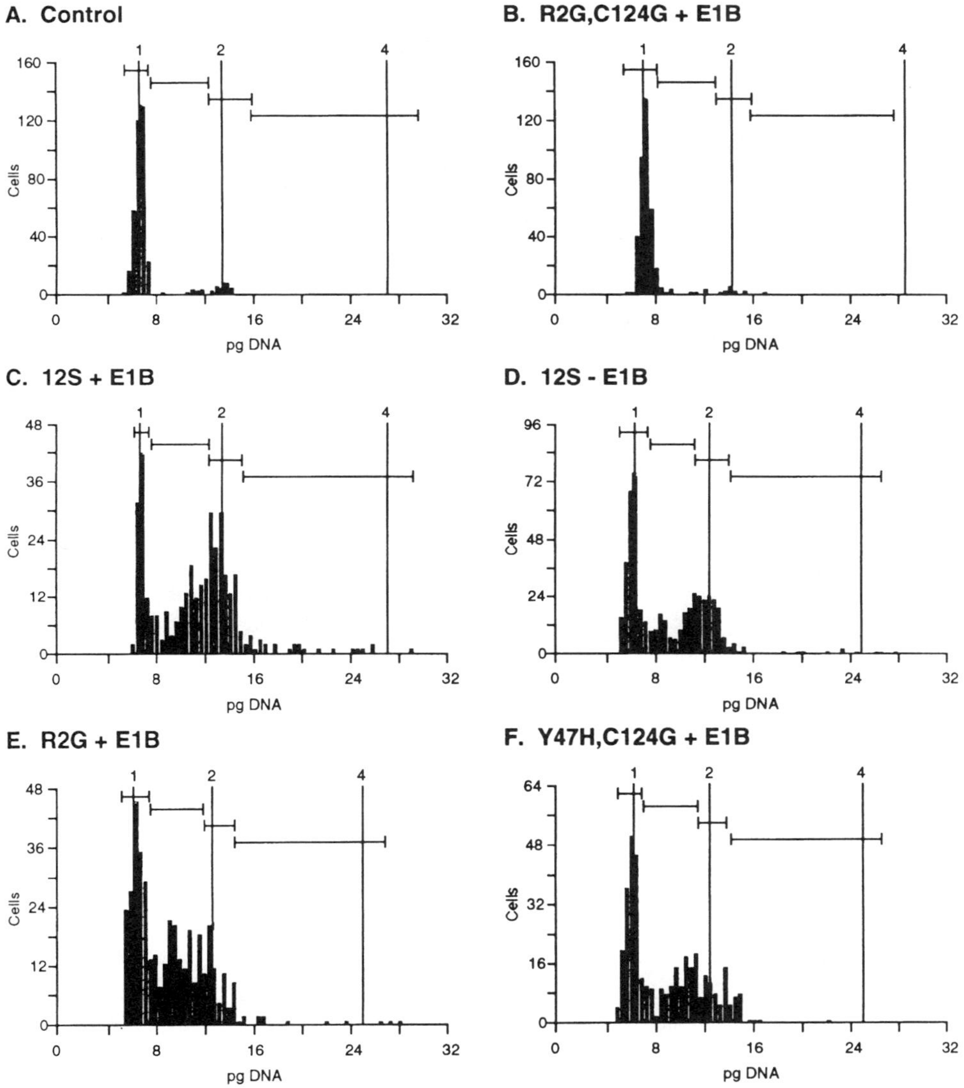

FIG. 4–5. Adenovirus E1A proteins reactive the cell cycle in cardiac myocytes. DNA content in cardiac myocytes was determined by Feulgen-staining of cardiac nuclei followed by detailed image analysis. (**A**) Uninfected control cells. (**B**) R2GC124G (inactive form of E1A). (**C**) 12SE1A+E1B. (**D**) 12SE1A-E1B. (**E**) R2G + E1B (p300-binding mutant of E1A). (**F**) Y47HC124G + E1B (pocket-protein-binding mutant of E1A). Adenovirus E1A proteins provoke cell reactivation with the accumulation of cells in the G2-M phase of the cell cycle and tetraploid 4N content of DNA of 14pg per nucleus.

To confirm that the DNA provoked by E1A proteins was due not to DNA damage or DNA repair but to cell cycle reactivation, we stained our neonatal cardiac nuclei with Feulgen stain followed by detailed image analysis to measure total DNA content. Shown in Fig. 4–5 are DNA histograms of neonatal cardiac nuclei that were normalized to normal diploid rat liver as an internal control. Uninfected control cells are shown in panel A. These cells displayed the normal diploid 2N content of DNA of 7pg per nucleus, with the predominant cell population in the G0–G1 phase of the cell cycle indicated by the single discrete peak. Similarly, cells infected with the inactive form of E1A are shown in panel B and were not significantly different from control cells. Thus, neither adenovirus infection, the presence of E1B, nor the inactive form of E1A had any effect on these parameters. In agreement with our DNA synthesis data, 80% of the cells infected with the wild-type 12E1A + E1B exited the G0–G1 phase of the cell cycle and accumulated in G2-M as indicated by the two individual peaks panel C. These cells displayed a tetraploid or 4N content of DNA of about 14pg of DNA per nucleus. Some S-phase cells with intermediate levels of DNA were also observed. Mutations of E1A that interfere with p300 binding or pocket protein binding were also sufficient to reactivate the cell cycle with the accumulation of cardiac muscle cells in G2-M. This established that E1A proteins induced DNA synthesis in cardiac muscle cells by reactivating the cell cycle.

SUMMARY AND CONCLUSIONS

We have demonstrated that adenovirus E1A proteins provoke three distinct events in cardiac muscle cells. In the first in the absence of E1B, E1A was cytotoxic, with features typical of apoptosis. Second in the presence of E1B, E1A preferentially inhibited transcription of cardiac-restricted α-actin promoters, and reactivated DNA synthesis in cardiac myocytes, without cell death. The reactivation of DNA synthesis in ventricular myocytes was substantiated by double immunocytochemistry for BrdU incorporation and sarcomeric myosin. Additionally, the increase in DNA synthesis was accompanied by a parallel increase in DNA content, as demonstrated by quantitative image analysis of Feulgen-stained cardiac nuclei. Lastly, mutations of E1A that abrogate binding to activities of the amino-terminus of E1A, versus conserved region 2, demonstrate that "pocket" proteins- and p300-binding domains of E1A suffice to repress cardiac gene transcription and provoke reentry into the S phase of the cell cycle in ventricular muscle cells.

To our knowledge these studies demonstrate for the first time the potential operation of a "pocket-protein" and a p300-dependent pathway in cardiac muscle cells. However, it remains to be proven whether these or alternative targets mediate the phenotype produced with E1A in cardiac muscle cells. Identifying the cellular targets for E1A in cardiac myocytes should provide further insight into the molecular events that govern the cardiac phenotype.

ACKNOWLEDGMENTS

I am grateful to E. Moran and E. White for viruses cited, S. Chakraborty for Feulgen staining, and M. D. Schneider for guidance and support. This work was funded by the Medical Research Council of Canada.

REFERENCES

1. Rumyantsev PP. Interrelations of the proliferation and differentiation processes during cardiac myogenesis and regeneration. *Int Rev Cytol* 1977;51:187–273.
2. Anversa P, Olivetti PG, Bracchi Loud AV. Postnatal development of the M-band in rat myofibrils. *Circ Res* 1981;48:561–568.
3. Anversa P, Capasso JM, Olivetti G, Sonnenblick EH. Myocyte cellular hypertrophy and hyperplasia in the heart during postnatal maturation and aging. *Acta Paediatr* 1991;383 (suppl):29–31.
4. Izumo S, Nadal-Ginard B, Mahdavi V. Protooncogene induction and reprogramming of cardiac gene expression produced by pressure overload. *Proc Natl Acad Sci USA* 1988;85:339–343.
5. Claycomb WC. Proliferative potential of the mammalian ventricular cardiac muscle cell. In: Oberpriller J, Oberpriller J, Mauro A, eds. *The development and regenerative potential of cardiac muscle.* New York: Harwood Academic, 1990.
6. Rakusan K. Cardiac growth, maturation and aging. In: Zak R, ed. *Growth of the heart in health and disease.* New York: Raven Press; 1984:25–40.
7. Lee EY, To H, Shew JY, Bookstein R, Scully P, Lee WH. Inactivation of the retinoblastoma susceptibility gene in human breast cancers. *Science* 1988;241:218–221.
8. DeCaprio JA, Ludlow JW, Lynch D, Furukawa Y, Griffin J, Worms HP, Huang CM, Livingston DM. The product of the retinoblastoma susceptibility gene has properties of a cell cycle regulatory element. *Cell* 1989;58:1085–1095.
9. Benediet WF, Murphree AL, Banerjee A, Spinae CA, Sparkes MC, Sparkes RS. Patient with 13 chromosome deletion: evidence that the retinoblastoma gene is a recessive cancer gene. *Science* 1983;219:973–975.
10. Lee EY, Chang CY, Hu N, Wang YC, Lai CC, Herrup K, Lee WH, Bradley A. Mice deficient for Rb are nonviable and show defects in neurogenesis and haematopoiesis. *Nature* 1992;359 288–294.
11. Horowitz JM, Park SH, Bogenmann E, Cheng JC, Yandell DW, Kaye FJ, Minna JD, Dryja TP, Weinberg RA. Frequent inactivation of the retinoblastoma anti-oncogene is restricted to a subset of human tumor cells. *Proc Natl Acad Sci USA* 1990;87:2775–2779.
12. Buchkovich K, Duffy LA, Harlow E. The retinoblastoma protein is phosphorylated during specific phase of the cell cycle. *Cell* 1989;58:1097–1105.
13. Chen PL, Scully P, Shew JY, Wang JY, Lee WH. Phosphorylation of the retinoblastoma gene product is modulated during the cell cycle and cellular differentiation. *Cell* 1989;58:1193–1198.
14. Nevins JR. E2F: a link between the Rb turnor suppressor protein and viral oncoproteins. *Science* 1992;258:424–429.
15. Zhu L, van den Heuvel S, Helin K, Fattaey A, Ewen M, Livingston D, Dyson N, Harlow E. Inhibition of cell proliferation by p 1 07, a relative of the retinoblastoma protein. *Genes Dev* 1993;7: 1111–1125.
16. Gu W, Schneider JW, Condorelli G, Kaushal S, Mahdavi V, Nadai-Ginard B. Interaction of myogenic factors and the retinoblastoma protein mediates muscle cell commitment and differentiation. *Cell* 1993;72:309–324.
17. Schneider JW, Gu W, Zhu L, Mahdavi V, Nadai-Ginard B. Reversal of terminal differentiation mediated by p107 in Rb(-/-) muscle cells. *Science* 1994;264:1467–1471.
18. Breitbart RE, Liang C-S, Smoot LB, Laheru DA, Mahdavi V, Nadal-Ginard B. A fourth human MEF2 transcription factor, hMEF2d, is an early marker of the myogenic lineage. *Development* 1993;118:1095–1106.
19. Kim KK, Soonpaa MH, Daud AI, Koh GY, Kim JS, Field LJ. Tumor suppressor gene expression during normal and pathologic myocardial growth. *J Biol Chem* 1994;269:22607–22613.

20. Ueno H, Perryman MB, Roberts R, Schneider MD. Differentiation of cardiac myocytes following mitogen withdrawal exhibits three sequential stages of the ventricular growth response. *J Cell Biol* 1988;107:1911–1918.
21. Parker TG, Packer SE, Schneider MD. Peptide growth factors can provoke "fetal" contractile protein gene expression in rat cardiac myocytes. *J Clin Invest* 1990;85:507–514.
22. Webster KA, Muscat GE, Kedes L. Adenovirus E1 A products suppress myogenic differentiation and inhibit transcription from muscle-specific promoters. *Nature* 1988;332:553–557.
23. Taylor DA, Kraus VB, Schwarz JJ, Olson EN, Kraus WE. E1A-Mediated inhibition of myogenesis correlates with a direct physical interaction of E1A12S and basic helix-loop-helix proteins. *Mol Cell Biol* 1993;13:4714–4727.
24. Moran E, Grodzicker T, Roberts RJ, Mathews MB, Zerier B. Lytic and transforming functions of individual products of the adenovirus E1 A gene. *Mol Cell Biol* 1986;57:765–775.
25. Wang H-GH, Rikitake Y, Carter MC, Yaciuk P, Abraham SE, Zerler B, Moran E. Identification of specific adenovirus-E1A N-terminal residues critical to the binding of cellular proteins and to the control of cell growth. *J Virol* 1993;67:476–488.
26. Field LJ. Atrial natriuretic factor-SV40 T antigen transgenes produce tumors and cardiac arrhythmias in mice. *Science* 1988;239:1029–1033.
27. Kirshenbaum LA, MacLellan WR, Mazur W, French BA, Schneider MD. Highly efficient gene transfer to adult rat ventricular myocytes by recombinant adenovirus. *J Clin Invest* 1993;92:381–387.
28. Moran E. Interaction of adenoviral proteins with pRB and p53. *FASEB J* 1993;7:880–885.
29. Eckner R, Ewen ME, Newsome D, Gerdes M, Decaprio JA, Lawrence JB, Livingston DM. Molecular cloning and functional analysis of the adenovirus E1A-associated 300-kD protein (P300) reveals a protein with properties of a transcriptional adaptor. *Genes Dev* 1994;8:869–884.
30. Kirshenbaum LA, Schneider MD. Adenovirus EI A represses cardiac gene transcription and reactivates DNA synthesis in ventricular myocytes, via alternative pocket protein- and p300-binding domains. *J Biol Chem* 1995;270:7791–7794.
31. Abdellatif M, MacLellan WR, Schneider MD. p21 Ras as a governor of global gene expression. *J Biol Chem* 1994;269:15423–15426.
32. Bader D, Masaki T, Fischman DA. Immunochemical analysis of myosin heavy chain during avian myogenesis in vivo. *J Cell Biol* 1982;95:763–770.
33. Rao L, Debbas M, Sabbatini P, Hockenberry D, Korsmeyer S, White E. The adenovirus E1 A proteins induce apoptosis, which is inhibited by the E1 B 19-kDa and Bcl-2 proteins. *Proc Natl Acad Sci USA* 1992;89:7742–7749.
34. Sen D, Dunnmon P, Henderson S, Gerard RD, Chien KR. Terminally differentiated neonatal rat myocardial cells proliferate and maintain specific differentiated functions following expression of SV40 large T antigen. *J Biol Chem* 1988;263:19132–19136.

The Developing Heart,
edited by Bohuslav Ošťádal et al.
Lippincott-Raven Publishers,
Philadelphia © 1997.

5

The Trabecular Component of the Embryonic Ventricle

Diego Franco, Jing Ya, Gerry T. M. Wagenaar, Wouter H. Lamers, and Antoon F. M. Moorman

Department of Anatomy and Embryology, Academic Medical Center, University of Amsterdam, Amsterdam, The Netherlands

The heart develops from a single tube into a four-chambered heart. During this process many changes in the pattern of gene expression are observed. In the tubular heart, five different compartments can be distinguished, based on morphological and functional characteristics—namely, inflow tract, atrium, atrioventricular canal, ventricle, and outflow tract (1). The atrial segment contracts and relaxes quickly, allowing it to function as the drainage pool of the embryo. The ventricle contracts quickly but shows a longer-lasting relaxation. These two segments are flanked by slow-conducting areas, the inflow tract, the atrioventricular junction, and the outflow tract (2). The functional differences are correlated with distinct molecular phenotypes (1).

Many proteins and their encoding mRNAs initially show gradients in expression along the cardiac tube (3–6). During subsequent development these gradients, such as those of the myosin heavy chain (MHC) and myosin light chain (MLC) isoforms, become specifically restricted to a single compartment (7,8). Other gene products such as α-smooth muscle actin are replaced by their cardiac or skeletal isoform during development (9). These changes occur gradually and are mostly completed after septation. A third category may comprise the regulatory ventricular MLC isoform (2V) that already becomes restricted to the ventricular compartment soon after its formation (10).

Interestingly, within the same cardiac compartment some proteins show differences in their expression pattern as well. The muscle-specific creatine kinase (MCK) isozyme in human embryos is more abundantly expressed in the embryonic left ventricle, whereas the brain isoform (BCK) is more expressed in the right ventricle (11). Similar observations have been reported for mouse MCK mRNA (8) and rat MCK protein (12).

The recent approach of making detailed topographical maps of the patterns of gene expression (for a review see ref. 1) has contributed substantially to our knowledge about the molecular basis of cardiac function. So far, within the ventricular compartment, the trabecular and compact components have not been distinguished systematically with respect to their molecular phenotype. In this study we analyzed and reviewed the expression patterns, at the mRNA and protein levels, of proteins involved in conduction, contraction–relaxation, energy metabolism, and cellular architecture during different stages of rodent cardiac development. The results suggest that the trabecular component shows an "atrial-like phenotype" for the contractile proteins, which may confer a faster contraction to the trabecular component than to the compact myocardium. Furthermore, the distribution of proteins involved in calcium clearance suggests that relaxation takes place first in the outer side of the ventricular compartment (i.e., compact myocardium) and later in the inner layer (i.e., the trabecular component).

MATERIALS AND METHODS

Embryos

Wistar rat embryos were obtained from timed-pregnant rats (12–20 embryonic days; ED). CD1 mouse embryos were collected from time-pregant mice (10–16 ED). Adult hearts of both species were also processed. All tissues were fixed either in 4% freshly prepared formaldehyde during 4 h (*in situ* hybridization) or overnight in methanol:acetone:water (2:2:1) at room temperature (immunohistochemistry). After dehydration in a graded series of ethanol and embedment in paraplast, serial sections were cut at 7 μm and mounted onto RNAse-free 3-aminopropyltriethoxysilane (AAS)-coated slides (*in situ* hybridization) or onto polylysine-coated slides (immunohistochemistry).

In Situ Hybridization

Complementary RNA probes of rat α-MHC mRNA (13,14), rat β-MHC mRNA (13), rat sarcoplasmatic reticulum calcium ATPase (SERCA2) mRNA (5,15), rat phospholamban (PLB) mRNA (5), mouse alkali atrial (MLC1A) and ventricular (MLC1V) myosin light chains mRNAs (16,17), mouse regulatory atrial (MLC2A) and ventricular (MLC2V) myosin light chain mRNAs (10,18), connexin 40 (Cx40) and connexin 43 (Cx43) mRNAs (19) were radiolabeled with ^{35}S-UTP by *in vitro* transcription according to standard procedures (20). Pretreatment and RNA–RNA hybridization conditions were performed as detailed elsewhere (5).

Immunohistochemistry

Specific primary monoclonal antibodies against rat α-smooth muscle actin (α-SMA; Sigma), human α-MHC (21), human β-MHC (21), human desmin (Sanbio), human muscle-specific creatine-kinase (MCK; 11), and human brain-specific creatine kinase isoform (BCK; 11) were used. After deparaffination in xylene, sections were hydrated in a graded series of ethanol, washed in phosphate-buffered saline (PBS), and treated with hydrogen peroxide (3% in BPS, 30 min) to reduce endogenous peroxidase activity. Subsequently, an incubation in TENG-T (10 mM EDTA, 150 mM NaCl, 0.25% gelatine, 0.05% Tween-20, pH = 8.0, 30 min) was performed to avoid nonspecific bindings. After pretreatment, sections were washed again in PBS and incubated overnight with the corresponding primary antibody diluted in PBS at the required concentration. First, antibody binding was detected by the uncoupled peroxidase–antiperoxidase method, as detailed elsewhere (11).

RESULTS

We analyzed the patterns of expression of several mRNAs encoding contractile proteins (MHC and MLC isoforms), proteins involved in calcium handling (SERCA2, PLB) and conduction (Cx40 and Cx43). At the protein level, we analyzed α-MHC, β-MHC, α-SMA, MCK, BCK, and desmin. The results are presented according to functional groups. Data were obtained from rat hearts, if not

TABLE 5–1. *Patterns of gene expression in the trabeculated and compact ventricular myocardium*

Probes[a]	Relative expression in the trabeculated versus compact component
mRNA level	
α-MHC[R,M]	TC > CC
β-MHC[R,M]	TC = CC
MLC1A[M]	TC > CC
MLC1V[R,M]	TC < CC
MLC2A[R,M]	TC > CC
MLC2V[R,M]	TC < CC
Cx40[R]	TC < CC[b]
Cx43[R]	TC > CC
SERCA2A[R]	TC < CC
PLB[R]	TC < CC
Protein level	
α-MHC[R,H]	TC > CC
β-MHC[R,H]	TC = CC
α-SMA[R,H]	TC > CC
MCK[R,H]	TC > CC[b]
BCK[R,H]	TC > CC[b]
Desmin[R,H]	TC > CC

Note: The levels of expression of proteins involved in contraction, relaxation, calcium clearance, energy metabolism, and intermediate filaments are given in the trabeculated component (TC) relative to the compact component (CC). It should be realized that the patterns are not in all stages equally clear but represent the predominant phenotype.

[a]Species analyzed: R = rat; M = mouse; H = human.

[b]Additional differences were observed among the right and left ventricular compartments (referred to the compact myocardium itself).

stated otherwise. Table 5–1 summarizes the patterns of expression in the trabecular versus the compact ventricular myocardium.

Morphological Characteristics of the Ventricular Compartment Development

Early in development (e.g., ED 10 rat), the heart tube shows an S-shape in which only two layers are recognizable (the endocardial and myocardial layers), separated by a thick acellular extracellular matrix, the cardiac jelly. Following the looping process, the myocardium expands in the direction of the arterial and venous poles. Eventually, five different compartments can be distinguished (i.e., inflow

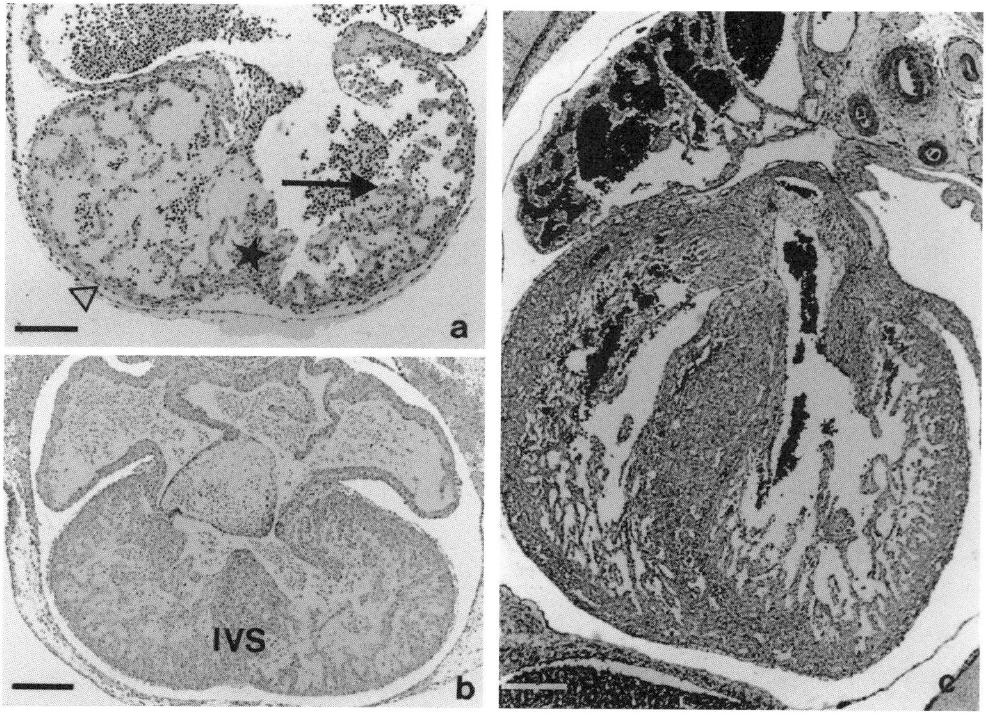

FIG. 5–1. Histologic sections of embryonic hearts showing the ventricular compartment at the level of the atrioventricular junction (**a, b**) and at the level of the right ventricular outflow (**c**). At 12ED (**a**), the outer ventricular myocardium (*arrowhead*) is very thin and no morphologic differences are observed as compared with the trabeculations (*arrows*). The IVS starts already to show a thicker morphology (*asterisk*). At 14ED (**b**), the ventricular free walls are thick and a compact myocardium morphology is clearly observed in the interventricular septum (IVS). At 16ED, a compact myocardial layer is visible in both ventricular free walls, being slightly more developed in the left ventricular component than in the right one. Hematoxiline–azofloxine. Bars **a**, 70 μm; **b**, 120 μm; **c**, 220 μm.

tract, atria, atrioventricular canal, ventricles, and outflow tract). The ventricles have, initially, a trabeculated morphology (22). At ED 12, the interventricular septum (IVS, Fig. 5–1a) is formed, representing the first ventricular structure that shows a compact myocardial morphology (Fig. 5–1b). When septation reaches completion, the free ventricular wall begins to develop a compact myocardial layer. This process starts in the IVS, expands earlier to the left ventricular free wall (ED 16 rat), and finally continues also (ED 18 rat) to the right ventricular wall (Fig. 5–1c). At birth only a few trabeculations are still present in the ventricles. Differences in the molecular phenotype of the myocytes occupying the trabeculations and the ventricular walls are, therefore, expected to arise after ED 12 in the rat.

Patterns of Expression in the Ventricular Compartment

Early in development (ED 10 rat), both MHCs protein isoforms are expressed in opposite gradients throughout the tubular heart. α-MHC is higher in the inflow tract and progressively decreases toward the outflow tract region. β-MHC is higher expressed mostly at the outflow tract/ventricle and decreases toward the inflow tract (3). The same pattern of expression for each MHC isoform is also observed at the mRNA level (data not shown). At ED 12 (rat), α-MHC mRNA has become restricted mostly to the atria, but the trabeculated ventricular component still shows a moderate intensity of expression. α-MHC has disappeared from the IVS and the free ventricular walls. On the other hand, β-MHC expression is restricted mostly to the ventricular compartment, but no differences between IVS and trabeculated ventricles can be observed. The same patterns are also observed at the protein level (α- and β-MHC) even later in development, both in rats and in human embryos (see, e.g., ref. 6). α-MHC mRNA and protein remain higher expressed in the trabeculated component compared to the developing compact myocardial layers (i.e., ventricular free walls).

The MLC isoforms become also specifically confined to a distinct compartment with development (ED 12–14). MLC1A and MLC2A mRNAs are almost entirely restricted to the atrial compartment, whereas MLC1V and MLC2V are mostly confined to the ventricular compartment. It is important to note that MLC1A and MLC2A mRNAs show higher expression in the trabeculation when compared to the IVS or the myocardium of the ventricular free wall (Fig. 5–2a). On the other hand, MLC1V and MLC2V showed a down-regulation in the trabecular component of the ventricles (Fig. 5–2b). Thus, the "atrial" contractile isoforms disappear from the compact myocardial layers and remain expressed in the trabeculations. This tendency confers an atrial-like phenotype to the trabecular component. The differences are observed even up to the fetal period in rats and mice, when the trabeculations are hardly recognizable as a distinct component.

α-SMA is initially observed along the entire cardiac myocardium (ED 12). Throughout development α-SMA protein starts to disappear gradually from the

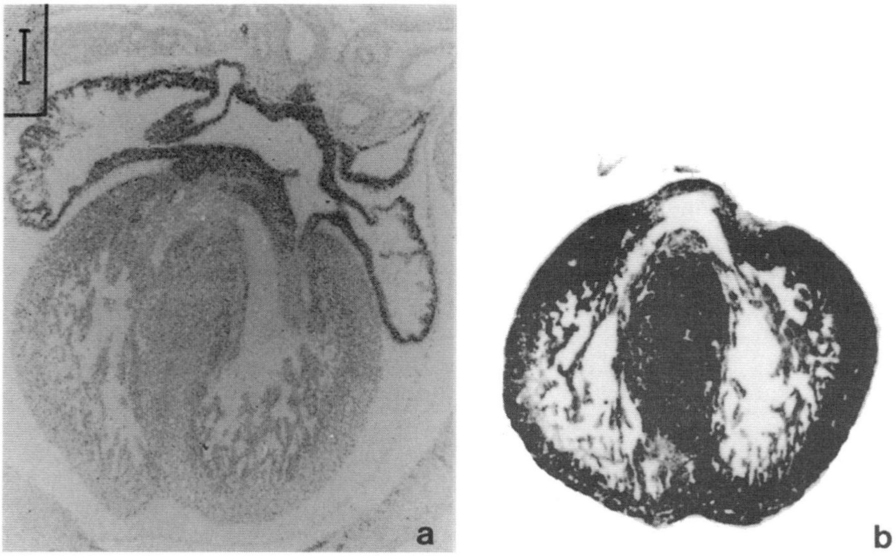

FIG. 5–2. Serial sections of 14ED mouse processed for *in situ* hybridization. Observe that MLC1A mRNA (**a**) is higher expressed in the atria than in the ventricles. Furthermore, the trabeculations show a higher expression than the compact myocardium. On the other hand, MLC2V is down-regulated in the trabeculated as compared to the ventricular compact myocardium (**b**). Bar 220 μm.

ventricles and later in development (ED 20 rat) from the atria (23). Interestingly, from ED 14 (rat) onward a difference in staining intensity in the trabeculations can be observed when compared to the compact myocardium. α-SMA protein is higher expressed in the trabecular component of the embryonic ventricular compartment, resembling, at this time point, the phenotypical appearance of the atrial myocardium. Moreover, the right ventricle shows more trabeculations than the left one, because the compact myocardium has not yet been fully developed.

From early in development (ED 12 rat) onward, the SERCA2 and PLB expression patterns are different. SERCA2 mRNA is higher expressed in the atria than in the ventricles, whereas PLB mRNA is higher in the ventricles than in the atria (5). However, both mRNAs are lower expressed in the ventricular trabeculations compared to the developing compact myocardial layer of the ventricular free walls or the IVS (Fig. 5–1). Hence, the expression of SERCA2 mRNA does not resemble an atrial-like phenotype in the trabecular component at any time point of cardiac development.

The mRNA encoding the gap junctional protein connexin 43 is higher expressed in the ventricles than in the atria. On the other hand, connexin 40 is higher expressed in the atria than in the ventricles. Interestingly, it also shows differences between right and left ventricular compartments. Connexin 43 mRNA is down-regulated, whereas connexin 40 mRNA is up-regulated in the trabecular compartment as compared to the compact myocardium. In both cases an atrial-like phenotype is observed in the fetal period (ED 16–20).

Two different creatine kinase isoforms are expressed in the developing heart. So far, it has been reported to show right/left differences and transmural gradients at the protein and mRNA level in different species (8,12,21). These transmural gradients appear to reflect merely differences in expression between the trabecular component and the developing compact myocardium (see, e.g., ref. 21).

Desmin is an intermediate filament protein present in rat cardiomyocytes and skeletal myocytes from early in development and remains up to adult stages (22). Intermediate filaments contribute to the structural organization of the cytoskeleton and have therefore been considered a differentiation marker. Throughout development, desmin is slightly higher expressed in the atrial compartment than in the ventricular compartment. Differences between the trabeculations and the compact myocardium (i.e., IVS) are observed up to ED 20 in rats. Later in development these differences are hardly visible.

DISCUSSION

The molecular phenotype of the trabecular component of the ventricular compartment suggests that the trabeculations have a faster contraction and impulse conduction during the embryonic and fetal period than the surrounding compact myocardium. This faster contraction of the trabeculated component will require a higher energy consumption, as reported in skeletal muscle (24–26). Furthermore, the molecular phenotype of the trabeculations suggests a slower relaxation in this component than in the compact myocardium.

The different phenotype of the trabeculations versus the compact myocardium of the ventricular compartment is seen from very early in development onward. The "atrial-specific" contractile isoforms maintain a higher expression in the trabeculations, whereas the "ventricular-specific" isoforms are down-regulated. The genes encoding proteins involved in calcium clearance, in contrast with the atrial-like phenotype of the contractile proteins, are expressed to a higher extent in the surrounding compact myocardium.

If we consider the anatomy of the heart it can be envisioned that the outer side (i.e., compact myocardium) has a longer curvature and thus is mechanically more stretched during the natural cardiac cycle than the inner side. The presence of atrial contractile isoforms in the trabecular component suggests that the inner side of the ventricle (i.e., trabecules) contracts quicker than the outer side (i.e., compact myocardium). These phenotypes are in line with reports on skeletal muscles subjected to stretch where a switch from the fast-twitch to a slow-twitch phenotype in the program of gene expression is observed (27,28). It can be envisioned that relaxation (calium clearance) occurs the other way around—that is, the relaxation of the compact myocardium precedes that of the inner trabecular component.

The analysis of other contractile protein, α-SMA, and intermediate filament, desmin, suggests that the trabeculations retain the characteristics of the primary myocardium. α-SMA and desmin protein are initially expressed throughout the entire heart and progressively disappear first from the compact ventricular myocardium and later from the trabeculations and atria (23).

Connexins are structural proteins forming the gap junctions and therefore responsible for a correct cell–cell communication. Within the heart, gap junctions are believed to play a crucial role in the conduction of the impulse: Gap junctions built up from connexin 43 are the predominant junctions. Differences between compact myocardium and trabeculations have been described at the mRNA and protein level (29). This author suggested that impulse conduction was driven via the trabecular component and then transmitted to the compact myocardium. Therefore, these data are also in favor of a fast conduction throughout the trabeculations matching with the notion of a faster contraction.

Our data support the hypothesis that the trabeculations play an important transient role by driving contraction and impulse conduction during the period that specialized conduction tissue and mature myocardial cells (i.e., free walls) are not yet fully formed. After those structures have been formed, the trabeculations will disappear as a distinct, functional component of the adult ventricular compartment.

In summary, the molecular phenotype of the trabecular component supports the notion that this component has a fast contraction and slow relaxation compared to the ventricular compact myocardium. This phenotype allows it to function in harmony with the surrounding ventricular compact myocardium.

SUMMARY

During the process of looping and septation of the cardiac tube, changes in the pattern of gene expression are observed that are correlated with differences in function. The embryonic ventricular cavity is characterized initially by a trabeculated morphology; with development, a compact myocardial layer is gradually developed. So far, differences in the molecular phenotype of the trabecular and compact components within the ventricular compartment have not been distinguished systematically, which is why it is addressed in the present study. We show that the trabecular component has a clear, atrial-like phenotype for the contractile proteins, which allows a faster contraction of the trabecular component than that of the compact myocardium. The molecular phenotype also indicates a quicker impulse conduction and a slower relaxation than the surrounding ventricular compact myocardium. The functional significance of this difference in phenotype between the trabeculations and the compact myocardium may be that it allows a coordinate contraction–relaxation of the ventricle, the contraction being initiated in the centrally localized trabeculations and the relaxation by the surrounding compact myocardium. Thus, the trabeculations must be considered as a distinct segment that functions in harmony with the surrounding ventricular compact myocardium.

ACKNOWLEDGMENTS

The authors are indebted to Kenneth H. Boheler (London, UK) for supplying cDNA probes to rat α-MHC, β-MHC, and phospholamban mRNAs; to Ketty Schwartz, for supplying the cDNA probe to sarcoplasmatic reticulum Ca^{2+} ATPase mRNA; to Margaret Buckingham (Paris, France), for supplying cDNA probes for MLC1A and MLC1V mRNAs; to Kenneth R. Chien (La Jolla, CA), for supplying cDNA probes to MLC2A and MLC2V mRNAs; and to David L. Paul (Boston, MA) for supplying the cDNA probes to connexin 40 and 43 mRNAs. This study was partially supported by the Spanish government. D. Franco is the recipient of EX93-27383269 fellowship grant from the DGICYT, Madrid, Spain.

REFERENCES

1. Moorman AFM, Lamers WH. Molecular anatomy of the developing heart. *Trends Cardiovasc Med* 1994;4:257–264.
2. De Jong F, Ophof T, Wilde AAM, Janse MJ, Charles R, Lamers WH, Moorman AFM. Persisting zones of slow impulse conduction in developing chicken hearts. *Circ Res* 1992;71:240–250.
3. De Groot IJM, Lamers WH, Moorman AFM. Isomyosin expression pattern during heart morphogenesis: an immunohistochemical study. *Anat Rec* 1989;224:365–373.
4. De Jong F, Geerts WJC, Lamers WH, Moorman AFM. Isomyosin expression pattern during formation of the tubular chicken heart: 3D immunohistochemical analysis. *Anat Rec* 1990;226:213–227.
5. Moorman AFM, Vermeulen JLM, Schwartz K, Lamers WH, Boheler KR. Patterns of expression of sarcoplasmic reticulum Ca^{++} ATPase and phospholamban mRNA during rat heart development. *Circ Res* 1995;76:616–625.
6. Wessels A, Vermeulen JLM, Viragh S, Kalman F, Lamers WH, Moorman AFM. Spatial distribution of "tissue-specific" antigens in the developing human heart and skeletal muscle. II. An immunohistochemical analysis of myosin heavy chain isoforms expression patterns in the embryonic heart. *Anat Rec* 1991;229:335–368.
7. De Jong F, Geerts WJ, Los JA, Moorman AFM. Isomyosin expression pattern in tubular stages of chicken heart development: a 3D immunohistochemical analysis. *Anat Embryol* 1987;177(1):81–90.
8. Lyons G. In situ analysis of the cardiac muscle gene program during embryogenesis. *Trends Cardiovasc Med* 1994;4(2):70–77.
9. Ruzicka DL, Schwartz RJ. Sequential activation during avian cardiogenesis: vascular smooth muscle alpha-actin gene transcripts mark the onset of cardiac differentiation. *J Cell Biol* 1988;107: 2575–2585.
10. Kubalak SW, Miller-Hance WC, O'Brien TX, Dyson E, Chien KR. Chamber specification of atrial myosin light chain-2 expression precedes septation during murine cardiogenesis. *J Biol Chem* 1994;269(24):1691–1697.
11. Wessels A, Vermeulen JLM, Viragh S, Moorman AFM, Lamers WH. Spatial distribution of "tissue-specific" antigens in the developing human heart and skeletal muscle. I. An immunohistochemical analysis of creatine kinase isoenzyme expression patterns. *Anat Rec* 1990;228:163–176.
12. Hasselbaink HDJ, Labruyère WT, Moorman AFM, Lamers WH. Creatine kinase isozyme expression in prenatal rat heart. *Anat Embryol* 1990;182:195–203.
13. Boheler KR, Chassage C, Martin X, Wisnewsky C, Schwart K. Cardiac expression of alpha and beta myosin heavy chains and sarcomeric alpha-actins are regulated through trabeculational mechanisms. *J Biol Chem* 1992;267(18):12979–12985.

14. Schiaffino S, Samuel JL, Sasson D, Lompre AM, Garner I, Marotte F, Buckingham M, Rappapert L, Schwart K. Nonsynchronous accumulation of alpha-skeletal actin and beta-myosin heavy chain mRNAs during early stages of pressure-overload-induced cardiac hypertrophy demonstrated by in situ hybridisation. *Circ Res* 1989;64:937–948.
15. Lompre AM, de la Bastie D, Boheler KR, Schwart K. Characterisation and expression of the rat heart sarcoplasmic reticulum Ca^{++}-ATPase mRNA. *FEBS Lett* 1989;249(1):35–41.
16. Barton PJR, Robert B, Cohen A, Garner I, Sassoon D, Weydert A, Buckingham M. Structure and sequence of the myosin alkali light chain gene expressed in adult cardiac atria and fetal striated muscle. *J Biol Chem* 1988;263(25):12669–12676.
17. Lyons GE, Schiaffino S, Sasson D, Barton P, Buckingham M. Developmental regulation of myosin expression in mouse cardiac muscle. *J Cell Biol* 1990;111:2427–2437.
18. Lee KJ, Ross RS, Rockman HA, Harris AN, O'Brien TX, Van Bilsen M, Shubetta HE, Kandolf R, Brem G, Price J, Evans SM, Zhu H, Franz WH, Chien KR. Myosin light chain-2 luciferase transgenic mice reveal distinct regulatory programs for cardiac and skeletal muscle-specific expression of a single contractile protein gene. *J Biol Chem* 1992;267:15875–15885.
19. Beyer EC. Molecular cloning and development expression of two chick embryo gap junctionals proteins. *J Biol Chem* 1990;265(43):14439–14443.
20. Melton DA, Krieg PA, Rebagliati MR, Maniatis T, Zinn K, Green MR. Efficient in vitro synthesis of biologically active RNA and RNA hybridization probes from plasmids containing a bacteriophage SP6 promoter. *Nucleic Acids Res* 1984;12(18):7035–7056.
21. Wessels A, Vermeulen JLM, Moorman AFM, Becker AE. Immunohistochemical detection of myosin heavy chain isoforms in large sections of whole human hearts. In: *Sarcomeric and non-sarcomeric muscles: basis and applied research prospects for the 90's.* Padova: Unipress; 1988:311–316.
22. Ben-Sahchar G, Arcilla RA, Lucas RV, Manasek FJ. Ventricular trabeculations in the chick embryo heart and their contribution to ventricular and muscular septal development. *Circ Res* 1985;57: 759–766.
23. Ya J, Markman MWM, Wagenaar GTM, Moorman AFM, Lamers WH. Expression of the intermediate filament protein desmin and the smooth-muscle proteins caldesmon, calponin and smooth-muscle actin in the prenatal rat heart as parameter of myocardial maturation (submitted to *Anat Rec*).
24. Booth FW, Thomason DB. Molecular and cellular adaptation of muscle in response to exercise: perspective of various models. *Physiol Rev* 1991;71(2):541–585.
25. Kushmerick MJ. Energetics studies of muscle of different types. *Basic Res Cardiol* 1987;82(suppl 2):17–30.
26. Rall JA. Energetics aspects of skeletal muscle contraction implications of fibers types. *Exerc Sport Sci Rev* 1985;13:33–74.
27. Kennedy JM, Kamel S, Tambone WW, Vrbova G, Zak R. The expression of myosin heavy chain isoforms in normal and hypertrophied chicken slow muscle. *J Cell Biol* 1986;103:977–983.
28. Reiser PJ, Greaser ML, Moss RL. Myosin heavy chain composition of single cells from avian slow skeletal muscle is strongly correlated with velocity of shortering during development. *Dev Biol* 1988;129:400–407.
29. Van Kempen MJA. *Distribution of gap junction mRNA and protein in the heart.* Amsterdam, The Netherlands: University of Amsterdam; 1994. PhD thesis.

PART III

Cardiac Growth and Development

The Developing Heart,
edited by Bohuslav Ošťádal et al.
Lippincott-Raven Publishers,
Philadelphia © 1997.

6

The Effect of Developmental Stage on Cardiac Growth Response

Karel Rakusan and Marcia I. Heron

Department of Physiology, Faculty of Medicine, University of Ottawa, Ottawa, Ontario K1H 8M5, Canada

Studies on cardiac growth and development have gone beyond natural curiosity. The simple task of "mapping new territory" by creating the developmental chart gained additional importance after the realization that the developmental stage can determine the cardiac response to various physiologic and pathologic stimuli (1). Moreover, even cardiac failure can be considered an abnormality of cardiac growth, as witnessed by a close relationship between pathologic cardiac growth and cardiac failure (2–4).

The importance of developmental aspects for subsequent health and disease of the individual was evident to embryologists, developmental physiologists, and pediatricians for a long time. This issue gained additional credence by the epidemiologic studies of Barker and his co-workers, which were recently summarized in a book entitled *Fetal and infant origins of adult disease* (5). These authors compared infant morbidity and mortality in the earlier part of this century with recent adult morbidity and mortality in the same geographical regions. Among many important conclusions arising from their studies is their finding that ischemic heart disease in adulthood is strongly correlated with both neonatal and postneonatal development. Thus, men with the lowest body weights at birth and at 1 year had the highest death rates from ischemic heart disease (6). Similarly, systolic blood pressure was inversely related to birth weight, supporting the hypothesis that the intrauterine environment influences blood pressure later in life (7). Similar effects were also found in the case of chronic bronchitis, stroke, and insulin-resistant type II diabetes.

In this article, we present some experimental correlates to the preceding observations. Alterations in early growth rate may be produced by manipulating the litter size in neonatal animals. By varying the number of newborn rats nursed by a signal dam, one can create litters of fast- and slow-growing animals. The effect of early postnatal growth on cardiac mass and on the number and size of cardiac myocytes is presented in the first part of this article. In the second part, we review our results on capillarization of human hearts in neonatal and adult cardiac hypertrophy. Finally, we summarize our studies on short and long-term effects of neonatal hypo- and hyperthyroidism.

THE EFFECT OF EARLY POSTNATAL GROWTH ON CARDIAC MYOCYTES

We studied the effects of different rates of postnatal body growth on cardiac growth and growth of cardiac myocytes in rats (8,9). Growth rates were altered by adjusting the number of newborn animals per litter to 4 (fast-growing), 8 (normal), or 16 (slow-growing). This manipulation resulted in large differences in body weight among experimental animals at the time of sacrifice, with fast-growing animals having more than double the body weight of slow-growing animals (23.8 g versus 50.9 g). Increases in heart weight were proportional to total body growth, thus keeping relative heart weight constant. Larger hearts in fast-growing animals not only had larger cardiac myocytes but also had a significantly higher total number of myocytes per organ when compared to the remaining groups. Slow-growing hearts had the smallest cardiac myocytes and the lowest total number. These re-

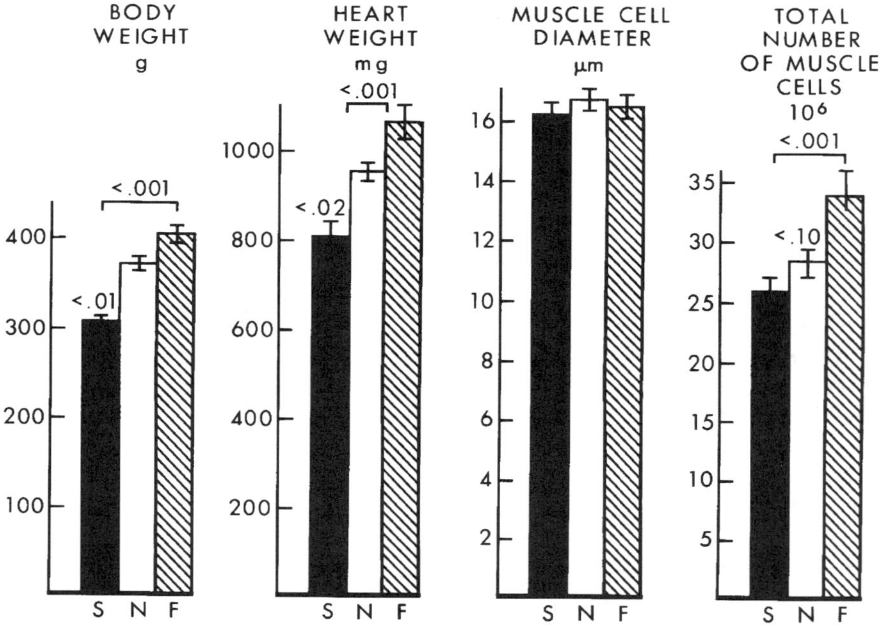

FIG. 6–1. The effect of litter size on body weight, heart weight, cardiac myocyte diameter, and total number of cardiac myocytes. Slow- (S), normal- (N) and fast- (F) growing rats.

sults demonstrate that accelerated cardiac growth during the early postnatal period is associated with increased proliferation of myocytes.

Some of the preceding changes are probably permanent. We transferred fast-, normal-, and slow-growing animals to a normal laboratory diet after the weaning period; 3 months later we obtained the following results (Fig. 6–1): (a) Differences in body weight and heart weight among the three experimental groups persist into adulthood, albeit on a much smaller scale. (b) Cardiac myocytes attain the same size in all experimental groups, suggesting that the total number of cardiac myocytes in fast-growing animals remained elevated. As a matter of fact, no additional myocyte hyperplasia was detected during subsequent growth from the age of 3 weeks to that of 3 months, as the total numbers of myocytes remained unchanged.

THE EFFECT OF AGE ON CAPILLARIZATION OF PRESSURE-OVERLOAD LEFT VENTRICULAR HYPERTROPHY IN HUMAN HEARTS

Recently, we studied the morphometry of human coronary capillaries during normal growth, as well as in two types of left ventricular pressure-overload hypertrophy (10). Results from left ventricular hypertrophy caused by congenital aortic

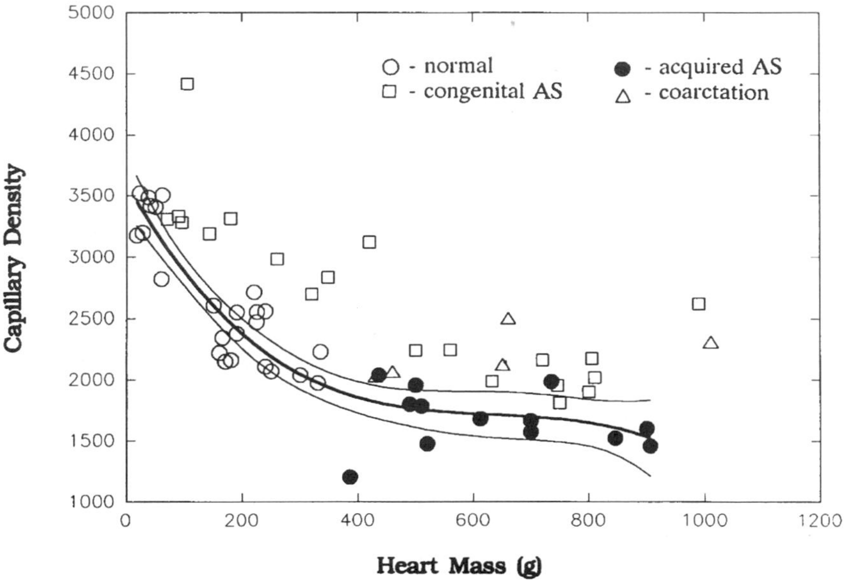

FIG. 6–2. Changes in capillary density with increasing cardiac weight in humans. Data for normal hearts and hearts with acquired aortic stenosis (AS) are best approximated as a single third-order polynomial (r = 0.93). Note that capillary density with congenital AS or with aortic coarctation is always higher than expected from the preceding relation. (Reprinted from ref. 10.)

valve stenosis or congenital aortic stenosis were compared to those in which the hypertrophy occurred as a result of rheumatic aortic valve stenosis in adulthood. The main results are summarized in Fig. 6–2, in which capillary density for each heart is plotted as a function of cardiac weight. Capillary density decreased exponentially with increasing cardiac weight in normal hearts. The relation of capillary density and heart weight in hearts hypertrophic because of aortic stenosis acquired later in life is in direct continuation of the preceding relationship. A single line may be used to approximate this relationship in both groups. In contrast, results obtained from cardiac hypertrophy caused by congenital aortic stenosis or coarctation lie above the line, indicating capillary densities higher than expected for a given heart weight. This was especially pronounced with cardiac hypertrophy in youngest age groups. Thus, pressure-overload hypertrophy with onset in childhood is structurally different from cardiac hypertrophy originating in adult patients. These results clearly demonstrate the importance of age and developmental stage in cardiac tissue response to growth stimuli.

THE EFFECT OF NEONATAL HYPO- AND HYPERTHYROIDISM ON CARDIAC TISSUE OF YOUNG AND ADULT RATS

Induction of hypo- and hyperthyroidism in neonatal rats was found not only to influence body and cardiac growth, but also to influence the postnatal growth of the coronary arteriolar network (11). Neonatal hypothyroid rats were developmentally delayed, exhibiting both attenuated cardiac and arteriolar growth, but not diminished capillary proliferation. The same arteriolar response was not observed in adult animals (12). In contrast, accelerated maturation and a significantly greater cardiac mass, matched by stimulated arteriolar and capillary proliferation, was observed in neonatal hyperthyroid rats. These findings are comparable to the response observed in adult hyperthyroid rats (e.g., 13,14).

Long-term effects of neonatal thyroid conditions were examined in weaned rats, 52 days after discontinuing treatment. Even though euthyroidism had been naturally reestablished at this time, both body and heart mass were significantly lower in previously hypo- and hyperthyroid rats compared to age-matched euthyroid controls. Interestingly, inhibition of subsequent arteriolar growth was noted in previously hyperthyroid rats, but not in previously hypothyroid rats. It thus appears that neonatal-onset hypo- and hyperthyroidism, although producing immediate effects on the developing arteriolar network, also induce long-term changes in subsequent arteriolar and cardiac growth.

SUMMARY

We have provided examples from humans and animals that serve to illustrate the importance of the developmental stage in the cardiac response to physiologic and pathologic stimuli, at the level of both the cardiomyocyte and the coronary microvasculature. We have also described instances whereby long-term changes in the adult organism have resulted from disturbances originating during early neonatal development. With increasing data from molecular biology studies suggesting regression to a fetal or neonatal phenotype in adult cardiac hypertrophy, and a growing body of evidence indicating the importance of developmental aspects in subsequent health and disease, a more detailed knowledge of all aspects of early postnatal growth and development is necessitated.

REFERENCES

1. Rakusan K. Postnatal growth and restructuring of mammalian hearts. In: Ostadal B, Dhalla NS, eds. *Heart function in health and disease.* Boston: Kluwer Academic Publishers; 1993:23–30.
2. Meerson FZ. Insufficiency of hypertrophied heart. *Basic Res Cardiol* 1976;71:343–354.
3. Katz AM. Is heart failure an abnormality of myocardial cell growth? *Cardiology* 1990;77:346–356.
4. Katz AM. Cardiomyopathy of overload: a major determinant of prognosis in congestive heart failure. *New Engl J Med* 1990;322:100–110.
5. Barker DJP, et al. *Fetal and infant origins of adult disease.* London: British Medical Journal, 1992.
6. Barker DJP, Winter PD, Osmond C, Margetts B, Simmonds SJ. Weight in infancy and death from ischemic heart disease. *Lancet* 1989;ii:577–580.
7. Law CM, Barker DJP, Bull AR, Osmond C. Maternal and fetal influences on blood pressure. *Arch Dis Child* 1991;66:1291–1295.
8. Rakusan K, Raman S, Layberry R, Korecky B. The influence of aging and growth on the postnatal development of cardiac muscle in rats. *Circ Res* 1978;42:212–218.
9. Rakusan K, Korecky B. The size and number of cardiac myocytes in young and adult rats of different growth rates. Abstract. *Fed Proc* 1978;37(1–3):86.
10. Rakusan K, Flanagan MF, Geva T, Southern J, Van Praagh R. Morphometry of human coronary capillaries during normal growth and the effect of age in left ventricular pressure-overload hypertrophy. *Circulation* 1992;86:38–46.
11. Heron MI, Rakusan K. Coronary microvasculature in neonatal hypo- and hyperthyroid rats. Changes in morphometry and cardiac function after return to euthyroidism. *J Mol Cell Cardiol* 1995;27(6):A230. Abstract.
12. Tomanek RJ, Barlow PA, Connell PM, Chen Y, Torry RJ. Effects of hypothyroidism and hypertension on myocardial perfusion and vascularization in rabbits. *Am J Physiol (Heart Circ Physiol)* 1993;34:H1638–H1644.
13. Chillian WM, Wangler RD, Peters KG, Tomanek RJ, Marcus ML. Thyroxine-induced left ventricular hypertrophy in the rat: anatomical and physiological evidence for angiogenesis. *Circ Res* 1985;57:591–598.
14. Heron MI, Rakusan K. Geometry of coronary capillaries in hyperthyroid and hypothyroid rat heart. *Am J Physiol (Heart Circ Physiol)* 1994;36:H1024–H1031.

The Developing Heart,
edited by Bohuslav Ošťádal et al.
Lippincott-Raven Publishers,
Philadelphia © 1997.

7

Cardiac Myocyte Growth in the Neonatal Mouse Heart

The Effect of Overexpression of the c-*myc* Proto-oncogene

Sanford P. Bishop, Noboru Machida, Nancy Brissie, and Catherine Sreenan

Department of Pathology, University of Alabama at Birmingham, Birmingham, AL 35294-0019

Cellular growth of the developing heart involves a complex series of poorly understood controls that promote cellular proliferation and differentiation to form the adult four-chambered heart of the mid-fetal period. Contractile proteins first appear at about 10 days of embryonic development in the rat, when the heart is still in the tubular stage (1); by 12 days of gestation in the rat, when septation is completed, sparse myofibrils are clearly present in myocytes. From day 12 at mid-gestation to birth there is rapid myocyte proliferation, gradual increase in blood pressure, and progression of cell differentiation to the point that myocytes are elongated with many easily recognizable, though incompletely developed, myofibrils. Depending on the species, sometime between birth and a few weeks after birth, myocytes normally undergo their last cellular division, and all further growth of the heart is by increase in cell volume, or hypertrophic growth. At the same time as the last cellular division and the initiation of hypertrophic cell growth, a number of other developmental structural, functional, and biochemical changes in the myocardium occur.

Previous studies in our laboratory (2–5) as well as from others (6–11) have described the morphologic changes that occur in cardiac muscle during the neonatal conversion from hyperplastic cell growth to hypertrophic growth. During the first week after birth in the rat heart, myocytes divide, on average, one more time, doubling the number of cells present at birth. Between 5 and 12 days of age in the rat heart, many cells undergo one more nuclear division without subsequent cytokine-

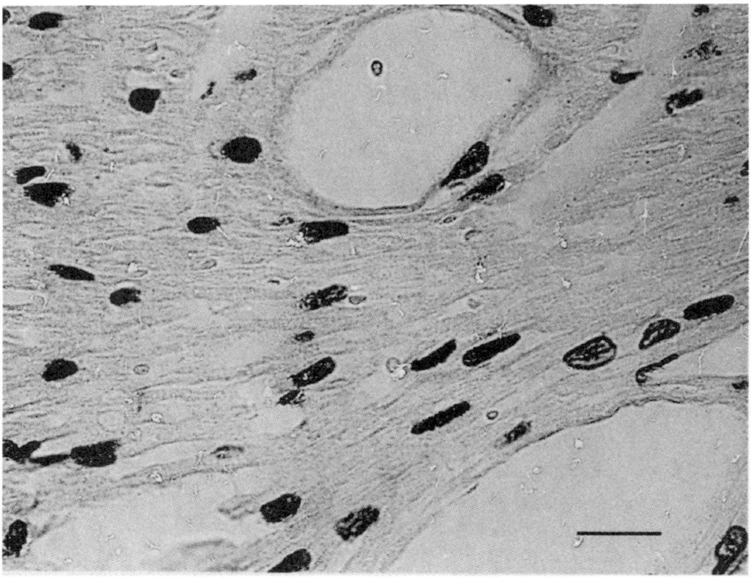

FIG. 7–1. BrdU incorporation into the nucleus of 7–day-old c-*myc* transgenic mouse neonatal cardiac muscle and nonmuscle cells. BrdU immunostain with no counterstain. Bar = 25 μm.

sis, and all subsequent growth of the myocyte occurs through hypertrophy (2). Data presented in this review show that the same time frame is applicable to the mouse heart. A small number of myocyte nuclei continue to undergo mitosis without subsequent cytokinesis until about 17 days of age in both the rat and the mouse.

During the first 2–3 weeks of postnatal life there is also rapid proliferation of the vascular system, and many labeled nuclei during this period are endothelial and smooth muscle cells. However, by 17–21 days in the rat heart, tritiated thymidine (^{3}H-Thd) uptake is very low (2,7,12,13), reflecting slow continued endothelial and other nonmyocyte proliferation. Bromodeoxyuridine (BrdU) is an analog of thymidine that is incorporated into the nucleus during the S phase of the cell cycle (Fig. 7–1). In the neonatal mouse heart during the first week after birth, approximately 10–12% of cardiac nuclei were labeled with BrdU, and about 25% of labeled nuclei were identified as myocytes, whereas approximately 75% were nonmyocytes. By 14–20 days of age, only 1–3% of cardiac cells were labeled with BrdU, and more than 97% of these were nonmyocytes.

CONTROL OF MYOCYTE PROLIFERATION IN THE NEONATE

Factors that control the conversion from proliferative myocyte growth to hypertrophic growth are not well understood. The time after birth for the final cell division may be altered by appropriate stimuli. Increased work on the late fetal or neonatal heart induced by iron deficiency anemia (14), carbon monoxide–induced volume overload (15), outflow track stenosis (16), or hypobaric oxygen at high altitude (17) have been shown to accentuate the hyperplastic phase of cell growth in animals. In the spontaneously hypertensive rat (SHR) there is increased systemic pressure at birth and more cells of the same size than in control WKY rats. Binucleation, an index of conversion to hypertrophic growth (2), occurs at an earlier time in SHR than in WKY, indicating accelerated conversion from hyperplastic to hypertrophic myocyte growth. However, by 15 days of age, cell number is equal in both strains (4). These studies from our laboratory, and by others, demonstrate that altering the hemodynamic load of the developing heart can influence morphologic development, principally by increasing the hyperplastic response of myocytes.

Several humoral factors, proto-oncogenes, and growth factors have also been implicated in the regulation of myocyte proliferation in the developing heart. Thyroxine, for instance, was shown to prematurely convert myocytes from hyperplastic growth to hypertrophic growth in neonatal rats (18), although a co-stimulatory effect on hypertrophic growth by catecholamines induced by thyroxine or other factors in the neonatal period cannot be ruled out (19–21). The proto-oncogenes c-*myc* and r-*fos* have been found to be present at high levels in fetal myocardium, and decrease to low levels during the early neonatal period at the time of the transition period to hypertrophic growth (22,23). On the other hand, TGF-β is present at low levels in the embryonic and fetal heart, but at the time of conversion to hypertrophic growth, it is present at high levels (24). Further, in newborn SHR, which have evidence of early conversion from hyperplastic to hypertrophic myocyte growth (vide supra) (4,25), TGF-β is present in greater amounts than in control WKY rats (24). While TGF-β is known to play a role in either promotion or inhibition of cell proliferation in various systems, it is not clear what role is played by this growth factor in the neonatal heart, though its appearance coincident with the end of the proliferative phase of myocyte growth suggests a role in inhibiting myocyte proliferation. It must be noted, however, that this is also the same time that there is an increase in fibroblast proliferation and collagen formation, as well as extensive angiogenesis.

CELL GROWTH, HYPERTROPHY, AND THE C-*MYC* PROTO-ONCOGENE

Several proto-oncogenes, which may be activated by a variety of mechanisms, can lead to unregulated cell growth and transformation (26–28). Although its precise function is unknown, the c-*myc* gene has been implicated in cellular transformation through the association of overexpression of this gene with continued cell proliferation and even tumor development. The c-*myc* proto-oncogene has been associated with proliferating cardiac myocytes prior to stages of final differentiation and is decreased in normal differentiated cells (22). In some nonmuscle cells, such as adipocytes (29) and chondroblasts (30), c-*myc* expression appears to prevent cell differentiation, but in skeletal and cardiac muscle, overexpression of c-*myc* does not prevent differentiation (31,32).

TRANSGENIC MOUSE MODEL OF C-*MYC* OVEREXPRESSION

The transgenic (TG) mouse model used in this study was originally prepared by using a recombinant fusion gene constructed from the 3′LTR of the Rous sarcoma virus and a DNA fragment from the mouse S107 plasmacytoma containing immunoglobulin sequences and a truncated c-*myc* gene. This fusion gene was used to produce transgenic mice on a CD1 stock. A male founder animal was identified through Southern blot analysis of DNA extracted from the tail (33,34). Subsequently, heterozygote male animals were transported to Birmingham and maintained in a barrier system. A nonbarrier colony was established from these males bred to CD1 females and Caesarian-derived pups raised by foster mothers. Subsequent matings were between heterozygote males, confirmed by PCR analysis of tail DNA, and either heterozygote TG or wild-type (WT) females derived from the original founder animals. The gene is transmitted as an autosomal dominant with parental imprinting, so that only the males transmit the gene with phenotypic expression to their progeny (33).

Body weight gain of surviving TG animals is not different from WT littermates, and many animals have survived to more than 2 years of age until used for study.

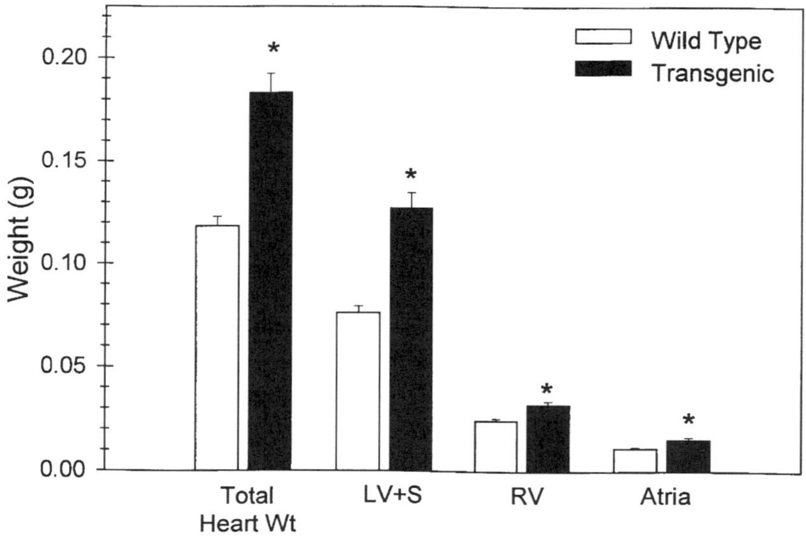

FIG. 7–2. Regional heart weights from a group of adult WT and TG mice. All regions of the heart are significantly enlarged. $n = 11$ WT and 8 TG. * = $p < 0.01$.

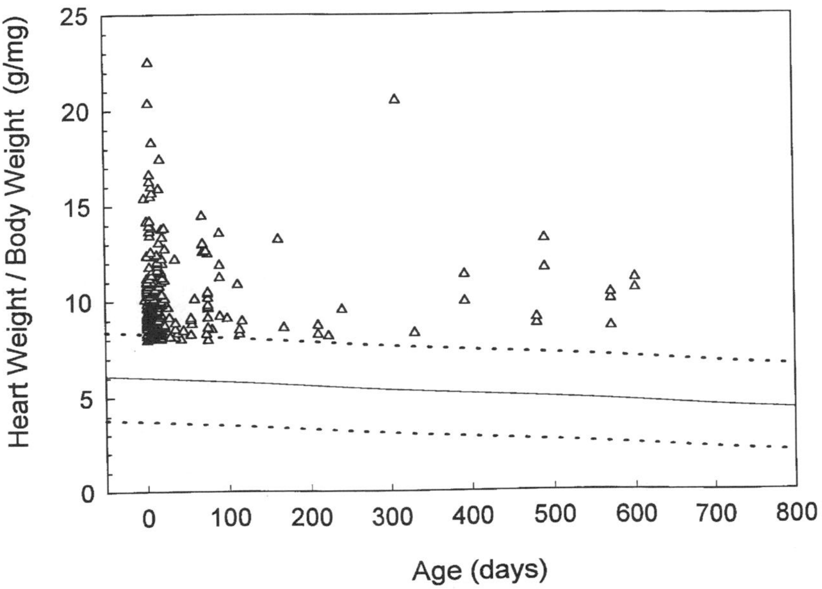

FIG. 7–3. Heart weight to body weight ratio of wild-type (WT; $n = 736$) and transgenic (TG; $n = 283$) mice from birth to 2 years of age. The mean value for wild-type mice is depicted as the solid line, and ±2SD are shown by the dotted lines. The open triangles are individual values for transgenic mice at various ages studied (selected for animals with HW/BW greater than 8.0 mg/kg). There is considerable variability in the ratio among TG mice, with many animals exceeding twice the normal wild-type value.

However, litter size from TG sires is usually smaller than normal, and the number of TG animals relative to WT animals is less than expected based on transmission as an autosomal dominant gene. Fetal deaths are often noted by examination of the pregnant uterus, and early neonatal deaths are common. Those that survive to weaning have normal growth and usually are active breeders.

The affected transgenic progeny (TG) have a 50% or more increase in cardiac mass compared to wild-type (WT) littermates or parent CD1 stock, both before and after birth (34). Hearts of TG mice have a characteristic phenotypic appearance, with a markedly enlarged left ventricle and prominent left ventricular apex), though the increase in mass affects all four chambers (Fig. 7–2). Measurement of heart weights from a large series of animals from birth to 2 years of age revealed that normal WT mice have a mean heart weight to body weight ratio (HW/BW) of 5.78 ± 1.14 (SD) mg/g. Animals with HW/BW of less than 8 mg/g seldom had positive c-*myc* DNA by PCR. As illustrated in Figure 7–3, most mice whose HW/BW exceeded the mean plus 2 SD had values between 8 and 11 mg/g, but many animals had values above 12 mg/g, twice the normal heart weight, and some were more than three times normal HW/BW.

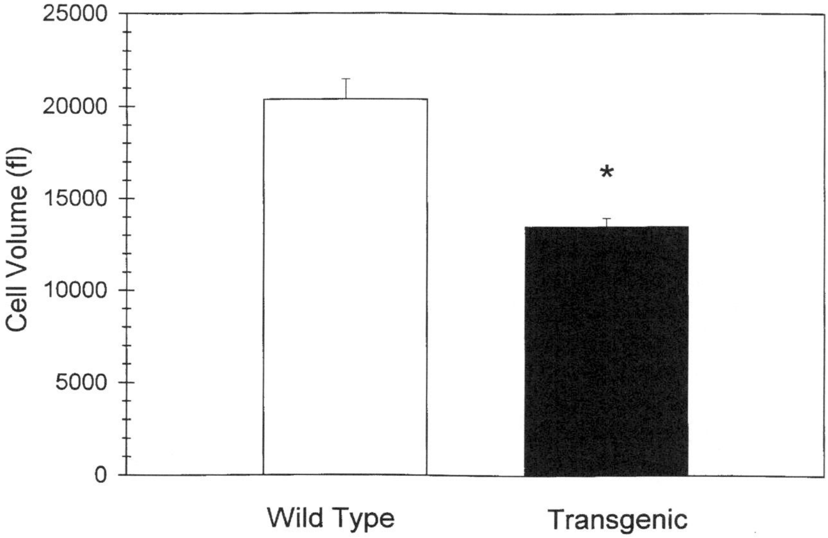

FIG. 7–4. Median cell volume of wild-type and transgenic mice as determined on isolated myocytes from adult littermate mice. Myocytes from TG mice are significantly smaller than those from WT mouse hearts. $n = 20$ WT and 9 TG. * = $p < 0.01$.

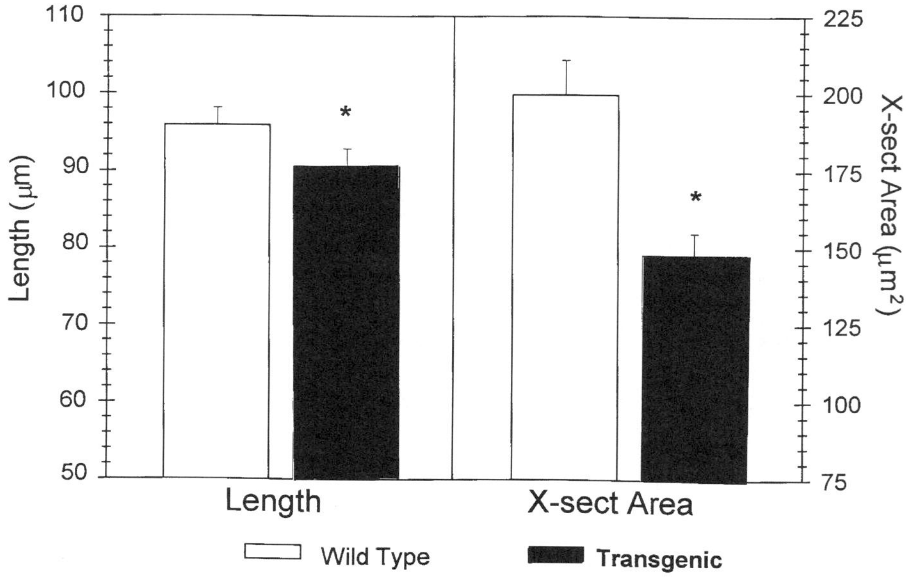

FIG. 7–5. Mean cell length and cross-sectional area of isolated myocytes from wild-type and transgenic mouse hearts. Myocytes from transgenic mice are shorter and have smaller cross-sectional area than wild-type littermate mice. * = $P < 0.01$.

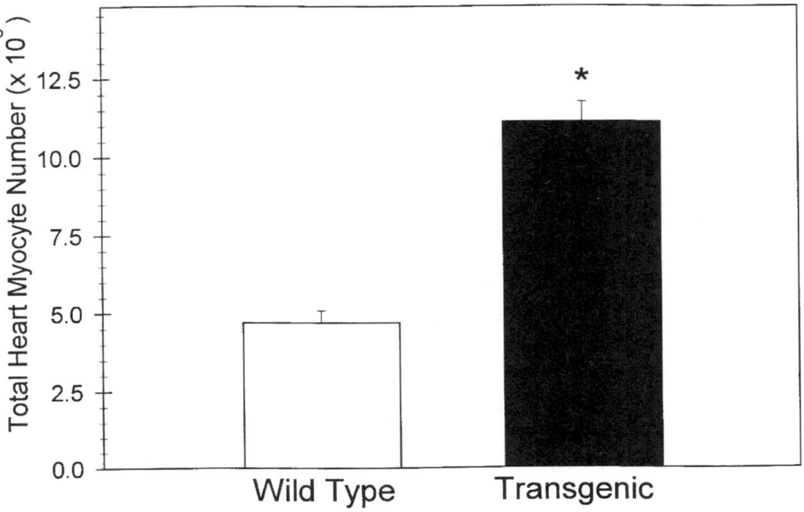

FIG. 7–6. Number of myocytes in wild-type and transgenic mouse hearts, calculated from the median cell volume of isolated myocytes and total ventricular weight. There are more than twice as many myocytes in the TG hearts as in WT hearts. * = $p < 0.01$.

Early studies demonstrated that DNA content was increased in TG hearts compared to WT, but these studies did not prove whether the cardiac enlargement was the result of cellular hypertrophy or hyperplasia. To more definitively address the question of hypertrophy/hyperplasia in the enlarged hearts of the transgenic mice, isolated myocytes were prepared by collagenase perfusion of the hearts from 3-month-old, 30-gram mice, and cell volume determined with a Coulter Counter system (34). Median cell volume was smaller in TG (13,491 ± 1465 fl) than in WT 20,517 ± 4896) ($p < 0.05$) (Fig. 7–4). Isolated myocyte length, measured directly by microscopy, and cell cross-sectional area (Coulter median volume/mean cell length) were also smaller (Fig. 7–5). Calculated total ventricular myocyte number was more than twice as great in TG (11.1×10^6 cells) as in WT (4.9×10^6) ($p < 0.05$) (Fig. 7–6). In summary, myocytes from TG mice are smaller and more than twice as numerous as in WT hearts, so that myocyte hyperplasia accounts for the 50% greater cardiac mass in TG mice.

MORPHOLOGIC CHARACTERIZATION OF THE C-*MYC* TRANSGENIC MOUSE MYOCARDIUM

Original founder animals and subsequent animals from our colony were perfusion fixed for light and electron microscopy or used for isolation of myocytes to confirm that myocyte hyperplasia persisted into later adulthood. Light microscopic examination of hearts from birth to more than 1 year of age has revealed no major architectural changes in myocyte and collagen connective tissue in TG mice, other than the smaller myocyte size, which can only be appreciated by quantitative evaluation. In TG mice more than 6 months of age, numerous left ventricular myocytes have very large and irregular nuclei, containing multiple nucleoli. Electron microscopy confirms multiple folding of the nuclear membrane. These nucleolar changes suggest active RNA synthesis, and the enlarged nuclei suggest polyploidy of DNA. These features have not been seen by us in normal aging rats or mice. Other ultrastructural features include occasional disoriented myofibrillar alignment, scattered cells with severe atrophy and loss of myofibrils, and occasional leptofibril structures associated with cell membranes, suggestive of myofibril formation. None of these changes is specific for any particular known abnormality, but they suggest abortive attempts of cellular hypertrophy.

EFFECT OF C-*MYC* OVEREXPRESSION IN MYOCYTE PROLIFERATION IN THE NEONATAL PERIOD

To determine the time during fetal and neonatal development that the increased myocyte proliferation occurred, we injected BrdU intraperitoneally in littermate mice from transgenic sires at 2–4-day intervals from birth to 20 days of age ($n = 3$ WT and 3 TG per age group). One hour later the animals were anesthetized with sodium pentobarbital, the thorax was opened, and the heart was perfused through the left ventricular apex with a 21-gauge needle using 10% phosphate buffered formalin. The fixed heart was then removed from the thorax, pulmonary and vascular tissue was trimmed, and the heart was weighed and immersed an additional day in fresh fixative. Paraffin-embedded sections of the left ventricle and interventricular septum were stained with hematoxylin to identify nuclei, and a serial section was stained by the avidin biotinylated peroxidase method using a BrdU primary antibody without any counterstain to identify cells in S phase.

Nuclear density of all hematoxylin stained cells (myocytes and nonmyocytes) and of all BrdU stained cells was determined with a video image analysis system (Image-1, Universal Imaging Corporation, West Chester, PA) using an Olympus AH3 microscope, a Dage CCD72 video camera, and an 80486 computer. The BrdU Labeling Index (LI) was calculated as the number of BrdU labeled cells/total nuclei $\times$ 100. Subsequently, the percentage of myocyte- and nonmyocyte-labeled nuclei was determined by counting 100 labeled nuclei in the left ventricular region of each animal.

Total nuclear density in TG mice was 6.8–31.2% greater in both LV and IVS than in WT at all ages, indicating a smaller cytoplasm per cell in TG mice, consistent with the smaller cell volume measured with the Coulter Counter in isolated myocytes of adult mice. In WT mice, the rate of BrdU incorporation in both LV and IVS remained almost constant at 11.2–12.5% LI until 7 days of age, was significantly reduced at 10 days of age, and fell to approximately 2% by 14 days of age. Thereafter, there was a further, gradual decrease in LI, reaching less than 0.5% by 20 days of age. In contrast, LI of TG that was not different from WT at 1–3 days after birth fell rapidly to 4.4 $\pm$ 0.29% and 4.6 $\pm$ 0.20% at 7 days and to 2.7 $\pm$

0.30% and 2.5 ± 0.10% at 10 days in LV and IVS, respectively. During the following 10 days, LI in both LV and IVS slowly declined to about 1.5% at 14 days of age and 0.4% at 20 days of age, similar to that in the WT mice. LI was markedly and significantly lower in TG than in WT animals at 5, 7, and 10 days of age, indicating an earlier cessation of DNA synthesis in the TG mice compared to WT mice. There were no differences between data derived from the two regions, LV and IVS, for any age studied. The percentage of labeled cells during the first 3 postnatal days was approximately 75% nonmyocytes and 25% myocytes in both groups. From 5 through 14 days of age, there was a significantly lower percentage of labeled myocytes in the TG mice than in WT mice, and by 16 days of age and later, less than 3% of labeled cells were myocytes in both groups.

The results of this study have demonstrated that in spite of the accelerated cell proliferation in the fetal period, the myocyte hyperplastic phase of cell growth is completed at an earlier age in c-*myc* TG mice than in WT mice. Thus, the increased myocyte number previously shown to be present in this model (34) is produced entirely within the prenatal period, and the myocytes enter the hypertrophic stage of cell growth approximately 5 days earlier in the TG mice than in WT mice. Second, the increased cell number and smaller myocyte size previously reported for adult TG c-*myc* mice is shown to be present at birth to 20 days of age by the increased nuclear density found at all ages studied.

SUMMARY

Results from this study demonstrate that the mouse has a very similar time course to the rat for conversion from hyperplastic to hypertrophic growth in the normal wild-type animal. DNA synthesis and myocyte proliferation continue at a constant level from birth to 5–7 days of age. Hypertrophic cell growth starts at 5–7 days as indicated by decreasing nuclear density, while DNA synthesis, representing karyokinesis not followed by cytokinesis, continues through 10 days of age and then rapidly declines. In the c-*myc* overexpressing transgenic mouse, however, DNA synthesis rapidly declines from the time of birth, and is significantly less than in WT mice at 5, 7, and 10 days of age, indicating an early transition from hyperplastic to hypertrophic cell growth in this animal model. The increased cellular proliferation previously identified in this model has been completed during the fetal stage of myocardial growth. This transgenic animal serves as a useful model for the study of factors that play a role in the differentiation and proliferation of cardiac myocytes.

ACKNOWLEDGMENTS

Supported in part by a grant-in-aid from the American Heart Association and by U.S. Public Health Service grant HL 36892. The authors acknowledge the expert technical contribution of Lisa Doss, Jeanette Bicknell, and Paul Norton.

REFERENCES

1. Chacko KJ. Observations on the ultrastructure of developing myocardium of rat embryos. *J Morphol* 1976;150:681–710.
2. Clubb FJ Jr, Bishop SP. Formation of binucleated myocardial cells in the neonatal rat: an index for growth hypertrophy. *Lab Invest* 1984;50:571–577.
3. Bishop SP. The myocardial cell: normal growth, cardiac hypertrophy and response to injury. *Toxicol Pathol* 1990;18:438–453.
4. Clubb FJ Jr, Bell PD, Kriseman JD, Bishop SP. Myocardial cell growth and blood pressure development in neonatal spontaneously hypertensive rats. *Lab Invest* 1987;56:189–197.
5. Bishop SP, Hine P. Cardiac muscle cytoplasmic and nuclear development during canine neonatal growth. In: Roy P, ed. *Recent advances in studies on cardiac structure and metabolism.* Vol 8, *The cardiac sarcoplasm.* Baltimore: University Park Press; 1975:77–98.
6. Zak R. Cell proliferation during cardiac growth. *Am J Cardiol* 1973;31:211–219.
7. Rumyantsev PP. DNA synthesis and nuclear division in embryonal and postnatal histogenesis of myocardium (autoradiographic study). *Fed Proc* 1965;24:T899–T902.
8. Erokhina IL, Rumyantsev PP. Proliferation and biosynthetic activities of myocytes from conductive system and working myocardium of the developing mouse heart: light microscopic autoradiographic study. *Acta Histochem* 1988;84:51–66.
9. Rumyantsev PP. Interrelations of the proliferation and differentiation processes during cardiac myogenesis and regeneration. *Int. Rev Cytol* 1977;51:187–273.
10. Anversa P, Vitali-Mazza L, Loud AV. Morphometric and autoradiographic study of developing ventricular and atrial myocardium in fetal rats. *Lab Invest* 1975;33:696–705.
11. Anversa P, Olivetti G, Loud AV. Morphometric study of early postnatal development in the left and right ventricular myocardium of the rat. I. Hypertrophy, hyperplasia and binucleation of myocytes. *Circ Res* 1980;46:495–502.
12. Claycomb WC. Biochemical aspects of cardiac muscle differentiation. *J Biol Chem* 1975;250: 3229–3235.
13. Sasaki R, Morishita T, Ichikawa S, Yamagata S. Autoradiographic studies and mitosis of heart muscle cells in experimental cardiac hypertrophy. *Tohoku J Exp Med* 1970;102:159–167.
14. Neffgen JF, Korecky B. Cellular hyperplasia and hypertrophy in cardiomegalies induced by anemia in young and adult rats. *Circ Res* 1972;30:104–113.
15. Clubb FJ Jr, Penney DG, Baylerian MS, Bishop SP. Cardiomegaly due to myocyte hyperplasia in perinatal rats exposed to 200 ppm carbon monoxide. *J Mol Cell Cardiol* 1986;18:477–486.
16. Archie JP, Fixler DE, Ullyot DJ, Buckberg GD, Hoffman JIE. Regional myocardial blood flow in lambs with concentric right ventricular hypertrophy. *Circ Res* 1974;34:143–154.
17. Pietschmann M, Bartels H. Cellular hyperplasia and hypertrophy, capillary proliferation and myoglobin concentration in the heart of newborn and adult rats at high altitude. *Respir Physiol* 1985;59:347–360.
18. Gerdes AM, Kriseman J, Bishop SP. Changes in myocardial cell size and number during the development and reversal of hyperthyroidism in neonatal rats. *Lab Invest* 1983;48(5):598–602.
19. Iwasaki T, Takino Y, Suzuki T. Effects of isoproterenol on the developing heart in rats. *Jpn Circ J* 1990;54:109–116.
20. Lau C, Slotkin TA. Accelerated development of rat sympathetic neurotransmission caused by neonatal triiodothyronine administration. *J Pharmacol Exp Ther* 1979;208(3):485–490.
21. Claycomb WC. Biochemical aspects of cardiac muscle differentiation. *J Biol Chem* 1976;251(19): 6082–6089.
22. Schneider MD, Payne PA, Ueno H, Perryman MB, Roberts R. Dissociated expression of c-myc and a fos-related competence gene during cardiac myogenesis. *Mol Cell Biol* 1986;6:4140–4143.
23. Zimmerman KA, Yancopoulos GD, Collum RG, Smith RK, Khol NE, Denis KA, Nau MM, Witte ON, Toran-Allerand D, Gee CE, Minna JD, Alt FW. Differential expression of myc family genes during murine development. *Nature* 1986;319:780–783.
24. Engelmann GL, Boehm KD, Birchenall-Roberts MC, Ruscetti FW. Transforming growth factor-beta 1 in heart development. *Mech Dev* 1992;38:85–97.
25. Engelmann GL, Gerrity RG. Biochemical characterization of neonatal cardiomyocyte development in normotensive and hypertensive rats. *J Mol Cell Cardiol* 1988;20(3):169–178.
26. Rollins BJ, Stiles CD. Regulation of c-*myc* and c-*fos* proto-oncogene expression by animal cell growth factors. *In Vitro Cell Dev Biol* 1988;24:81–84.

27. Bishop JM. Viral oncogenes. *Cell* 1985;42:23–38.
28. Adamson ED. Oncogenes in development. *Development* 1987;99(4):449–471.
29. Freytag SO. Enforced expression of the c-myc oncogene inhibits cell differentiation by precluding entry into a distinct pre-differentiation state in G_0/G_1. *Mol Cell Biol* 1988;8(4):1614–1624.
30. Farquharson C, Hesketh JE, Loveridge N. The proto-oncogene c-myc is involved in cell differentiation as well as cell proliferation: studies on growth plate chondrocytes in situ. *J Cell Physiol* 1992;152:135–144.
31. Endo T, Nadal-Ginard B. Transcriptional and posttranscriptional control of c-myc during myogenesis: its mRNA remains inducible in differentiated cells and does not suppress the differentiated phenotype. *Mol Cell Biol* 1986;6:1412–1421.
32. Schneider MD, Perryman MB, Payne PA, Spizz G, Roberts R, Olson EN. Autonomous expression of c-*myc* in BC3H1 cells partially inhibits but does not prevent myogenic differentiation. *Mol Cell Biol* 1987;7:1973–1977.
33. Swain JL, Stewart TA, Leder P. Parental legacy determines methylation and expression of an autosomal transgene: a molecular mechanism for parental imprinting. *Cell* 1987;50:719–727.
34. Jackson T, Allard MF, Sreenan CM, Doss LK, Bishop SP, Swain JL. The c-myc proto-oncogene regulates cardiac development in transgenic mice. *Mol Cell Biol* 1990;10:3709–3716.

The Developing Heart,
edited by Bohuslav Ošťádal et al.
Lippincott-Raven Publishers,
Philadelphia © 1997.

8

The Cardiac Extracellular Matrix During Development

Ian M. C. Dixon and Haisong Ju

Molecular Cardiology Laboratory, Institute of Cardiovascular Sciences, St. Boniface General Hospital Research Centre, University of Manitoba, Winnipeg, Manitoba, R2H 2A6 Canada

In any given organ, the volume displaced by constitutive cells may account for a fraction of the total volume of the tissue. That is, a substantial amount of organ volume is occupied by a complex network of macromolecules that are collectively defined as the extracellular matrix; this matrix forms physical connections among the constitutive cells. In most organs, the extracellular matrix is composed of a variety of polysaccharides and proteins that are secreted by fibroblast cells present among the primary cell types (1). The major components of the extracellular matrix include (a) structural proteins, such as collagen and elastin; (b) cell adhesive or antiadhesive molecules, including fibronectin, vitronectin, laminin, and tenascin; and (c) proteoglycans, which are a complex array of proteins linked to glycosaminoglycans side-chains. Another distinct class of proteins, known as integrins, serves as matrix receptors and is synthesized by various cells in the heart. Cardiac myocytes occupy ~75% of the total tissue space but represent only one-third of the total cell number. The nonmyocyte cells reside in the cardiac interstitium and account for about two-thirds of the total cell population. These cell types include cardiac fibroblasts, endothelial cells, and vascular smooth muscle cells. Cardiac fibroblasts exist in large numbers in the heart and form the largest group among cardiac nonmyocyte cells (2–3). The components of the extracellular matrix have been shown to influence phenotypic and genetic changes in the development of tissues. Recent data indicate that the cardiac extracellular matrix plays a critical role in growth and development. It is becoming clear that extracellular matrix proteins are not merely involved in serving only as the cellular scaffolding for the myocardium per se; they may significantly contribute to heart development, growth, and cardiac function by direct modulation of the behavior of cells that contact it (4–6). Because some recent biochemical and molecular studies have led to a burgeoning knowledge of the general characteristics of the cardiac stromal tissue and because much recent work in various experimental models has addressed the role of extracellular matrix in the developing heart, we have undertaken a review of these topics. Cardiovascular development is the net result of a complex genetic program subject to regulation by signals transmitted among cardiac cells and its extracellular environment. The role of the extracellular matrix in heart development during embryonic, fetal, and neonatal stages includes signaling necessary for cell migration, cell sorting, adhesion, differentiation, angiogenesis, and valve formation (7,8). Our review will summarize the structure and function of cardiac extracellular matrix, and the role of the extracellular matrix in heart during development.

COLLAGEN IN THE HEART DURING DEVELOPMENT

At least five collagen isoforms—including types I, III, IV, V, and VI—are present in the adult myocardium (6,9–11). Collagen types I and III are the most abundant forms of collagen, and together they represent more than 90% of all collagen proteins within the myocardium (5). Mature collagen types I and III are composed of three different chains or identical chains, respectively; collagen type IV is a dimer of different chains and is present in the basement membrane of myocytes and all other cell types. All types of collagen (with the exception of collagen type IV) are synthesized and metabolized exclusively by cardiac fibroblasts. Using Northern blot analysis and in situ hybridization techniques, Eghbali et al. (12,13) made the seminal observation that types I and III mRNAs exist predominantly in the space adjacent to myocytes as well as in the interstitium, which is commonly populated by cardiac fibroblasts. Moreover, the mRNAs for all three collagen types were observed to be present in the isolated fibroblasts, whereas collagen type IV mRNA was identified within both the myocytes and fibroblast cells. The function of cardiac collagen in adult heart in physiological and pathological conditions has been reviewed by the authors (14).

In addition to the collagen subtypes mentioned earlier, collagen types II and VIII are known to be transiently expressed during cardiac development and growth; the proportion of each collagen type is distinct from the normal distribution pattern in adult heart. For example, in mammalian neonatal hearts, type III collagen constitutes about one-third of the total collagen complement (15). Therefore, the ratio of collagen type I to type III is significantly lower than that of the adult heart. In healthy adult cartilaginous tissue, collagen type II is highly expressed. During early embrogenesis, collagen types I, II, V, and VIII have been detected in the atrioventricular region (an area associated with the formation of cardiac valves) of embryonic avian and mouse heart, suggesting these collagens might play a role in valve formation. Staining with antibodies against interstitial collagen types I and III demonstrated the presence of these collagens in the valvular regions in 19-day fetal rat heart (4). In another study, immunoreactive type VIII collagen was detected on day 11 in the developing mouse embryo (16). The distribution of this protein is known to be rapidly modulated during cardiac morphogenesis. Initially, type VIII collagen was associated with cardiac myoblasts. From days 15–18 the immunoreactive component was observed in the subendocardial layer of the atrioventricular canal and again later in the myocardial basement membrane. This result suggested that the contribution of this collagen type to cardiac morphogenesis may contribute to the partial regulation of the differentiation of the myocardium and formation of the cardiac valves. In the neonatal growth stage, fibrillar collagen subtypes also exhibited dynamic changes in expression patterns. It has been reported that collagen types I and III mRNA abundance is rapidly increased after birth and that expression of these types peaked at 3–5 days (17). These data support the hypothesis that synthesis and organization of extracellular matrix components are regulated, in part, by mechanical stimulation of heart cells during this period of development. Type VI collagen is typically found in the basement membrane and acts as an anchor linking the myocardial cell basement membrane to the extracellular matrix and to cardiac interstitial cells, thus contributing to coordination of force generation and mechanical stress throughout the myocardium (10); integrin proteins are another notable matrix receptor in the heart, partially fulfilling a similar function.

Recent experiments provide evidence supporting the hypothesis that cardiac collagen plays a vital role in the maintenance of myofibrillogenesis (18). Treatment of embryonic cardiac myocytes *in vitro* with two different kind inhibitors of collagen synthesis, *cis*-hydroxy-L-proline and ethyl-3,4-dihydroxy-benzoate, effectively inhibits collagen secretion. Inhibition of collagen secretion disrupts myofibrillogenesis and results in the inhibition of expression of muscle-specific genes (myosin heavy chain and troponin T), suggesting that collagen synthesis plays an essential role in maintaining the differentiated phenotype of cardiac myocytes (18). There is also some evidence to support the hypothesis that collagen is essential for the survival and growth of cardiac myocytes *in vitro*. It is well known that coating culture plates with specific extracellular matrix proteins is an essential step to culture both neonatal and adult myocytes. Neonatal myocytes attach well to collagen types I, II, III, IV, and V; adult myocytes only attached well to type IV collagen under culture condition (19–22).

FIBRONECTIN IN THE HEART DURING DEVELOPMENT

Fibronectin is another important cardiac extracellular matrix protein, and it is homogeneously distributed throughout the extracellular space in which elements such as the T-tubule network of cardiac myocytes and collagens are located (23). Fibronectin is a dimeric glycoprotein and has binding sites for collagen, heparin, fibrin, and proteoglycans (24). Because of alternative mRNA splicing, fibronectin has three forms, EIIIA, EIIIB and V; both EIIIA and EIIIB are present in heart tissue (25,26). Cardiac myocytes adhere to the cardiac extracellular matrix via matrix-specific receptors, including those specific for fibronectin. Thus, these receptors serve as a bridge for the structural connection between myocytes and extracellular matrix (5).

Fibronectin influences a variety of cell behaviors, including cell growth, adhesion, migration, and wound healing (25). The fibronectin mRNA was found abundant in day 14 of fetal rat heart, and rapidly decreased during cardiac physiologic growth. The percentages of fibronectin transcripts containing of EIIIA or EIIIB exons are very high in the early fetal heart but are known to decrease thereafter (26). During the chicken embryo development, two waves of cell migration have been described during the cardiogenesis (8). The first wave occurs during gastrulation and involves a subset of mesodermal cells that regroup in a particular region of the embryo to form the precardiac cells. These cells subsequently move anteriorly to reach the midline of the embryo, where they differentiate into two endocardial tubes, which fuse later to form the beating tubular heart (8). An increased concentration of fibronectin proteins has been detected along the migratory route of the precardiac mesoderm, suggesting that the precardiac cells may migrate by moving along the substratum toward areas of greater adhesiveness. Thus, the gradient of adhesiveness to the substrate is involved in the directionality of migration of these cells (27). This result supports the hypothesis that fibronectin may be involved in regulation of cell migration during development. To test the role of fibronectin in the migration of precardiac cells, chick embryos were incubated with different concentrations of antibody against fibronectin (28). Cardiac development was subsequently arrested in the presence of high concentration of antifibronectin antibody. These results support the hypothesis that fibronectin is a major component in the migratory pathway and plays a role in the directional migration of precardiac cells to the embryonic midline.

The second wave of cell migration takes place after the heart tube has formed. The inner endocardium layer becomes separated from the myocardium by an expanded extracellular matrix, the so-called cardiac jelly (8). A number of endocardiac cells from the atrioventricular zone soon break away from the endocardium and migrate into the cardiac jelly to form the heart septa and the valves. The early chick heart tube consists of myocardium and endothelium separated by a myocardial derived basement membrane. As development proceeds, the endothelium undergoes a transition into mesenchyme only in the atrioventricular area and outflow tract, but the ventricular endothelium is not transformed into mesenchyme (the progenitor of heart septa and valves) (29). Embryonic heart regions cultured on three-dimensional collagen gels showed that atrioventricular endothelium could only form mesenchyme if co-cultured with atrioventricular myocardium. Fibronectin appeared in a gradient of decreasing concentration extending from the myocardium toward the endothelium. These results show that a regionally specific interaction of the myocardium with the endothelium is required to initiate the formation of prevalvular mesenchyme and serves as a haptotactic mechanism for migration of cells. A progressive decrease in fibronectin mRNA abundance was noted at 11 days postconception and showed a steady decrease thereafter. The fibronectin gene is specifically expressed in the heart early in embryogenesis, without preferential selection at the level of EIIIA and EIIIB splicing and without detectable fibronectin protein in the extracellular matrix (30). This result suggests that fibronectin is probably not involved in the later stages of cardiac organogenesis or in the maintenance of the differentiated tissue (30). In contrast, some studies that focused on earlier time points showed that fibronectin protein was abundant at 5 days postpartum and was maintained until day 20 postpartum (31). A different *in vivo* study also has confirmed that fibronectin plays a certain role in cardiac development, wherein defects in mesoderm, the heart, and embryonic vessels were present in studies utilizing the fibronectin gene knock-out mouse model (32).

It has been reported that several receptors—including those for laminin, fibronectin, and hyaluronic acid—display specific expression patterns during cardiac development. For example, it is known that blockage of the fibronectin receptor results in aberrant heart formations. These observations support the hypothesis that morphogenesis requires specific cell adhesion molecules that are expressed in precisely choreographed programs (33). In addition to regulating the development of heart, fibronectin influences vascular development. Vasculogenesis begins early in development by the formation of the blood island in the yolk sac (34). These blood vessels grow toward various tissues in a directed way guided by factors including fibronectin.

LAMININ IN THE HEART DURING DEVELOPMENT

Laminin is composed of three subunits, a 400-kDa A-chain and two 200-kDa B-chains. The B1- and B2-chains are homologous to each other and to two-thirds of the N-terminal protein of A-chain (35). Laminin is a large glycoprotein and resides in the basement membrane of both cardiac myocytes and fibroblasts and is known to bind to collagen type IV as well as to struts composed of collagen types I and III (21). In adult hearts, laminin was found along the entire length of the basement membrane and was most abundant in areas of morphologic specialization, such as Z-bands, where collagen bundles are known to contact the sarcolemmal membrane (36). Laminin is the most extensively characterized member of a family of basement membrane glycoproteins. The functions of laminin include mediation of adhesion, migration, growth, and differentiation of cells.

During fetal development laminin is localized in sarcolemma; distribution of laminin in neonatal tissue is marked by increased absolute amount and is associated with the developing basement membrane (36). Analysis of the interaction between cardiac myocytes and the basement membrane proteins has led to the recognition and in vitro application of extracellular matrix components that are important for survival of cardiac myocytes in culture conditions (21–22). This experiment was performed by measuring cell attachment to various matrix substrate moieties. The results showed that neonatal myocytes attached well to all types of collagen, as well as to fibronectin and laminin, and that adult myocytes attached efficiently to laminin and collagen type IV. On the other hand, adult myocytes were seen to attach weakly to fibronectin within 1–4 hours from seeding the cells (21–22). It was also revealed that only collagen type IV and laminin could support adequate survival of attached myocytes when examined after 2 weeks in culture conditions (21–22). Recent studies have shown that different matrix molecules interact with each other and with their specific receptors on cell surfaces (37). Extracellular signals are transmitted across the cell membrane via the transmembrane receptors such as the integrin receptor that recognizes extracellular matrix molecules (38). Changes in these receptors, triggered by ligand binding, may cause rearrangement of the cytoskeletal network and the intracellular cascade of mechanotransduction leading to changes in gene expression and therefore the growth and differentiation state of the cells (38). Because the cardiac extracellular matrix is a complex and highly organized composite that is specifically anchored to cardiac myocytes, it can be seen that mechanical stimulation of cellular gene expression via the matrix may play a role in the regulation of matrix development and growth through these specific extracellular matrix receptors. The role laminin plays in histogenesis and organogenesis during *Drosophila* development and morphogenesis has been investigated (39). This study showed that in laminin A–deficient embryos, the heart is "broken" as a result of dissociation of the pericardial cells. This result indicates that laminin is required for the heart development in the *Drosophila* embryo.

INTEGRIN IN THE HEART DURING THE DEVELOPMENT

Integrins were named by R.O. Hynes in 1987 for the family of integral membrane receptors through to "integrate" the cytoskeleton of one cell with that of another cell or with extracellular matrix (40). Integrins are a family of proteins that are localized in the cell membrane of both cardiac myocytes and cardiac fibroblasts in the heart. All integrins are $\alpha\beta$ heterodimers, and it is known that various combinations of different isoforms of each subunit exist in different organ. The α subunits vary in size between 120 and 180 kDa and are each noncovalently associated with β subunits (90–110 kDa). Specific integrins such as $\alpha 1/\beta 1$, $\alpha 2/\beta 1$, $\alpha 3/\beta 1$ serve as a receptor in the cell membrane and have been demonstrated to bind to collagen, laminin, and fibronectin (37). The predominant isoform present in the adult moycardium is $\alpha 1$, $\alpha 3$, $\alpha 5$, and $\beta 1$ (41). The heterodimers of integrin form a transmembrane complex linking the extracellular matrix outside of the cell to the cytoskeleton on the cytosolic side of the membrane (42). The intracellular domain of the integrin proteins is believed to be linked to the contractile apparatus by several cytoskeletal proteins such as talin, vinculin, and α-actinin (43,44). Many integrins that bind to matrix molecules recognize the tripeptide sequence Arg-Gly-Asp (RGD). These RGD sequences are found within a number of matrix proteins, including fibronectin, laminin, vitronectin, and type I collagen (45).

The β-1 integrin is predominantly found in regions of remodeling (trabeculae) in the early heart (10–13 days of gestation). After 15 days of gestation, β-1 integrin is abundant in regions containing an elaborate extracellular matrix, such as the valves (46). These results support the hypothesis that the expression of integrins and extracellular matrix proteins are coordinately regulated in the developing heart. In the neonatal myocytes, β1 integrin was abundantly stained along the Z-bands. It has also been reported that integrin has an influence on myocyte behavior, and specifically on myofibrillogenesis and cytoarchitecture (41). This hypothesis also was supported by the observation that the addition of anti-β1 integrin antibodies to primary myocyte seeded to either fibronectin, laminin, or collagen-coated plates blocked the outward spread of cells on the substrates and altered normal myofibrillogenesis. The expression of α-integrin is known to vary with different stages of development. The presence/expression of the α1-chain was also associated with developmental stages when collagen synthesis was increased, especially during fetal and neonatal growth, as well as during the development of cardiac hypertrophy (41). The expression of the α1-chain was prominently associated with the recognition of interstitial collagens. This study indicates that integrins play a major role in the regulation of interaction between cardiac myocytes and the extracellular matrix during development and in disease processes. Immunohistochemical localization with an antibody against β1-integrin demonstrated that this protein is localized in Z lines of cardiac myocytes, and this finding led to the suggestion that the presence of β1-integrin is crucial in myofibrillogenesis during development (47).

OTHER EXTRACELLULAR MATRIX COMPONENTS

In addition to the extracellular matrix proteins mentioned earlier, many other kinds of cardiac matrix molecules were involved in the regulation of heart development. Fibulins-1 and -2 are two recently characterized extracellular matrix proteins. A striking co-distribution of fibulin-1 and -2 was seen at all stages in the development of the endocardial cushion tissue (ECT). Fibulin-2 was found to be a more specific marker for the embryonic ECT than fibulin-1, which was also transiently expressed in cardiac muscle (48). The neural cell adhesion molecule (NCAM) is present in several nonneuronal tissues, including heart. Cardiac myocytes expressed NCAM in newborn rat heart, whereas NCAM was absent from myocytes in young adult heart (49). NCAM is a transmembrane protein, and the extracellular portion of the molecule is known as the muscle-specific domain (MSD) (50). Immunohistochemical studies have shown that NCAM molecules containing the MSD region are colocalized with sarcomeric Z discs in day 18 of embryonic development, and it was suggested that this form of NCAM is involved in early myofibrillogenesis (50). Vascular cell adhesion molecule 1 (VCAM-1) is a cytokine-induced cell surface protein capable of mediating adhesion to leukocytes expressing α-4 integrin. A recent study showed that VCAM-1 deficient mouse embryos displayed several abnormalities in the ventricular myocardium and intraventricular septum (51). These hearts also contained significant amounts of blood in the pericardial space and lacked an epicardium. The results of this study led the investigators to suggest that VCAM-1 may play an important role in cardiac development.

SUMMARY

The cardiac extracellular matrix (ECM) contains collagen subtypes, glycoproteins, and proteoglycans. Some ECM components are expressed throughout heart development, but other ECM molecules exhibit a transit spatial and temporal distribution in the heart. Recent studies indicated that ECM plays an important role in signaling cell migration, sorting, proliferation, differentiation, morphology, and adhesion in the early stages during embyronic and late fetal as well as early neonatal stages in the development of the heart. This review summarizes the recent findings of the role of various ECM molecules during the development of heart.

ACKNOWLEDGMENTS

This work was supported by the Medical Research Council of Canada and the Manitoba Health Research Council. Dr. I. M. C. Dixon is a scholar of the Medical Research Council of Canada/PMAC program (with funding provided by Astra Pharma, Inc). Dr. H. Ju is a recipient of a Manitoba Health Research Council Studentship.

REFERENCES

1. Lin CQ, Bissell MJ. Multi-faceted regulation of cell differentiation by extracellular matrix. *FASEB J* 1993;7:737–743.
2. Zak R. Cell proliferation during cardiac growth. *Am J Cardiol* 1973;31:211–219.
3. Frank JS, Langer GA. The myocardial interstitium: its structure and its role in ionic exchange. *J Cell Biol* 1974;60:586–601.
4. Borg TK, Raso DS, Terracio L. Potential role of the extracellular matrix in postseptation development of the heart. *Ann NY Acad Sci* 1990;588:87–92.
5. Pelouch V, Dixon IMC, Golfman L, Beamish RE, Dhalla NS. Role of extracellular matrix proteins in heart function. *Mol Cell Biochem* 1993;129:101–120.
6. Weber KT, Sun Y, Tyagi SC, and Cleutjens JPM. Collagen network of the myocardium: function, structural remodeling and regulatory mechanisms. *J Mol Cell Cardiol* 1994;26:279–292.
7. Damsky CH, Werb Z. Signal transduction by integrin receptors for extracellular matrix: cooperative processing of extracellular information. *Curr Opin Cell Biol* 1992;4:772–781.
8. Duband J-L, Dufour S, Thiery JP. The instructive role of fibronectins in cell migration during embryonic development. *Ann NY Acad Sci* 1990;588:273–280.
9. Chapman D, Weber KT, Eghbali M. Regulation of fibrillar collagen type I and type III and basement membrane type IV: collagen gene expression in pressure overloaded rat myocardium. *Circ Res* 1990;67:787–794.
10. Bashey RI, Martinez-Hernandez A, Jimenez SA. Isolation, characterization, and localization of cardiac collagen type VI: association with other extracellular matrix components. *Circ Res* 1992;70: 1006–1017.
11. Speiser B, Riess CF, Schaper J. The extracellular matrix in human myocardium. Part 1: collagens I, III, IV, and VI. *Cardioscience* 1991;2:225–232.
12. Eghbali M, Czaja MJ, Zeydel M, Weiner FR, Zern MA, Seifter S, Blumenfeld OO. Collagen chain mRNAs in isolated heart cells from young and adult rats. *J Mol Cell Cardiol* 1988;20:267–276.
13. Eghbali M, Blumenfeld OO, Seifter S, Buttrick PM, Leinwand LA, Robinson TF, Zern MA, Giambrone MA. Localization of type I, III and IV collagen mRNAs in rat heart cells by in situ hybridization. *J Mol Cell Cardiol* 1989;21:103–113.

14. Ju H, Dixon IMC. Cardiac extracellular matrix and its role in the development of heart failure. In: Singal PK, Dixon IMC, Beamish RE, Dhalla NS, eds. *Mechanisms of heart failure.* Boston: Kluwer Academic Publishers; 1995:75–90.
15. Medugorac I. Myocardial collagen in different forms of heart hypertrophy in the rat. *Res Exp Med (Berl)* 1980;177:201–211.
16. Iruela-Arispe ML, Sage EH. Expression of type VIII collagen during morphogenesis of the chicken and mouse heart. *Dev Biol* 1991;144:107–118.
17. Carver W, Terracio L, Borg TK. Expression and accumulation of interstitial collagen in the neonatal rat heart. *Anat Rec* 1993;236:511–520.
18. Fisher SA, Periasamy M. Collagen synthesis inhibitors disrupt embryonic cardiocyte myofibrillogenesis and alter the expression of cardiac specific genes in vitro. *J Mol Cell Cardiol* 1994;26:721–731.
19. Borg TK, Rubin K, Lundgren E, Borg K, Öbrink B. Recognition of extracellular matrix components by neonatal and adult cardiac myocytes. *Dev Biol* 1984;104:86–96.
20. Borg TK, Johnson LD, Lill PH. Specific attachment of collagen to cardiac myocytes: in-vivo and in-vitro. *Dev Biol* 1983;97:417–423.
21. Lundgren E, Gullberg D, Rubin K, Borg TK, Terracio MJ, Terracio L. In vitro studies on adult cardiac myocytes: attachment and biosynthesis of collagen type IV and laminin. *J Cell Physiol* 1988;136:43–53.
22. Lundgren E, Terracio L, Mardh S, Borg TK. Extracellular matrix components influence the survival of adults cardiac myocytes in vitro. *Exp Cell Res* 1985;158:371–381.
23. Speiser B, Weihrauch D, Reiss CF, Schaper J. The extracellular matrix in human cardiac tissue. Part II: vimentin, laminin, and fibronectin. *Cardioscience* 1992;3:41–49.
24. Casscells W, Kimura H, Sanchez JA, Yu ZX, Ferrans VJ. Immunohistochemical study of fibronectin in experimental myocardial infarction. *Am J Pathol* 1990;137:801–810.
25. Farhadian F, Contard F, Corbier A, Barrieux A, Rappaport L, Samuel JL. Fibronectin expression during physiology and pathological cardiac growth. *J Mol Cell Cardiol* 1995;27:981–990.
26. Farhadian F, Barrieux A, Lortet S, Marotte F, Oliviero P, Rappaport L, Samuel JL. Differential splicing of fibronectin pre-messenger ribonucleic acid during cardiac ontogeny and development of hypertrophy in the rat. *Lab Invest* 1994;71:552–559.
27. Linask KK, Lash JW. Precardiac cell migration: fibronectin localization at mesoderm–endoderm interface during directional movement. *Dev Biol* 1986;114:87–101.
28. Linask KK, Lash JW. A role for fibronectin in the migration of avian precardiac cells. *Dev Biol* 1988;129:315–323.
29. Mjaatvedt CH, Lepera RC, Markwald RR. Myocardial specificity for initiating endothelial–mesenchymal cell transition in embryonic chick heart correlates with a particulate distribution of fibronectin. *Dev Biol* 1987;119:59–67.
30. Samuel JL, Farhadian F, Sabri A, Marotte F, Robert V, Rappaport L. Expression of fibronectin during rat fetal and postnatal development: an in situ hybridization and immunohistochemical study. *Cardiovasc Res* 1994;28:1653–1661.
31. Borg TK, Gay R, Johnson LD. Changes in the distribution of fibronectin and collagen during development of the neonatal rat heart. *Collagen Rel Res* 1982;2:211–218.
32. George EL, Georges-Labouesse EN, Patel-King RS, Rayburn H, Hynes RO. Defects in mesoderm, neural tube and vascular development in mouse embryos lacking fibronectin. *Development* 1993;119:1079–1091.
33. Buck CA, Baldwin HS, DeLisser H, Mickanin C, Shen HM, Kennedy G, Chen A, Edelman JM, Albelda SM. Cell adhesion receptors and early mammalian heart development: an overview. *Crit Rev Acad Sci III* 1993;316:838–859.
34. Risau W, Lemmon V. Changes in the vascular extracellular matrix during embryonic vasculogenesis and angiogenesis. *Dev Biol* 1988;125:441–450.
35. Kreis T, Vale R. *Guidebook to the extracellular matrix and adhesion proteins.* New York: Oxford University Press; 1993:66.
36. Price RL, Nakagawa M, Terracio L, Borg TK. Ultrastructural localization of laminin on in vivo embryonic, neonatal, and adult rat cardiac myocytes and in early rat embryos raised in whole-embryo culture. *J Histochem Cytochem* 1992;40:1373–1381.
37. Hynes RO. Integrins: versatility, modulation, and signaling in cell adhesion. *Cell* 1992;69:11–25.
38. Nowak R. Cell biologists get the message in New Orleans. *Science* 1994;263:30–31.
39. Yarnitzky T, Volk T. Laminin is required for heart, somatic muscles, and gut development in the Drosophila embryo. *Dev Biol* 1995;169:609–618.

40. Hynes RO. Integrins: a family of cell surface receptors. *Cell* 1987;48:549–554.
41. Terracio L, Rubin K, Gullberg D, Balog E, Carver W, Jyring R, Borg TK. Expression of collagen binding integrins during cardiac development and hypertrophy. *Circ Res* 1991;68:734–744.
42. Clark EA, Brugge JS. Integrins and signal transduction pathways: the road taken. *Science* 1995;268:233–239.
43. Eng C, Zhao M, Factor SM, Sonnenblick EH. Post-ischemic cardiac dilation and remodeling: reperfusion injury of the interstitium. *Eur Heart J* 1993;14(suppl A):27–32.
44. Wang N, Butler JP, Ingber DE. Mechanotransduction across the cell surface and through the cytoskeleton. *Science* 1993;260:1124–1127.
45. Ruoslahti E, Pierschbacher MD. New perspectives in cell adhesion: RGD and integrins. *Science* 1987;238:491–497.
46. Carver W, Price RL, Raso DS, Terracio L, Borg TK. Distribution of β-1 integrin in the development rat heart. *J Histochem Cytochem* 1994;42:167–175.
47. Hilenski LL, Ma XH, Vinson N, Terracio L, Borg TK. The role of beta 1 integrin in spreading and myofibrillogenesis in neonatal rat cardiomyocytes in vitro. *Cell Motil Cytoskeleton* 1992;21:87–100.
48. Zhang HY, Chu ML, Pan TC, Sasaki T, Timpl R, Ekblom P. Extracellular matrix protein fibulin-2 is expressed in the embryonic endocardial cushion tissue and is a prominent component of valves in adult heart. *Dev Biol* 1995;167:18–26.
49. Linnemann D. Reexpression of the neural cell adhesion molecule (NCAM) on cardiac myocytes in aging rat heart. *Acta Histochem* 1994;96:349–354.
50. Byeon MK, Sugi Y, Markwald RR, Hoffman S. NCAM polypeptides in heart development: association with Z discs of forms that containing the muscle-specific domain. *J Cell Biol* 1995;128:209–210.
51. Kwee L, Baldwin HS, Shen HM, Stewart CL, Buck C, Buck CA, Labow MA. Defective development of the embryonic and extraembryonic circulatory systems in vascular cell adhesion molecule (VCAM-1) deficient mice. *Development* 1995;121:489–503.

The Developing Heart,
edited by Bohuslav Ošťádal et al.
Lippincott-Raven Publishers,
Philadelphia © 1997.

9

Regulation of Coronary Vessel Formation in Embryonic and Fetal Hearts

Robert J. Tomanek and Anna Ratajska

Department of Anatomy and The Cardiovascular Center, University of Iowa, Iowa City, IA 52242

During early development the heart chambers are sufficiently thin; therefore, a coronary circulation is unnecessary. The inner portion of the ventricles is spongy because of the extensive trabeculation of the myocardium. In mammals, unlike some lower animals, this spongy myocardium is replaced with a compact layer (for review see refs. 1–3). As this compact region expands via myocyte proliferation, precursor cells from the epicardium differentiate into endothelial cells and migrate and form vascular tubes, a process called vasculogenesis. Formation of these microvascular tubes is the first stage in the formation of the coronary vascular system. Subsequently, these vascular channels expand by migration and proliferation of their endothelial cells, a process known as angiogenesis. Figure 9–1 summarizes these processes. From this microvascular network spring the veins and arteries.

Although a number of studies have described the formation of various components of the coronary circulation (see refs. 4 and 5 for review), this important phenomenon has not been well understood. For example, proof that the left and right coronary arteries arise by ingrowth into the aorta rather than by an outgrowth from the aorta has only been provided during the last decade (6–8). Moreover, the putative factors that regulate coronary vasculogenesis and angiogenesis are only now being investigated.

This communication highlights some of the more recent work regarding the formation of the coronary vasculature and the factors that regulate this process. Our focus is on recent studies that have addressed the influence of the extracellular matrix, hormones, nerves, and growth factors.

ORIGIN AND MIGRATION OF PRECURSOR ENDOTHELIAL CELLS

Proepicardial tissue, which consists of glandular-like structures, lies between the sinus horns and the liver primordium and provides the angioblasts, fibro-

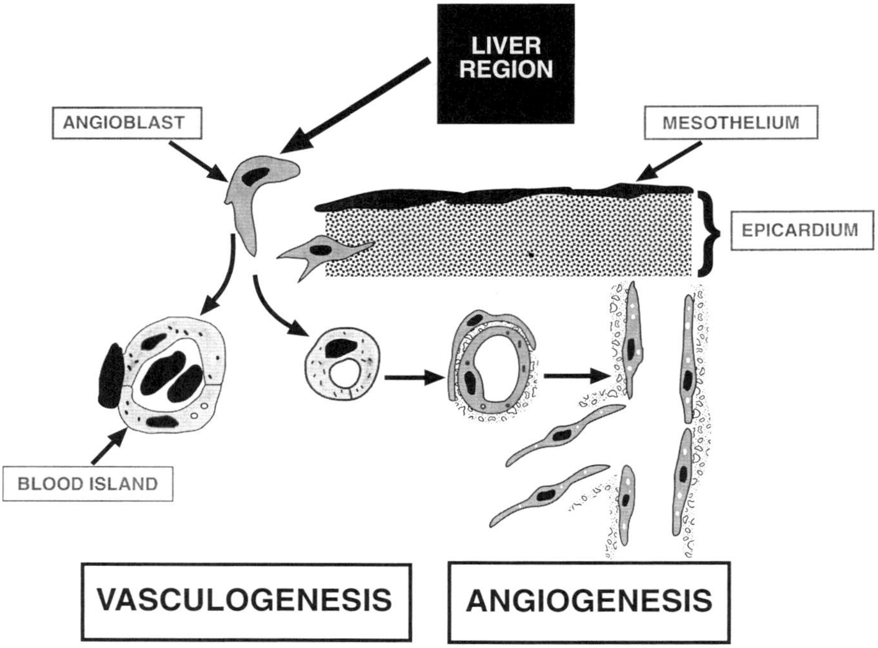

FIG. 9–1. Coronary vascular channels are formed from angioblasts which migrate to the epicardium. Vasculogenesis occurs as these cells (a) associate in clusters with red blood cells to form blood island-like structures or (b) simply form small tubes. The vascular tubes (capillaries) mature as they secrete a basement membrane and are joined by pericytes on their albuminal surface. These vessels then continue to grow by sprouting (angiogenesis). (This figure reprinted from ref. 49, with permission.)

blasts, and blood cells that form the epicardium (9). Scanning microscopy of chick embryonic hearts reveals that the appearance of pericardial villi, which bridge the pericardial cavity, coincides with the time the epicardium forms (10). Mikawa and Fischman (7) used a retrovirus to demonstrate that endothelial precursor cells migrate to the heart, with mesothelial cells forming the epicardium. They also noted that none of the endothelial cells forming the endocardium were labeled, thus suggesting that this cell layer is of independent origin. The origin of angioblasts that form coronary vessels was demonstrated a year later when Poelmann and colleagues (11) identified endothelial cells and their precursors with anti-MB1 antibody in quail-chicken chimeras. Endothelial cells were not found in the heart when pure epicardial primordia were transplanted from quail to chick embryos. In contrast, endothelial cells populated the heart when a liver graft, either alone or in combination with epicardial primordium, was performed, indicating that the endothelial cell precursors arise from the liver region.

THE VASCULARIZATION PROCESS

The first signs of coronary vessel formation are the presence of endothelial tubes or blood islandlike structures in the subepicardium (12–14). The latter consist of endothelial precursor cells in conjunction with erythroblasts and erythrocytes. As vascularization procedes, a subepicardial plexus covers the surface of the heart; subsequently, capillaries can be seen within the myocardium. Over time capillaries mature as evidenced by thinning of the endothelial cytoplasm, the development of specialized junctions, and an increase in plasmalemmal vesicles (14,15).

Although veins have been historically described as arising from the sinus venosus, Poelmann and colleagues (11) used quail-chicken chimeras to demonstrate that endothelial precursor cells appeared in the myocardium before their incorporation into the sinus venosus. Thus, venules and veins have their origins from precursor cells in the myocardium and are not direct outgrowths of the sinus venosus. The continuity of the venous system with the sinus venosus occurs prior to perfusion of the myocardium from the aorta via the coronary arteries. Several studies have shown that a capillary plexus encircles the aorta at its root and that, subsequently, components of this plexus coalesce and penetrate the aorta to form the two major coronary arteries. This phenomenon was first shown by Bogers and colleagues (6), who used the monoclonal anti-endothelium antibody in quail. They were unable to trace the migration of endothelial precursors toward the aorta from the epicardium. This conclusion was confirmed by Waldo et al. (8), who injected ink intravascularly and demonstrated ingrowth of the capillaries into the aorta, and by Mikawa and Fischman (7), who injected a retrovirus into chick embryos and observed discontinuous colonies of microvessels that subsequently formed arteries.

Up to the time just described, the coronary vascular system consists of endothelial tubes and pericytes. The tunica media first occurs as the vascular plexus coalesces and penetrates the aorta; its development proceeds from the ventricle's base to its apex (16,17). As noted in our studies on rat heart development (17), coronary arteries persist as an anastomotic network, even at the time of birth. Therefore, postnatal vascular remodeling must occur to establish the treelike branching system characteristic of the adult coronary arterial tree.

Thus, the vascularization process proceeds in a predictable sequence. First, simple endothelial tubes are formed and grow toward each other. Second, the tubes branch and anastomase. Third, venous vessels are formed and attach to the sinus venosus. Finally, a capillary plexus at the root of the aorta coalesces, penetrates the aortic wall, and then develops a medium as smooth muscle cells become attached to the endothelial tube. The remainder of this chapter considers the factors that may regulate these events.

EXTRACELLULAR MATRIX

Extracellular matrix (ECM) molecules are recognized for their role in providing a substratum for migration and orientation of vascular endothelial cells, regulating their proliferation and enabling their differentiated state (18–22). For example, fibronectin has been shown to provide a migratory pathway for endothelial cells, while laminin coincides with tube formation and is linked with the vessel maturation (21). Based on the rationale that ECM molecules have been implicated in the vascularization process, we employed immunohistochemical techniques to determine the temporal and spatial relationship of selected ECM molecules and coronary vessel formation during development in the rat (18). Microvessels were visualized by labeling with the lectin Griffonia Simplicifolia I or by immunolabeling endothelial cells with platelet endothelial cell adhesion molecule. The same sections were double-labeled for fibronectin, laminin, or collagen I, III, or IV. Our findings indicate that fibrinoectin precedes coronary vasculogenesis and that laminin deposition coincides with tube formation. The appearance of collagen IV closely follows that of laminin. Collagens I and III were not related to tube formation, nor were they found in association with capillaries. Staining for these collagens was limited to the adventitia of vessels larger than capillaries and in septa and the epicardium. These findings suggest that in the developing heart (a) the major scaffolding for migration of endothelial cells and their precursors is provided by fibronectin, (b) laminin and collagen IV correlate with tube formation, and collagens I and III are unrelated to cell migration and tube formation. The temporal relationship of these ECM molecules is consistent with that found in vessels developing in the chick chorioallantoic membrane (23), and the distribution of specific molecules in the adult rat is consistent with earlier findings (24).

GROWTH FACTORS

Most of our knowledge regarding the role of growth factors in vascular growth is based on in vitro approaches (endothelial cell cultures) and studies on vascularization of tumors. The two growth factors that have received the most attention relative to their effects on the coronary vasculature are basic fibroblast growth factor (bFGF) and vascular endothelial growth factor (VEGF). Both bFGF (25) and VEGF (26) were shown to increase myocardial collateral flow by enhancing development of collaterals in dogs with experimentally included ischemia. Moreover, VEGF expression is induced by myocardial ischemia (27). During development, both acidic (28–30) and basic (17,31–33) FGF are widespread in the rat heart. Moreover, bovine bFGF levels have been shown to be much higher during the prenatal and neonatal periods than in the adult (34). VEGF is considered to be of special significance in vascular development because its receptors are found only on endothelial cells. Binding of VEGF to receptors on blood vessels during rat embryonic development has been documented (35). Moreover, flk-1 receptor tyrosine kinase mRNA expression, demonstrated by in situ hybridization, has been found to be up-regulated in sprouting vessels in mouse embryos (36). VEGF has a high affinity for this receptor and was found to correlate with the spatial and temporal pattern of flk-1.

To determine the role of VEGF and bFGF in vascularization of the developing heart, we have used both in vivo and in vitro models. To test the hypothesis that these growth factors stimulate (a) cell migration and (b) assembly into cordlike structures in embryonic rat heart, we cultured explanted atria and ventricles on collagen gels for 5 days (37). Western blot analysis demonstrated that endogenous VEGF was present in the tissues during incubation. When bFGF was added to avascular 12-day explants, cell migration distance increased significantly. In contrast, addition of VEGF had no effect. Neither growth factor stimulated tube or cord formation of migrating cells in the 12-day explants. However, addition of VEGF, but not bFGF, to 14-day explants, in which vasculogenesis is under way, caused the formation of cordlike branching structures. Many of the structures were tubes as documented by serial sectioning and electron microscopy. These experiments indicate that in this model system, VEGF and bFGF play distinct roles, at specific time points, in coronary vascular tube formation in the developing heart.

Our *in vivo* experiments in rats also implicate VEGF and bFGF in coronary development. Immunohistochemical data have documented a virtual homogeneity of staining for bFGF of cardiocytes and an intense staining of the media of arterioles (17). Using *in situ* hybridization we found that bFGF mRNA expression was homogeneous throughout the myocardium during development (17). We then used a quantitative approach (grain counting) to assess changes in mRNA and found the highest expression during the early period of vascularization (embryonic days 14 and 15) and the early neonatal period (1–6 days after birth), which corresponds to a period of substantial microvascular growth.

Using immunostaining, we have shown that VEGF shows a temporal–spatial relationship in the developing rat heart (38). In embryonic day 13 (E13) hearts immunoreactivity is virtually limited to the epicardial region, while in E16 hearts it occurs throughout the myocardium. This pattern corresponds to the gradient of vascularization (i.e., the onset is epicardial and subsequently includes deeper layers of the myocardium). In postnatal rats the staining is limited to microvessels or their extracellular regions, a finding consistent with growth by angiogenesis, which is probably the major type of vascular growth occurring postnatally. Accordingly, these findings demonstrate that VEGF is appropriately positioned to stimulate the formation of microvessels during development. This finding precipitates the question: What is the stimulus for VEGF expression? Considering that hypoxia up-regulates VEGF mRNA (39), we proposed the hypothesis that cardiocytes along the epicardial surface are faced with decreasing levels of O_2 as the ventricular wall thickens and the distance between these cells and the sinusoids increases (4). This hypothesis fits with the observation that VEGF first appears along the epicardium and then spreads throughout the myocardium.

A role for FGF in coronary vessel formation has been suggested by Mikawa (40), who introduced a retrovirus endocrine FGF and a reporter gene into the intracellular space of chick epicardial primordium at in ovo day 3. This precocious expression of endogenous precursor cells resulted in abnormal branching patterns of the coronary vasculature. Thus, there is some direct evidence that FGF can have an influence on coronary vessel development. However, the precise role that this growth factor plays in coronary vasculogenesis and angiogenesis is not clear. Part of the difficulty in evaluating FGF in vivo is that it affects several cell types and plays a key role in myocyte hyperplasia (41). Therefore, the influence of this growth factor could be secondary to its effects on other cells (e.g., cardiocytes). Nevertheless, *in vitro* studies have clearly shown both aFGF and bFGF to be endothelial cell mitogens (42). Moreover, the chick chorioallantoic membrane assays verify this effect in vivo (42). Accordingly, it is likely that FGF influences coronary vascular growth. The key questions yet to be answered relate to its specific effects, its window of influence along the temporal scale, and the stimulus for its synthesis.

VEGF is less problematic because its receptors are limited to endothelial cells. The developmental expression of its binding sites in rat embryos suggests a role for this growth factor in vasculogenesis and angiogenesis (35). Transcripts for its flk-1 receptor were found to be abundant in proliferating endothelial cells of mouse embryos (36). Moreover, the importance of VEGF in embryonic development is indicated by recent experiments on mice deficient in the flk-1 receptor (43). In these mice yolk sac blood islands and vessels fail to develop.

A number of other angiogenic peptides have been characterized (see ref. 42 for review). Growth factors that are expressed during development include platelet-derived endothelial growth factor, platelet-derived growth factor, and transforming growth factor–beta. The first two are both angiogenic and chemoatactic; the latter is important in regulating extracellular matrix formation and proteolysis (44). Although a role for these polypeptides in vasculogenesis/angiogenesis of the developing heart is not evident at this time, their influence cannot be ruled out. It is plausible that these growth factors act synergistically or activate heparin-binding growth factors.

NEURAL AND HUMORAL INFLUENCES

Many extrinsic factors—humoral, neural, and mechanical—could influence vasculogenesis and angiogenesis in the heart. To test hypotheses regarding the first two, we grafted E12 embyronic rat hearts into the anterior eye chamber of adult rat hosts. We had previously demonstrated that E12 hearts are vascular and that the coronary vasculature that develops in this in oculo system originates from the graft and not from the host (14). Because fetal cardiocytes have receptors and are responsive to thyroid hormone modulation, and because thyroid hormone–induced hypertrophy in young and adult rats is associated with marked coronary angiogenesis, we tested the hypothesis that this hormone plays a role in early vascularization of embryonic and fetal hearts (45). Host rats were treated with T_4, propylthiouracil (PTU), or saline for 21 days, after which time the heart implants growing in oculo were analyzed with transmission electron microscopy and the volume densities of vessels, cardiocytes, and the extracellular matrix were quantified by stereology. Neither an excess of T_4 nor its virtual elimination by PTU treatment affected the volume density of vessels or any other tissue component. Thus, we concluded that thyroxine is not an essential regulator of vascular growth in the embryonic/fetal heart. Because these hearts are not loaded, although they continue to beat, we conclude that the angiogenic effect of thyroxine in postnatal hearts (46) is secondary to increased work-related events.

The in oculo model was also utilized to test the hypothesis that coronary vasculogenesis/angiogenesis is independent of sympathetic nerves (47). We grafted E12 rat hearts into the anterior eye chamber of host rats that had undergone unilateral superior cervical gangliectomies (innervation to the contralateral eye chamber remained intact and served as a control). We harvested the grafts 14 or 35 days later and determined volume densities of vessels and other tissue components, as described earlier. In another set of rats, graft perfusion and metabolism were assessed with thallium 201 and 2-[^{14}C]deoxy-D-glucose uptake, respectively. None of the parameters investigated were altered by sympathectomy, indicating that sympathetic innervation during this time period does not affect the growth of the microvasculature, or myocardial perfusion or metabolism of the embryonic/fetal heart, at least in the unloaded state.

PHYSICAL FORCES

There is evidence that physical forces (i.e., increased blood flow and the associated shear stress, wall tension, and stretch) can stimulate vascular growth (for review see ref. 48). For example, Ingber and Folkman (49) showed that expansion of the substratum can increase endothelial cell proliferation, and Bishop et al. (50) noted that cyclic stretch of fibroblasts caused a release of growth factors. Because the embryonic heart grows rapidly and pump function increases to meet the demands of the growing organism, coronary vascularization occurs during a period of changing cardiac dynamics. As we have observed with the electron microscope (unpublished data), and as noted by others (8,12), coronary vasculogenesis begins at approximately Hamburger-Hamilton heart stage 23 in the chick heart. This stage is included in a time period (stages 21–29) during which ventricular work and mass increase dramatically (51). To test the hypothesis that the formation of microvessels in the myocardium adapts to the increased ventricular mass due to increased ventricular pressure, we constricted the outflow track of chick hearts at stage 21 and studied the hearts at stages 29 and 33 (52). Despite the fact that heart mass was 73% greater in the banded chicks than in the shams already at stage 29, vascular volume percent (mean $\pm$ S.E.) was virtually identical in the two groups (sham = 12.33 $\pm$ 1.20; constricted = 12.67 $\pm$ 1.20). Moreover, the values were similar at stage 33. These data indicate that during embryonic development the increased ventricular mass in response to chronically elevated ventricular pressure is fully compensated by an acceleration of growth of the microvasculature.

Because coronary flow from the aorta does not occur until HH stages 32–34 in the chicken and embryonic days 16–17 in the rat, the initial microvascular bed forms in the absence of intraluminal hemodynamic forces. Thus, during this period extravascular forces are the primary mechanical influences on the vasculature. Once flow is established, hemodynamic forces may influence vascular growth. This transition has not been studied, but it may constitute an important period for the determination of the anatomic and geometric properties of the arterial and possibly the venous systems.

SUMMARY AND CONCLUSIONS

Vasculogenesis and angiogenesis in the embryonic and fetal heart occur in an environment of rapid growth characterized by proliferation of myocytes, changes in ventricular geometry and physical forces, and influence of a variety of molecules (e.g., growth factors and extracellular matrix components). Early capillary formation occurs via vasculogenesis and subsequently involves angiogenesis. The formation of capillary plexuses contributes to the establishment of larger vessels. In the latter the tunica media is formed as myocytes differentiate in a base to apex progression.

VEGF and bFGF are two growth factors implicated in coronary vascularization. However, the precise roles of these polypeptides have yet to be determined. A central question regarding the role of angiogenic growth factors concerns stimuli that up-regulate their mRNA and/or increase their receptors. The proliferation and maturation of cardiocytes could in and of themselves provide signals for these events. In view of the evidence that VEGF mRNA is up-regulated by hypoxia, we suggest this as a plausible stimulus in the expanding ventricular wall. Similarly, mechanical factors such as stretch may provide a stimulus for the expression of growth factors.

Various signaling mechanisms are likely to play a role in coronary vascular growth. Many questions regarding this developmental process remain unanswered. For example, what regulates the differential development of veins and arteries from simple endothelial channels, and what signal directs these channels to attach so precisely to the coronary sinus and aorta? Future studies need to utilize novel approaches to answer these and other related questions.

REFERENCES

1. Agnisola C, Tota B. Structure and function of the fish cardiac ventricle: flexibility and limitations. *Cardioscience* 1994;5:145–153.
2. Ostádal B, Rychter Z, Poupa O. Comparative aspects of the development of the terminal vascular bed in the myocardium. *Physiol Bohemslov* 1970;19:1–7.
3. Tota B, Cimini V, Salvatore G, Zummo G. Comparative study of the arterial and lacunary systems of the ventricular myocardium of elasmobranch and teleost fishes. *Am J Anat* 1983;167:15–32.
4. Tomanek RJ, Ratajska A. Vasculogenesis and angiogenesis in the developing heart. In: Burggren W, Keller B, eds. *Development of cardiovascular systems: molecules to organisms.* New York: Cambridge University Press (in press).
5. Tomanek RJ. Formation of the coronary vasculature: a brief review. *Cardiovasc Res* 1996;31: E46–E51.

6. Bogers AJJC, Gittenberger-de-Groot AC, Poelmann RE, Péault BM, Huysmans HA. Development of the origins of the coronary arteries, a matter of ingrowth or outgrowth? *Anat Embryol* 1989; 180:437–441.
7. Mikawa T, Fischman D. Retroviral analysis of cardiac morphogenesis: discontinuous formation of coronary vessels. *Proc Natl Acad Sci USA* 1992;89:9504–9508.
8. Waldo KL, Wilner W, Kirby ML. Origin of the proximal coronary artery sterns and a review of ventral vascularization in the chick embryo. *Am J Anat* 1990;188:109–120.
9. Virágh S, Gittenberger-deGroot AC, Poelmann RE, Kalman F. Early development of quail heart epicardium and associated vascular and glandular structures. *Anat Embryol* 1993;188:381–393.
10. Manner J. The development of pericardial villi in the chick embryo. *Anat Embryol* 1992;186:379–385.
11. Poelmann RE, Gittenberger-deGroot AC, Metink MMT, Bökenkamp R, Hogers B. Development of the cardiac vascular endothelium, studied with anti-endothelial antibodies in chicken-quail chimeras. *Circ Res* 1993;73:559–568.
12. Hiruma T, Hirakow R. Epicardial formation in embryonic chick heart: computer-aided reconstruction, scanning, and transmission electron microscopic studies. *Am J Anat* 1989;184:129–138.
13. Hutchins GM, Kessler-Hanna A, Moore GW. Development of the coronary arteries in the embryonic human heart. *Circulation* 1988;77:1250–1257.
14. Rongish BJ, Torry RJ, Tucker DC, Tomanek RJ. Neovascularization of embryonic rat hearts cultured in oculo closely mimics in utero coronary vessel development. *J Vasc Res* 1994;31:205–215.
15. Porter GA, Bankston PW. Maturation of myocardial capillaries in the fetal and neonatal rat: an ultrastructural study with a morphometric analysis of the vesicle populations. *Am J Anat* 1987;178: 116–125.
16. Hood LC, Rosenquist TH. Coronary artery development in the chick: origin and development of smooth muscle cells, and the effect of neural crest ablation. *Anat Rec* 1992;234:291–300.
17. Tomanek RJ, Haung L, Suvarna P, O'Brien LC, Ratajska A, Sandra A. Coronary vascularization during development in the rat and its relationship to basic fibroblast growth factor. *Cardiovasc Res* 1996;31:E116–E126.
18. Rongish BJ, Hinchman G, Doty MK, Baldwin HS, Tomanek RJ. Relationship of the extracellular matrix to coronary neovascularization during development. *J. Molec Cell Cardiol* 1996;28:2203–2215.
19. Carey DJ. Control of growth and differentiation of vascular cells by extracellular matrix proteins. *Annu Rev Physiol* 1991;53:161–177.
20. Grant DS, Kleinman HK, Martin GR. The role of basement membranes in vascular development. *Ann NY Acad Sci* 1990;588:61–72.
21. Ingber DE, Folkman J. How does extracellular matrix control capillary morphogenesis? *Cell* 1989;58:803–805.
22. Risau W, Lemmon V. Changes in the vascular extracellular matrix during embryonic vasculogenesis and angiogenesis. *Dev Biol* 1988;125:441–450.
23. Ausprunk DA, Dethlefsen SM, Higgens ER. Distribution of fibronectin, laminin, and type IV collagen during development of blood vessels in the chick choriollantoic membrane. In: Feinberg RN, Sherer GK, Auerbach R, eds. *The development of the vascular system.* Basel: Karger; 1991:93–108.
24. Bashey RI, Martinez-Hernandez A, Jemenez SA. Isolation, characterization, and localization of cardiac collagen type VI: associations with other extracellular matrix components. *Circ Res* 1992; 70:1006–1017.
25. Unger EF, Banai S, Shou M, Lazarous DF, Jaklitsch MT, Scheinowitz M, Correa R, Klingbeil C, Epstein SE. Basic fibroblast growth factor enhances myocardial collateral flow in a canine model. *Am J Physiol* 1994;266:H1588–H1595.
26. Banai S, Jaklitsch MT, Shou M, Lazarous DF, Scheinowitz M, Biro S, Epstein SE, Unger EF. Angiogenic-induced enhancement of collateral blood flow to ischemic myocardium by vascular endothelial growth factor in dogs. *Circulation* 1994;89:2183–2189.
27. Hashimoto E, Ogita T, Nakaoka T, Matsuoka R, Takao A, Kira Y. Rapid induction of vascular endothelial growth factor expression by transient ischemia in rat heart. *Am J Physiol* 1994;267:H1948–H1954.
28. Engelmann GL, Dionne CA, Jaye MC. Acidic fibroblast growth factor and heart development: role in myocyte proliferation and capillary angiogenesis. *Circ Res* 1993;72:7–19.
29. Fu YM, Spirito P, Yu Z-X, Biro S, Sasse J, Lei J, Ferrans V, Epstein SE, Casscells W. Acidic fibroblast growth factor in the developing rat embryo. *J Cell Biol* 1991;114:1261–1273.
30. Spirito P, Fu Y-M, Zu Z-X, Epstein SE, Casscells W. Immunohistochemical localization of basic and acidic fibroblast growth factors in the developing rat heart. *Circulation* 1991;84:322–332.

31. Consigli SA, Joseph-Silverstein J. Immunolocalization of basic fibroblast growth factor during chicken cardiac development. *J Cell Physiol* 1991;146:379–385.
32. Joseph-Silverstein J, Consigli SA, Lyser KM, Ver Pault C. Basic fibroblast growth factor in the chick embryo: immunolocalization to striated muscle cells and their precursors. *J Cell Biol* 1989; 108:2459–2466.
33. Parlow MH, Bolender DL, Kokan-Moore NP, Lough J. Localization of bFGF-like proteins as punctate inclusions in the preseptation myocardium of the chick embryo. *Dev Biol* 1991;146:139–147.
34. Cummins P, Logan A, Cummins B. Basic fibroblast growth factor in the developing bovine heart. *Biochem Soc Trans* 1991;19:79S.
35. Jakeman LB, Armanini M, Phillips HS, Ferrara N. Developmental expression of binding sites and messenger ribonucleic acid for vascular endothelial growth factor suggests a role for this protein in vasculogenesis and angiogenesis. *Endocrinology* 1993;133:848–859.
36. Millauer B, Wizigmann-Voos S, Schnurch H, Martinez R, Moller NPH, Risau W, Ulrich A. High affinity VEGF binding and developmental expression suggest Flk-1 as a major regulator of vasculogenesis and angiogenesis. *Cell* 1993;72:835–846.
37. Ratajska A, Torrey RJ, Kitten GT, Kolker SJ, Tomanek RJ. Modulation of cell migration and vessel formation by vascular endothelial growth factor and basic fibroblast growth factor in cultured embyronic heart. *Dev Dyn* 1995;203:399–407.
38. Ratajska A, Kitten GT, Tomanek RJ. Vascular endothelial growth factor during coronary vessel development in rats. *Circulation* 1994;90:1–470.
39. Schweiki D, Itin A, Soffer D, Keshet E. Vascular endothelial growth factor induced by hypoxia may mediate hypoxia-initiated angiogenesis. *Nature* 1992;359:843–845.
40. Mikawa T. Retroviral targeting of FGF and FGFR in cardiomyocytes and coronary vascular cells during heart development. *Ann NY Acad Sci USA* 1995;752:506–515.
41. Mima T, Ueno H, Fischman DA, Williams LT, Mikawa T. Fibroblast growth factor receptor is required for in vivo cardiac myocyte proliferation at early embryonic stages of heart development. *Proc Natl Acad Sci USA* 1995;92:467–471.
42. Folkman J, Shing Y. Angiogenesis. *J Biol Chem* 1992;267:10931–10934.
43. Shalaby F, Rossant J, Yamaguchi TP, Gertsenstein M, Wu XF, Breitman ML, Shulz AC. Failure of blood-island formation and vasculogenesis in Flk-1 deficient mice. *Nature* 1995;376:62–66.
44. Schott RJ, Morrow LA. The role of growth factors in angiogenesis. In: Cummins P, ed. *Growth factors and the cardiovascular system.* Boston: Kluwer Academic Publishers; 1993:148–168.
45. Rongish BJ, Torry RJ, Tomanek RJ. Coronary neovascularization of embyronic rat hearts cultured in oculo is independent of thyroid hormones. *Am J Physiol* 1995;268:H811–H816.
46. Chilian WM, Wangler RD, Peters KG, Tomanek RJ, Marcus ML. Thyroxine-induced left ventricular hypertrophy in the rat: anatomical and physiological evidence for angiogenesis. *Circ Res* 1985; 57:591–598.
47. Torry RJ, Rongish BJ, Tucker DC, Kostreva DR, Tomanek RJ. Influence of graft innervation on neovascularization of embryonic heart tissue grafted in oculo. *Am J Physiol* 1996;270:H33–H37.
48. Hudlicka O, Brown M. Physical forces and angiogenesis. In: Rubanyi GM, ed. *Mechanoreception by the vascular wall.* Mount Kisco, NY: Futura; 1993:197–241.
49. Ingber DE, Folkman J. Regulation of endothelial growth factor action: solid state control of extracellular matrix. *Prog Clin Biol Res* 1987;249:273–282.
50. Bishop JE, Absher M, Mitchell J, Woodstock MJ, Baldor L, Low RB. Release of growth factors by cyclically stretched fibroblasts. *J Cell Biol* 1989;109:2429.
51. Hu H, Clark EB. Hemodynamics of the stage 12 to stage 29 chick embryo. *Circ Res* 1989;65: 1665–1670.
52. Tomanek RJ, Phan BP, Hu N, Clark EB. Myocardial vascularization is accelerated in chick embryos with increased afterload and ventricular mass. *FASEB J* 1996;10:A579.

The Developing Heart,
edited by Bohuslav Ošt'ádal et al.
Lippincott-Raven Publishers,
Philadelphia © 1997.

10

Distribution of Tyrosine Hydroxylase in Relation to Calcitonin Gene–Related Peptide-Containing Neurons in the Developing Rat Right Atrium

*J. Slavíková and **A. Dahlström

**Department of Physiology, Medical Faculty, Charles University, Plzeň, Czech Republic **Institute of Neurobiology, University of Göteborg, Göteborg, Sweden.*

The autonomic innervation in the rat heart is immature at birth and becomes functional during the first 3 weeks of life (for reviews see refs. 1–4). The previous studies of autonomic innervation in developing heart focused on the development of its adrenergic (cardioexcitatory) and cholinergic (cardioinhibitory) components (5–14), releasing neurotransmitters noradrenaline (NA) and acetylcholine (ACh) acting in a reciprocal manner (5–18). The results of more recent studies have demonstrated the presence of purine-, biogenic amine-, and neuropeptide-containing nerve cell bodies, fibers, and terminals within the heart of several species (for review see ref. 19). The neuropeptide-containing nerves, whose origin is extrinsic, are thought to be either postganglionic sympathetic motor fibers co-storing NA and neuropeptide Y (NPY) (20,21), or primary sensory afferent neurons, co-storing calcitonin gene-related peptide (CGRP), substance P (SP), and related neurokinins (for reviews see refs. 22, 23). Postganglionic parasympathetic motor neurons, whose origin is intrinsic, contain VIP and somatostatin in addition to ACh (24). Furthermore, evidence has accumulated that the cardiac tissue in many species may contain intrinsic intraganglionic neurons and/or small intensely fluorescent (SIF) cells (25–30).

Morphologic studies of the development of the innervation of the heart have been limited to sections of myocardial tissue. The anatomic distribution of the autonomic innervation in the heart as a whole has not yet been investigated, because of technical limitation. However, confocal laser scanning microscopy (CFLM) suitable for the use of whole-mount preparations has recently been introduced, and it was used in this study. A modification of the whole-mount preparation procedure described by Costa et al. (31) was adopted and the presence, distribution, and density of nerve fibers with tyrosine hydroxylase (TH)- and CGRP-like immunoreactivities (LI) were studied.

TH is the rate-limiting enzyme in the biosynthesis of the neurotransmitters dopamine (DA) and noradrenaline (NA) in catecholaminergic neurons and adrenal medullary cells (32). Thus, the rabbit–anti-TH antiserum used specifically localizes catecholaminergic neural tissue (29,33,34).

CGRP is a 37-amino-acid peptide produced by alternative processing of the calcitonin gene (35–38) that is supposed to function as a neurotransmitter of nonadrenergic noncholinergic (NANC) primary sensory neurons in the heart of several mammals (23,39–54). The distribution of the synaptic vesicle antigens SV2 and synaptophysin (p38) was also studied and compared to the TH- and CGRP-LI in double incubation studies. Immunofluorescence was recorded using CFLM, which enabled us to observe the complete pattern of innervation within the right atria of all examined ages, since we could scan the thick whole-mount of the tissue with high resolution at all planes of focus. Although morphologic developmental studies of sympathetic innervation in the rat heart sections have been reported (55–58), in all previous reports the morphologic and functional studies concerning CGRP have been limited to the heart from adult animal. The complete developmental pattern has not been established yet. Moreover, the definite function has not been fully clarified. Since CGRP likely affects other autonomic neural tissue (53), the developmental pattern changes might modulate the functional onset of nervous control of the heart. On the other hand, the developmental imbalance in cardiac nervous system might play a role in the pathologic status.

MATERIALS AND METHODS

Sprague-Dawley rats of both sexes were used. At the ages of 1, 10–11, 18–20, and 40 days the animals were anesthetized with ether and decapitated. The heart was isolated, quickly cleaned in saline, and dissected as previously described (29). The preparations were mounted posterior side up and pinned flat. The procedure for fixation and immunoincubation of whole-mount stretch preparations as described by Costa et al. (31) was used: the atria were fixed in a mixture of picric acid (15%) and paraformaldehyde (4%) in 0.1 M phosphate buffer, pH 7.3 at 4°C for 2 hours (for TH) or 18 hours (for CGRP), respectively. After fixation the tissues were washed in 80% ethanol and left in phosphate buffered saline, pH 7.4 (PBS), (20 mM phosphate buffer and 0.15 M NaCl) overnight. On the following day the specimens were dehydrated in ethanol (80%, 95%, 100%), for 30 min each, cleared in xylene, and rehydrated in a descending series of ethanol and stored in PBS at 4°C until incubated.

IMMUNOHISTOCHEMICAL PROCEDURE

After 30 min of preincubation with normal goat serum (diluted 1:50) or normal swine serum (diluted 1:30) and/or normal horse serum (diluted 1:50), the preparations were incubated using the following antisera: rabbit anti-TH (produced with TH from rat PC12 cells (59) antiserum (diluted 1:400 with PBS), rabbit anti-CGRP (Cambridge) antiserum (diluted 1:200 with PBS) overnight at room temperature in a moist chamber. After thorough washing in PBS (3 × 10 min), the primary antibody was visualized in two different ways: (a) incubation for 1 hour in biotinylated goat-anti-rabbit-IgG (1:100, Vektor Lab., Burlingame, USA) followed by streptavidin conjugated to fluorescein isothiocyanate (FITC) (1:100, Vektor Lab., Burlingame, USA) for 1 hour, or (b) directly labeled with swine-anti-rabbit-IgG (SWAR) conjugated to FITC. Such directly labeled specimens were also used for double incubations with the mouse monoclonal antibody 10H, recognizing the 94-kDa integral vesicle membrane glycoprotein named SV2 (60), or with the mouse monoclonal anti-p38 antiserum, recognizing the integral vesicle membrane glycoprotein named *synaptophysin* (61). Following incubations with either 10H or anti-p38 antisera at room temperature overnight, the second incubation was carried out with biotinylated goat-anti-mouse IgG (1 hour, ambient temperature, diluted 1:200) followed by Texas red labeled streptavidin (1 hour, ambient temperature, diluted 1:100, Vektor Burlingame, USA). After washing, the preparations were mounted in glycerol, buffered at pH 8.6 with diazobicyclooctan (DABCO, Sigma Chemical Co., St. Louis, USA) added to prevent fading. Fluorescence was examined in a CFLM (MRC 500, Lasersharp, Cambridge, UK).

RESULTS

The specimens were scanned at 1–2 μm incremental levels, their whole thickness was between 0.2 and 0.8 mm. The scanned frames were then projected linearly to yield a combined picture of the innervation throughout the specimens.

Ontogeny of TH- and CGRP-LI

At birth, there were already many TH-positive (Fig. 10–1A) nerve fibers forming thick bundles that appeared to enter the right atrium from the epicardial surface along the superior caval vein. Stained individual fibers exhibited fine varicose immunopositive appearance. Incoming Th-positive nerve fibers continued from the opening of the superior caval vein in smaller bundles or in single fibers, which formed a nerve terminal network with the highest density adjacent to the sinoatrial (SA) node (Fig. 10–1B) and continued along the muscle strands toward the atrioventricular (AV) opening (Fig. 10–1C). Also, strongly TH-positive nerve cell bodies were found on the epicardial surface of the atrial myocardium at birth (Fig. 10–1D). The relatively dense network, clearly visible on the whole epicardial surface of the right auricle, originated from either the plexuses near the opening of the superior caval vein, or from the inferior caval vein (Fig. 10–1E). The density of innervation decreased from the epicardial surface to the endocardium, an observation that was confirmed in immunoincubated cross sections of the wall.

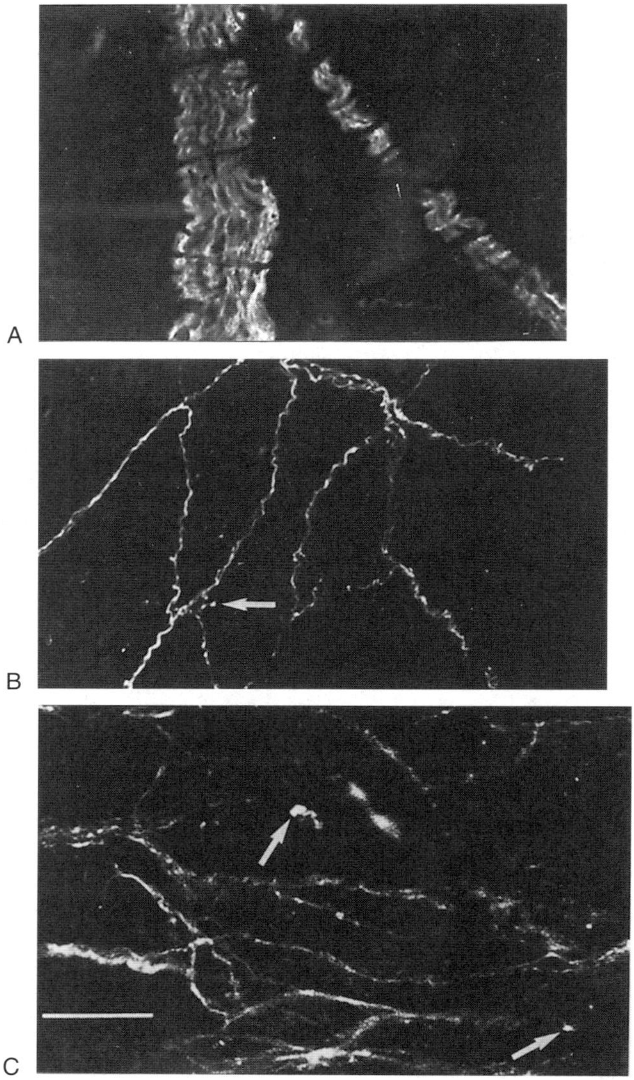

FIG. 10–1. Whole-mount preparations of newborn rat right atrium incubated with anti-TH antiserum. Confocal laser scanning pictures. (**A**) Near the orifice of the superior caval vein a thick bundle of TH-positive axons is seen entering the heart and giving off fluorescent branches. The bundle is composed of many TH-positive axons with wavy appearance in *X-Y* and *Z* planes. Dark bands perpendicular to the fibers are caused by the fibers extending into non-scanned incremental *Z* planes. (**B**) Near the sinoatrial node and (**C**) in the area of the atrioventricular node, TH-immunoreactive nerve fibers, single and in bundles, are present. Growth conelike structures are indicated by arrows. (Bars are 50 μm.) (**D**) Also, groups of very strongly TH-positive cell bodies with short processes on the epicardial surface adjacent to the sinoatrial node are seen. (**E**) The relatively dense network of TH-positive bundles, fibers, and terminals forming epicardial plexus on the right auricle is shown. (Bar is 50 μm.)

D

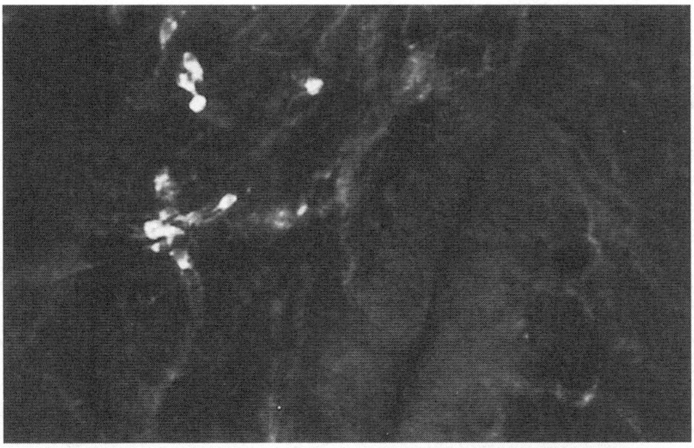

E

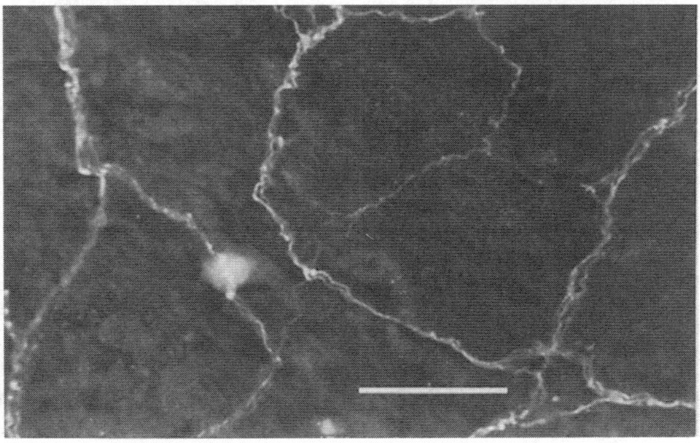

FIG. 10–1. *Continued*

CGRP-immunoreactive nerve fibers were found within the pericardium (Fig. 10–2A) at birth as individual axons with relatively large varicosities. Near the opening of the superior caval vein these axons with scattered varicosities formed bundles (Fig. 10–2B) consisting of sparse immunoreactive fibers coursing together with nonstained nerve processes. Numerous CGRP-positive nerve fibers forming bundles primarily composed of CGRP-LI appeared near the opening of the superior caval vein into the right atrium at the age of 10-day-old animal (Fig. 10–3A). These fibers branched into smaller bundles or fibers forming terminal network. Individual fibers contained clear, beadlike varicosities along their lengths and formed plexuses that seemed to course along the internodal pathways toward the AV opening (Fig. 10–3B). In the right atria from 10- to 20-day-old animals the TH- and CGRP-positive branches were arranged in a sizable plexus of nerve terminals with more varicosities and stronger fluorescence intensity in all regions mentioned earlier (Fig. 10–4A,B, 10–5A,B). At this age an extensive net-

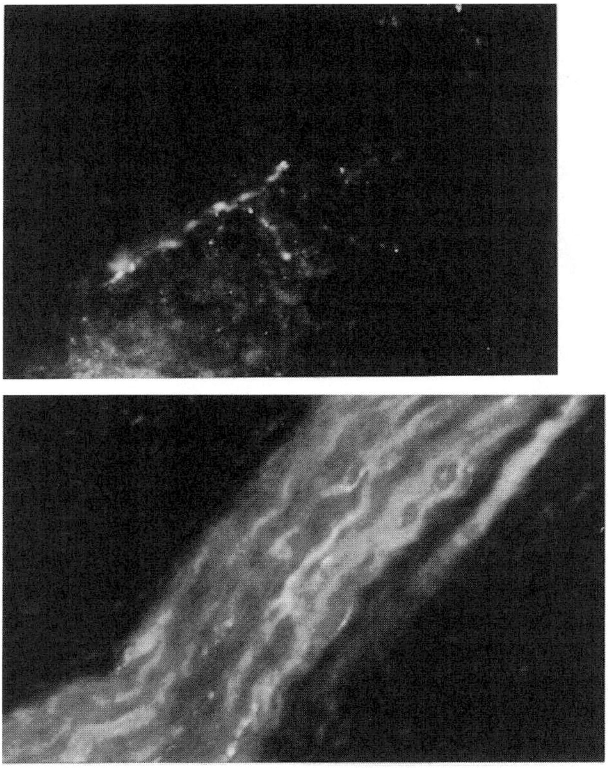

A

B

FIG. 10–2. Whole-mount preparations of newborn rat pericardium (**A**) and newborn rat right atrium (**B**) incubated with anti-CGRP antiserum. Confocal laser scanning pictures. (**A**) Stained individual axon containing enlargements of the axoplasm resembling varicosities along its length is seen. (**B**) Near the opening of the superior caval vein into the right atrium, bundles composed of sparse CGRP-positive fibers with scattered varicosities running in parallel together with nonstained nerve processes are seen.

work of TH- and CGRP-positive nerve fibers was also seen along all the larger vessels examined, including the coronary artery, parts of which were sometimes present in the preparations (Fig. 10–4A,B, 10–5B). However, in comparison to TH-LI, no CGRP-immunoreactive cell bodies were found within the right atrium at any age examined.

Progressive increase in thickness of TH- and CGRP-positive nerve fiber bundles together with an increase in fluorescence was clearly seen up to the age of 40 days (Fig. 10–6A,B).

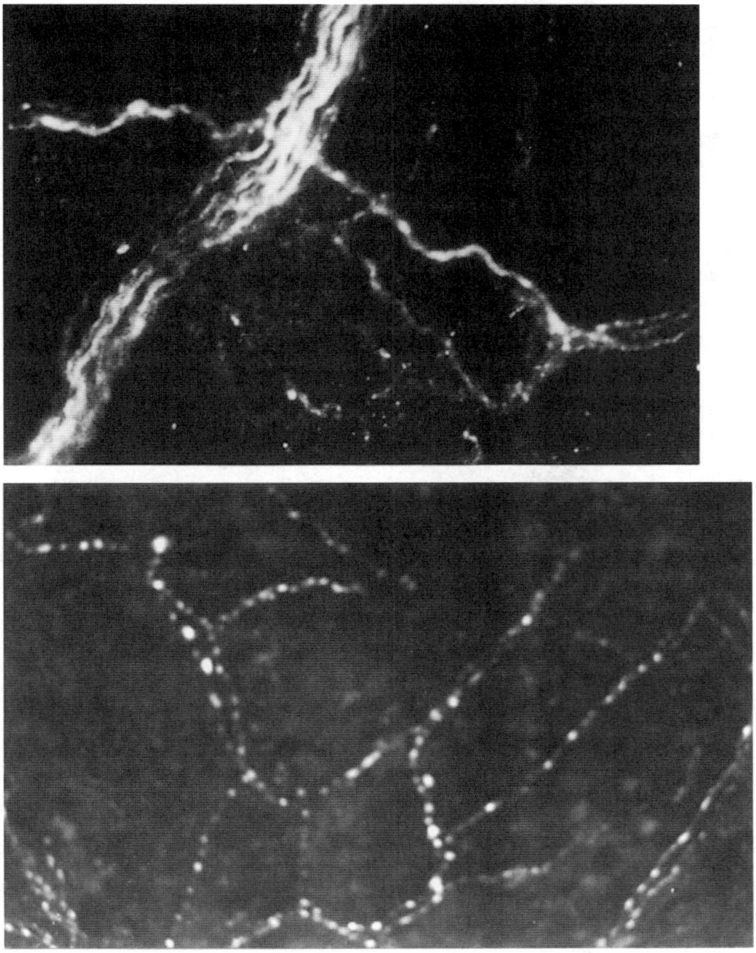

A

B

FIG. 10–3. Whole-mount preparations of rat right atria of 10–day-old animals, incubated with anti CGRP-antiserum. Confocal laser scanning pictures. (**A**) From the epicardial surface, incoming nerve fibers forming bundles composed primarily of strongly CGRP-positive processes are seen. Nerve bundles branch into smaller bundles or fibers forming epicardial plexus and penetrating myocardium. (**B**) Also, individual CGRP-positive fibers in deeper layers of musculature, containing clear, beadlike varicosities of different size surrounding musculature are present.

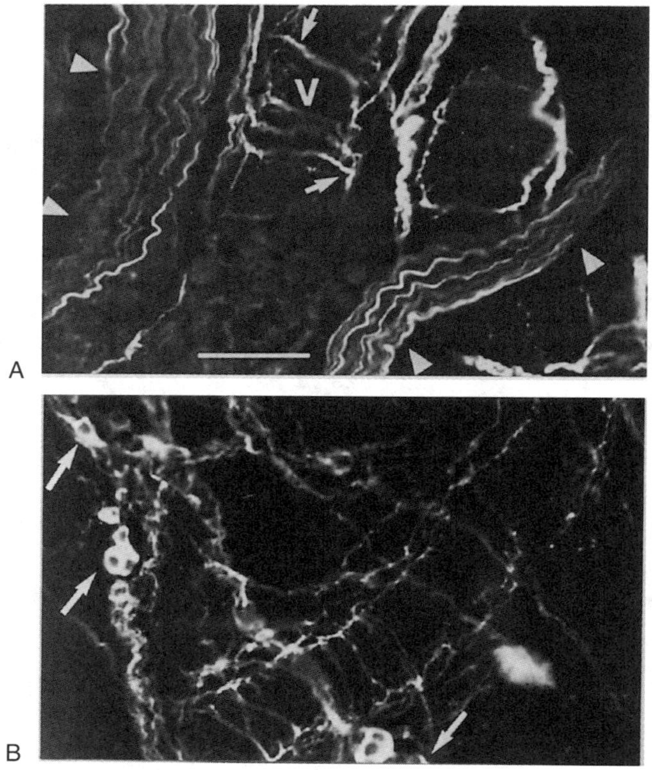

FIG. 10–4. Whole-mount preparations of right atria of an 11-day-old rat (**A**) and a 20-day-old rat (**B**). All atria were incubated with anti-TH antiserum. Confocal laser scanning pictures. (**A**) TH-positive nerve fiber bundles (arrowheads) along a vessel (V), which also has many TH-immunoreactive nerve terminals in the wall (arrow) are present. (Scale bar is 50 m m.) (**B**) Near the orifice of the inferior caval vein. A dense plexus of TH-positive nerve terminals and bundles of fibers is seen mainly surrounding vessels. Also bundles of nerve fibers and groups of strongly TH-positive nerve cell bodies are present (arrows).

Vesicle Markers in Relation to TH and CGRP

The nerve terminals in the right atrial wall were clearly SV2-positive at birth (Fig. 10–7) and had the same distribution as nerve terminals with TH-LI, but it could not be established if the SV2-containing terminals were more numerous than the TH-positive fibers. An extensive network of SV2-positive terminals was seen in the right atria from 11-day-old animal, and there was a clear co-localization with TH-immunoreactive terminals (Fig. 10–8A,B). Furthermore, in most areas the delicate varicose SV2-positive nerve terminals appeared to be more numerous than

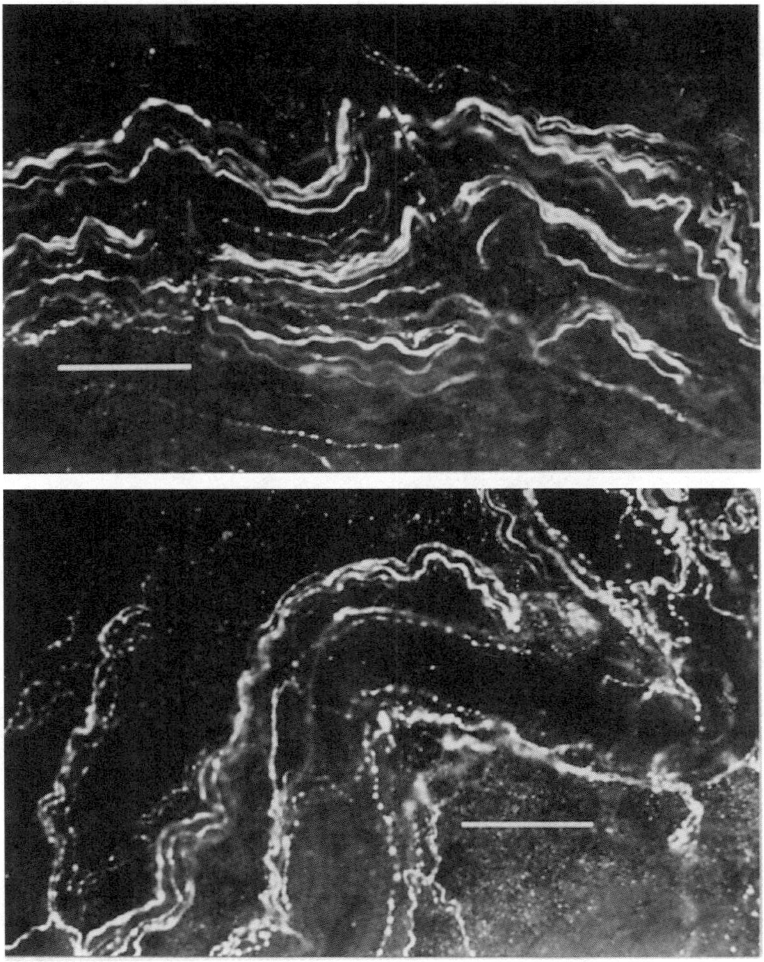

A

B

FIG. 10–5. Whole-mount preparations of rat right atria of an 18-day-old animals. All atria were incubated with anti-CGRP antiserum. Confocal laser scanning pictures. (**A**) CGRP-positive nerve fibers with more varicosities and stronger fluorescence intensity are seen at the orifice of the superior caval vein. (**B**) Strongly CGRP-positive nerve terminals are also present, surrounding vessels with more or less thick fiber bundles forming network in deeper layers musculature. (Bars are 5 m m.)

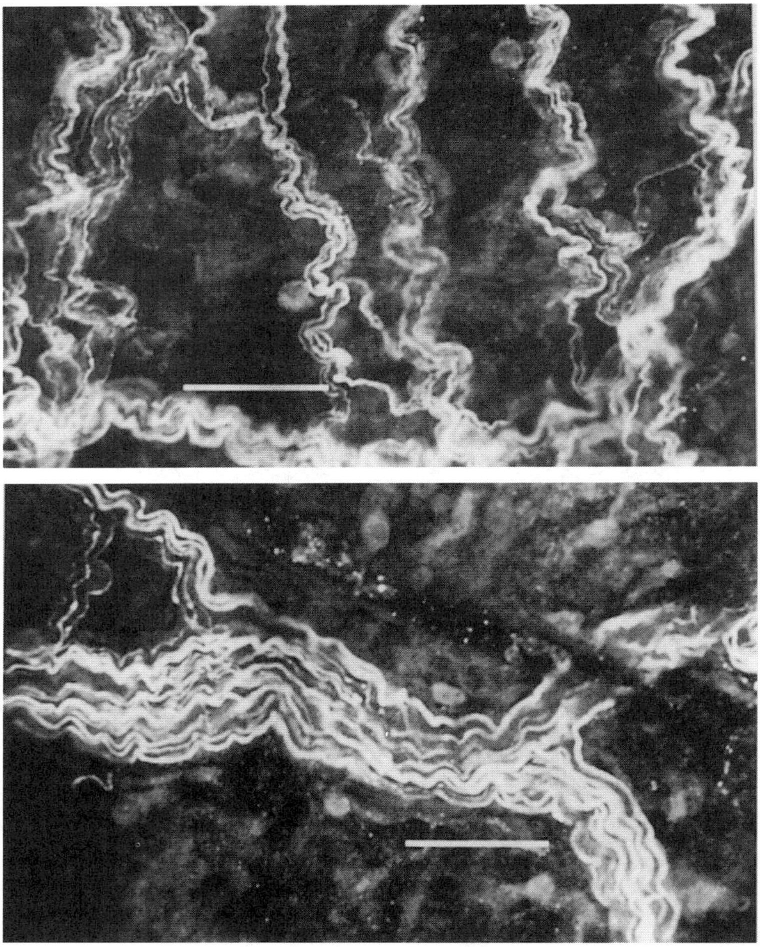

FIG. 10–6. Whole-mount preparation of right atria of a 40-day-old rat. Atria were incubated with anti-TH antiserum (A) and anti-CGRP antiserum (B). Confocal laser scanning pictures. (A) Near the opening of the superior caval vein, progressive increase in the thickness of TH-positive nerve fiber bundles forming dense epicardial plexus together with an increase in fluorescence intensity is seen. (B) Also, the thick bundles of CGRP-immunoreactive nerve fibers are present near the opening of the superior caval vein. Immunopositivity of individual fibers is strong and almost homogeneous. (Bars are 50 μm.)

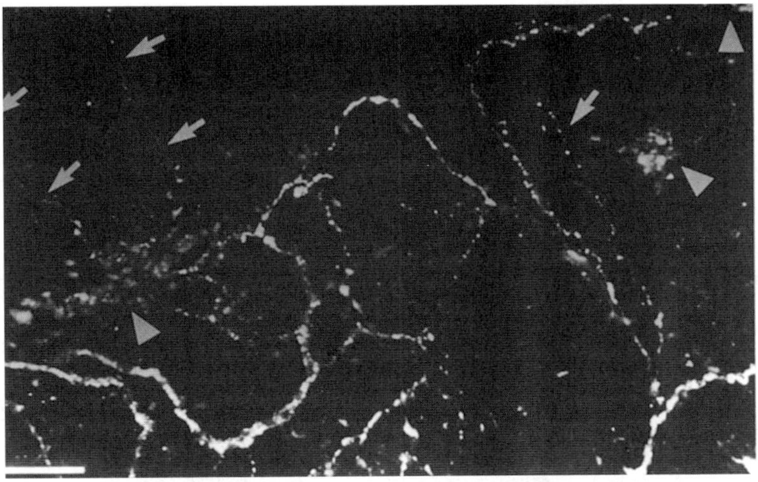

FIG. 10–7. Whole-mount preparation of right atrium of newborn rat, incubated with antibody 10H, directed toward the transmembrane synaptic vesicle marker SV2. Confocal laser scanning picture. A plexus of SV2-positive terminals, with a thin varicose appearance can be observed. Some terminals are very delicate (*arrows*). Red blood cells (*arrowheads*) in vessels are weakly labeled by the secondary antiserum (present also in control incubated specimens). (Bar is 100 μm.)

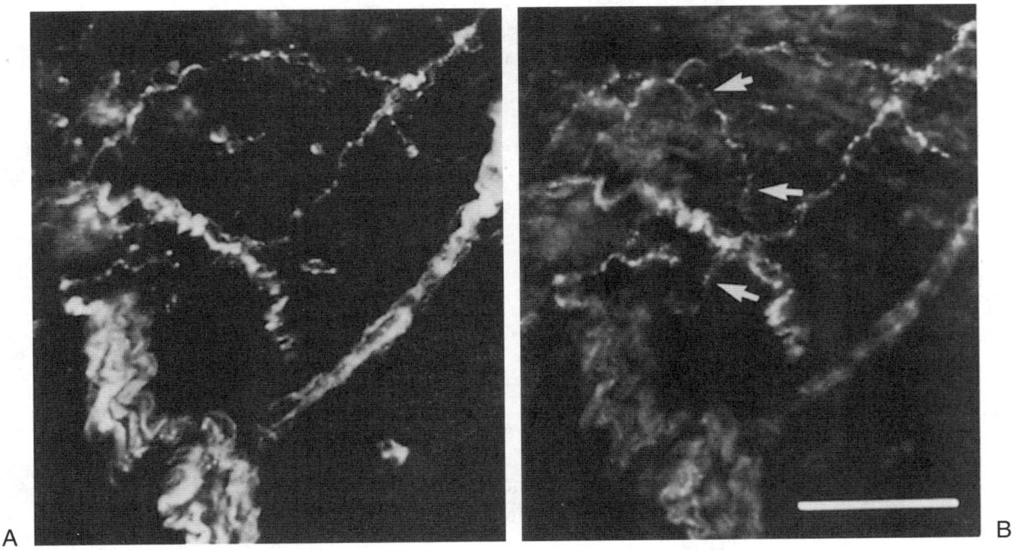

FIG. 10–8. Whole-mount preparation of right atrium of an 11-day-old rat, double-incubated with anti-TH antiserum and swine anti-rabbit-IgG-FITC (**A**) and the mouse monoclonal antibody 10H (directed toward the synaptic vesicle marker SV2) visualized by incubation with biotinylated horse-anti-mouse IgG and Texas red labeled streptavidin (**B**). Near the orifice of the superior caval vein the nerve fiber bundles have a strong TH-immunoreactivity, but only weak SV2-immunoreaction. In most terminals there appears to be co-localization of TH-LI and SV2, but in some nerve terminal structures only SV2 can be observed (*arrows*). Confocal laser scanning picture, dual channel setting. (Bar is 50 μm.)

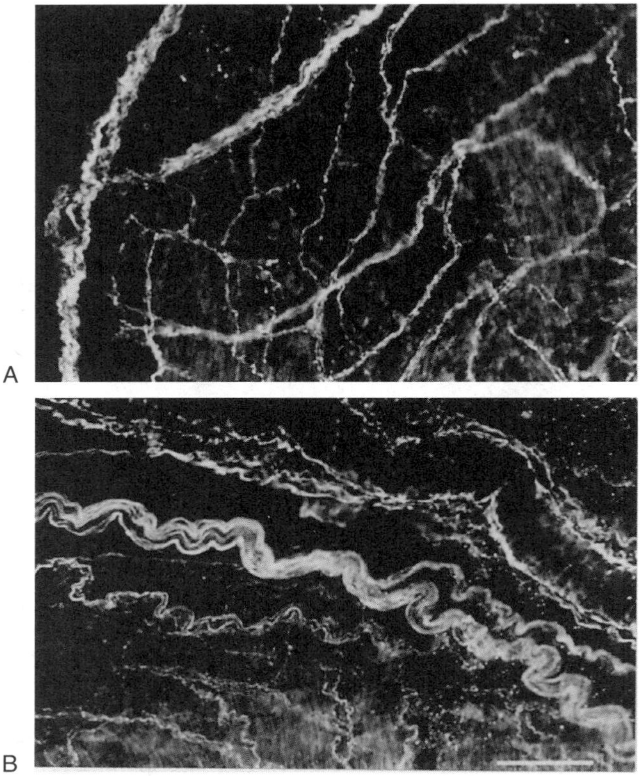

FIG. 10–9. Whole-mount preparations of right atria of an 11-day-old rat (**A**), and a 20-day-old rat (**B**). Atria were incubated with anti-p38 antiserum. Confocal laser scanning pictures. (**A**) A dense network of strong p38-LI nerve bundle, fibers, and terminals is visible on the whole epicardial surface of the right auricle. (**B**) Near the internodal pathways, a dense plexus of strong p38-positive nerve bundles, fibers, and terminals is seen. The terminals have finely granular pattern. Also, p38-LI nerve fibers surrounding vessels are present.

the TH-positive nerve terminals, indicating that SV2 antigen is present also in non-TH-LI nerves.

A dense network of strong p38-LI nerve terminals, fibers, and bundles was clearly visible on the whole epicardial surface, including the right auricle at the age of 11-day-old animal (Fig. 10–9A). Progressive increases in the thickness and density of the nerve terminals, together with an increase in immunofluorescence intensity, were seen up to the age 20 days. Also p38-LI nerve fibers surrounding vessels were present (Fig. 10–9B).

CGRP does not co-localize in the same preparation with p38 antigen, as could be observed using double immunostaining method. On one specimen stained for both antigens different immunopositivities were present in different intramural nerve

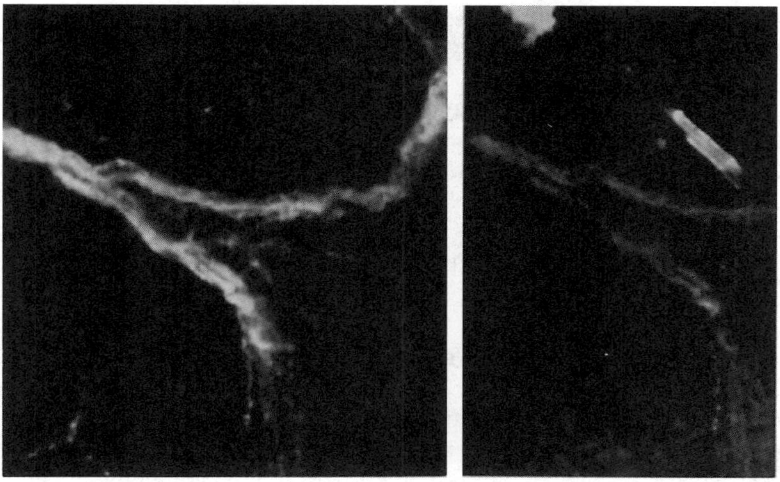

FIG. 10–10. Whole-mount preparation of right atrium of a 10–day-old rat, double-incubated with anti-CGRP antiserum and swine anti-rabbit-IgG-FITC (**A**), and the mouse monoclonal anti-p38 antiserum (directed toward the synaptic vesicle marker p38) visualized by incubation with biotinylated horse–anti mouse–IgG and Texas red–labeled streptavidin (**B**). Confocal laser scanning pictures. Near the orifice of the superior caval vein the nerve fiber bundles and terminals have a strong and clear CGRP-LI (**A**), but only weak or no p38-LI (**B**).

fibers and terminals. The nerve fiber bundles and terminals near the orifice of the superior caval vein in the right atria from 10-day-old rat examined strong and clear CGRP-positivity, but only weak or none p38-LI (Fig. 10–10A,B).

DISCUSSION

The total pattern of distribution of catecholaminergic neurons in relation to primary sensory afferents in the different parts of the rat heart during the postnatal development has not yet been studied. In the present investigation we examined the postnatal developmental pattern of TH- and CGRP-positive innervation in rat right atria in whole-mount preparations, using indirect immunofluorescence. The age stages examined were based on previous knowledge of the developmental physiologic changes of the sympathetic innervation after birth (4,62,63). We chose to investigate the right atrium because SA node is a primary pacemaker controlling the beat rate of the entire heart. It is known that atria are densely innervated by both divisions of the autonomic nervous system with dual efferent motor and afferent sensory activity. The use of whole-mount stretch preparations facilitated the study of the entire distribution of nerve cell bodies, fibers, bundles, branches, and terminals, from the epicardial surface to the endocardium; using CFLM, the delicate networks surrounding muscle strands in deeper layers of myocardium were visible.

Thus, the great advantage of the CFLM is the possibility of obtaining a precise picture of the innervation from all levels of the preparation.

Most TH-immunoreactive neural tissue is present within nerve processes. Stained nerve fibers present already at birth entered the right atrium along the superior caval vein in thick bundles (Fig. 10–1A). The fibers are probably adrenergic axons, but they may represent cholinergic nerves that later resume adrenergic characteristics (64,65). The postganglionic sympathetic axons, representing efferent motor cardioexcitatory division of autonomic innervation, originate in the stellate and cervical ganglia. In addition to the stained axons, minor component of immunofluorescence was localized within strongly TH-positive nerve cell bodies with short stained processes (Fig. 10–1D). They were located mainly adjacent to the orifice of the superior caval vein and near the AV opening on the epicardial surface. The presence of NA-containing cell bodies was described under the pericardium near the base of the rat heart (66). The aminergic intrinsic neurons were first documented near the atrioventricular junction in the rat adult heart (67). The authors proposed that these neurons may be involved in modulation of neurotransmission. Intrinsic neurons resemble small, intensely fluorescent cells (SIF) described within autonomic ganglia of many different species (27,28,68,69). We found these intracardiac "short" TH-positive neurons in right atria already at birth (Fig. 10–1D), as well as in 20-day-old animal (Fig. 10–4B) in contrast to recent work (58), in which only NPY-positive neurons in the rat atrial intrinsic ganglia, present on the second postnatal day, were described, but these neurons never exhibited TH-immunoreactivity.

Near the opening of the superior caval vein into the right atrium, the TH-positive nerve fibers branched into thinner bundles forming a typical ground plexus (70,71). From the network near the opening of the inferior caval vein, thin fibers were observed running in the opposite direction. The fibers that entered the atrium along the superior caval vein formed the densest network in the area of the SA-node (Fig. 10–1B) and projected, surrounding fascicles of the atrial musculature toward the AV opening (Fig. 10–1C). The network spread to the cranial part of the right auricle, forming a rather dense epicardial network of TH-positive terminals (Fig. 10–1E). Also the AV node was found to be supplied by a dense and delicate network of TH-positive nerve fibers (Fig. 10–1C).

At birth TH-positive nerve fibers were already visible as epicardial plexuses and as networks surrounding atrial musculature throughout the whole thickness of the myocardium. Thus, the basic pattern of innervation of the atria seen in 40-day-old animals was qualitatively present at birth. Previous investigators found that the innervation of NA-fluorescent nerve terminals at birth was very low (5,55,66,72). Our observation that a nerve terminal plexus with TH-LI is present at birth suggests that the catecholamine-synthetic enzyme is present in nerve terminals, which are probably at least partly sympathetic, adrenergic before the capacity to take up and store catecholamines develops to significant levels (72).

The synaptic vesicle antigen SV2 was also present in terminals at birth (see Fig. 10–7), which may indicate transmitter storage and release functions, since these antigens have been closely linked to mature synaptic vesicles (60,61). Although co-localization studies appeared to indicate a spatial association between TH-LI and SV2 in most nerve fibers, the SV2 was observed in some TH-negative structures may have been present in parasympathetic fibers, known to run in parallel with sympathetic fibers.

At all stages examined, the epicardial aspect had a greater density of innervation than the endocardial area. This is not due to poor diffusion of the antibodies used for incubation, because a similar pattern was observed in cryostat cross sections of the atrial wall. Rather, it may be because the innervating nerve fibers grow into the atria from the outside, as suggested previously (73).

It is interesting that the basic pattern of sympathetic motor innervation of the right atria is present at birth, long before neuroeffector mechanisms can be recorded (1,4). One may speculate if these early nerves have other, nontransmissive, tasks during the postnatal development (e.g., secretion of trophic substances to support the growing heart muscle).

In our present study, the pattern of TH-LI distribution was compared with the pattern of CGRP-LI in the rat right atria during postnatal development. Immunocytochemical studies have demonstrated that CGRP-LI is widely distributed in the primary afferents in the viscera and cardiovascular system, particularly in the heart in several species (74). The sensory origin of CGRP and its colocalization with substance P in the cardiovascular system has been substantiated by using selective neurotoxin capsaicin, which treatment of guinea pigs and rats leads to marked loss of CGRP- and substance P-immunoreactivity (75–77).

The reports that concern the presence and functional significance of CGRP in guinea pig heart are numerous (74), but those in rat heart are few, and to our knowledge no immunocytochemical report concerning newborn heart, the developmental changes of CGRP in neural tissue, the pattern of its distribution in the tissue as a whole, and its relation to synaptic vesicle markers has been published. The distribution of CGRP in the cardiovascular tissue of the rat investigated by radioimmunoassay was described in all regions of the heart, particularly in association with coronary arteries, within the papillary muscles, and in SA and AV nodes (43).

In contrast to TH-LI immunoreactivity, in our present study, CGRP-LI was identified exclusively within the enlargements resembling varicosities along the lengths of nerve processes at all stages examined. Since these enlargements differed in size, no immunoreactive cell bodies were found within the rat atrial myocardium, in contrast to observations in guinea pig atrium (45), in which infrequent CGRP-immunoreactive perikarya in ganglionic structure were found. Our observations suggest that CGRP-immunoreactive nerve supply to the heart is of extrinsic origin, which is in agreement with findings in dog hearts (53).

CGRP-LI at birth was scattered, localized in individual nerve axons in pericardium (Fig. 10–2A). Incoming sparse stained fibers formed bundles together with nonstained processes near the opening of the superior caval vein into the right atrium (Fig. 10–2B). The bundles composed mainly of CGRP-positive nerve processes were identified within the atrial myocardium of 10–day-old animal (Fig.

10–3A). These fibers branched into smaller bundles, giving rise to individual fibers and terminals penetrating musculature (Fig. 10–3B). In the right atria from 10- to 40-day-old animals, changes of CGRP-LI could be considered as quantitative; the density of innervation as well as the intensity of fluorescence increased (Fig. 10–5A,B). The distribution of CGRP-positive fibers gives a picture similar to TH-positive nerve fibers. They seem to come along the superior caval vein, forming thick bundles near its opening (Fig. 10–2B). In this part of the right atrium, from the epicardial surface, the bundles branched into thinner bundles and fibers, forming epicardial plexus. Nerve fibers and terminals penetrate the atrial musculature and run along the muscle strands, establishing a fine terminal plexus, surrounding coronary vessels also (Fig. 10–3A,B; 10–5A,B). The highest density of the terminal network was seen in the nodal regions (Fig. 10–5B).

CGRP exerts both positive chronotropic and inotropic effects on the rat heart and is likely to function as neurotransmitter of NANC nerves (48–50). Our results with double labeling procedure support this origin. CGRP-LI was not co-localized with p-38 antigen (Fig. 10–10A,B), which is present in small synaptic vesicles of classical innervation. The potent effect of exogenous CGRP on heart rate (78), and the effect of transmural nerve stimulation on chronotropic and contractile response of rat atria (49,50) suggest that this innervation may still be of importance. Sensory substances thus antidromically released at perifery are agents for pre- and postsynaptic modulatory actions (79). The presence of CGRP even in the newborn animals, the extent and the distribution of the right atrium innervation, and its quantitative changes postnatally seem likely a developmental role of NANC innervation in the onset of the nervous control of the heart.

SUMMARY

The developmental pattern and distribution of tyrosine hydroxylase (TH) and calcitonin gene-related peptide (CGRP) immunoreactive nerves in the rat heart has been studied by indirect immunofluorescence. Anti-TH, -CGRP, and monoclonal antibodies against small synaptic vesicle antigens SV2 and synaptophysin-p38 were applied to whole-mount stretch preparations of the right atria from hearts of newborn to 40-day-old animals. Immunofluorescence was studied with confocal laser scanning microscopy (CFLM). Nerve fibers with TH- and CGRP-like immunoreactivities (TH- and CGRP-LI) were present throughout the atria already at birth. That most fibers within large bundles entered the right atrium along the superior caval vein suggested that both types of innervation are extrinsic in origin. The postnatal changes of innervation were basically quantitative, in the density and number of varicosities. With increasing age, the intensity of fluorescence increased, while the basic pattern of innervation was essentially unchanged. The highest density of TH- and CGRP-LI was found around the sinoatrial (SA) node. Also, TH-positive ganglionic cells were present around the openings of the caval veins, in contrast to CGRP-LI located exclusively within nerve processes. TH was co-localized in most nerve terminal arborizations with the synaptic vesicle marker

SV2. In comparison with TH-positive fibers, SV2- positive nerve terminal fibers were more delicate, and the number of fibers was larger in all areas studied. In axon bundles, TH-LI was very prominent, while the SV2-LI was weak. In contrast, CGRP was not co-localized in the same preparations with p38 antigen supporting nonadrenergic noncholinergic (NANC) origin of CGRP. The results show that TH-positive, possibly adrenergic, nerve fibers are distinct from CGRP-positive fibers, NANC, and that both innervations are present at birth. The distribution of TH-LI and CGRP-LI at birth was qualitatively similar to that observed in adults. TH-positive ganglionic cells are short intrinsic neurons probably involved in modulation of neurotransmission in cardiac intramural ganglia.

ACKNOWLEDGMENTS

Supported by the Swedish MRC (2207), by I.-B. and A. Lundbergs Stiftelse, The Ministry of Education in Prague (J.S.), and The Swedish Institute, Stockholm (J.S.). We thank Kerstin Lundmark and Anne Kling-Petersen for excellent technical assistance.

REFERENCES

1. Cohen HL. Development of autonomic innervation in mammalian myocardium. In: Gootman PM, ed. *Developmental neurobiology of the autonomic nervous system.* Clifton, NJ: Humana Press; 1986:159–161.
2. Gootman PM. Postnatal development of central nervous system regulation of cardiovascular function. In: Gootman N, Gootman PM, eds. *Perinatal cardiovascular function.* New York: Dekker; 1983:265–328.
3. Gootman PM. Development of central autonomic regulation of cardiovascular function. In: Gootman PM, ed. *Developmental neurobiology of the autonomic nervous system.* Clifton, NJ: Humana Press; 1983:279–325.
4. Slotkin TA. Endocrine control of synaptic development in the sympathetic nervous system. In: Gootman PM, ed. *Developmental neurobiology of the autonomic nervous system.* Clifton, NJ: Humana Press; 1986:97–130.
5. Lipp JAM, Rudolp AM. Sympathetic nerve development in the rat and guinea pig heart. *Biol Neonate* 1972;21:76–82.
6. Kent KM, Epstein SE, Cooper T, Jacobowitz DM. Cholinergic innervation of the canine and human ventricular conducting system. *Circulation* 1974;50:948–955.
7. Atwood GF, Kirschner N. Postnatal development of catecholamine uptake and storage of the newborn rat heart. *Develop Biol* 1976;49:532–538.
8. Kuntscherová J, Slavíková J, Vlk J. Postnatal development of cholinergic innervation in the heart pacemaker of rats. *Physiol Bohemoslov* 1977;26:264.
9. Seidler FJ, Slotkin TA. Presynaptic and postsynaptic contributions to ontogeny of sympathetic control of heart rate in the preweanling rat. *Br J Pharmacol* 1979;65:531–534.
10. Marwin WJ, Jr, Hermsmeyer K, McDonald RI, Roskoski LM, Roskoski R, Jr. Ontogenesis of cholinergic innervation in the rat heart. *Circ Res* 1980;46:690–695.
11. Bareis DL, Morgan RE, Lau C, Slotkin TA. Maturation of sympathetic neurotransmission in rat heart. IV. Effects of guanethidine-induced sympathectomy on neonatal development of synaptic vesicles, synaptic terminal function and heart growth. *Dev Neurosci* 1981;4:15–24.
12. Smith PG, Slotkin TA, Mills E. Development of sympathetic ganglionic neurotransmission in the neonatal rat: pre- and postganglionic nerve response to asphyxia and 2-deoxyglucose. *Neuroscience* 1982;7:501–507.

13. Slavíková J, Tuček S. Postnatal changes of the tonic influence of the vagus nerves on the heart rate, and of the activity of choline acetyltransferase in the heart atria of rats. *Physiol Bohemoslov* 1982;31:113–120.
14. Neef KJ, Versprille A, Wise ME, Jansen JRC. Functional development of the parasympathetic innervation of the sino-auricular node in newborn rabbits, cats and guinea pigs. *Pflugers Arch* 1983; 398:73–77.
15. Levy MN, Martin P. Neural regulation of the heart beat. *Annu Rev Physiol* 1981;43:443–458.
16. Levy MN, Martin P. Parasympathetic control of the heart. In: Randall WC, ed. *Nervous control of cardiovascular function.* New York: Oxford; 1984:68–94.
17. Randall WC. Selective autonomic innervation of the heart. In: Randall WC, ed. *Nervous control of cardiovascular function.* New York: Oxford; 1984:44–67.
18. Loffelholz K, Pappano AJ. The sympathetic neuroeffector junction of the heart. *Pharmacol Rev* 1985;37:1–24.
19. Burnstock G. The changing face in autonomic neurotransmission. *Acta Physiol Scand* 1986; 126:67–91.
20. Haass M, Cheng B, Richardt G, Lang RE, Schomig A. Characterization and presynaptic modulation of stimulation-evoked co-release of noradrenaline and neuropeptide Y in guinea pig heart. *Naunyn Schmiedebergs Arch Pharmacol* 1989;339:71–78.
21. Warner MR, Levy MN. Role of neuropeptide Y in neural control of the heart. *J Cardiovasc Electrophysiol* 1990;1:80–91.
22. Maggi CA, Meli A. The sensory-efferent function of capsaicin-sensitive sensory neurons. *Gen Pharmacol* 1988;19:1–43.
23. Rubino A. Non-adrenergic non-cholinergic (NANC) neural control of the atrial myocardium. *Gen Pharmacol* 1993;24:539–545.
24. Della NG, Papka RE, Furness JB, Costa M. Vasoactive intestinal peptide immunoreactivity in nerves associated with the cardiovascular system in guinea-pigs. *Neuroscience* 1983;9:605–619.
25. Sato H. Innervation of heart in dog. *Tohoku J Exp Med* 1954;59:343–356.
26. Moravec M, Moravec J, Forsgren S. Catecholaminergic and peptidergic nerve components of intramural ganglia in the rat heart. *Cell Tissue Res* 1990;262:315–327.
27. Kriebel RM, Angel A, Parsons RL. Biogenic amine localization in cardiac ganglion intrinsic neurons: electron microscopic histochemistry of SIF cells. *Brain Res Bull* 1991;27:175–179.
28. Konopka LM, Merriam LA, Hardwick JC, Parsons RL. Aminergic and peptidergic elements and actions in a cardiac parasympathetic ganglion. *Can J Physiol* 1992;70:S32–S43.
29. Slavíková J, Goldstein M, Dahlstrom A. The postnatal development of tyrosine hydroxylase immunoreactive nerves in rat atrium, studied with immunofluorescence and confocal laser scanning microscopy. *J Auton Nerv Syst* 1993;43:159–170.
30. Horackova M, Armour JA. Role of peripheral autonomic neurones in maintaining adequate cardiac function. *Cardiovasc Res* 1995;30:326–335.
31. Costa M, Buffa R, Furness JB, Solcia E. Immunohistochemical localization of polypeptides in peripheral autonomic nerves using whole-mount preparations. *Histochemistry* 1980;65:157–165.
32. Molinoff PB, Axelrod J. Biochemistry of catecholamines. *Annu Rev Biochem* 1971;40:465–500.
33. Goldstein M, Fuxe K, Hokfelt T. Characterization and tissue localization of catecholamine synthesising enzymes. *Pharmacol Rev* 1972;24:293–309.
34. Pickel VM, Joh TH, Field PM, Becker CG, Reis DJ. Cellular localization of tyrosine hydroxylase by immunohistochemistry. *J Histochem Cytochem* 1975;23:1–12.
35. Amara SG, Jonas V, Rosenfeld MG, Ong ES, Evans RM. Alternative RNA processing in calcitonin gene expression generates mRNA encoding different products. *Nature* 1982;298:240–244.
36. Craigh RK, Hall L, Edbrook MR, Allison J, MacIntyre I. Partial nucleotide sequence of human calcitonin precursor mRNA identifies flanking cryptic peptide. *Nature* 1982;295:345–347.
37. Rosenfeld MG, Mermod JJ, Amara SG, et al. Production of a novel neuropeptide by the calcitonin gene via tissue specific RNA processing. *Nature* 1983;304:129–132.
38. Nelkin BD, Rosenfeld KJ, de Bustros A, Leong SS, Roos BA, Baylin SB. Structure and expression of a gene encoding human calcitonin gene-related peptide. *Biochem Biophys Res Commun* 1984;123:648–655.
39. Alter WA, Weiss GK, Priola DV. Vagally induced tachycardia in atropinized dogs: effect of beta-adrenergic blockade. *Eur J Pharmacol* 1973;24:329–333.
40. Rigel DF, Lipson D, Katon PG. Excess tachycardia: heart rate after antimuscarinic agents in conscious dogs. *Am J Physiol* 1984;246:H168–H173.

41. Tippins JR, Morris HR, Panico M, et al. The myotropic and plasma-calcium modulating effects of calcitonin gene-related peptide. *Neuropeptides* 1984;4:425.
42. Gennari C, Fischer JA. Cardiovascular action of calcitonin gene-related peptide in humans. *Calcif Tissue Int* 1985;37:581.
43. Mulderry PK, Ghatei MA, Rodrigo J, Allen JM, Rosenfeld MG, Polak JM, Bloom SR. Calcitonin gene-related peptide in cardiovascular tissues of the rat. *Neuroscience* 1985;14:947–954.
44. Lundberg JM, Saria A, Franco-Cereceda A, Hokfelt T, Terenius L, Goldstein M. Differential effects of reserpine and 6-hydroxydopamine on neuropeptide Y and noradrenaline in peripheral neurons. *Nauyn Schmiedebergs Arch Pharmacol* 1985;328:331–340.
45. Gerstheimer FP, Metz J. Distribution of calcitonin gene-related peptide-like immunoreactivity in the guinea pig heart. *Anat Embryol* 1986;175:255–260.
46. Saito A, Kimura S, Goto K. Calcitonin gene-related peptide as potential neurotransmitter in guinea pig right atrium. *Am J Physiol* 1986;250:H693–H698.
47. Saito A, Ishikawa T, Kimura S, Goto K. Role of calcitonin gene-related peptide as cariotonic neurotransmitter in guinea pig left atria. *J Pharmacol Exp Ther* 1987;243:731–736.
48. Sigrist S, Franco-Cereceda A, Muff R, Henke H, Lundberg JM, Fischer JA. Specific receptor and cardiovascular effects of calcitonin gene-related peptide. *Endocrinology* 1986;119:381–389.
49. Wharton J, Gulbenkian S, Muldberry PK, Ghatei MA, McGregor GP, Bloom SR, Polak JM. Capsaicin induces a depletion of calcitonin gene-related peptide (CGRP)-immunoreactive nerves in the cardiovascular system of the guinea pig and rat. *J Auton Nerv Syst* 1986;16:289–309.
50. Goto K, Ishikawa T, Kimura S, Saito A. Intramural nerve-mediated inotropic responses of left atria of rats and guinea pigs: demonstration of alpha adrenergic and nonadrenergic noncholinergic responses in guinea pigs. *J Pharmacol Exp Ther* 1987;243:723–730.
51. Miyauchi T, Ishikawa T, Sugishita Y, Saito A, Goto K. Effects of capsaicin on nonadrenergic noncholinergic nerves in the guinea pig atria: role of calcitonin gene-related peptide as cardiac neurotransmitter. *J Cardiovasc Pharmacol* 1987;10:675–682.
52. Miyauchi T, Ishikawa T, Sugishita Y, Saito A, Goto K. Effects of piperine on calcitonin gene-related peptide (CGRP)- containing nerves in the isolated rat atria. *Neurosci Lett* 1988;91: 222–227.
53. Ursell PC, Ren CL, Albala A, Danilo P Jr. Nonadrenergic noncholinergic innervation. *Circ Res* 1991;68:131–140.
54. Dubois-Randé LC, Merlet P, Benvenuti C, et al. Effects of calcitonin gene-related peptide on cardiac contractility, coronary hemodynamics and myocardial energetics in idiopathic dilated cardiomyopathy. *Am J Cardiol* 1992;70:906–912.
55. Schiebler TH, Heene R. Nachweis von Katecholaminen in Rattenherzen wahrend der Entwicklung. *Histochemie* 1968;14:328–334.
56. Winckler J. Uber die adrenergen Herznerven bei Ratte und Meer schweinchen. *Z Zellforsch* 1969;98:106–121.
57. Lipp JM, Rudolph AM. Sympathetic nerve development in the rat and guinea-pig heart. *Biol Neonate* 1972;21:76–82.
58. Nyquist-Battie C, Cochran PK, Sands SA, Chronwall BM. Development of neuropeptide Y and tyrosine hydroxylase immunoreactive innervation in postnatal rat heart. *Peptides* 1994;15:1461–1469.
59. Goldstein M, Fuxe K, Hökfelt T. Characterization and tissue localization of catecholamine synthesizing enzymes. *Pharmacol Rev* 1972;24:293–309.
60. Buckley K, Kelly RB. Identification of a transmembrane glycoprotein specific for secretory for vesicles of neural and endocrine cells. *J Cell Biol* 1985;100:1284–1294.
61. Vlk J, Vincenzi FF. Functional autonomic innervation of mammalian cardiac pacemaker during the perinatal period. *Biol Neonate* 1977;31:19–26.
62. Smith PG, Mills E, Slotkin TA. Maturation of sympathetic neurotransmission in the efferent pathway to the rat heart: ultrastructural analysis of ganglionic synaptogenesis in euthyroid and hyperthyroid neonates. *Neuroscience* 1981;6:911–918.
63. Landis SC, Jackson PC, Frendieu JR, Thibault J. Catecholaminergic properties of cholinergic neurons and synapses in adult rat ciliary ganglion. *J Neurosci* 1987;7:3574–3587.
64. Wolinsky EJ, Landis SC, Patterson PM. Expression of noradrenergic and cholinergic traits by sympathetic neurons cultured without serum. *J Neurosci* 1985;5:1497–1508.
65. Owman C, Sjoberg N-O, Swedin G. Histochemical and chemical studies on pre- and postnatal development of the different systems of "short" and "long" adrenergic neurons in peripheral organs of the rat. *Z Zellforsch* 1971;116:319–341.

66. Moravec M, Coutalon A, Moravec J. Intrinsic neurosecretory neurons of the rat heart atrioventricular junction: possibility of local neuromuscular feedback loops. *J Mol Cell Cardiol* 1986;18:357–367.
67. Taxi J, Derer M, Domick A. Morphology and histopathology of SIF cells in the autonomic ganglia. In: Elfvin L-G, ed. *Autonomic ganglia.* New York: Wiley; 1983:67–95.
68. Williams T, Jew J. Monoamine connections in sympathetic ganglia. In: *Elfvin L-G, ed.* Autonomic ganglia. New York: Wiley; 1983:235–264.
69. Hillarp N-A. Structure of the synapse and peripheral innervation apparatus of the autonomic nervous system. *Acta Anat* 1946;4(suppl):1–153.
70. Hillarp N-A. The construction and functional organization of the autonomic innervation apparatus. *Acta Physiol Scand* 1959;46:1–38.
71. Sachs C, de Champlain J, Malmfors T, Olson L. The postnatal development of noradrenaline uptake in the adrenergic nerves of different tissues from the rat. *Eur J Pharmacol* 1979;9:67–79.
72. Volknandt W. The synaptic vesicle and its targets. *Neuroscience* 1995;64:277–300.
73. Hoar R, Hall JL. The early pattern of cardiac innervation in fetal guinea pig. *Am J Anat* 1970; 128:494–508.
74. Wharton J, Gulbenkian S. Peptides in the mammalian cardiovascular system. *Experientia* 1987; 47:821–832.
75. Furness JB, Elliot JM, Murphy R, Costa M, Chalmers JP. Baroreceptor reflexes in conscious guinea-pig are unaffected by depletion of cardiovascular substance P nerves. *Neurosci Lett* 1982; 32:285–290.
76. Duckles SP, Levitt B. Specificity of capsaicin treatment in the cerebral vasculature. *Brain Res* 1984;308:141–144.
77. Papka RE, Furness JB, Della NG, Murphy R, Costa M. Time course of effect of capsaicin on ultrastructure and histochemistry of substance P-immunoreactive nerves associated with the cardiovascular system of the guinea pig. *Neuroscience* 1984;12:1277–1292.
78. Fisher LA, Kikkawa DO, Rivier JE, et al. Stimulation of noradrenergic sympathetic outflow by calcitonin gene-related peptide. *Nature* 1983;305:534–536.
79. Cuello AC. Peptides as neuromodulators in primary sensory neurons. *Neuropharmacology* 1987; 26:971–979.

The Developing Heart,
edited by Bohuslav Ošťádal et al.
Lippincott-Raven Publishers,
Philadelphia © 1997.

11

Dystrophin and the Heart

Susan Y. Fu, Jacqueline Hance, and Marek Michalak

*Department of Biochemistry, University of Alberta,
Edmonton, Alberta, T6G 2S2, Canada*

Duchenne muscular dystrophy (DMD) is an X-linked, degenerative muscle disorder (1–4), affecting about one in 3,300 male births (5). Progressive muscle weakness starts to become noticeable during early childhood. Loss of ambulation usually occurs near the end of the first decade. Death due to respiratory and/or cardiac failure often happens by the end of the second decade. DMD is histologically characterized by progressive degeneration of muscle fibers. Although skeletal muscle weakness is the predominant symptom, cardiomyopathy is not uncommon and can be severe (6). In addition to muscle pathology, mental retardation of different degrees is present in about 30% of all DMD patients (7,8). Cardiomyopathy is also a predominant clinical problem in Becker muscular dystrophy (BMD), a milder variant of the DMD (9–11). Clinical manifestation includes weakness of proximal limb girdle muscles, hypertrophy of calf muscles, and high levels of serum creatine kinase in addition to cardiomyopathy (9–13). BMD patients are usually able to walk and have a normal life span.

DMD GENE

The gene responsible for DMD and BMD has been identified and its protein product is called dystrophin (14). Several isoforms of dystrophin have been identified (15). Three promoters located in the 5′ region of the dystrophin gene give rise to muscle type, brain type, and Purkinje-cell-type isoforms of the full-length transcription of a 14-kb mRNA (1). Each of these three promoters is linked to a unique first exon for transcription of each of the three different isoforms in a tissue-specific manner. In addition, alternatively spliced isoforms of the carboxyl-terminal (C-terminal) region of dystrophin have been identified in many other tissues (16,17). Another promoter located in the 5′ region of dystrophin gene, 750-kb upstream of the muscle promoter, is recently described and found to be active in lymphoblastoid cells (18).

Three promoters located at the 3′end of the dystrophin gene control expression of tissue-specific, alternative DMD gene products (16,17,19), including Dp140 expressed in the central nervous system, Dp116 expressed in Schwann cells of the peripheral nerves, and Dp71 expressed in many tissues such as smooth muscle, embryonic skeletal muscle, and cardiac muscle. A novel dystrophin isoform, Dp260, is recently identified in the retina and is likely driven by another promoter (20). In addition to this array of dystrophin isoforms, a homolog of dystrophin, dystrophin-related protein (DRP), or utrophin, is encoded by a gene on chromosome 6 (21,22). DRP is similar to dystrophin in both structure and amino acid sequence and is suggested to have a similar function. The presence of DRP at the neuromuscular junction indicates its potential role in synaptic formation and/or maintenance (21–23).

DYSTROPHIN

The muscle form of dystrophin is a 427-kDa protein (3685 amino acids in length) and is organized into four distinct structural domains. The N-terminal domain binds to actin and shows amino acid sequence similarity to the actin-binding domain of α-actinin. The next and the largest domain of dystrophin, approximately 3000 residues in length, comprises a repeating sequence of 109 amino acids that can be aligned with a consensus sequence of triple-helical repeats (106 amino acids) identified in spectrin. Dystrophin, like spectrin, probably has an elongated rod shape and may also be dimerized in an antiparallel fashion. This region of dystrophin also contains some proline-rich sequences that may lead to a breakdown in its repetitive, spectrin like organization. It has been postulated that these proline-rich "hinge" sequences may confer flexibility on the central, rodlike structure. The third domain is the cysteine-rich domain (Cys-rich), which is homologous to the C-terminal end of the slime mold α-actinin with two potential calcium binding sites. In fact, this domain of dystrophin does bind calcium in vitro when expressed in bacteria as a function protein (24). The C-terminal region of dystrophin consists of 325 amino acids. Many potential phosphorylation sites are found in the C-terminal region of dystrophin, which is recently shown to be a substrate of endogenous protein kinases (25–27).

DYSTROGLYCAN AND SARCOGLYCAN: THE DYSTROPHIN-ASSOCIATED PROTEINS

Dystrophin is a membrane cytoskeletal protein as based on its localization, biochemical properties, and structural similarities to other cytoskeletal proteins. In skeletal muscle, dystrophin is associated with a complex of membrane (glyco) proteins (156, 59, 50, 43, 35, and 25 kDa, respectively), originally referred to as dystrophin-associated proteins (DAP) (1,28–31). Tight association of this complex with dystrophin is demonstrated by their co-purification from rabbit skeletal muscle fiber membrane, co-sedimentation, immunoprecipitation, co-localization to muscle fiber sarcolemma, and protein cross-linking experiments. Figure 11–1 depicts the location of the DAP complex and other dystrophin-associated proteins.

There are five integral membrane proteins in the DAP complex: α-sarcoglycan (adhalin, 50 kDa), β-dystroglycan (43 kDa), β-sarcoglycan (43-kDa glycoprotein), γ-sarcoglycan (35-kDa glycoprotein), and 25-kDa protein (3,28,29) (Fig. 11–1). In addition, two peripheral membrane proteins belong to the complex: α-dystroglycan (156 kDa) and a syntrophin triplet (59 kDa) (see Fig. 11–1). Both α- and β-dystroglycans are derived from a common precursor protein (32).

The α-dystroglycan plays a critical role in connecting sarcolemma to the extracellular matrix by binding merosin, a muscle isoform of laminin, with high affinity and in a calcium-dependent manner (33–36). In muscle cells, dystrophin is linked to sarcolemma via interaction between its Cys-rich region and β-dystroglycan (33). A syntrophin triplet is also directly associated with dystrophin's C-terminal domain (residues 3447–3481) (Fig. 11–1) (32,33,37). Dystrophin's N-terminal domain binds to F-actin (38,39), providing a link between subsarcolemmal cytoskeleton and sarcolemma. Importantly, phosphorylation of dystrophin by cAMP-dependent protein kinase enhances its binding to actin (39), supporting the hypothesis (26) that phosphorylation of dystrophin may be crucial for the regulation of its interaction with other proteins. Figure 11–1 illustrates these findings, which together can be deemed to suggest that dystrophin has a structural role in skeletal muscle fibers, providing a mechanism for "anchoring" muscle cells to the extracelular matrix. The link between cytoskeletal protein and the extracellular

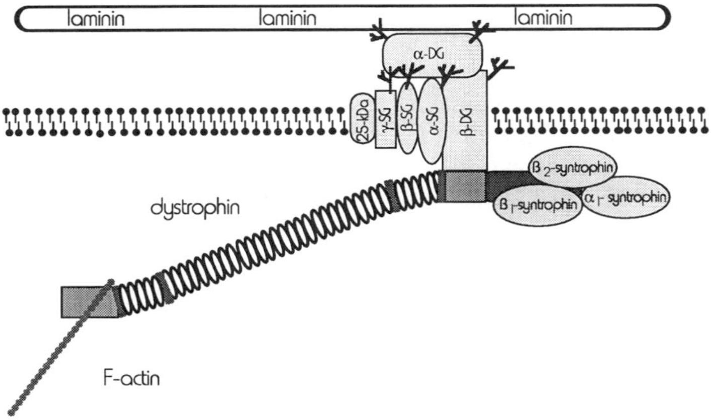

FIG. 11–1. Schematic illustration of dystrophin-glycoprotein complex. α-DG: α-dystroglycan (156 kDa); β-DG: β-dystroglycan (43 kDa); α-SG: α-sarcoglycan (adhalin, 50-kDa;); β-SG: β-sarcoglycan (43-kDa glycoprotein); γ-SG: γ-sarcoglycan (35-kDa glycoprotein). α-DG is associated with extracellular matrix protein laminin. Cysteine-rich region of dystrophin is associated with β-DG. N-terminal domain of dystrophin binds to F-actin.

matrix may stabilize muscle fiber membrane and protect it from the mechanical stress developed during muscle contraction.

Dystrophin normally resides in skeletal, cardiac, and smooth muscles and is also present in much lower amounts in the brain and peripheral nerves of several species (1,3,14,28,29,40–43). In both muscle and neuron, dystrophin is found in the plasma membrane (1,3,28,29,40–43) and is apparently enriched at the myotendinous junction and the postsynaptic membrane of the neuromuscular junctions (3,29). In DMD, dystrophin is absent from skeletal and cardiac muscles as revealed by both immunocytochemical and Western blot analysis of skeletal muscle biopsy (8,44,45). In 80% of BMD, dystrophin is expressed in mutant, truncated forms and is detected as a protein of smaller size on Western blots (46). The dystrophin gene in more than half of both DMD and BMD patients has partial deletions, with the majority of deletions occurring in a 2-kb region in the middle (47,48). Deletion size has no direct correlation with the clinical severity of the disease. Deletions of dystrophin gene in BMD, on the other hand, maintain the open reading frame for amino acid and are predicted to make shorter, lower-molecular-weight proteins with internal deletions. These smaller dystrophin gene products are presumably semifunctional and result in milder clinical phenotypes.

With few exceptions, deletions of both the N-terminal and C-terminal domains of dystrophin result in a more severe form of DMD (3,28,29). Quantities of the DAP complex are drastically reduced in DMD patients when dystrophin lacks the Cys-rich region and the C-terminal domains despite correct localization of the truncated dystrophin to the sarcolemma (3,28,29,42). Recently, two research groups have used transgenic *mdx* mice, which have a nonsense mutation in the dystrophin gene, resulting in absence of dystrophin to express variants of Dp71 (the truncated C-terminal region of dystrophin expressed primarily in nonmuscle tissues) under a muscle-specific promoter (49,50). Overexpression of Dp71 restores levels of the DAP complex to normal, suggesting that the C-terminal of dystrophin is critical for binding the DAP complex. However, the restored levels of the DAP complex in the transgenic *mdx* mouse fail to prevent muscle fibers from degeneration and necrosis. These results strongly suggest that association of dystrophin to cell membrane and extracellular matrix via its Cys-rich region may not be enough to exert its function. Dystrophin may function only when it is associated with both cytoskeletal actin and extracellular matrix proteins.

THE HEART

The majority of studies on dystrophin have focused on the understanding of its structure and function in skeletal muscle, probably because skeletal muscle is the most severely affected organ in DMD and BMD patients. Although respiratory failure is the most common cause of death in DMD patients, virtually every DMD patient eventually develops cardiomyopathy (51,52). Since the life span of DMD patients has significantly increased as a result of improved health management, cardiomyopathy has become an increasingly important cause of morbidity, responsible for 40% of deaths (53). In BMD patients, although skeletal muscle lesions are mild compared to those of DMD, severe cardiomyopathy may develop in the later stages of the disease in a large percentage of patients (11). Thus, understanding the function of dystrophin in cardiac muscle is equally important to that in skeletal muscle. Here we will focus on a possible role that dystrophin may play in physiology and pathophysiology of the heart.

DYSTROPHIN AND CARDIAC DEVELOPMENT

During development of cardiac muscle, dystrophin expression is regulated differently from that of skeletal muscle. During mouse embryogenesis, dystrophin is not detectable in heart before day 9, when cardiac muscle already contracts. Thereafter, the amount of dystrophin increases and reaches its maximal level by day 14 but wanes to a lower level after birth (54). Similarly, in developing rat myocardium, dystrophin is not detected immunohistochemically by day 15 (55), when the heart is able to beat spontaneously (56). By day 17, dystrophin starts to be expressed on the cell membrane of cardiac myocyte. These results are confirmed by Western blot analysis (55). In humans, the heart begins to beat by the twenty-sixth day of gestation (57), long before dystrophin is expressed at the sixth to eighth week of gestation (58). Because dystrophin is not expressed before contractile proteins (actin and myosin) are expressed and initiation of heartbeat, it is unlikely that dystrophin is necessary for the initial development and maintenance of myocardial function.

Dystrophin in mouse skeletal muscle is first detectable at nearly the same time as that in the heart during development (54). Expression of contractile proteins such as myosin heavy chain also begins at this time. The observation that expression of dystrophin starts at the same time or even precedes expression of contractile proteins suggests a crucial role of dystrophin for the initial development of the function of skeletal muscle fibers.

The amount of dystrophin in rat cardiac myocyte increases during the perinatal period, reaching its maximal level 2 weeks after birth (55). In humans, the amount of dystrophin also increases after its first appearance of 6–8 weeks of gestation (58). During the perinatal period, there are increases in contractile protein content, sarcoplasmic reticulum function (59–61), and membrane Ca^{2+} channel density (62). Consequently, there are increases in maximum heartbeat rate, contractile force, and velocity in the developing heart (61,63,64). In addition, sympathetic acceleration of the heart starts during the early neonatal period (63,65). All these changes enhance myocardial performance during the perinatal period. The developmental increase in dystrophin expression accompanies these changes, suggesting that dystrophin may be required in myocardia for rapid and powerful contraction.

LOCALIZATION OF DYSTROPHIN IN THE HEART

When dystrophin is first detected in cardiac myocytes, its immunoreactivity is diffuse, suggesting cytoplasmic localization, similar to that in skeletal muscle (57,66). With progression of development, dystrophin begins to distribute only in the inner surface of the cell membrane. The localization of dystrophin in skeletal muscle follows the same pattern as in cardiac muscle (58). In mature cardiac muscle, many studies have shown that dystrophin is localized entirely to the inner surface of the sarcolemma (45,55,67–69). Dystrophin in cardiac muscle is also associated with a group of membrane-associated glycoproteins as found in skeletal muscle (70,71), suggesting that dystrophin may function in a similar pattern in both types of muscles. In addition, dystrophin may be also present at the T-tubular membrane in cardiac myocyte. Some earlier experiments show that dystrophin is present only in the inner surface of sarcolemma in cardiac muscle, using antibodies against distal rod region of dystrophin but not in the T-tubular or the intercalated disk membrane (55,68,72), even with immunoelectron-microscopic localization (70). However, other studies show co-localization of dystrophin and dystrophin-related proteins not only in the free surface of sarcolemma but also in T-tubular membrane using polyclonal antibodies against the C-terminal region of dystrophin (71,73,74). It has been suggested that the additional staining by the C-terminal antibody used in these studies over that of the antibody against distal rod region of dystrophin used in earlier studies may be explained by the presence of a C-terminal transcript of dystrophin, Dp-71, which is normally present in cardiac muscle. Nonetheless, a recent study has confirmed the finding that muscle isoform of dystrophin is present in the T-tubular membrane in cardiac muscle using antibodies against the rod domain of dystrophin and Western blot analysis (75). The presence of dystrophin in T-tubular membrane suggests that dystrophin may function differently in cardiac muscle. The observation that dystrophin is absent from the membrane of intercalated disks is surprising because intercalated disks are force-transducing structures that are essentially membrane apposed Z-lines (76). If the function of dystrophin in cardiac muscle is the same as that proposed for skeletal muscle, dystrophin should be present in the intercalated disk of cardiac myocyte.

In the development of heart conduction systems, dystrophin first appears in the myocyte of the ventricle conduction system around the eighth week of gestation and is mainly distributed in the sarcoplasma of myocyte (77). Dystrophin starts to localize in the sarcolemma by the thirteenth week of gestation in myocytes of the ventricle conduction system. In adult, multiple dystrophin isoforms are found in cardiac Purkinje fibers (78), which are primarily localized in cell membrane. One of the dystrophin isoforms is found to be predominant in the brain (79,80). In the cardiac muscle of DMD patients, dystrophin is absent from the myocyte of conduction systems, which may be responsible for the observed cardiac conduction defects in DMD patients (78).

In addition to the muscle-specific isoform of dystrophin mentioned earlier, other types of dystrophin, including the brain type and Dp71, are normally present in cardiac muscle, though in much lower quantity (80–82).

CARDIOMYOPATHY IN DMD AND BMD PATIENTS

In DMD patients, dystrophin is completely absent from the surface membrane of cardiac myocyte (73) and Purkinje fibers (78). In BMD, dystrophin immunoreactivity is patchy and discontinuous inside the surface membrane (83–85), similar to that of skeletal muscle (73,85). This immunostaining pattern may result from the smaller size of dystrophin, which is too short to form continuous lattice network under the cell membrane (73,85). These dystrophin abnormalities are the primary cause of cardiomyopathy in DMD/BMD patients.

Pathologic basis of cardiac involvements in DMD and BMD lies in the occurrence of muscle fiber degeneration, necrosis, and interstitial fibrosis. Histochemical examination of cardiac biopsy often reveals degenerative changes in cardiac muscle fibers and small foci of fibrosis in ventricles, atria, and the specific conduction system (86–92). Muscle degeneration and fibrosis are most pronounced in the posterobasal region and the adjacent lateral wall of the left ventricle. Scarring of the posterobasal portion of the left ventricle is found in 90% of the DMD patients and results in a loss of posteriorly directed electrical current in the electrocardiogram (86,87).

One of the earliest and very sensitive indicators of myocardial involvement is alternations in electrocardiogram (ECG) (6,93). Preclinical cardiomyopathy is featured on ECG by shortened PQ segment (PQs), prolonged QT interval, and increased QT/PQ ratio (cardiomyopathy index) (89,93,94). In the early stage of clinically dilated cardiomyopathy, ECG shows a characteristic change consisting of tall right precordial R waves (R/S ratio greater than 1 in V1) and deep but narrow Q waves (greater than 3 mm) in the left precordial and limb leads, which is a result of fibrosis of the posterior and lateral wall of the left ventricle (86,87). This characteristic ECG change has been found in 90% of DMD patients (86,87). The epicardial half of the posterior wall is found to be the earliest site of myocardial involvement by both morphologic and metabolic analyses (88,93). Perfusion defect in cardiac muscle is very common in DMD, affecting as many as 96% of the patients (93,95). The perfusion defect, likely a result of cardiac muscle fibrosis, spreads from the lateral wall of the left ventricular to the anterior wall and/or interventricular septum (96). As the disease progresses, cardiac involvement becomes more generalized and dilated cardiomyopathy may eventually develop. Echocardiography is a useful method for providing information on ventricular size and function (86,97).

Abnormalities in heart rate, rhythm, and conduction can also be observed. The average pulse rate in DMD children after 5 years of age is much higher (100/min) than a corresponding value (77/min) in age-matched control children (86,89). A study of cardiac rhythm in DMD patients has shown persistent or labile sinus tachycardia, sinus arrhythmias, infrequent atrial ectopic beats, atrial ectopic rhythms, and ventricular premature complexes (93). In addition, abnormalities in cardiac conduction systems are found in about 50% of DMD patients. Intra-atrial conduction defects are common, infranodal conduction defects appear in 10% and more than one type of defects occur in one-third of the patients (89,93). Many rhythmic and conduction abnormalities of the heart observed in DMD are also present in BMD patients (98).

Cardiac involvement in DMD appears later in life than clinically apparent skeletal muscle damage and nearly inevitably starts as preclinical cardiomyopathy with symptoms or overt clinical signs (6). Subsequently, preclinical cardiomyopathy tends to evolve toward stages of clinically evident cardiac diseases that are more frequently represented by dilated cardiomyopathy. Among DMD patients, clinically apparent cardiomyopathy is first evident after 15 years of age and is present in all DMD patients older than 18 years of age (6). Cardiac involvement in BMD usually follows the same evolution as in DMD (11,90), but cardiomyopathy can sometimes appear as the first manifestation of the disease (7,8,99). Other forms of cardiomyopathy include hypertrophic cardiomyopathy and arrhythmogenic myocardial abnormality (11,98). Damage of the right ventricle is more often observed in young patients, while impairment of the left ventricle occurs in older patients (98). However, there is no correlation between the severity of cardiac involvement and the severity of skeletal muscle damage (11,98). Equal amounts of dystrophin are found in skeletal and cardiac muscles in normal individuals (8). Thus, it is difficult to comprehend why these two types of striated muscles, which seem to require the same amount of dystrophin for their normal functions, have such marked differences in their extent and onset of dysfunction in the absence of dystrophin.

Cardiac muscle is known to differ from skeletal muscle in many aspects. First, the manner of proliferation and differentiation during development is different. Cardiac muscle cells undergo proliferation and differentiation at the same time during early development. Skeletal muscle cells halt DNA replication and cell proliferation early in differentiation, and then fuse into multinucleated myotubes before initiating their terminal differentiation program (100). Second, cardiac myocytes are mononucleated and branched, while skeletal myocytes are multinucleated and linear. Third, skeletal muscle in adult has satellite cells that differentiate into myotubes and are able to regenerate after injury; on the other hand, adult cardiac myocytes are not thought to have any regenerative capacity (101). Last, connective tissue in cardiac muscle is different from that in skeletal muscle. Endomysium is the connective tissue between skeletal muscle fibers and contains very few cells and only trace amounts of collagen. In contrast, connective tissue in the heart is much more developed, containing more cells, extensive network of collagen fibers, fine microfibrils, and microthread, all of which may play important roles in force transmission (102).

These intrinsic differences between cardiac and skeletal muscles may be one of the factors responsible for the observed difference in their functional response to the absence of dystrophin. For example, it has been hypothesized that because of differences in the morphology of muscle fibers and the amount of connective tissue, forces produced by skeletal myocytes are almost entirely directed along their longitudinal axes, whereas forces produced by cardiac myocytes, though primarily axial, are more broadly distributed (103). It is therefore suggested that the degree of longitudinal axil stress may be positively correlated to the extent of muscle damage during contraction. Alternatively, dystrophin in cardiac muscle may play a different role from that in skeletal muscle, since dystrophin is absent from the intercalated disk and may be present in the T-tubule system in cardiac muscle.

CORRELATION BETWEEN DYSTROPHIN GENE DEFECT AND SEVERITY OF CARDIOMYOPATHY

Although cardiomyopathy frequently occurs in both DMD and BMD patients, associated with a spectrum of dystrophin gene deletions, no apparent relationship has been identified between the region of dystrophin gene deletion and the severity of cardiac involvement (90,104).

Clinically evident cardiomyopathy is, however, more frequently observed in both DMD and BMD patients when deletions involve exons 48–49 (105,106). High frequency of severe cardiomyopathy in both BMD and DMD patients is observed when deletions involve exons 48–49 as compared to other types of deletions (106). In agreement, exon 49 deletion is found to be invariably associated with cardiac involvement and exon 48 deletion relates to cardiomyopathy in most of the BMD patients (98). Deletion of exons 45–48 also leads to severe dilated cardiomyopathy, with very mild involvement of skeletal muscle (107). It is, therefore, hypothesized that a regulatory function may be present in genomic region encompassing exons 48–49 or in an adjacent region that is removed together with these exons (106).

Deletions in other regions of the dystrophin gene, nonetheless, also cause severe cardiomyopathy (106,108,109). Deletion at exon 1 has been reported to result in fatal cardiomyopathy despite the absence of significant skeletal muscle weakness (110). In addition, predominant cardiomyopathy has been observed in BMD patients with deletions of exon 45–47 (109,111). More recently, a male patient 14 years of age who died of dilated cardiomyopathy with very mild signs of skeletal muscle involvement was linked to dystrophin gene deletion at the N-terminal region (112). In the skeletal muscle of this patient, a smaller dystrophin that lacks the N-terminal region of the protein is detected using immunohistochemical staining and Western blotting analysis. PCR reaction reveals a deletion of the dystrophin gene from exons 6 to 13. Thus, a deletion in the dystrophin gene has shortened the dystrophin protein by removing a segment near its N-terminal region. Because the patient shows very little skeletal muscle involvement but severe cardiomyopathy, it is suggested that the deleted region of dystrophin may be more important for cardiac function than for the function of skeletal muscle. However, the definite cause of cardiomyopathy in this patient cannot be determined because the protein expression in cardiac muscle was not assessed.

Based on these observations, it is very difficult at this stage to draw any conclusion about the correlation between cardiomyopathy and the region of gene deletion. It seems that deletions at many different regions of dystrophin gene can lead to cardiomyopathy, although cardiomyopathy is more often associated with deletions in 48 and 49 of dystrophin gene due to unknown reasons.

DYSTROPHIN DEFICIENCY AND X-LINKED DILATED CARDIOMYOPATHY

X-linked dilated cardiomyopathy (XLDCM) is an X-chromosome-linked dominant disorder with symptoms of congestive heart failure, cardiomegaly, pulmonary edema, and ventricular dilation (113). In males, it occurs in early age, ranging from late teens to early 20s, and progresses rapidly, with death due to heart failure within 1–2 years. In manifesting female carriers, the disease is usually milder and has a much later onset, usually in the fifth decade of life. The progression of the disease is also much slower. Skeletal muscle myopathy is absent in these patients. However, almost all patients have elevated muscle creatine kinase.

A recent study of two pedigrees has mapped the gene responsible for XLDCM to the 5′ region of the dystrophin gene at Xp21.2 locus. XLDCM in these two families is associated with a cardiac dystrophin defect in its N-terminal region (114). The amount of dystrophin is significantly reduced in cardiac muscle of these patients. In contrast, dystrophin is present in normal quantities in skeletal muscles and patients are devoid of skeletal muscle pathology. It is suggested that the disease may be due to (a) mutation in the 5′ region of the dystrophin gene-coding regions preferentially affecting cardiac function, (b) mutation of an unknown cardiac promoter that affects expression of dystrophin specifically in cardiac muscle, and (c) abnormal splicing of the dystrophin gene resulting in a nonfunctional protein in cardiac muscle. However, because the type of mutation in dystrophin gene is not identified in this study, the cause for the selective reduction of dystrophin in cardiac muscle remains unknown. It appears, therefore, that XLDCM is an extreme form of BMD in which only cardiac muscle is affected. However, the question remains why mutations of dystrophin gene result in severe cardiomyopathy, but it has no detrimental effect on the skeletal muscle.

In one-X-linked pedigree, a deletion leading to removal of the dystrophin muscle promoter region, including the first muscle exon and part of intron 1, causes dilated cardiomyopathy without muscle weakness (115). Dystrophin, however, is present in normal amounts in skeletal muscle. In addition, normal expression and localization of dystrophin associated proteins are found in skeletal muscle. Transcription experiments show that dystrophin present in skeletal muscle is not the muscle-specific isoform. Instead, it originates from the brain and Purkinje cell isoforms that are upregulated in skeletal muscle (116). In contrast to skeletal muscle, dystrophin gene transcription and expression are absent in the heart with the exception of the distal Dp71 dystrophin isoform that is normally present in the heart (117). Also, the 43- and 50-kDa dystrophin-associated proteins (α-sarcoglycan and β-sarcoglycan) are severely reduced in the heart despite the presence of Dp71. Thus, absence of dystrophin and severe reduction in two dystrophin-associated proteins are suggested to be responsible for severe cardiomyopathy. Lack of skeletal muscle involvement in this patient is likely due to compensatory expression of dystrophin isoforms that are normally expressed in brain and Purkinje cells, which are able to functionally replace the muscle-type dystrophin in skeletal muscle. However, it is not known why deletions in this region specifically compromise the expression of other major dystrophin isoforms in addition to the muscle isoform in cardiac muscle. It has been suggested that different transcriptional "pathways" may be responsible for dystrophin expression in skeletal muscle and the heart; deletion in the muscle promoter region may specifically remove the cardiac-specific regulatory sequence (117).

SUMMARY

Dystrophin is normally localized in the inner surface of sarcolemma and in cardiac myocyte and Purkinje cells as well as T-tubular membrane but absent from the intercalated disk between cardiac myocytes. It is absent in the cardiac muscle of DMD patients and present in smaller size in BMD patients. The defect of dystrophin in cardiac muscle leads to many different phenotypes of cardiomyopathy, ranging from nonsymptomatic preclinical cardiac involvement to fatal dilated cardiomyopathy. Cardiac involvement usually evolves with age and progression of the pathology in both DMD and BMD patients. There is no positive correlation between the degree of skeletal muscle damage and the severity of cardiomyopathy, nor is there an obvious relationship between the region of dystrophin gene deletion and the severity of cardiomyopathy.

ACKNOWLEDGMENT

The work was supported by the Muscular Dystrophy Association of Canada.

REFERENCES

1. Fabbrizio E, Pons F, Robert A, Hugon G, Bonet-Kerrache A, Monret D. The dystrophin superfamily: variability and complexity. *J Muscle Res Cell Motility* 1994;15:595–606.
2. Matsumura K, Campbell KP. Dystrophin-glycoprotein complex: its role in the molecular pathogenesis of muscular dystrophies. *Muscle Nerve* 1994;17:2–15.
3. Tinsley JM, Blake DJ, Zuelling RA, Davies KE: Increasing complexity of the dystrophin-associated protein complex. *Proc Natl Acad Sci USA* 1994;91:8307–8313.
4. Worton R. Muscular dystrophies: diseases of the dystrophin-glycoprotein complex. *Science* 1995; 270:755–756.

5. Emery AEH. *Duchenne muscular dystrophy.* 2nd ed. New York: Oxford University Press; 1988:1–137.
6. Nigro G, Comi L, Politano L, Bain R: The incidence and evolution of cardiomyopathy in Duchenne muscular dystrophy. *Int J Cardiol* 1990;26:271–277.
7. Moser H. Duchenne muscular dystrophy: pathogenetic aspects and genetic prevention. *Hum Genet* 1984;66:17–40.
8. Hoffmann EP, Hudecki MS, Rosenberg PA, Pollina CA, Kunkel LM. Cell and fibre-type distribution of dystrophin. *Neuron* 1988;1:411–420.
9. Sakata C, Yamada H, Sunohara N, Arahata K, Nonaka I. Cardiomyopathy in Becker muscular dystrophy. *Rinsho Shinkeigaku* 1990;30:952–955.
10. De Vissier M, De Voogt W, Riviere GV. The heart in Becker muscular dystrophy, facioscapulohumeral dystrophy, and Bethlem myopathy. *Muscle Nerve* 1992;15:591–596.
11. Nigro G, Comi L, Politano L, et al. Evaluation of the cardiomyopathy in Becker muscular dystrophy. *Muscle Nerve* 1995;18:283–291.
12. Emery AEH, Dreifuss FE. Unusual type of benign X-linked muscular dystrophy. *J Neurol Neurosurg Psychiatry* 1966;29:338–342.
13. Ringel SP, Carroll JE, Schold SC. The spectrum of mild X-linked recessive muscular dystrophy. *Arch Neurol* 1977;34:408–416.
14. Worton RG, Thompson MW. Genetics of Duchenne muscular dystrophy. *Annu Rev Genet* 1988; 22:601–629.
15. Ahn AH, Kunkel LM. The structural and functional diversity of dystrophin. *Nature Genet* 1993; 3:283–291.
16. Fabbrizio E, Nude U, Hugon G, Robert A, Pones E, Mornet D. Characterisation and localisation of a 77 kDa protein related to the dystrophin gene family. *Biochem J* 1994;299:359–365.
17. Lidov HGW, Selig S, Kunkel LM. 1995. Dp140: a novel 140 kDa CNS transcript from the dystrophin locus. *Hum Mol Genet* 1995;4:329–335.
18. Nishio H, Takeshima Y, Narita N, et al. Identification of a novel first exon in the human dystrophin gene and of a new promoter located more than 500 kb upstream of the nearest known promoter. *J Clin Invest* 1994;94:1037–1042.
19. Byers TJ, Lidov HGW, Kunkel LM. An alternative dystrophin transcript specific to peripheral nerve. *Nature Genet* 1993;4:77–81.
20. D'Souza VN, Thi Man N, Morris GE, Karges W, Pillers DM, Ray P. A novel dystrophin isoform is required for normal retinal electrophysiology. *Hum Mol Genet* 1995;4:837–842.
21. Love DR, Hill DF, Dickson G, et al. An autosomal transcript in skeletal muscle with homology to dystrophin. *Nature* 1989;339:55–58.
22. Khurana TS, Hoffman EP, Kunkel LM. Identification of a chromosome 6-encoded dystrophin-related protein. *J Biol Chem* 1990;265:16717–16720.
23. Campanelli J, Roberds S, Campbell K, Scheller R. A role for dystrophin-associated glycoproteins and utrophin in agrin-induced AchR clustering. *Cell* 1994;77:663–674.
24. Milner RE, Busaan JL, Michalak M. Isolation and characterization of different C-terminal fragments of dystrophin expressed in *Escherichia coli. Biochem J* 1992;288:1037–1044.
25. Luise M, Presotto C, Senter L, et al. Dystrophin is phosphorylated by endogenous protein kinases. *Biochem J* 1993;293:243–247.
26. Milner RE, Bussan JL, Holmes CFB, Wang JG, Michalak M. Phosphorylation of dystrophin. The carboxyl-terminal region of dystrophin is a substrate for in vitro phosphorylation by $p34^{cdc2}$ protein kinase. *J Biol Chem* 1993;268:21901–21905.
27. Madhaven R, Jarrett HW. Calmodulin-activated phosphorylation of dystrophin. *Biochemistry* 1995;33:5797–5804.
28. Monaco AO, Kunkel LM. Cloning of the Duchenne/Becker muscular dystrophy locus. *Adv Hum Genet* 1988;17:61–98.
29. Hoffman EP, Schwartz L. Dystrophin and disease. *Mol Aspects Med* 1991;2:175–194.
30. Ervasti JM, Ohlendieck K, Kahl SD, Campbell KP. Deficiency of glycoprotein components of dystrophin complex in dystrophic muscle. *Nature* 1990;345:315–319.
31. Ervasti JM, Campbell KP. Membrane organization of the dystrophin-glycoprotein complex. *Cell* 1991;66:1121–1131.
32. Ibraghimov-Beskrovnaya O, Ervasti JM, Leveille CJ, Slaughter CA, Sernett SW, Campbell KP. Primary structure of dystrophin-associated glycoproteins linking dystrophin to the extracellular matrix. *Nature* 1992;355:696–702.
33. Suzuki A, Yoshida M, Hasyashi K, Mizuno Y, Hagiwara Y, Ozawa E. Molecular organization at the glycoprotein-complex-binding site of dystrophin. *Eur J Biochem* 1994;220:283–292.

34. Gee SH, Blacher RW, Douville PJ, Provost PR, Urchenco PD, Carbonetto S. Laminin-binding protein 120 from brain is closely related to the dystrophin-associated glycoprotein, dystroglycan, and binds with high affinity to the major heparin binding domain of laminin. *J Biol Chem* 1993; 268:14972–14980.
35. Sunada Y, Bernier SM, Kozak CA, Yamada Y, Campbell KP. Deficiency of merosin in dystrophic *dy* mice and genetic linkage of laminin M chain gene to *dy* locus. *J Biol Chem* 1994;269: 13729–13732.
36. Ervasti JM, Campbell KP. A role for the dystrophin-glycoprotein complex as a transmembrane linker between laminin and actin. *J Cell Biol* 1993;122:809–823.
37. Yang B, Jung D, Rafael JA, Chamberlain JS, Campbell KP. Identification of α-syntrophin binding to syntrophin triplet, dystrophin, and utrophin. *J Biol Chem* 1995;270:4975–4978.
38. Jarrett HW, Foster JL. Alternate binding of actin and calmodulin to multiple sites on dystrophin. *J Biol Chem* 1995;270:5578–5586.
39. Senter L, Ceoldo S, Meznaric Petrusa M, Salviati G. Phosphorylation of dystrophin: effects on actin binding. *Biochem Biophys Res Commun* 1995;206:57–63.
40. Anderson MS, Kunkel LM. The molecular and biochemical basis of Duchenne muscular dystrophy. *Trends in Biochem Sci* 1992;17:289–292.
41. Hoffman EP, Kunkel LM. Dystrophin abnormalities in Duchenne/Becker muscular dystrophy. *Neuron* 1989;2:1019–1029.
42. Hoffman EP. 1994. Dystrophin associated proteins fail in filling dystrophin's shoes. *Nature Genet* 8:311–312.
43. Boyce FM, Beggs AH, Kunkel LM. Muscular dystrophy research: what have we learned and where do we go from here? In: McHugh PR, McKusick VA, eds. *Genes, brain, and behavior.* New York: Raven Press; 1991:121–127.
44. Patel K, Voit T, Dunn MJ, Strong PN, Dubowitz V. Dystrophin and nebulin in the muscular dystrophies. *J Neurol Sci* 1988;87:315–326.
45. Arahata K, Ishihara T, Kamakura K, et al. Dystrophin and Duchenne's muscular dystrophy. *Nature* 1989;321:398–399.
46. Hoffman EP, Fischbeck K, Brown RH, et al. Characterization of dystrophin in muscle-biopsy specimens from patients with Duchenne's muscular dystrophy. *N Engl J Med* 1988;318:1363–1368.
47. Koenig M, Hoffman EP, Bertelson CJ, Monaco AP, Feener C, Kunkel LM. Complete cloning of the Duchenne muscular dystrophy (DMD) cDNA and preliminary genomic organization of the DMD gene in normal and affected. *Cell* 1987;50:509–517.
48. Forrest SM, Cross GS, Flint T, Speer A, Robson KJH, Davis KE. Further studies of gene deletions that cause Duchenne and Becker muscular dystrophies. *Genomics* 1988;2:109–114.
49. Cox GA, Sunada Y, Campbell KP, Chamberlain JS. Dp71 can restore the dystrophin-associated glycoprotein complex in muscle but fails to prevent dystrophy. *Nature Genet* 1994;8:333–339.
50. Greenberg DS, Sunada Y, Campbell KP, Yaffe D, Nudel U. Exogenous Dp71 restores the levels of dystrophin associated proteins but does not alleviate muscle damage in *mdx* mice. *Nature Genet* 1994;8:340–344.
51. Tanaka H, Nishi S, Katanasako H. Natural course of cardiac myopathy in Duchenne muscular dystrophy. *Jpn Circ J* 1979;43:974–984.
52. Nigro G, Comi LI, Politano L, Bain RJI. The incidence and evolution of cardiomyopathy in Duchenne muscular dystrophy. *Int J Cardiol* 1990;26:271–277.
53. Mukoyama M, Kondo K, Hizawa K, Nishitani H. Life span of Duchenne muscular dystrophy patients in the hospital care program in Japan. *J Neurol Sci* 1987;81:155–158.
54. Houzelstein D, Lyons GE, Chamberlain JK, Buckingham ME. Localisation of dystrophin gene transcripts during mouse embryogenesis. *J Cell Biol* 1992;119:811–821.
55. Tanaka H, Ozawa E. Expression of dystrophin mRNA and the protein in the developing rat heart. *Biochem Biophys Res Commun* 1990;172:824–829.
56. Bernard C. Establishment of ionic permeabilities of the myocardial membrane during embryonic development of the rat. In: Liebermann M, Sano T, eds. *Developmental and physiological correlates of cardiac muscle.* New York: Raven Press; 1976:169–184.
57. O'Rahilly R, Muller F. *Developmental stages in human embryos.* Carnegie Institution of Washington, 1987.
58. Chevron MP, Cirard F, Claustres M, Demaille J. Expression and subcellular localization of dystrophin in skeletal, cardiac and smooth muscles during the human development. *Neuromuscul Disord* 1994;4:419–432.

59. Hirakow R, Gotoh T. A quantitative and ultrastructural study on the developing rat heart. In: Liebermann M, Sano T, eds. *Developmental and physiological correlates of cardiac muscle.* New York: Raven Press; 1975:37–49.
60. Hirakow R, Gotoh T, Watanabe T. Quantitative studies on the ultrastructural differentiation and growth of mammalian cardiac muscle. *Acta Anat (Basel)* 1980;108:144–152.
61. Tanaka H, Shigenobu K. Effect of ryanodine on neonatal and adult rat heart: developmental increase in sarcoplasmic reticulum function. *J Mol Cell Cardiol* 1989;21:1305–1313.
62. Kojima M, Ishima T, Taniguchi N, Kimura K, Sada H, Sprerelakis N. Developmental changes in beta-adrenoceptors, muscarinic cholinoceptors and Ca^{2+} channels in rat ventricular muscles. *Br J Pharmacol* 1990;99:334–339.
63. Tucker DC, Johnson AK. Development of autonomic control of heart rate in genetically hypertensive and normotensive rats. *Am J Physiol* 1984;246:R570.
64. Shigenobu K, Tanaka H, Kasyta Y. Changes in sensitivity of rat heart of norepinephrine and isoproterenol during pre- and postnatal development and its relation to sympathetic innervation. *Dev Pharmacol Ther* 1988;11:226–236.
65. Seidler FJ, Slotkin TA. Presynaptic and postsynaptic contributions to ontogeny of synaptic control of heart rate in the preweanling rat. *Br J Pharmacol* 1979;65:431–434.
66. Wessels A, Ginjaar IB, Moorman AFM, Van Ommen GJB. Different localisation of dystrophin in developing and adults human muscle. *Muscle Nerve* 1991;14:1–7.
67. Arahata K, Hoffman EP, Kunkel LM, et al. Dystrophin diagnosis: comparison of dystrophin abnormalities by immunofluorescence and immunoblot analysis *Proc Natl Acad USA* 1989;86:7154–7158.
68. Uchino M, Araki S, Mike T, Teramoto H, Nakamura T, Yasutake T. Localization and characterization of dystrophin in muscle biopsy specimens from Duchenne muscular dystrophy and various neuromuscular disorders. *Muscle Nerve* 1989;12:1009–1016.
69. Byers TJ, Kundel LM, Watkins SC. The subcellular distribution of dystrophin in mouse skeletal, cardiac and smooth muscle. *J Cell Biol* 1991;115:411–421.
70. Matsumura K, Ervasti JM, Ohlendieck K, Kahl SD, Campbell K. Association of dystrophin-related protein with dystrophin-associated proteins in *mdx* mouse muscle. *Nature* 1992;360:588–591.
71. Klietsch R, Ervasti JM, Arnold W, Campbell KP, Jorgensen AO. Dystrophin-glycoprotein complex and laminin colocalize to the sarcolemma and transverse tubules of cardiac muscle. *Circ Res* 1993;72:349–360.
72. Arahata K, Ishiura S, Ishiguro T, et al. Immunostaining of skeletal and cardiac muscle surface membrane with antibody against Duchenne muscular dystrophy peptide. *Nature* 1988;333:861–866.
73. Frank JS, Mottino G, Chen F, Peri V, Holland P, Tuana BS. Subcellular distribution of dystrophin in isolated adult and neonatal cardiac myocytes. *Am J Physiol* 1994;C1707–C1716.
74. Roberds SL, Ervasti JM, Anderson RD, et al. Disruption of the dystrophin-glycoprotein complex in the cardiomyopathic Hamster. *J Biol Chem* 1993;268:11496–11499.
75. Pons F, Robert A, Fabbrizio E, et al. Untrophin localization in normal and dystrophin-deficient heart. *Circulation* 1994;90:369–374.
76. Junquiera LC, Carniero J, Long JA, eds. *Muscle tissue in basic histology.* Norwalk, CT: Appleton-Century-Crofts; 1986:5:234–254.
77. Ginjaar IB, Vragh S, Markman MWM, van Ommen GJB, Moorman AFM. Dystrophin expression in the developing conduction system of the human heart. *Microsc Res Tech* 1995;30:458–468.
78. Bies RD, Freidman D, Roberts R, Perryman MB, Caskey CT. Expression and localization of dystrophin in human cardiac Purkinje fibers. *Circulation* 1992;86:147–153.
79. Feener CA, Koenig M, Kunkel LM. Alternative splicing of human dystrophin mRNA generates isoforms at the carboxyl terminus. *Nature* 1989;338:509–511.
80. Bies RD, Phelps SF, Cortez MD, Roberts R, Caskey CT, Chamberlain JS. Human and murine dystrophin mRNA transcripts are differentially expressed during skeletal muscle, heart and brain development. *Nucleic Acids Res* 1992;20:1725–1731.
81. Muntoni F, Melis MA, Granau A, Dubowitz. Transcription of the dystrophin gene in normal tissue and in skeletal muscle of a family with X-linked dilated cardiomyopathy. *Am J Hum Genet* 1995;56:151–157.
82. Fabbrizio E, Harricane MC, Pons F, Leger J, Mornet D. Properties of chicken cardiac dystrophin. *Biol Cell* 1992;6:167–174.
83. Anan R, Higuchi I, Ichinari K, et al. Myocardial patchy staining of dystrophin in Becker's muscular dystrophy associated with cardiomyopathy. *Am Heart J* 1992;123:1088–1089.
84. Schmidt-Achert M, Fisher P, Pongratz D. Myocardial evidence of dystrophin mosaic in a Duchenne muscular dystrophy carrier. *Lancet* 1992;340:1235–1236.

85. Maeda M, Nakao S, Miyazata H, et al. Cardiac dystrophin abnormalities in Becker muscular dystrophy assessed by endomyocardial biopsy. *Am Heart J* 1995;129:702–707.
86. Farah MG, Evans EB, Vignos PJ. Echocardiographic evaluation of left ventricular function in Duchenne's muscular dystrophy. *Am J Med* 1980;69:248.
87. Perloff JK, Roberts WC, de Leon AC, O'Doherty D. The distinctive electrocardiogram of Duchenne's progressive muscular dystrophy: an electrocardiographic-pathologic correlative study. *Am J Med* 1967;42:179.
88. Sanyal SK, Johnson WW, Thaper MK, Pitner SE. An ultrastructural baiss for electrocardiographic alterations associated with Duchenne's progressive muscular dystrophy. *Circulation* 1978;57:1122.
89. Sanyal SK, Johnson WW. Cardiac conduction abnormalities in children with Duchenne's progressive muscular dystrophy: electrocardiographic features and morphologic correlates. *Circulation* 1982;66:863.
90. Steare SE, Dubowitz V, Benatar A. Subclinical cardiomyopathy in Becker muscular dystrophy. *Br Heart J* 1992;68:304–308.
91. Perloff JK. Neurological disorders and heart disease. In: Braunwald E, ed. *Heart disease.* Philadelphia: WB Saunders; 1988:1782–1786.
92. Nomura H, Hizawa K. Histopathological study of the conduction system of the heart in Duchenne progressive muscular dystrophy. *Acta Pathol Jpn* 1982;32:1027–1032.
93. Perloff JK. Cardiac rhythm and conduction in Duchenne's muscular dystrophy: a prospective study of 20 patients. *J Am Coll Cardiol* 1984;3:1263–1268.
94. Nigro G, Comi LI, Politano L, et al. Electrocardiographic evaluation of the P-type stage of dystrophic cardiomyopathy. *Cardiomyology* 1984;3:45–58.
95. Yamamoto S, Matsushima H, Suzuki A, Sotobata I, Indo T, Matsuoka Y. A comparative study of thallium-201 single-photon emission computed tomography and electrocardiography in Duchenne and other types of muscular dystrophy. *Am J Cardiol* 1988;61:836–843.
96. Tamura T, Shibuya N, Hashiba K, Oku Y, Mori H, Yano K. Evaluation of myocardial damage in Duchenne's muscular dystrophy with thallium-201 myocardial SPECT. *Jpn Heart J* 1992;34:51–61.
97. Hunsaker RH, Fulkerson PK, Barry FJ, Lewis RP, Leier CV, Unverferth DV. Cardiac function in Duchenne's muscular dystrophy: results of 10-year follow-up study and noninvasive tests. *Am J Med* 1982;73:235–238.
98. Melacini P, Fanin M, Danieli GA, et al. Cardiac involvement in Becker muscular dystrophy. *J Am Coll Cardiol* 1993;22:1927–1934.
99. Yazawa M, Ikeda S, Owa M, et al. A family of Becker's progressive muscular dystrophy with severe cardiomyopathy. *Eur Neurol* 1987;27:13–19.
100. Claycomb WC, Lanson NA Jr. Proto-oncogene expression in proliferating and differentiating cardiac and skeletal muscle. *Biochem J* 1987;247:701–706.
101. Kardami E. Stimulation and inhibition of cardiac myocyte proliferation in vitro. *Mol Cell Biochem* 1990;92:129–135.
102. Braunwald E, Sonnenblick EH, Ross J Jr. Mechanisms of cardiac contraction and relaxation. In: Braunwald E, ed. *Heart disease: a textbook of cardiovascular medicine.* Philadelphia: WB Saunders; 1988:385.
103. Cziner DG, Levin RI. The cardiomyopathy of Duchenne's muscular dystrophy and the function of dystrophin. *Med Hypotheses* 1993;40:169–174.
104. Beggs AH, Hoffman EP, Snyder JR, et al. Exploring the molecular basis for variability among patients with Becker muscular dystrophy: dystrophin gene and protein studies. *Am J Hum Genet* 1991;49:54–67.
105. Politano L, Colonna Romano S, Esposito MG, et al. Genotype-phenotype correlation in patients with deletion of Duchenne/Becker gene. *Acta Cardiomiol* 1991,III;2:239–244.
106. Nigro G, Politano L, Nigro V, Petretta VR, Comi LI. Mutation of dystrophin gene and cardiomyopathy. *Neuromuscul Disord* 1994;4:371–379.
107. Siciliano G, Fanin M, Angelini G, et al. Prevalent cardiac involvement in dystrophin Becker type mutation. *Neuromuscul Disord* 1994;4:381–386.
108. Gold R, Kress W, Meuers B, Meng G, Reichmann H, Muller CR. Brief communication. Becker muscular dystrophy: detection of unusual disease course by combined approach to dystrophin analysis. *Muscle Nerve* 1992;15:214–216.
109. Bushby KMD, Gardner-Medwin D, Nicholson LVB, et al. The clinical, genetic and dystrophin characteristics of Becker muscular dystrophy. II. Correlation of phenotype with genetic and protein abnormalities. *J Neurol* 1993;240:105–112.

110. Yoshida K, Ikeda S, Kakamura A, et al. Molecular analysis of Duchenne muscular dystrophy gene in patients with Becker muscular dystrophy presenting with dilated cardiomyopathy. *Muscle Nerve* 1993;16:1161–1166.
111. Palmucci L, Doriguzzi C, Mongini T, et al. Dilating cardiomyopathy as the expression of Xp21 Becker type muscular dystrophy. *J Neurol Sci* 1992;111:218–221.
112. Oldfors A, Eriksson BO, Kyllerman M, Martinsson T, Wahlström J. Dilated cardiomyopathy and dystrophin gene: an illustrated review. *Br Heart J* 1994;72:344–348.
113. Berko BA, Swift M. X-linked dilated cardiomyopathy. *N Engl J Med* 1987;316:1186–1191.
114. Towbin JA, Hejtmancik JF, Brink P, et al. X-linked dilated cardiomyopathy-molecular genetic evidence of linkage to the Duchenne muscular dystrophy (dystrophin) gene at the Xp21 locus. *Circulation* 1993;87:1854–1865.
115. Muntoni F, Cau M, Congiu R, et al. Deletions of dystrophin muscle-promoter region associated with X-linked dilated cardiomyopathy. *N Engl J Med* 1993;329:921–925.
116. Muntoni F, Melis MA, Ganau A, Dubowitz V. Transcription of the dystrophin gene in normal tissues and in skeletal muscle of a family with X-linked dilated cardiomyopathy. *Am J Hum Genet* 1995;56:151–157.
117. Muntoni F, Wilson L, Marrosu G, et al. A mutation in the dystrophin gene selectively affecting dystrophin expression in the heart. *J Clin Invest* 1995;96:693–699.

The Developing Heart,
edited by Bohuslav Ošťádal et al.
Lippincott-Raven Publishers,
Philadelphia © 1997.

12

Basement Membrane–Associated Proteins During the Development of the Myocardium

Jane-Lyse Samuel and Lydie Rappaport

INSERM U127, IFR Circulation, Université D. Diderot, 75010 Paris, France

Extracellular matrix (ECM) and basement membrane (BM) components are essential for morphogenesis. ECM interacts with cell surface by binding to specific receptors, integrins, and dystroglycans. BM constitutes the substrate for cell migration and is required for the polarization of cells. The ECM–cell interactions initiate a flow of information that regulates fundamental processes that modulate growth, differentiation programs, and cell migration (1).

The role of FN in anchoring cells to the ECM depends on the multiple ligand domains of the protein with components of both the ECM and the basement membrane (laminin and collagen type IV mainly) and with cell transmembrane receptors, such as integrins. These transmembrane receptors, when stimulated by interactions with FN or proteins of the basement membrane, connect the ECM and the cytoskeleton, the cellular architecture upon which biochemical signal transduction pathways are overlaid (2).

The aim of this review was to analyze the expression of some of these proteins in the cardiovascular system and its regulation during development of the heart. In the heart, FN and the collagens are synthetized by smooth muscle cells and fibroblasts (3,4), whereas laminin is synthetized and secreted by the contractiles cells. Both laminin and fibronectin have been implicated in embryogenesis and tissue differentiation (3,5–7).

FIBRONECTIN, COLLAGENS, AND LAMININ

1-Fibronectin is a heterodimer expressed by a single gene. It exists as a soluble form, which polymerizes when exsudated from the plasma and as a cellular form secreted *in situ* by numerous cell types.

Multiple FN isoforms differ by their primary structure secondary to posttranscriptional modifications and by alternative processing of a common RNA precursor. The splicing is cell specific. FN-EIIIA and -EIIIB exons are facultative, and type III homology regulating processing is likely to involve different mechanisms (8). Fibronectin is expressed in a highly specific fashion during embryogenesis (6,9,10). FN mRNA splicing is developmentally regulated (11), and tissue-specific alternative splicing of the primary transcript may constitute an important mechanism of genetic regulation during development, as it has been proposed for other genes (12). Indeed, the two exons coding for the FN-EIIIA and -EIIIB domains are coexpressed in the early embryo and are spliced out in a tissue-specific manner after the completion of embryogenesis and organogenesis (10,11,13,14). The regulated expression of fibronectin together with the ability of the protein to affect cell adhesion (15), migration, and cytodifferentiation in vitro suggest that fibronectin is implicated in organogenesis (5,16,17). According to Armstrong and Armstrong (18), the composition of the interstitial matrix exerts an important influence on the mutual organization of mesenchymal tissues and their adjacent tissues; tissue segregation is promoted if the mesenchyme contains a well-developed adhesive interstitial matrix, whereas a poor development of that matrix establishes conditions that favor tissue invasion.

In the rat fetal heart, fibronectin is present whatever the age of the fetus and distributed in a reticular pattern suggestive of a pericellular or interstitial localization (7). Fibronectin, which is synthetized predominantly by cardiac mesenchymal cells, is particularly abundant at the crest of the developing interventricular septum. It has been implicated in the regulation of precardiac cell migration and epithelial–mesenchymal transformation and thus in the formation of the heart tube, as well as in the remodeling of the heart tube into a multichambered organ (19,20). In the developing mouse heart at days 11 and 13 in utero, pFN is present in the outflow tract and in the outer layer of the visceral pericardium (19). Recently, we analyzed precisely the temporal pattern of the fibronectin expression during cardiac development in the rat (21,22), and showed: (a) a progressive decrease in the amount of total FN mRNA and (b) a parallel and harmonious decrease in the percentage in FN mRNA containing EIIIA or EIIIB exons. Taken together these data indicate that the coupling of EIIIA and EIIIB splicing is independent of fibronectin mRNA accumulation during normal cardiac development (21). Qualitative and spatial analyses reveal that at 11 days post coïtum (pc), FN mRNA is highly expressed in the entire heart tube; later, the hybridization signal progressively decreases, FN-mRNA being absent from the differentiated myocardium but highly expressed in the pericardium and the ventricular trabeculae area rich in nonmuscle cells. The cardiac distributions of FN mRNA, whether or not they contain EIIIA and/or EIIIB exons, are identical, indicating that there is no preferential splicing in specific areas of the developing myocardium (22). Furthermore, c-FN protein is undetectable by immunolabeling, suggesting that during this period the protein is poorly synthesized or secreted. Thus, c-FN does not play a major role during cardiac differentiation (22). Just before birth, when the coronary vessels are well developed (23), both FN mRNA and protein are expressed throughout the coronary artery wall. In the adult, FN mRNA is no more detectable but c-FNprotein is present in the basal lamina of the endothelium (4,22,24). Thus, after an initial high level of coexpression in the cardiac tube, each FN transcript decreases progressively according to the same pattern, suggesting a single cell-specific and stage-specific coordinated regulation of FN transcription and splicing in the rat developing heart. Our results and those of others (18,19) favor the idea that c-FN is not directly involved in cardiac differentiation, and no clue exists today that permits the assessment that FN expression is involved, directly or indirectly, in the phenotypic changes in either the contractile or nonmuscle cells that occur during the advanced phase of cardiac organogenesis (25). Thus, only p-FN that accumulates in the interstitial space (19,22) would be involved at this stage in the morphologic changes of the heart. Further evidence that p-FN rather than locally synthetized c-FN is required for cardiac development is provided by abnormal cardiac development either in the chicken embryo exposed to antibodies directed against FN (26) or in the mutated murine embryo whose only source of FN is from maternal blood (20).

FN transcription is induced by serum, epidermal growth factor, platelet growth factor (PDGF), transforming growth factor (TGFβ), c-AMP, and angiotensin II (27,28). In vitro, serum and c-AMP stimulations of the FN gene expression are mediated through different c-AMP response elements (CRE). One high-affinity and two low-affinity CREs mediate the c-AMP response through the binding of three proteins, PEA2, CREB, and an unidentified factor (28). A glucocorticoid (dexamethasone) stabilizes FN mRNA, whereas forskolin, an activator of adenyl cyclase, and TGFβ increase its transcription (29). FN is also involved in the organization of the extracellular matrix via its interactions with the collagens and the proteoglycans and binds to basal membrane proteins such as the laminins.

2-Collagen type IV is a major component of vertebrate BM. Six genes encoding α1–α6 collagen IV chains have been described, the form α5 (IV) being expressed at high levels in the heart, and a switch to collagen α3–α5 (IV) expression occurs during development (30).

3-Laminins consist of 3 associated α,β,γ-chains, and eight genetically distinct laminin chains with different assembly forms are known so far. The most extensively characterized form, the laminin-1 (α1β1γ1), shows calcium-dependent self-assembly and heterotypic binding to matrix and BM components, thus suggesting a crucial role in the supramolecular organization of BM. Laminins possess binding sites for at least six different integrin receptors and are thus involved in many cell–matrix interactions that have been shown to be important during embryonic development (31), signal transduction, and cell growth (32). Laminin-2 (formerly merosin) is a homolog of the prototypical laminin-1 form that includes an α2-chain isoform. In contrast to the α1 chain, this chain is expressed in most cells of mesenchymal origin (33).

Laminin isoform expression is regulated during cardiac ontogenic development and varies according to the cell type (34–38). The mRNA content in the forms of two laminin subunits (α2,β2) is abundant around birth and, as that of collagen type IV, progressively decreases, at the end of the postnatal growth period (39).

In humans, maturation of arterial SMCs is accompanied by a switch from expression of α1β1γ1 to α1β2γ1 laminin (34). In adult heart the myocytes, endothelial cells, and smooth muscle cells (SMC) synthesize laminin (38,40). The expression of laminin chains is specific for each type of cell; the laminin-3 (α1β2γ1) is particularly expressed in smooth muscle cells, whereas the laminin-2 (merosin) (α2β1γ1) is expressed in cardiac muscle (37). However, the exact number of isoforms expressed in the cardiovascular system is not yet defined. A novel α4 chain has been described recently in humans and is said to be present in the heart in adults and in the smooth muscle in fetuses (41).

THE INTEGRINS

The emerging concept is that integrins can transduce informational signals related to growth and gene expression, as well as structural messages related to organization of internal and external cytoarchitecture (42–44). The specific response of cells to integrin engagement depends on the types of cell, integrin, and ligand.

Integrins belong to a family of heterodimeric transmembrane receptors (αβ) composed of more than 20 functional members, many of which have overlapping and competing affinities for individual ECM ligands. A large extracellular domain binds to various ECM proteins, and a short intracellular domain interacts with the cytoskeleton. The "ECM contacts" consist of clustered integrin receptors binding to fibrils of ECM, especially fibronectin, with distinct cytoskeleton association (2). Experiments with chimeric integrins demonstrated that β subunits are necessary and sufficient for targeting integrins to sites of cell matrix adhesion in a ligand-independent manner; subunits mostly determine the specificity of the ligand binding (45–47). Indeed, integrins can transmit signals by modulating the organization of the cytoskeleton, which is directly linked to the nuclear matrix through the nuclear lamins (48). The resulting restructure of the nuclear matrix would initiate changes in DNA-binding activity and therefore gene expression. The existence of more than 20 distinct integrins raises the likelihood of individualization of signaling pathways, and each of the numerous isoforms of FN and laminin may be linked differently to the various integrins and, therefore, trigger various modulations of cell phenotype. It was suggested that among the β1 isoforms the β1B isoform may function as a "des-adhesion" integrin receptor during embryogenesis (49) while the β1C form expression markedly inhibits DNA synthesis and causes growth arrest at the late G1 phase of the cell cycle (50). Recently, a fourth variant of β1 integrin β1D was described as a muscle-specific isoform, replacing the common β1A isoform in terminally differentiated striated muscles (51). In cardiac muscle, this form was localized at the intercalated disks and the major cell–cell contact structures of cardiomyocytes and was associated essentially with the α7B integrin subunit. This α7β1D appears to be the major integrin receptor involved in cytoskeleton–matrix interactions of differentiated striated muscle (51). Stimulated integrins are necessary for myodifferentiation and the formation of sarcomeric architecture (52,53).

TABLE 12–1. *Expression of integrin subunits during the development of the cardiovascular system*

		Fetus		Newborn		Adult	
Integrin subunits	Ligands	Heart	Aorta[34]	Heart	Aorta[34]	Heart	Aorta[34]
α1[60]	coll I, III, IV, laminin	+++	++	++	++	–	++
α2	coll I, III, IV, laminin	nd	–	nd	–	nd	–
α3[60]	FN, laminin coll I, III, IV	+++	+	++	++	++	++
α4	FN	+	nd	nd	nd	nd	nd
α5[60,19]	FN	+++	++	++	++	–	++
α6[58]	Laminin	++	–	+	–	++	–
β1[60]		+++	++	++	++	+++	++

+++ very abundant; ++ abundant; + poorly abundant; – absent; nd - not determined.

As a result of binding to ECM components, integrins can function in additive or synergistic fashion with growth factors (54), and optimal induction likely requires the cooperative action of integrins and growth factor receptors (55). Indeed, molecules such as $p^{125\text{-fak}}$ can be phosphorylated via both integrin and growth factor pathways and may be key regulator components at one of the junctions between different signaling pathways (56).

Integrins are important regulators in early cardiac development, providing positional information for migrating and differentiating cells (3,19,57–60). In human aorta integrins α1β1 and α3β1 are the major binding proteins (34), whereas in heart α3β1 and α6β1 are the major potential receptors for ECM protein. The latter isoform that also associates to laminin was recently described as being both temporally and spatially regulated in the developing heart (Table 12–1). It first appears in 8.5 dpc embryos and is segregated in the myocardium, showing a gradient of expression, increasing from the outer to the inner layers of the myocardium (58). These localized patterns of expression suggest a specialized role for this integrin in cardiogenesis, perhaps regulating the positional relationship of differentiating myocytes with laminin-containing ECM (59).

SUMMARY

It is now understood that many ECM molecules, when interacting with one or more receptors on the cell surface, can trigger transmembrane signaling events that lead to second messenger activities and cytoskeletal rearrangements and that, consequently, influence gene expression. The molecular basis by which cells respond to ECM is still at an early stage. The next few years should provide much greater insights into these processes, particularly with respect to cell surface complexity and second messenger pathways.

ACKNOWLEDGMENT

The authors thank Gwenaelle Ondola for her secretarial help.

REFERENCES

1. Roskelley CD, Srebrow A, Bissel MJ. A hierarchy of ECM-mediated signalling regulates tissue-specific gene expression. *Curr Opin Cell Biol* 1995;7:736–747.
2. Yamada KM, Miyamoto S. Integrin transmembrane signaling and cytoskeletal control. *Curr Opin Cell Biol* 1995;7:681–689.
3. Borg TK, Terracio L. Interaction of the extracellular matrix with cardiac myocytes during development and disease. In: Stolte H, Kinne RKH, Bach PH, eds. *Cardiac myocyte–connective tissue interactions in health and disease.* New York: Karger AG; 1990:113–129.
4. Samuel JL, Barrieux A, Dufour S, et al. Accumulation of fetal fibronectin mRNAs during the development of rat cardiac hypertrophy induced by pressure overload. *J Clin Invest* 1991;88:1737–1746.
5. Hay E. Collagen and other matrix glycoproteins in embryogenesis. In: Hay ED, ed. *Cell biology of extracellular matrix.* New York: Plenum Press; 1991:419–456.
6. Thiery JP, Duband JL, Dufour S, Savagner P, Imhof BA. Roles of fibronectins in embryogenesis. In: Mosher DF, eds. *Fibronectin.* New York: Academic Press; 1989:181–212.
7. Ahumada GG, Rennard SI, Figueroa AA, Silver MH. Cardiac fibronectin: developmental distribution and quantitative comparison of possible sites of synthesis. *J Mol Cell Cardiol* 1981;13:667–678.
8. Barone MV, Henchcliffe, Baralle FE, Paolella G. Cell type specific trans-acting factors are involved in alternative splicing of human fibronectin pre-mRNA. *EMBO J* 1989;8:1079–1085.
9. Vartio T, Laitinen L, Narvanen O, Cutolo M, Thornell LE, Zardi L, Virtanen I. Differential expression of the ED sequence-containing form of cellular fibronectin in embryonic and adult human tissues. *J Cell Sci* 1987;88:419–430.
10. Bennett VD, Pallante KM, Adams SL. The splicing pattern of fibronectin mRNA changes during chondrogenesis resulting in an unusual form of the mRNA in cartilage. *J Biol Chem* 1991;266:5918–5924.
11. Hynes RO. In: Rich A, ed. *Fibronectins.* Berlin: Springer Verlag; 1990:1–545.
12. Patton JG, Mayer SA, Nadal Ginard B. Characterization and molecular cloning of polyprimidine tract-binding protein: a component of a complex necessary for pre-mRNA splicing. *Gene Dev* 1991;1237–1251.
13. French-Constant C, Van De Water L, Dvorak HF, Hynes RO. Reappearance of an embryonic pattern of fibronectin splicing during wound healing in the adult rat. *J Cell Biol* 1989;109:903–914.
14. Glukhova MA, Frid MG, Shekhonin BV, Vasilevkaya TD, Grunwald J, Saginati M, Koteliansky VE. Expression of extradomain A fibronectin sequence is phenotype dependent. *J Cell Biol* 1989;109:357–366.
15. Akiyama SK, Yamada SS, Chen WT, Yamada KM. Analysis of fibronectin receptor function with monoclonal antibodies: roles in cell adhesion, migration, matrix assembly, and cytoskeletal organization. *J Cell Biol* 1989;109:863–875.
16. Hedin U, Bottger BA, Forsberg E, Johansson S, Thyberg J. Diverse effects of fibronectin and laminin on phenotypic properties of cultured arterial smooth muscle cells. *J Cell Biol* 1988;107:307–319.
17. Hedin U, Bottger BA, Luthman J, Johansson S, Thyberg J. A substrate of the cell-attachment sequence of fibronectin (Arg-Gly-Asp-Ser) is sufficient to promote transition of arterial smooth muscle cells from a contractile to a synthetic phenotype. *Dev Biol* 1989;133:489–501.
18. Armstrong PB, Armstrong MT. An instructive role for the interstitial matrix in tissue patterning: tissue segregation and intracellular invasion. *J Cell Biol* 1990;110:1439–1455.
19. Roman J, McDonald JA. Expression of fibronectin, the integrin alpha5, and alpha-smooth muscle actin in heart and lung development. *Am J Respir Cell Mol Biol* 1992;6:472–480.
20. George EL, Georges-Labouesse EN, Patel-King RS, Rayburn H, Hynes RO. Defects in mesoderm, neural tube and vascular development in mouse embryos lacking fibronectin. *Development* 1993; 119:1079–1091.
21. Farhadian F, Barrieux A, Lortet S, Marotte F, Oliviero P, Rappaport L, Samuel JL. Differential splicing of fibronectin pre-mRNA during cardiac ontogeny and development of hypertrophy in the rat. *Lab Invest* 1994;71:552–559.

22. Samuel JL, Farhadian F, Sabri A, Marotte F, Robert V, Rappaport L. Expression of fibronectin during rat fetal and postnatal development: an in situ hybridisation and immunohistochemical study. *Cardiovasc Res* 1994;28:1653–1661.
23. Rakusan K, Turek Z. Protamine inhibits capillary formation in growing rat heart. *Circ Res* 1985;85:393–398.
24. Contard F, Sabri A, Glukhova M, et al. Arterial smooth muscle cell phenotype in stroke-prone spontaneously hypertensive rats. *Hypertension* 1993;22:665–676.
25. Lompré AM, Mercadier JJ, Schwartz K. Changes in gene expression during cardiac growth. *Int Rev Cytol* 1991;124:137–186.
26. Linask KK, Lash JW. A role for fibronectin in the migration of avian precardiac cells. I. Dose-dependent effects of fibronectin antibody. *Dev Biol* 1988;129:315–323.
27. Ignotz RA, Massague J. Transforming growth factor-β stimulates the expression of fibronectin and collagen and their incorporation into the extracellular matrix. *J Biol Chem* 1986;261:4337–4345.
28. Dean DC, McQuillan JJ, Weintraub S. Serum stimulation of fibronectin gene expression appears to result from rapid serum-induced binding of nuclear proteins to a cAMP response element. *J Biol Chem* 1990;265:3522–3527.
29. Dean DC, Newby RF, Bourgeois S. Regulation of fibronectin biosynthesis by dexamethasone, transforming growth factor β, and cAMP in human cell lines. *J Cell Biol* 1988;106:2159–2170.
30. Miner JH, Sanes JR. Collagen iv α3, α4, and α5 chains in rodent basal laminae: sequence, distribution, association with laminins, and developmental switches. *J Cell Biol* 1994;127:879–891.
31. Timpl R, Brown JC. The laminins. *Matrix Biol* 1994;14:275–281.
32. Kubota S, Tashiro K, Yamada Y. Signaling site of laminin with mitogenic activity. *J Biol Chem* 1992;267:4285–4288.
33. Vuolteenaho R, Nissinen M, Sainio K, et al. Human laminin M chain (merosin): complete primary structure, chromosomal assignment, and expression of the M and A chain in human fetal tissues. *J Cell Biol* 1994;124:381–394.
34. Glukhova M, Koteliansky V, Fondacci C, Marotte F, Rappaport L. Laminin variants and integrin laminin receptors in developing and adult human smooth muscle. *Dev Biol* 1993:157;437–447.
35. Huner DD, Porter BE, Bulock JW, Adams SP, Merlie JP, Sanes JR. Primary sequence of a motor neuron–selective adhesive site in the synaptic basal lamina. *Cell* 1989;59:905–913.
36. Wewer U, Engvall E, Paulsson M, Yamamda Y, Alberechtsen R. Laminin A B1, B2, S and M subunits in the postnatal rat liver development and after partial hepatectomy. *Lab Invest* 1992; 66:378–389.
37. Engvall E, Earwicker D, Haaparanta T, Ruoslahti E, Sanes JR. Distribution and isolation of four laminin variants; tissue restricted distribution of heterotrimers assembled from five different subunits. *Cell Regul* 1990;1:731–740.
38. Tryggvason K. The laminin family. *Curr Opin Cell Biol* 1993;5:877–882.
39. Farhadian F, Oliviero P, Marotte F, Rappaport L, Samuel JL. Expression of laminin variant mRNA during normal and pathological cardiac growth in the rat. *J Mol Cell Cardiol* 1995;27:A78.
40. Speiser B, Weihrauch D, Riess CF, Schaper J. The extracellular matrix in human cardiac tissue. Part II: vimentin, laminin and fibronectin. *Cardioscience* 1992;3:41–49.
41. Iivanainen A, Sainio K, Sariola H, Tryggvason K. Primary structure and expression of a novel human laminin a4 chain. *FEBS Lett* 1995;365:183–188.
42. Hynes RO. Integrins: versatility, modulation, and signaling in cell adhesion. *Cell* 1992;69:11–25.
43. Juliano RL, Haskill S. Signal transduction from the extracellular matrix. *J Cell Biol* 1993; 120:577–585.
44. Damsky CH, Werb Z. Signal transduction by integrin receptors for extracellular matrix: cooperative processing of extracellular information. *Curr Opin Cell Biol* 1992;5:772–781.
45. Hayashi Y, Haimovich B, Reszka A, Boettiger D, Horwitz AF. Expression and function of chicken integrin β1 subunit and its cytoplasmic domain mutants in mouse NIH 3T3 cells. *J Cell Biol* 1990;100:175–182.
46. LaFlamme SE, Akiyama SK, Yamada KM. Regulation of fibronectin receptor distribution. *J Cell Biol* 1992;177:437–447.
47. Ylanne J, Chen TE, O'Toole TE, Loftus JC, Takada Y, Ginsberg MH. Distinct roles of integrin α and β subunit cytoplasmic domains in cell spreading and formation of focal adhesions. *J Cell Biol* 1993;122:223–233.
48. Wang N, Butler JP, Ingber DE. Mechanotransduction across the cell surface and through the cytoskeleton. *Science* 1993;260:1124–1127.

49. Balzac F, Retta SF, Albini A, Melchiorri A, Koteliansky VE, Geuna M, Silengo L, Tarone. Expression of β1B integrin isoform in CHO cells results in a dominant negative effect on cell adhesion and mobility. *J Cell Biol* 1994;127:557–565.
50. Meredith J, Takada Y, Fornaro M, Languino LR, Schwartz MA. Inhibition of cell cycle progression by the alternative spliced integrin β1C. *Science* 1995;269:1570–1572.
51. Belkin AM, Zhidkova N, Balzac F, Altruda F, Tomatis D, Maier A, Tarone G, Koteliansky V, Burridge K. β1D integrin displaces the β1A isoform in striated muscles: localization at junctional structure and signaling potential in nonmuscle cells. *J Cell Biol* 1996;132:211–226.
52. Menko AS, Boettiger D. Occupation of the extracellular matrix receptor, integrin, is a central point for myogenic differentiation. *Cell* 1987;51:51–57.
53. Volk T, Fessler LI, Fessler JH. A role for integrin in the formation of sarcomeric cytoarchitecture. *Cell* 1990;63:525–536.
54. Arora PD, Ma J, Min W, Cruz T, McCulloch CAG. Interleukin-1–induced calcium flux in human fibroblasts is mediated through focal adhesions. *J Biol Chem* 1995;270:6042–6049.
55. McNamee HP, Ingber DE, Schwartz MA. Adhesion to fibronectin stimulates inositol lipid synthesis and enhances PDGF-induced inositol lipid breakdown. *J Cell Biol* 1993;121:673–678.
56. Richardson A, Parson JT. Signal transduction through integrins; a central role for focal adhesion kinase? *Bioessays* 1995;17:229–236.
57. Litvin J, Montgomery M, Gonzalez-Sanchez A, Bisaha JG, Bader D. Commitment and differentiation of cardiac myocytes. *Trends Cardiovasc Med* 1992;2:27–32.
58. Buck CA, Baldwin HS, DeLisser H. Cell adhesion receptors and early mammalian heart development: an overview. *Crit Rev Acad Sci (III)* 1993;316:849–859.
59. Collo G, Domanico SZ, Klier G, Quaranta V. Gradient of integrin a6A distribution in the myocardium during early heart development. *Cell Adhes Commun* 1995;3:101–113.
60. Teraccio I, Rubin K, Gullberger D, Balog F, Carver W, Syring R, Borg TK. Expression of collagen binding integrins during cardiac development and hypertrophy. *Circ Res* 1991;68:734–744.

PART IV

Development of Excitation–Contraction Coupling

The Developing Heart,
edited by Bohuslav Ošťádal et al.
Lippincott-Raven Publishers,
Philadelphia © 1997.

13

Developmental Changes in Ionic Currents of the Heart

Nicholas Sperelakis, Yasuhiro Katsube, *Hideaki Sada, and **Hiroshi Masuda, USA

*Department of Molecular and Cellular Physiology, College of Medicine, University of Cincinnati, Cincinnati, OH 45267 *Pharmacology Department, Yamaguchi University, Japan, and **Pediatrics Department, Hiroshima University, Japan*

The electrophysiology of the heart changes dramatically during development, during both the embryonic/fetal period and the neonatal period. These changes in electrical properties are caused by changes in the number (density) and types of ion channels, with resultant changes in the magnitude and kinetic properties of the various types of ionic currents. The alterations in the ion channels are responsible for the changes in the resting potential and characteristics of the action potentials that occur during cardiac development. Changes in excitation–contraction coupling also occur during development of the heart. This review-type article will summarize the major changes in the ionic currents of the ventricular myocardial cells that have been reported to occur, with special emphasis on chick and rat. For the specific references on each topic, the reader is referred to some of the review-type articles in the reference section (1–11).

RESTING POTENTIAL AND ACTION POTENTIALS

Resting Potential

The resting potential (RP) of the ventricular cells in the early embryonic/fetal period is low (e.g., −40 to −50 mV), and there is a progressive increase in RP during embryonic life, so that in the late embryonic period the RP has attained nearly the adult level (e.g., −75 to −85 mV). The increased RP is due to a decrease in the ratio of permeabilities to Na^+ and K^+ (P_{Na}/P_K ratio) (see later).

In the early embryonic period, the low RP of the ventricular cells is not stable, but exhibits a spontaneous depolarization, the pacemaker potential (phase 4 diastolic depolarization). The slope of the pacemaker potential progressively decreases during embryonic development and disappears. Thus, automaticity of the ventricular cells is lost by the middle embryonic period. One factor in the loss of automaticity is the increase in the RP (more hyerpolarized), which takes the membrane potential (E_m) out of the range over which automaticity is possible. Another factor is the loss of the hyperpolarization-activated inward current (I_h or I_f) (see later).

The low RP cannot be accounted for by changes in the intracellular ion concentrations—for example, $[K]_i$ is already high in the early embryonic period (12). Although the (Na, K)-ATPase/pump-specific activity was found to be low in the early embryonic period (13), and increased progressively during embryonic life, the Na–K pump is sufficient to maintain a high $[K]_i$ and low $[Na]_i$ because the cell membrane is less leaky (i.e., high resistance) (12).

Action Potentials

The action potentials (APs) get larger and faster-rising during embryonic development. They get bigger because of the larger RP and because the overshoot increases (most prominent in chick) (e.g., to about +30 mV).

The maximum rate of rise of the AP (max *dV/dt*) increases dramatically during embryonic development, from about 20 V/sec to about 200 V/sec in the late embryonic stage (to about the adult level). This increase in rate of rise is produced by a much greater number (density) of TTX-sensitive fast Na^+ channels (see later).

The duration of the AP (e.g., at 50% repolarization, APD_{50}) does not change much in the chick during development. In the rat, however, there is a large decrease in APD_{50}, beginning in the late fetal period and extending through the first 3 weeks of neonatal life, after which the adultlike brief APs are attained (14). Several factors contribute to this marked abbreviation of the AP, including increase in the transient outward current (I_{to}) carried primarily by K^+ ions. Any increase in outward K^+ current acts to hyperpolarize (toward E_K, the K^+ equilibrium potential) and to shorten the AP plateau.

Cyclic Nucleotides

Prominent changes in the levels of the cyclic nucleotides also occur during development of the heart. Cyclic AMP was found to be very high in early embryonic stages and to decrease rapidly over the next few days to nearly the adult level (15). In contrast, cyclic GMP changed almost reciprocally. Cyclic GMP was found to be very low in early embryonic stages and to increase rapidly over the next few days to about the adult level (16). Since these cyclic nucleotides act to regulate, among other things, the activity of the L-type Ca^{2+} channels, this is relevant to the theme of the present article.

IONIC CURRENTS

Inwardly Rectifying K^+ Current (I_{K1})

It was demonstrated that I_{K1} of ventricular cells increases markedly during development in both embryonic chick hearts (17,18) and fetal/neonatal rat hearts (19). Figure 13–1 illustrates the increase in I_{K1} for rat heart development. The increase in I_{K1} is likely to be the major factor responsible for the increase in RP (hyperpolarization) that occurs during development, concomitant with a decrease in membrane resistivity (R_m) and in membrane time constant ($t_m = R_m C_m$) (12). The increase in I_{K1} channels also can account for the decrease in the P_{Na}/P_K ratio that occurs during development (12)—namely, it results in an increase in the K^+ permeability P_K. This is summarized in Table 13–1.

Hyperpolarization-Activated Inward Current (I_h or I_f)

The I_h channel is a nonselective cation (e.g., Na^+, K^+) channel that is turned on (activated) by hyperpolarization (toward the RP) and turned off by depolarization (e.g., during the AP) and is thought to contribute to automaticity of heart cells (20). But since the I_h channel current turns on very slowly (long t), it may be involved in automaticity primarily of Purkinje fiber and not of SA nodal cells (21). At poten-

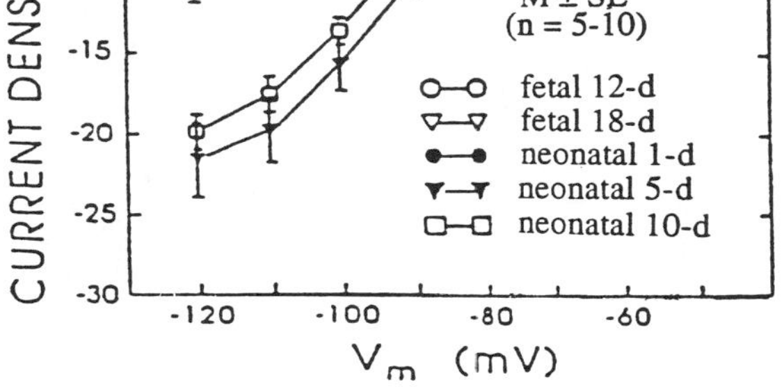

FIG. 13–1. Developmental changes of the inwardly rectifying K^+ current (I_{K1}) in rat ventricular myocytes. Current/voltage relations at the different developmental stages (from fetal day 12 to neonatal day 10). Currents were elicited from a HP of −40 mV. Data points were shown as mean ± SEM. (Taken from ref. 19, with permission.)

TABLE 13–1. *Summary outline of the various ionic currents that change during development of the heart and the associated figures that illustrate these currents and their developmental changes*

I_{K1} increases	Fig. 13–1
inc. RP	
dec. R_m and τ_m	
dec. P_{Na}/P_K	
I_h (I_f) decreases	Fig. 13–2
dec. automaticity	
$I_{Na(f)}$ increases	Fig. 13–3
inc. AP max *dV/dt*	Fig. 13–4
inc. propag. vel.	
$I_{Ca(L)}$ decreases in chick	Fig. 13–5
increases in rat	
$I_{Ca(L)}$ stim. by β-agonists	Fig. 13–6
	Fig. 13–7
Long openings of Ca^{2+} channels decrease	Fig. 13–8
chick	Fig. 13–9
rat	
$I_{Ca(L)}$ inhib. by cGMP/PK-G	Fig. 13–10
	Fig. 13–11
$I_{Ca(T)}$ decreases (chick)	
$I_{Ca(F)}$ decreases (rat)	Fig. 13–12
	Fig. 13–13
I_{ti}, DADs, and triggered automaticity	Fig. 13–14
	Fig. 13–15
Excitation–contraction coupling	Fig. 13–16

tials near the RP (or maximum diastolic potential, MDP), the main current of the I_h channel is *inward* and carried by Na^+ influx (because the Na^+ electrochemical driving force [$E_m - E_{Na}$] is so much greater than the K^+ driving force [$E_m - E_K$]). Therefore, the I_h current is depolarizing and contributes to the pacemaker potential depolarization (diastolic or phase 4 depolarization). It was found that I_h is present in young embryonic chick heart cells and disappears during subsequent development (22,23). This is illustrated in Fig. 13–2 and is summarized in Table 13–1. Therefore, the presence of I_h in young embryonic/fetal heart (ventricular) cells can account for their automaticity, at least in part.

Transient Outward Current (I_{to})

A substantial amount of transient outward current (I_{to}), presumably carried primarily by K^+ ions, was observed in early embryonic chick ventricular cells (Sada, unpublished observations; 24). In neonatal and young rats (5–21 days old), a prominent I_{to} was found in isolated ventricular cells that was completely blocked by 3 mM 4-AP (4-amino-pyridine) (Conforti & Sperelakis, unpublished observations).

In neonatal rat ventricular cells, the density of I_{to} was reported to increase about fourfold between day 1 and day 10 (about 7 pA/pF) (25). Since the reversal poten-

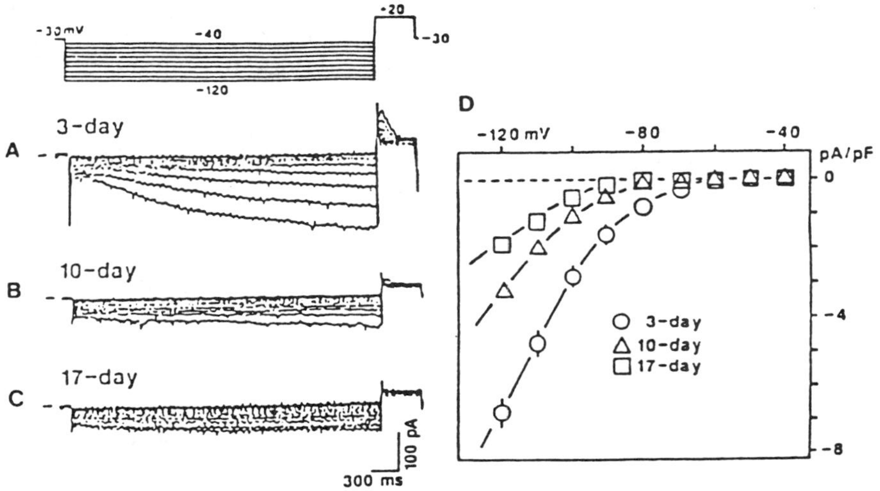

FIG. 13–2. Developmental changes of the hyperpolarization-activated inward current (I_h) in young embryonic chick ventricular cells. Test pulses were applied between −40 and −120 mV, in 10-mV increments, from a HP of −30 mV. (**A**) Presence of I_h in a 3-day-old cell. Note the presence of the large inward current slowly activated by hyperpolarization. (**B**) Smaller I_h in a 10-day-old cell. (**C**) Absence of I_h in a 17-day-old cell. (**D**) Current/voltage relations for I_h current density at the three developmental stages. The values plotted are mean ± SEM. (Taken from ref. 23, with permission.)

tial for I_{to} increased from about −30 mV on day 1 to −55 mV on day 10, the increase in current density was attributed primarily to a change in ion selectivity of the channel, namely, an increase in K^+ permeability and decrease in Na^+ permeability. In another study on rat ventricular myocytes, I_{to} was reported to increase from about 2 pA/pF on neonatal day 1 to 4 pA/pF on day 20, and to 6 pA/pF at adult (26). This current was blocked by 2 mM 4-AP.

In canine ventricular cells, it was reported that I_{to} was absent in neonatal cells (days 0–14) and present in adult cells (about 20 pA/pF at +20 mV) (27). In its place, the neonatal cells possessed a similar outward current that was not 4-AP (2 mM) sensitive and decayed very slowly (about 20 pA/pF at +20 mV).

In mouse embryonic stem cells differentiated in vitro for 10 days, an outward K^+ current that decayed rapidly and was blocked by 4-AP (2 mM) was exhibited (about 20 pA/pF at +20 mV). In normal adult human atrial cells, an I_{to} (about 2.5 pA/pF at +20 mV) was found that was sensitive to 2 mM 4-AP (28). I_{to} was lower in cells from diseased hearts.

The acetycholine-activated outward K^+ current ($I_{K(ACh)}$) has not been observed in ventricular cells but is present in atrial cells and in nodal cells. In the latter cells, ACh shortens the AP.

The ATP-inhibited K^+ channel ($I_{K(ATP)}$) is present in adult rat and guinea pig ventricular cells and atrial cells. This channel serves as an important protection mechanism for the heart under conditions of hypoxia or regional ischemia (29,30). That is, this channel is "masked" under normal conditions but becomes unmasked (activated or derepressed) when the ATP concentration is lowered in pathophysiologic conditions and acts to shorten the cardiac AP duration. The latter turns off the slow Ca^{2+} channels and current prematurely, and thereby reduces Ca^{2+} influx and contraction, and hence conserves ATP. Thus, the myocardial cells can recover when the blood flow returns to normal. This mechanism assists the primary mechanism for protection of the heart, namely, the ATP dependence and the pH dependence of the activity of the slow Ca^{2+} channels (30).

Fast Na^+ Current ($I_{Na(f)}$)

The TTX-sensitive fast Na^+ current in ventricular cells increases markedly during development by a factor of more than 10 in both chick and rat hearts (31–39). These changes are illustrated in Fig. 13–3. Consistent with this, it was shown that the specific binding of saxitoxin (STX, like TTX, a specific blocker of fast Na^+ channels) increases markedly during development of embryonic chick hearts (40). The large increase in number (density) of fast Na^+ channels accounts for the large increase in max *dV/dt* of the AP that occurs during development. It also may contribute to the increase in AP overshoot that occurs during development (very prominent in chick). The increase in $I_{Na(f)}$ also is a major factor responsible for the increase in propagation velocity that occurs during development. (We have recently found that fast Na^+ channels are present at high concentration in the intercalated disk [junctional] membranes of rat hearts [Ferguson et al., unpublished], and we believe that these enable and facilitate transfer of excitation from one cell to the next by the electric field that develops in the junctional cleft [41].)

The increase in cell size (both diameter and length) that occurs during heart development would also contribute to the increase in propagation velocity. Although rate of size of the AP is independent of cell size, from the cable equation, propagation velocity (θ) is directly proportional to the square root of fiber radius (42). In addition, it has been demonstrated that almost all propagation time is consumed at the cell junctions (intercalated disks), that is, the entire length of the cell fires the AP virtually simultaneously (for references, see 43). Therefore, both cell length and cell diameter are important determinants of propagation velocity in cardiac muscle.

The sensitivity to TTX of fast Na^+ channels varies greatly, depending on the channel isoform. For example, the TTX sensitivity of avian cardiomyocytes (in the *nanomolar* range) was about 1000 times greater than that for mammalian hearts like guinea pig, which are in the *micromolar* range (44). This finding is in agreement with previous reports of high sensitivity to TTX of embryonic chick

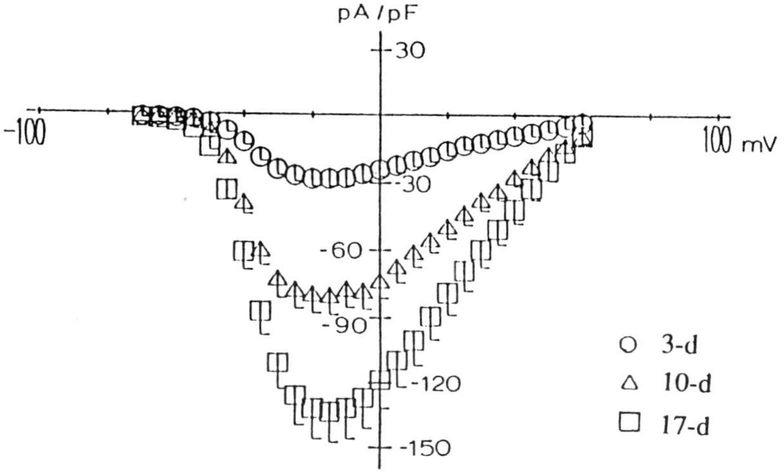

FIG. 13–3. Developmental increase of $I_{Na(f)}$ in embryonic chick hearts. Current/voltage relations at three developmental stages: 3-day, 10-day, and 17-day. Currents were elicited from a HP of −90 (mV). Data points are shown as mean ± SEM. (Taken from ref. 39, with permission.)

hearts (33,45,46). In addition, we reported that the activation of $I_{Na(f)}$ of chick cardiomyocytes followed the classical Hodgkin-Huxley m^3 kinetics for squid giant axon rather than m^1 kinetics (47). This is consistent with the high neuron-type sensitivity to TTX, because it has been proposed (48,49) that Na^+ channels following m^3 kinetics should have high sensitivity to TTX, and those following m^1 kinetics should have low TTX sensitivity. Some types of Na^+ channels are more resistant to TTX, and some types are actually insensitive to TTX. The TTX-insensitive Na^+ channels are kinetically slower, exhibiting slower activation and inactivation, and are therefore known as slow Na^+ channels and current ($I_{Na(s)}$) (50–54).

$I_{Na(f)}$ also has a slow component, in that a small fraction of this current is sustained for periods of more than 100 msec; that is, there is a very slowly inactivating component of $I_{Na(f)}$. This small, slow component of $I_{Na(f)}$ contributes to the formation of the AP plateau (55). Thus, if TTX is added, the APD_{50} is substantially shortened. Reopening of some of the fast Na^+ channels during a long depolarizing clamp step is one explanation for the small sustained component (47,56). As stated earlier, the AP becomes greatly abbreviated in length during development (late fetal and neonatal) in the case of rat heart; and that one factor responsible is an increase in I_{to} carried primarily by K^+. Another factor that may contribute to the shortening of the APD_{50} is the loss of the slow component. As shown in Fig. 13–4A, on fetal day 18, the AP still has a prominent plateau component, and there is a slowly inactivating component of $I_{Na(f)}$. However, by neonatal day 1, the slow component has disappeared (Fig. 13–4B).

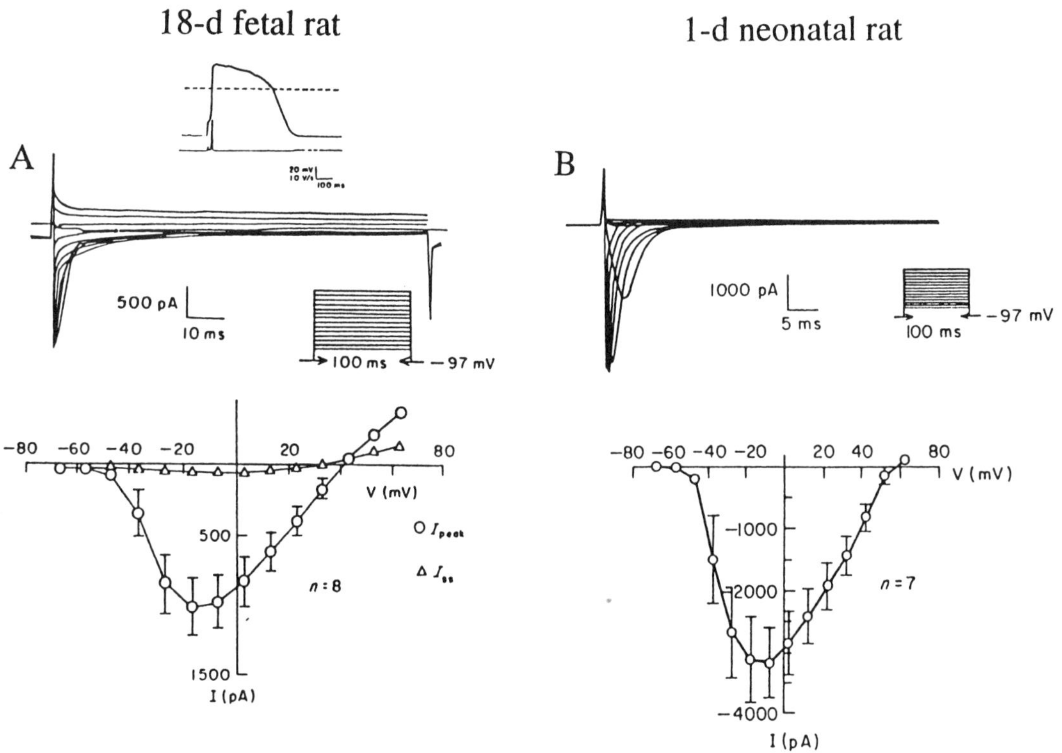

FIG. 13–4. Developmental changes of $I_{Na(f)}$ in fetal/neonatal rats. (**A** inset) A representative action potential elicited by a 2-ms duration stimulus in a fetal rat (18-day) ventricular myocyte using the current clamp method. The broken line indicates the zero potential level. (**A**) Membrane currents recorded from fetal rat (18-day) ventricular myocytes using voltage-clamp. *Top:* Representative family of membrane currents elicited by 100-ms depolarizing test pulses from −67 mV to 63 mV, in 10-mV increments, from a HP of −97 mV. *Bottom:* Current/voltage relationship for the peak (*circles*) and late (triangles, at the end of the test pulse [I_{ss}]) membrane currents. Data presented as mean ± SEM. (**B**) $I_{Na(f)}$ from 1-day-old neonatal rat ventricular cardiomyocytes. *Top:* Na^+ currents in response to several depolarizing steps (only the first 50 ms shown). *Bottom:* *I/V* relationship for the peak Na^+ current (mean ± SEM). The reversal potential was 53 ± 3 mV. (Taken from ref. 38, with permission.)

Slow Ca^{2+} Current ($I_{Ca(L)}$)

Changes in the slow (L-type) Ca^{2+} current also occur during development of the heart. However, the direction of the change is opposite in avian versus mammalian hearts. In rat heart, $I_{Ca(L)}$ increases during development (57), whereas in chick heart it actually decreases (58). These changes are illustrated in Fig. 13–5. Note that these data are presented as current densities (in pA/pF) (i.e., normalized for changes in cell size that occur during development). The intensity of $I_{Ca(L)}$ is, of course, important in determining the force of contraction of the heart.

Stimulation of $I_{Ca(L)}$ by the β-adrenergic agonist, isoproterenol (Iso), does not occur during the mid-fetal period of mammalian hearts. For example, in rat heart, Iso has almost no effect on fetal days 12–18 (59,60). However, on fetal day 20 and later, Iso exerts it usual large stimulating effect (Figs. 13–6 and 13–7). A similar pattern was found for forskolin (Fig. 13–7), a direct stimulator of adenylate cyclase. Thus, some component of the β-receptor/G_s-coupling protein/adenylate cyclase/cAMP/PK-A cascade is missing in the midfetal myocardial cell.

Long Openings of Slow Ca^{2+} Channels

In whole-cell voltage clamp of an isolated single cardiomyocyte, the magnitude of the peak $I_{Ca(L)}$ measured (the "macroscopic" current recorded from an assembly of channels) is a function of the current (i_{Ca}) through a single channel (which is a function of the single-channel conductance [e.g., 24 pS] times the electrochemical driving force [$E_m - E_{Ca}$]), times the number of channels (N), times the average open probability (P_o) of the channels.

$$I_{Ca} = i_{Ca} N P_o$$

The P_o value is a function of the number of channel openings (e.g., during a clamp period of 300 msec) and the mean open time (t_o) (i.e., the channel opens and closes, then reopens and recloses in a repeated or bursting fashion). Therefore, if some channels possessed a gating behavior that gave rise to prolonged openings ("mode 2" behavior in the case of the Ca^{2+} channel agonist, Bay-K-8644), then P_o is increased, causing a larger I_{Ca}.

We found that long openings of the slow Ca^{2+} channels occur relatively frequently in young embryonic chick heart cells (58,61) and in fetal rat heart cells (57). This phenomenon is illustrated in Fig. 13–8 for chick cells (embryonic day 3) and in Fig. 13–9 for rat cells (fetal day 12). The upper part of Fig. 13–8 shows successive sweeps of current recorded from a single Ca^{2+} channel (cell-attached patch configuration). Note that in some sweeps, the P_o value was close to 1.0. The lower part of Fig. 13–8 is a frequency histogram of the various P_o values. In old embryonic chick hearts (e.g., day 17), the right-hand portion of the histogram, with P_o values above 0.25, is essentially gone.

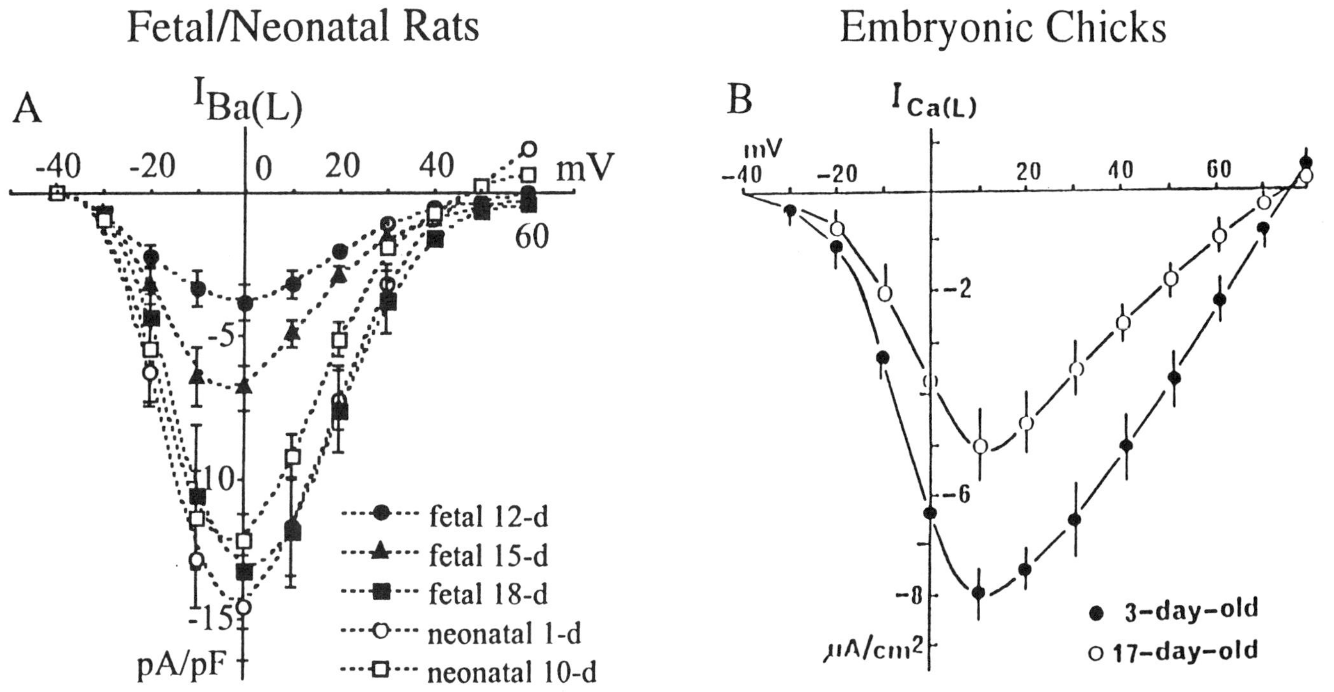

FIG. 13–5. Developmental changes of $I_{Ca(L)}$ in fetal/neonatal rats (**A**) and embryonic chicks (**B**). (**A**) $I_{Ba(L)}$ currents were elicited by depolarizing steps, from a HP of −40 mV. *I/V* curves (normalized as current density (mean ± SEM)) shown for the different developmental stages (from d-12 fetal to d-10 neonatal). (Taken from ref. 57, with permission.) (**B**) Changes in the density of $I_{Ca(L)}$ in isolated embryonic chick heart cells (mean ± SEM). Extracellular Ca^{2+} concentration was 1.8 mM, and the temperature was 35°C. Note that the Ca^{2+} current density was greater in the 3-day cells than in the 17-day cells. (Taken from ref. 58, with permission.)

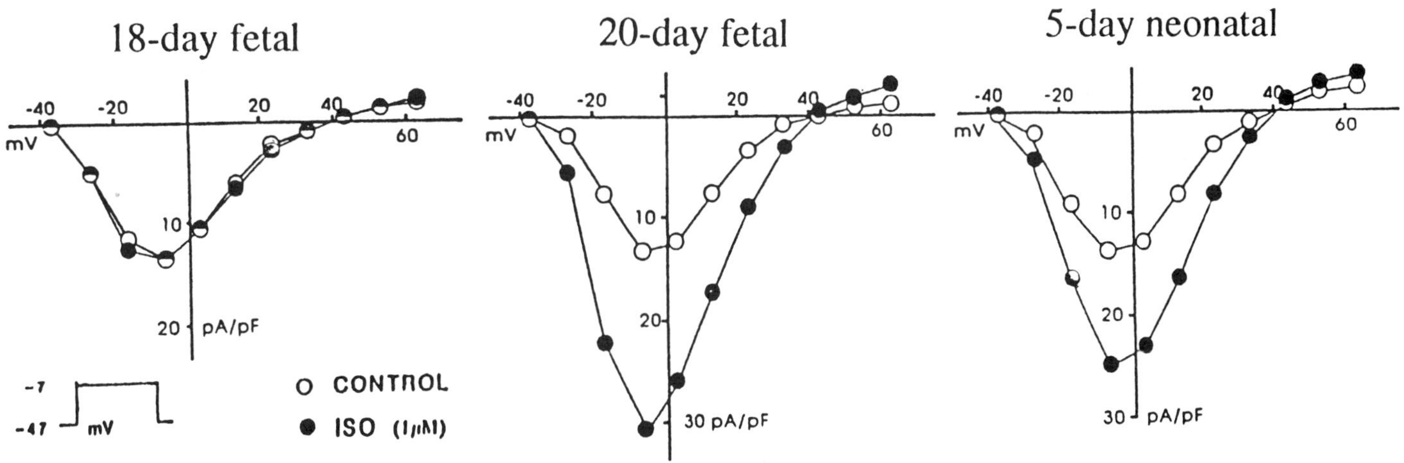

FIG. 13–6. Developmental changes in response to isoproterenol (ISO). *I/V* relationships for rat ventricular cardiomyocytes in the presence (filled circles) and absence (unfilled circles) of 1 μM ISO on one cell from three different developmental stages (18-d and 20-d fetal, and 5-d neonatal). Currents (carried by Ba^{2+} ions) are normalized as pA/pF. (Taken from ref. 60, with permission.)

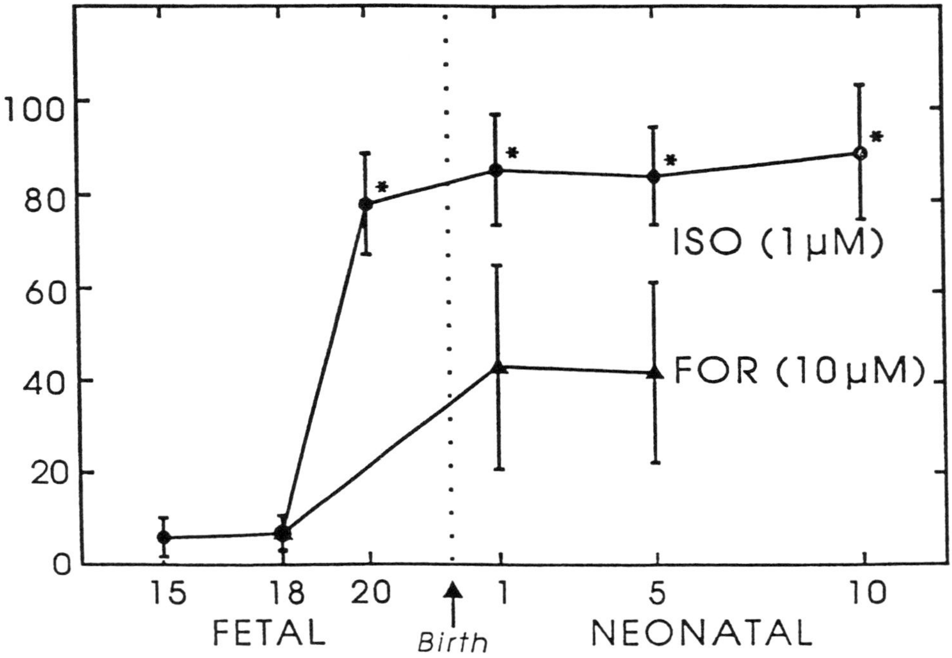

FIG. 13–7. Graphic summary of the developmental changes in response to isoproterenol (ISO) and forskolin (FOR). Percent increases in $I_{Ba(L)}$ produced by 1 μM ISO (circles) and 10 μM FOR (triangles) plotted for different developmental stages (mean ± SEM). Asterisks denote statistical significance ($p < 0.05$). Note the sharp jump in sensitivity to ISO between fetal days 18 and 20. (Taken from ref. 60, with permission.)

A similar pattern of long openings, but not as dramatic, was found for rat heart (Fig. 13–9). The upper part of Fig. 13–9 shows sample current records (cell-attached patch) from one cell on fetal day 12 and one cell on neonatal day 5. On neonatal day 5, the openings are generally brief (only one long opening in the third sweep down) and in a bursting pattern. In contrast, on fetal day 12, the channel exhibits a mixture of brief and long openings, the long openings being more prominent in part B than in part A. The lower part of Fig. 13–9 illustrates the *I/V* curves for the two developmental stages and shows that the single-channel conductance (23 pS) was not changed.

Regulation of Slow Ca^{2+} Channel Activity

The activity of the slow Ca^{2+} channels is regulated by several factors, *intrinsic* and *extrinsic* to the myocardial cell. Intrinsic factors involved include pH_i, $[ATP]_i$, $[Ca]_i$, [cAMP], and [cGMP]. The acidosis produced during ischemia causes a rapid

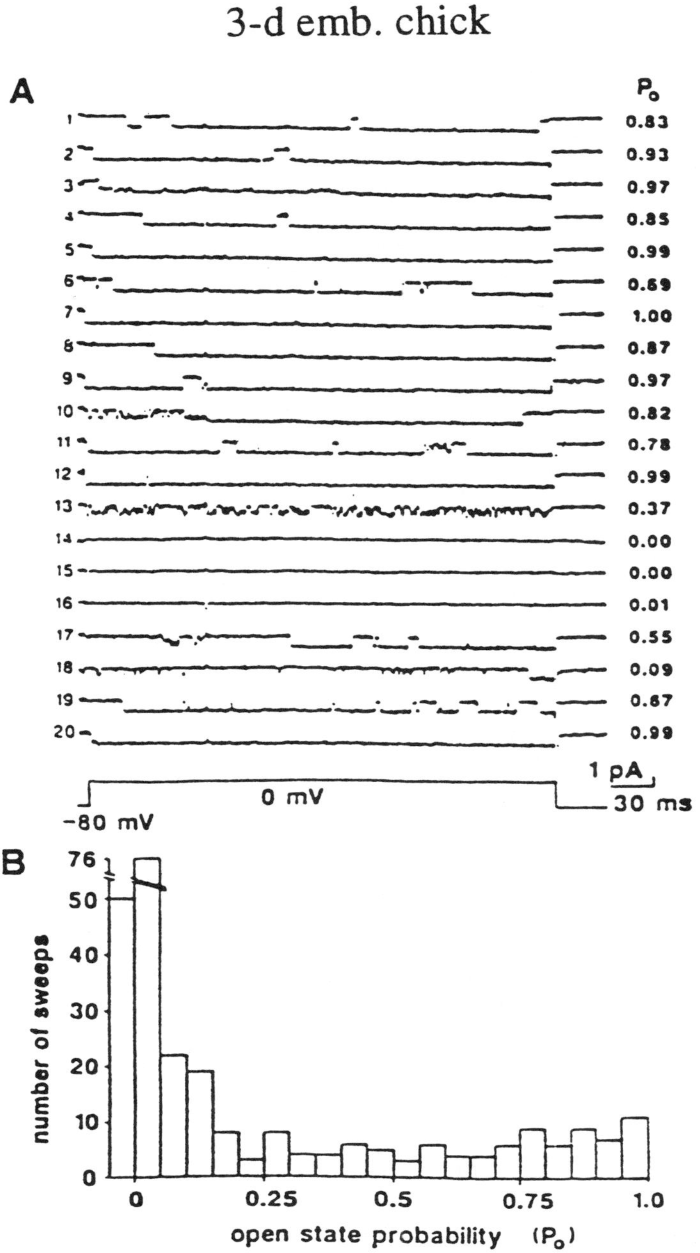

FIG. 13–8. Long openings of Ca^{2+} channels in 3-day embryonic chick heart cells. (**A**) Single-channel activity elicited by consecutive command pulses to 0 mV (from a HP of −80 mV) every 2 sec. The sweep-to-sweep variations of the probability of channel opening (P_o) are given in the right-hand column. (**B**) A histogram of P_o data taken from 9 cells (30 sweeps each). Note bimodal distribution of P_o. (Taken from ref. 61, with permission.)

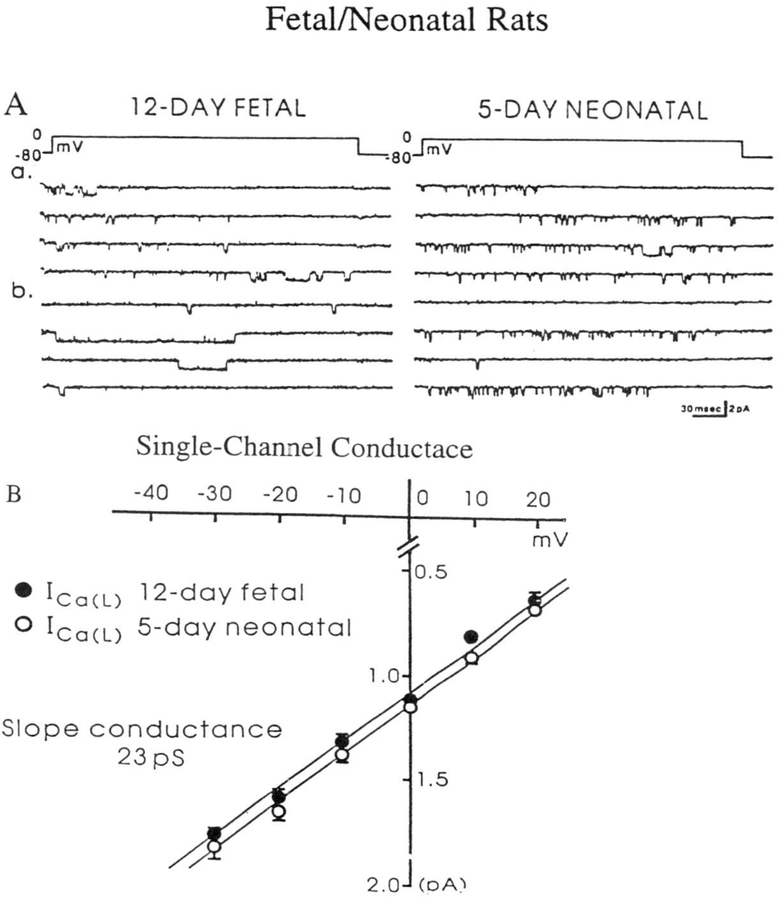

FIG. 13–9. Long openings of Ca^{2+} channels in fetal/neonatal rat heart cells. Single-channel data recorded (cell-attached configuration) from Ca^{2+} channels in day-12 fetal and day-5 neonatal ventricular myocytes. (**A**) Typical single-channel currents for a day-12 fetal cell (a, b) and a day-5 neonatal cell. Records in a and b were taken from two different cells to illustrate a patch with primarily brief openings (a) and one with primarily long openings (b). (**B**) *I/V* relationships of single-channel $I_{Ca(L)}$ currents for day-12 fetal (filled circles) and day-5 neonatal (open circles) myocytes. Data points are shown as mean ± SEM. (Taken from ref. 57, with permission.)

(and reversible) inhibition of the slow Ca^{2+} channels, without having much effect on the fast Na^+ channels and delayed-rectifier K^+ channels (62,63). Binding of ATP to the slow Ca^{2+} channel appears to be required for the channel to exhibit activity (64,65). There is also regulation by $[Ca]_i$, namely, a rise in $[Ca]_i$ inhibits the activity of the Ca^{2+} channel. The mechanism of this inhibition is not known but could be due to binding of Ca^{2+} ion to a negatively charged site on the inner surface of the channel.

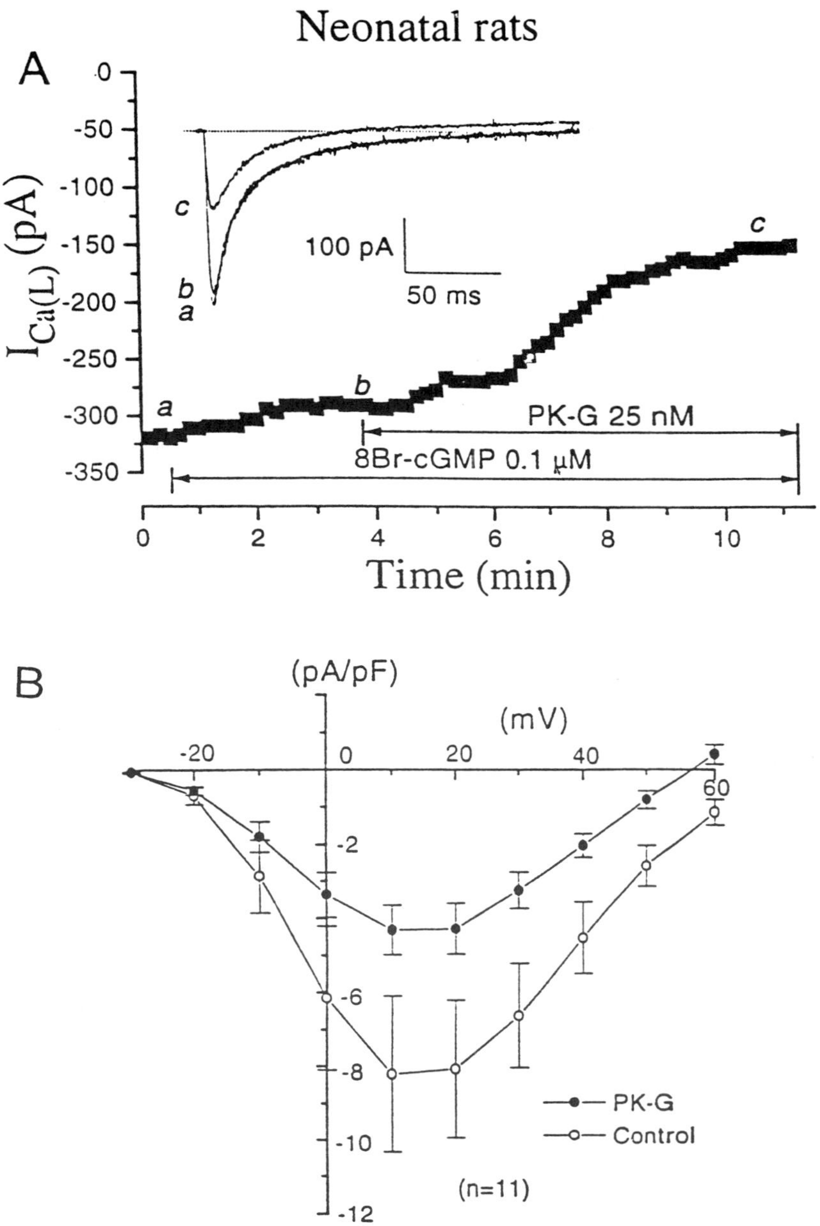

FIG. 13–10. PK-G inhibition of $I_{Ca(L)}$ in neonatal rat heart cells. (**A**) Time course of the effect of PK-G (25 nM) and low subthreshold dose of cGMP (100 nM) applied using the perfusion patch pipette technique on basal (not stimulated) $I_{Ca(L)}$ in a single ventricular myocyte (neonatal day-4). As shown, 8Br-cGMP had almost no effect; subsequent addition of PK-G rapidly produced inhibition. **Inset:** Selective current traces of $I_{Ca(L)}$ (a, b, and c) at points denoted on the time course curve. (**B**) The inhibitory effect of PK-G on the *I/V* relation for basal $I_{Ca(L)}$ in ventricular myocytes from neonatal rats (HP = −40 mV). *I/V* curves of peak $I_{Ca(L)}$ (normalized as pA/pF) for control (unfilled circles) and after application of PK-G (filled circles). Data points are shown as mean ± SEM. (Taken from ref. 67, with permission.)

The slow Ca^{2+} channels are regulated by the cyclic nucleotides and phosphorylation. Extrinsic factors, like neurotransmitters, hormones, and autacoids act, via membrane receptors and G-proteins to increase cAMP, cGMP, or diacylglycerol (DAG) levels, which in turn activate PK-A, PK-G, or PK-C, respectively. These protein kinases phosphorylate, among other proteins, the slow Ca^{2+} channels (or associated regulatory proteins), and thereby modulate their activity. cAMP/PK-A stimulates the slow Ca^{2+} channels of myocardial cells, whereas cGMP/PK-G inhibits their activity (66–68). The inhibition produced by cGMP/PK-G is illustrated at the whole-cell (macroscopic) current level (Fig. 13–10) and single-channel (microscopic) current level (Fig. 13–11). As shown in Fig. 13–11, 8 Br-cGMP (1 mM) added to the bath completely inhibited the activity of slow Ca^{2+} channels of young (day 3) embryonic chick cells (69). Phosphorylation by PK-C has been reported to stimulate $I_{Ca(L)}$ of myocardial cells (70).

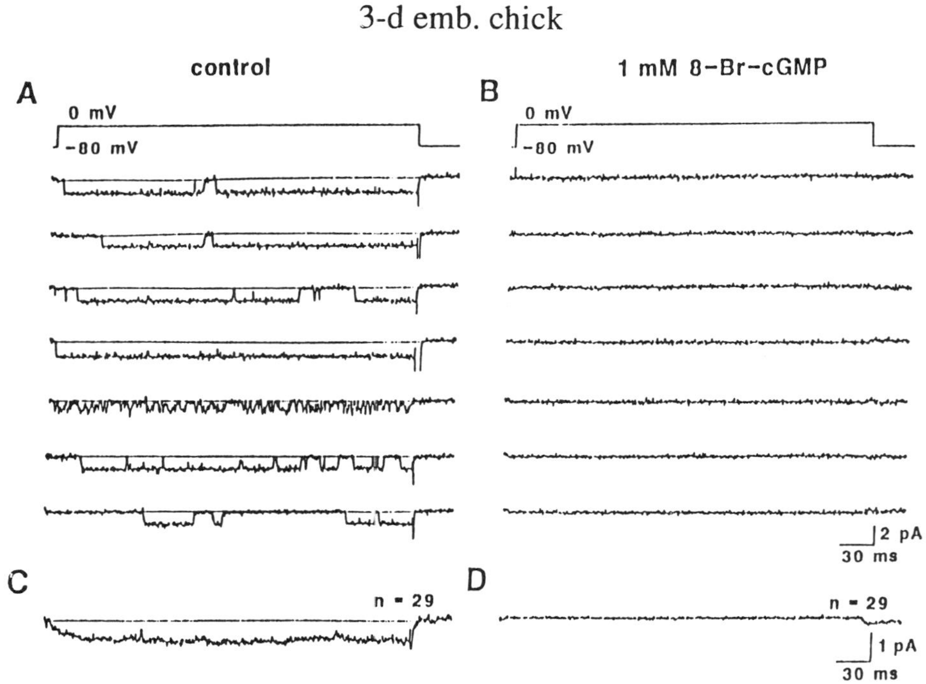

FIG. 13–11. cGMP inhibition of a single Ca^{2+} channel in a 3-day embryonic chick heart cell. Cell-attached patch configuration was used. Currents were evoked by depolarizing voltage pulses to 0 mV from a HP of −80 mV at a repetition rate of 0.5 Hz and duration of 300 msec. Examples of original current recordings from the same patch before (**A**) and after (**B**) superfusion with 1.0 mM 8Br-cGMP. (**C, D**) Ensemble-averaged currents calculated from 29 original current recordings. (Taken from ref. 69, with permission.)

Fast Ca^{2+} Current ($I_{Ca(T)}$)

It was found that the fraction of fast (T-type) Ca^{2+} current in young embryonic chick hearts is relatively high and decreases during subsequent development (71). That is, in old embryonic and adult hearts, the fraction of $I_{Ca(T)}$ of the total I_{Ca} is relatively small. Although the significance of the large $I_{Ca(T)}$ in young embryonic heart cells is not known, it has been suggested that $I_{Ca(T)}$ is a significant contributor to the pacemaker potential. In addition, the Ca^{2+} triggering of Ca^{2+} release from the SR is thought to be a function of $d[Ca]_i/dt$ (Fabiato), and so Ca^{2+} entering via the fast Ca^{2+} channels could be more effective for inducing Ca^{2+} release from the SR.

Fetal Type Ca^{2+} Channels ($I_{Ca(F)}$)

It was found that a large fraction of the total Ca^{2+} current in fetal rat heart cells is resistant to nifedipine and other Ca^{2+} channel blockers (Fig. 13–12) (72). This

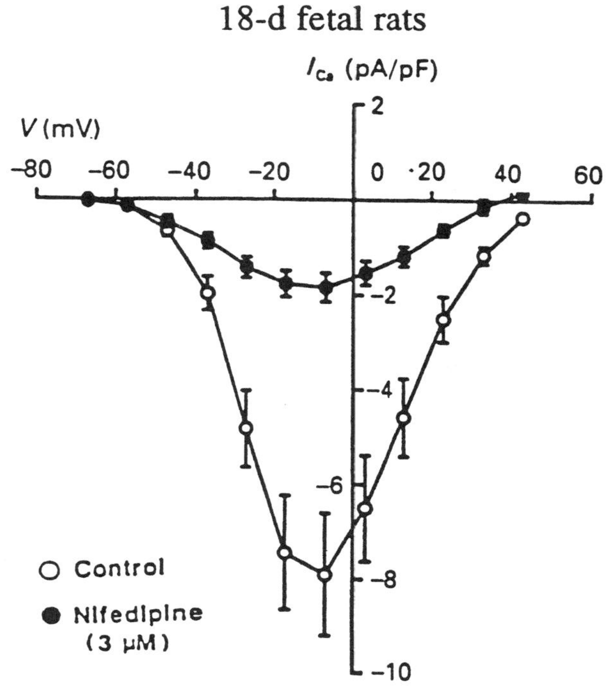

FIG. 13–12. Presence of the fetal-type Ca^{2+} current ($I_{Ca(F)}$) in 18-day fetal rat cardiomyocytes. *I/V* (current density) relationship data points are mean ± SEM. Nifedipine (3 μM) did not completely block the Ca^{2+} current. This nifedipine-resistant current represents $I_{Ca(F)}$. (Taken from ref. 72, with permission.)

nifedipine-resistant current was not blocked by an N-type Ca^{2+} channel blocker, ω-conotoxin, and was only partially inhibited by 30 μM Ni^{2+} ion, which is a blocker of T-type Ca^{2+} channels. Therefore, this channel was called a fetal-type (F-type) Ca^{2+} channel. $I_{Ca(F)}$ is absent in adult heart cells. The voltage for half-inhibition of $I_{Ca(F)}$ is about −58 mV compared to −42 mV for $I_{Ca(L)}$; that is, the inactivation curve for $I_{Ca(F)}$ is shifted to the left (hyperpolarizing direction) by about 16 mV (Fig. 13–13).

I_{ti}, DADs, and Triggered Automaticity

The transient inward current I_{ti}, is already present in young embryonic heart cells. This is evident by addition of ouabain, which induces delayed after-depolarizations (DADs) and oscillatory after-potentials (OAPs) (Fig. 13–14, top). When the DADs are large enough to reach threshold, they trigger action potentials (APs); this phenomenon is known as triggered automaticity and causes arrhythmias. Sometimes

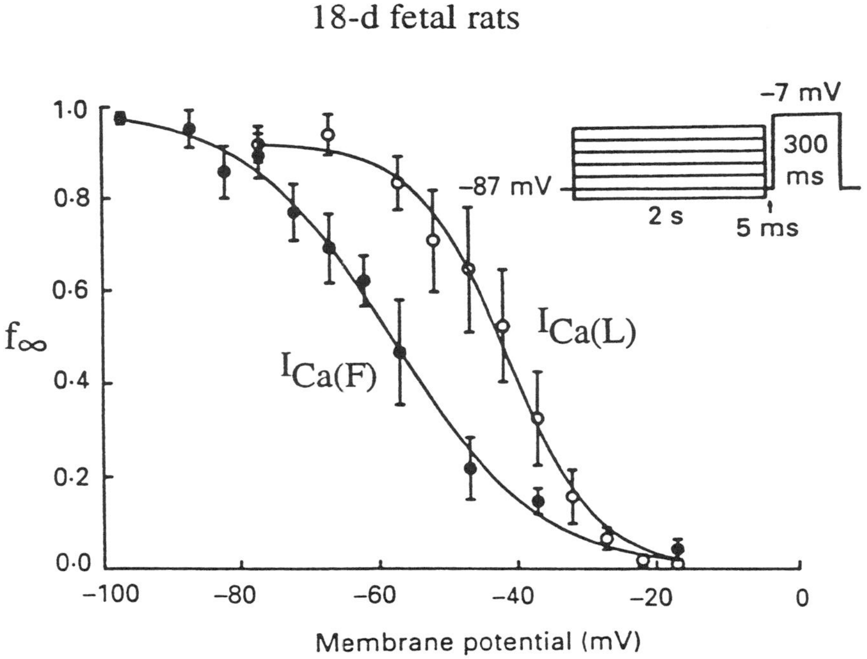

FIG. 13–13. Steady-state inactivation (f_{∞}) curves of the nifedipine (3 μM)-sensitive current ($I_{Ca(L)}$) and the nifedipine-resistant current $I_{Ca(F)}$. The inset shows the voltage protocol used. Test pulses were applied to −7 mV from various conditioning pulse levels, with a 5-ms interval interposed in which the membrane potential was returned to −87 mV. Data are shown as mean ± SEM. Both curves were fitted by the Boltzmann equation. The half-inactivation potential ($V_{0.5}$) was −42.0 mV and −58.4 mV for $I_{Ca(L)}$ and $I_{Ca(F)}$, respectively. Note the 16-mV shift of the curve for $I_{Ca(F)}$ in the hyperpolarized direction. (Taken from ref. 72, with permission.)

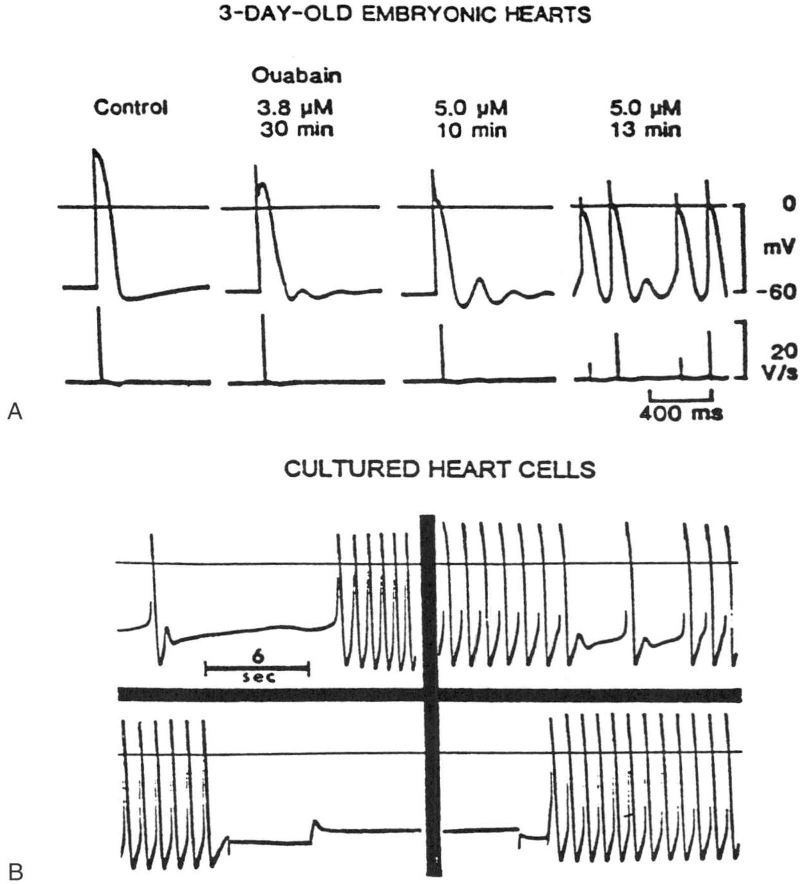

FIG. 13–14. Delayed after-depolarizations (DADs) and triggered automaticity in embryonic chick heart cells. **(A)** Ouabain (3.8 μM, 5.0 μM) induction of DADs in an organ-cultured 3-day embryonic chick heart. The preparation was stimulated at a rate of 0.5 Hz. (Taken from Kojima from ref. 75, with permission.) **(B)** Spontaneous production of DADs and triggered automaticity observed during intracellular microelectrode recordings in one cell of a monolayer culture of embryonic chick ventricular cells (upper row). In the bottom row, a hyperpolarizing current pulse was applied that turned off the train of action potentials. A hyperpolarizing pulse of greater intensity retriggered the train because of anodal-break excitation. (Taken from ref. 76, with permission.)

the DADs and triggered APs occur spontaneously (i.e., in absence of ouabain or other inducing agents such as β-adrenergic agonists) (Fig. 13–14, bottom).

The relationship between I_{ti} and DADs is summarized in Fig. 13–15. As depicted, I_{ti} can be produced by two different currents: (a) current from a Ca^{2+}-activated nonselective cation channel ($I_{Na,\ K(Ca)}$) and (b) the Na/Ca exchange current ($I_{Na/Ca}$). The relative importance of these two currents in the production of I_{ti} and DADs varies from one species to another. However, the common thread to both currents is the release of Ca^{2+} from the SR stores. This released Ca^{2+} can activate the nonselective cation channel and it can stimulate the Na/Ca exchange current (3 Na_o: 1 Ca_i) in the forward mode of operation (i.e., net inward current carried by Na^+ ion). The main current through the nonselective cation channel is an inward Na^+ current, because the electrochemical gradient for Na^+ is much greater than that for K^+ at the resting potential. Thus, both mechanisms result in a net inward Na^+ current, which is depolarizing and produces the DAD.

Also as depicted in Fig. 13–15, ischemia (and hypoxia) can induce I_{ti}, with resultant DADs, triggered APs, and tachyarrhythmias. As stated earlier, DADs can be produced by cardiac glycosides, β-agonists, and high (drive) heart rates. That is, anything that raises $[Na]_i$, and hence $[Ca]_i$ (via Na/Ca exchanger), and overloads the SR, will produce I_{ti} and resultant DADs and triggered automaticity.

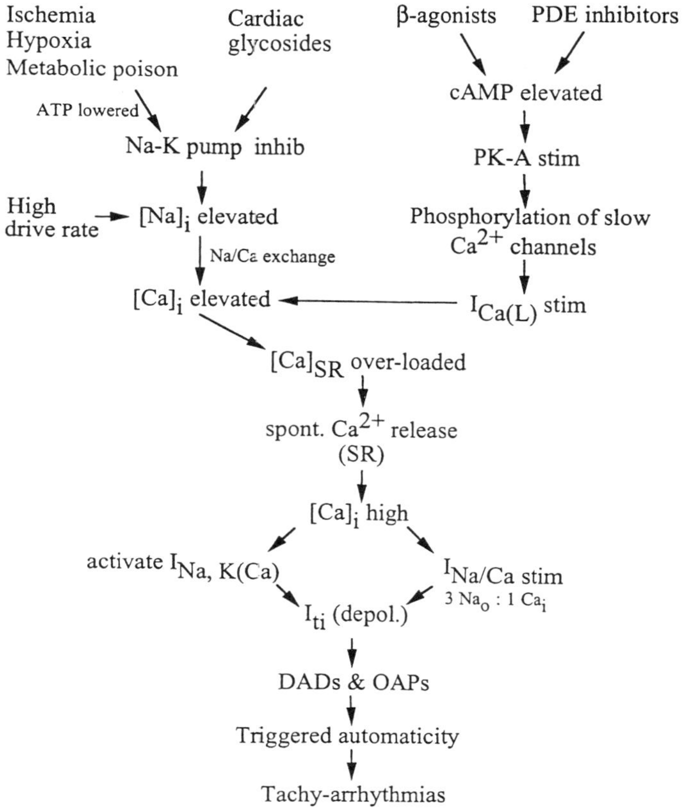

FIG. 13–15. Summary diagram of the mechanisms for generation of the arrhythmogenic transient inward current (I_{ti}). See text for a detailed explanation.

Excitation–Contraction Coupling

Changes in the excitation–contraction coupling process also occur during development of the heart. As depicted in Fig. 13–16 top, the source of Ca^{2+} ions for producing contraction is altered during development (73). In the fetal heart cells, the role of the SR is minimal, so that most of the Ca^{2+} necessary for contraction comes from Ca^{2+} influx through the voltage-dependent Ca^{2+} channels ($I_{Ca(L)}$ and $I_{Ca(T)}$). In the newborn heart cells, the SR begins to play a more prominent role; that is, the source of Ca^{2+} for contraction is about equally split between Ca^{2+} influx and Ca^{2+} release from the SR stores (via Ca^{2+} triggering of Ca^{2+} release through the Ca^{2+}-

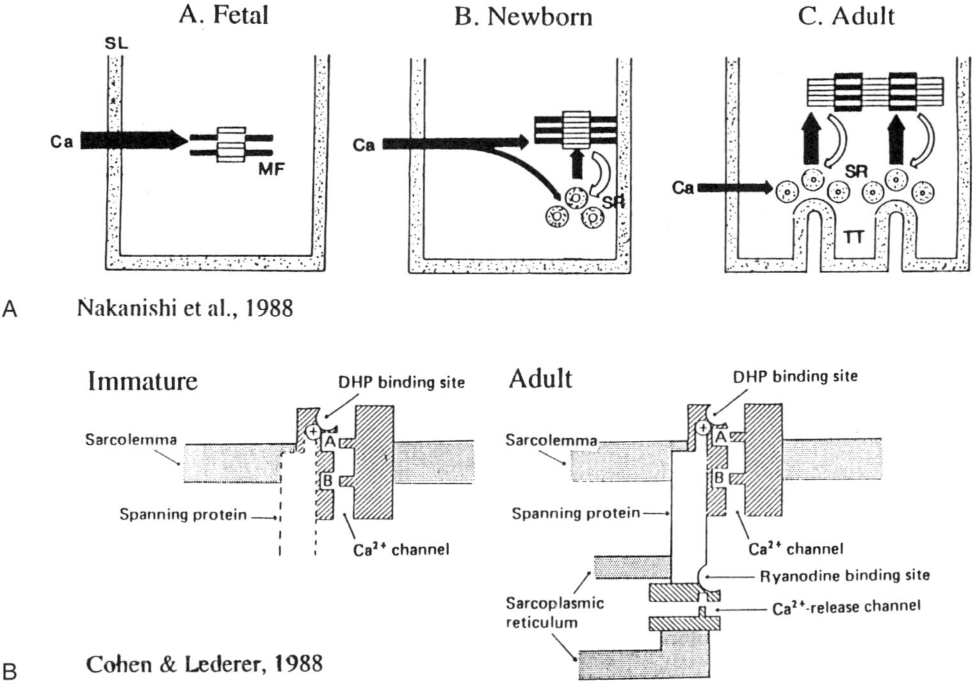

FIG. 13–16. Developmental changes in excitation–contraction coupling. **(A)** Schematic diagrams showing developmental changes in the excitation–contraction coupling. The arrows represent Ca^{2+} ion movements. In the early fetus (panel A), Ca^{2+} entering the cell across the sarcolemma (SL) directly activates the myofilaments (MF). In the newborn (panel B), Ca^{2+} influx across the SL induces some Ca^{2+} release from the sarcoplasmic reticulum (SR), which then contributes to the activation of the MFs. In the adult (panel C), the amount of Ca^{2+} released from SR is greater and most important. (Taken from ref. 73, with permission.) **(B)** Model of excitation–contraction coupling mechanisms in immature and adult heart cells. In the immature cells (left), the protein linking the Ca channel in the SL with the Ca-release channel in the SR appears to be absent. In the adult cells (right), the spanning protein is present, allowing Ca^{2+} release from the SR. (Taken from ref. 74, with permission.)

release channels of the SR). In the adult heart cells, most of the Ca^{2+} for contraction comes from the SR stores (e.g., 80–90%). However, it is the Ca^{2+} influx that is the determining factor of force of contraction, because the Ca^{2+} influx controls the Ca^{2+} release.

As depicted in Fig. 13–16 bottom, it has been proposed (74) that the "spanning protein" that couples the L-type Ca^{2+} channel in the T-tubule wall membrane to the Ca^{2+}-release channel in the SR membrane is absent in the immature fetal heart. If so, then the release of Ca^{2+} from any SR that may be present is prevented. Thus, Ca^{2+} influx would be the main source of Ca^{2+} for contraction.

SUMMARY

In summary, many changes in the electrophysiologic properties of the heart cells occur during development. These changes are caused by changes in the number (density) and types of ion channels. In the young embryonic/fetal heart cell (a) the number of I_{K1} channels is low and explains the low RP, the low P_K, and the high R_m and t_m; (b) the number of I_h channels is high, contributing to the high automaticity of the immature ventricular cells; (c) the number of $I_{Na(f)}$ channels is very low, explaining the low rate of rise of the AP and slow propagation velocity; (d) the number of $I_{Ca(T)}$ channels is high, and this may contribute to automaticity; (e) the number of L-type Ca^{2+} channels is relatively high, but with development, further increases in density in the rat, whereas it slightly decreases in the chick; (f) the L-type Ca^{2+} channels exhibit long openings in both the chick and rat; (g) ISO and forskolin on fetal day 18 and lower do not significantly stimulate $I_{Ca(L)}$ in the rat, indicating that some component is missing in the cascade for the indirect pathway (β-ag→ G_s→ ad. cyclase→ cAMP→ PK-A→ Ca^{2+} channel phosphorylation); (h) regulation of the L-type Ca^{2+} channels by cAMP/PK-A and cGMP/PK-G is already present in the early embryonic period; (i) fetal-type Ca^{2+} channels ($I_{Ca(F)}$) are present; (j) I_{ti} and DADs can be elicited in the immature heart cells; (k) the source of Ca^{2+} for contraction is primarily the Ca^{2+} influx via the voltage-dependent Ca^{2+} channels (i.e., the role of the SR is not significant).

REFERENCES

1. Sperelakis N, Shigenobu K, McLean MJ. Membrane cation channels: changes in developing hearts, in cell culture, and in organ culture. In: Lieberman M, Sano T, eds. *Developmental and physiological correlates of cardiac cells.* New York: Raven Press; 1976:209–234.
2. Sperelakis N, Bkaily G, Sada H, Kojima M. Development of conduction and contraction systems in the heart. In: Jones C, ed. *Fetal and neonatal development.* Ithaca, NY: Perinatology Press; 1987; *J Dev Physiol* 1988;113–124.
3. McLean MJ, Renaud JF, Niu MC, Sperelakis N. Membrane differentiation of cardiac myoblasts induced in vitro by an RNA-enriched fraction from adult heart. *Exp Cell Res* 1977;110:1–14.
4. Sperelakis N, McLean MJ. The electrical properties of embryonic chick cardiac cells. In: Longo LD, Reneau DD, eds. *Fetal and newborn cardiovascular physiology. Vol 1, developmental aspects.* New York: Garland Press; 1978:191–236.

5. Sperelakis N. Changes in membrane electrical properties during development of the heart. In: Zipes DP, Bailey JC, Elharrar E, eds. *The slow inward current and cardiac arrhythmias.* The Hague: Martinus Nijhoff; 1980:221–262.
6. Sperelakis N. Developmental changes in electrical activity and ion channels in the heart. In: Meisami E, Timiras PS, eds. *CRC handbook of human growth and developmental biology,* vol III, part B. Boca Raton, FL: CRC Press; 1990:51–67.
7. Sperelakis N, Pappano AJ. Physiology and pharmacology of developing heart cells. In: Papp JG, ed. *International encyclopedia of pharmacology and therapeutics.* Oxford: Pergamon Press; *Pharmacol Ther* 1983;22:1–39.
8. Sperelakis N, Haddad GE. Developmental changes in membrane electrical properties of the heart. In: Sperelakis N, ed. *Physiology and pathophysiology of the heart,* 3d ed. Boston: Kluwer Academic Publishers; 1994:669–700.
9. Kojima M, Sperelakis N, Johnson G, Ehhreich S, Balazs T. Age-dependent changes in electrophysiologic characteristics of fast and slow action potentials in rat papillary muscle. *Can J Physiol Pharmacol* 1983;61:1509–1515.
10. Kojima M, Sperelakis N, Sada H. Ontogenesis of transmembrane signaling systems for control of cardiac Ca^{2+} channels. Review article. *J Dev Physiol* 1990;14:181–219.
11. Sada H, Sada S, Sperelakis N. Reactivation processes of three inward current systems involved in the rising phase of the action potentials in embryonic chick hearts. *Can J Physiol Pharmacol* 1986;64:125–132.
12. Sperelakis N, Shigenobu K. Changes in membrane properties of chick embryonic hearts during development. *J Gen Physiol* 1972;60:430–453.
13. Sperelakis N, Lee EC. Characterization of (Na^+, K^+)-ATPase isolated from embryonic chick hearts and cultured chick heart cells. *Biochem Biophys Acta* 1971;233:562–579.
14. Kojima M, Sada H, Sperelakis N. Developmental changes in beta-adrenergic and cholinergic interactions on calcium-dependent slow action potentials in rat ventricular muscles. *Br J Pharmacol* 1990;99:327–333.
15. McLean MJ, Lapsley RA, Shigenobu K, Murad F, Sperelakis N. High cyclic AMP levels in young chick embryonic hearts. *Dev Biol* 1975;42:196–201.
16. Thakkar JK, Sperelakis N. Changes in cyclic nucleotide levels during embryonic development of chick hearts. *J Dev Physiol* 1987;9:497–505.
17. Josephson IR, Sperelakis N. Two types of outward K^+ channel currents in early embryonic chick ventricular myocytes. *J Dev Physiol* 1989;12:201–207.
18. Josephson IR, Sperelakis N. Developmental increases in the inwardly rectifying K^+ current of embryonic chick ventricular myocytes. *Biochim Biophys Acta* 1990;1052:123–127.
19. Masuda H, Sperelakis N. Inwardly-rectifying potassium current in rat fetal and neonatal ventricular cardiomyocytes. *Am J Physiol* 1993;265:H1107–H1111.
20. DiFrancesco D, Ferroni A, Mazzanti M, Tromba C. Properties of the hyperpolarizing-activated current (I_f) in cells isolated from the rabbit sino-atrial node. *J Physiol (Lond)* 1986;337:61–88.
21. Noma A, Morad M, Irisawa H. Does the pacemaker current generate the diastolic depolarization in rabbit SA node cells. *Pflugers Arch* 1983;397:190–194.
22. Satoh H, Sperelakis N. Identification of the hyperpolarization-activated inward current in young embryonic chick heart myocytes. *J Dev Physiol* 1991;15:247–252.
23. Satoh H, Sperelakis N. Hyperpolarization-activated inward current in embryonic chick cardiac myocytes: developmental changes and modulation by isoproterenol and carbachol. *Eur J Pharmacol* 1993; 240:283–290.
24. Satoh H, Sperelakis N. Identification of and developmental changes in transient outward current in embryonic chick cardiomyocytes. *J Dev Physiol* 1994;20:149–154.
25. Kilborn MJ, Fedida D. A study of the developmental changes in outward currents of rat ventricular myocytes. *J Physiol (Lond)* 1990;430:37–60.
26. Wahler GM, Dallinger SJ, Smith JM, Flemal KL. Time course of postnatal changes in rat heart action potential and in transient outward current is different. *Am J Physiol* 1994;267:H1157–H1166.
27. Jeck CD, Boyden PA. Age-related appearance of outward currents may contribute to developmental differences in ventricular repolarization. *Circ Res* 1992;71:1390–1403.
28. Mansourati J, Le Grand B. Transient outward current in young and adult diseased human atria. *Am J Physiol* 1993;265:H1466–H1470.
29. Noma A. ATP regulated K^+ channels in cardiac muscle. *Nature* 1983;305:147–148.
30. Sperelakis N. Defining ischemia. *Br Med J* 1995;311:890–891.

31. Sada H, Kojima M, Sperelakis N. Fast inward current properties of voltage-clamped ventricular cells of embryonic chick heart. *Am J Physiol* 1988;255:H540–H553.
32. Fujii S, Ayer RK Jr, DeHaan RL. Differentiation of transmembrane ionic currents in the early embryonic chick heart. *Prog Dev Biol (Part A)* 1986:353–356.
33. Fujii S, Ayer RK Jr, DeHaan RL. Development of the fast sodium current in early embryonic chick heart cells. *J Membr Biol* 1988;101:209–223.
34. McLean MJ, Sperelakis N. Rapid loss of sensitivity to tetrodotoxin of chick ventricular myocardial cells after separation from the heart. *Exp Cell Res* 1974;86:351–364.
35. Shigenobu K, Sperelakis N. Failure of development of fast Na^+ channels during organ culture of young embryonic chick hearts. *Dev Biol* 1974;39:326–330.
36. Jourdon P, Sperelakis N. Electrical properties of cultured heart cell reaggregates from newborn rat ventricles: comparison with intact non-cultured ventricles. *J Mol Cell Cardiol* 1980;12:1441–1458.
37. Frelin C, Cognad C, Vigne P, Lazdunski M. Tetrodotoxin-sensitive and tetrodotoxin-resistant Na^+ channels differ in their sensitivity to Cd^{2+} and Zn^{2+}. *Eur J Pharmacol* 1986;122:245–250.
38. Conforti L, Tohse N, Sperelakis N. Tetrodotoxin-sensitive sodium current in rat fetal ventricular myocytes: contribution to the plateau phase of action potential. *J Mol Cell Cardiol* 1993;25:159–173.
39. Sada H, Ban T, Fujita T, Ebina Y, Sperelakis N. Developmental change in fast Na channel properties in embryonic chick ventricular heart cells. *Can J Physiol Pharmacol* 1995;73:1475–1484.
40. Renaud JF, Romey G, Lombet A, Lazdunski M. Differentiation of the fast Na^+ channel in embryonic heart cells: interaction of the channel with neurotoxins. *Proc Natl Acad Sci* 1981;78:5348–5352.
41. Sperelakis N, Mann JE Jr. Evaluation of electric field changes in the cleft between excitable cells. *J Theor Biol* 1977;64:71–96.
42. Sperelakis N. *Electrogenesis of biopotentials in the cardiovascular system.* Boston: Kluwer Academic Publishers, 1995.
43. Sperelakis N, Ortiz-Zuazaga H, Picone JB. Fast conduction in the electric field model for propagation in cardiac muscle. *Innov Technol Biol Med* 1991;12:404–414.
44. Sada H, Ban T, Sperelakis N. Avian cardiac cells with neuronal type sensitivity to tetrodotoxin (submitted).
45. Iijima T, Pappano AJ. Ontogenetic increase of the maximal rate of rise of the chick embryonic heart action potential: relationship to voltage, time and tetrodotoxin. *Circ Res* 1979;44:358–367.
46. Marcus NC, Fozzard H. Tetrodotoxin sensitivity in the developing and adult chick heart. *J Mol Cell Cardiol* 1981;13:335–340.
47. Sada H, Ban T, Fujita T, Ebina Y, Sperelakis N. Role of the steady-state Na^+ channel current in pacemaker depolarizations in young embryonic chick ventricular myocytes. *Jpn J Pharmacol* 1995;69:159–166.
48. Mitsuiye T, Noma A. Exponential activation of the cardiac Na^+ current in single guinea-pig ventricular cells. *J Physiol (Lond)* 1992;453:261–277.
49. Ogata N, Tatebayashi H. Kinetic analysis of two types of Na^+ channels in rat dorsal root ganglia. *J Physiol (Lond)* 1993;466:9–37.
50. Sperelakis N, Lehmkuhl D. Insensitivity of cultured chick heart cells to autonomic agents and tetrodotoxin. *Am J Physiol* 1965;209:693–698.
51. Shigenobu K, Sperelakis N. Development of sensitivity to tetrodotoxin of chick embryonic hearts with age. *J Mol Cell Cardiol* 1971;3:271–286.
52. McLean MJ, Shigenobu K, Sperelakis N. Two pharmacological types of slow Na^+ channels as distinguished by verapamil blockade. *Eur J Pharmacol* 1974;26:379–382.
53. Bkaily G, Jacques D, Yamamoto T, Sculptoreanu A, Payet MD, Sperelakis N. Three types of slow inward currents as distinguished by melittin in 3-day-old embryonic heart. *Can J Physiol Pharmacol* 1988;66:1017–1022.
54. Bkaily G, Jacques D, Sculptoreanu A, Yamamoto T, Carrier D, Vigneault D, Sperelakis N. Apamin, a highly potent blocker of the TTX- and Mn^{2+}-insensitive fast transient Na^+ current in young embryonic heart. *J Mol Cell Cardiol* 1991;23:25–39.
55. Carmeliet E. Slow inactivation of the sodium current in rabbit Purkinje fibres. *Pflugers Arch* 1987;408:18–26.
56. Josephson IR, Sperelakis N. Tetrodotoxin differentially blocks peak and steady-state sodium channel currents in early embryonic chick ventricular myocytes. *Pflugers Arch* 1989;414:354–359.
57. Masuda H, Sumii K, Sperelakis N. Long openings of calcium channels in fetal rat ventricular cardiomyocytes. *Pflugers Arch* 1995;429:595–597.
58. Tohse N, Meszaros J, Sperelakis N. Developmental changes in long-opening behavior of L-type Ca^{2+} channels in embryonic chick heart cells. *Circ Res* 1992;71:376–384.

59. Kojima M, Ishima T, Taniguchi N, Kimura K, Sada H, Sperelakis N. Developmental changes in beta-adrenoceptors, muscarinic cholinoceptors and Ca^{2+} channels in rat ventricular muscles. *Br J Pharmacol* 1990;99:334–339.
60. Masuda H, Sumii K, Sperelakis N. Developmental changes in β-adrenergic and muscarinic modulations of Ca^{2+} currents in fetal and neonatal ventricular cardiomyocytes of rat. *Reprod Fertil Dev* 1996;8:129–135.
61. Tohse N, Sperelakis N. Long-lasting openings of single slow (L-type) Ca^{2+} channels in chick embryonic heart cells. *Am J Physiol* 1990;259:H639–H642.
62. Vogel S, Sperelakis N. Blockade of myocardial slow inward current at low pH. *Am J Physiol* 1977;233:C99–C103.
63. Irisawa H, Sato R. Intra- and extracellular actions of proton on the calcium current of isolated guinea pig ventricular cells. *Circ Res* 1986;59:348–355.
64. Sperelakis N, Schneider JA. A metabolic control mechanism for calcium ion influx that may protect the ventricular myocardial cell. *Am J Cardiol* 1976;37:1079–1085.
65. O'Rourke B, Backx PH, Marban E. Phosphorylation-independent modulation of L-type calcium channels by magnesium–nucleotide complexes. *Science* 1992;257:245–248.
66. Haddad GE, Sperelakis N, Bkaily G. Regulation of calcium channel by cyclic GMP-dependent protein kinase in chick heart cells. *Mol Cell Biochem* 1995;148:89–94.
67. Sumii K, Sperelakis N. Cyclic GMP-dependent protein kinase regulation of the L-type calcium current in rat ventricular myocytes. *Circ Res* 1995;77:803–812.
68. Tripathi O, Sperelakis N. Effects of 8-bromo cyclic GMP on slow channel mediated action potentials of 3-days-old embryonic chick ventricle. *J Dev Physiol* 1991;16:309–316.
69. Tohse N, Sperelakis N. cGMP inhibits the activity of single calcium channels in embryonic chick heart cells. *Circ Res* 1991;69:325–331.
70. Dösemeci A, Dhallan RS, Cohen NM, Lederer WJ, Rogers TB. Phorbol ester increases calcium current and stimulates the effects of angiotensin II on cultured neonatal rat heart myocytes. *Circ Res* 1988;62:347–357.
71. Creazzo TL, Burch J. Calcium current development in the embryonic chick heart. *Biophys J* 1994;66:A423 (abst).
72. Tohse N, Masuda H, Sperelakis N. Novel isoform of Ca^{2+} channel in rat fetal cardiomyocytes. *J Physiol (Lond)* 1992;451:295–306.
73. Nakanishi T, Seguchi M, Takao A. Development of the myocardial contractile system. *Experientia* 1988;44:936–944.
74. Cohen NM, Lederer WJ. Changes in the calcium current of rat heart ventricular myocytes during development. *J Physiol (Lond)* 1988;406:115–146.
75. Kojima M, Sperelakis N. Properties of oscillatory afterpotentials in young embryonic chick hearts. *Circ Res* 1984;55:497–503.
76. Lehmkuhl D, Sperelakis N. Electrical activity of cultured heart cells. In: Tanz RD, Kavaler F, Roberts J, eds. *Factors influencing myocardial contractility,* New York: Academic Press, 1967: 245–278.

The Developing Heart,
edited by Bohuslav Ošťádal et al.
Lippincott-Raven Publishers,
Philadelphia © 1997.

14

Electrophysiologic Changes in the Mammalian Heart During Postnatal Development

Anton Lukas

Institute of Cardiovascular Sciences, St. Boniface General Hospital Research Centre, and Department of Physiology, University of Manitoba, Winnipeg, Manitoba, R2H 2A6 Canada

The mammalian heart undergoes a number of remarkable changes after birth with respect to electrical activity. They include a decrease in heart rate, an increase in the PR and QT intervals of the electrocardiogram (ECG), and a prolongation or shortening of the ventricular action potential, depending on species. This chapter highlights the major alterations in electrophysiology and ionic currents that occur during postnatal development of the heart. The discussion focuses on results from ventricular tissues and myocytes isolated from rat, guinea pig, rabbit, dog, and human hearts whenever possible.

In the adult heart, significant heterogeneity exists across the ventricular wall in terms of the action potential morphology and response to heart rate (1–3). A prominent notch in the epicardial action potential (between phase 0 and 2) distinguishes it from endocardium in the rabbit (4), feline (5,6), canine (7), and human heart (8). Moreover, the midmyocardium contains a unique subtype of myocardial cells (M cells) that exhibit electrophysiologic features intermediate between those of muscle and conducting cells (9–11). Deceleration of the simulation rate produces much greater prolongation of action potentials in midmyocardium than in epicardium or endocardium. Because of the diverse electrophysiologic properties of the ventricular wall, the age-related changes in the different ventricular layers are discussed separately.

In this chapter, epicardium refers to the myocardial cells within the subepicardial layer of the ventricle. The term *endocardium* includes myocardial cells in the subendocardial ventricular layer, papillary muscles, and ventricular trabeculae. Midmyocardium encompasses the remaining muscle cells between the epicardial and endocardial layers.

POSTNATAL CHANGES IN ACTION POTENTIAL CONFIGURATION IN THE VENTRICLE

Epicardium

Very little information is available about the changes in electrophysiology of the epicardium during postnatal development in most mammals. Wahler et al. (12) reported that the epicardial action potential in the rat ventricle is shorter than the endocardial response at any given age past 1 day (Fig. 14–1). However, this study focused on changes in endocardium, so quantitative data are unavailable for epicardium. The epicardial action potential is thought to shorten markedly during postnatal development, as is the case for the endocardial response (see the following section entitled "Endocardium"). However, this hypothesis requires experimental confirmation.

To date, only one study has specifically examined changes in electrophysiology of the rabbit ventricular epicardium with age. Sanchez-Chapula et al. (13) compared epicardium from neonatal (1–3-day-old) and adult rabbits and found no significant differences in resting membrane potential, action potential amplitude (APA), and action potential duration at 30% and 90% of repolarization (APD_{30} and APD_{90}). The rabbit epicardium is atypical of other mammalian hearts in that its action potential characteristics do not change during postnatal growth. However, these authors did find that an increase in stimulation rate (from 0.1 to 1.0 Hz) significantly shortened APD_{90} in adult epicardium, but APD_{90} remained unchanged in neonatal epicardium. Possible explanations for the blunted frequency response in neonatal epicardium are explored in the section entitled "The Transient Outward Current." All other developmental studies of action potential changes in rat, guinea pig, and rabbit have used endocardium or myocytes of unspecified origin (not from a specific ventricular layer).

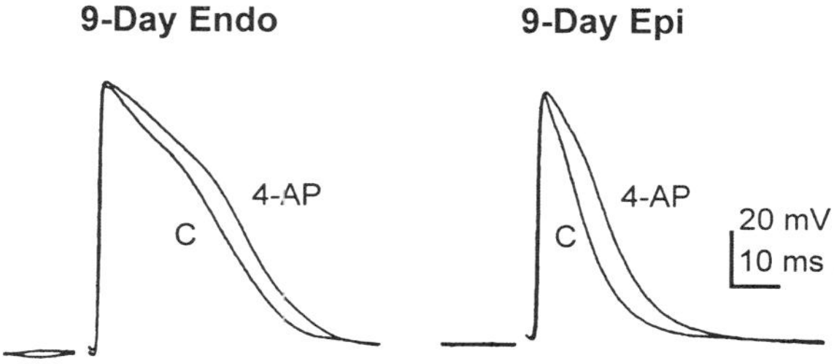

FIG. 14–1. Effect of 4-AP on action potentials recorded from the endocardial (left) and epicardial (right) surfaces of adjacent sections of right ventricle obtained from a 9-day-old neonatal rat heart. C, control; 4-AP, 4-aminopyridine (2 mM). The ventricular strips were stimulated at 0.5 Hz and maintained at 37°C. Note that the epicardial action potential is already significantly shorter than the endocardial action potential at this early age. (Reprinted with permission from ref. 12.)

At birth, the electrophysiology of the canine heart is fairly homogeneous, with the epicardial action potential resembling that of endocardium. Soon after, a notch begins to form following the action potential upstroke in epicardium to produce a characteristic "spike and dome" morphology (Fig. 14–2). The notch is absent in fetal (Fig. 14–2A) and neonatal (<2 weeks) canine epicardial tissue (3,14), but begins to appear within 10 weeks of age (Fig. 14–2B). The notch (phase 1) continues to increase progressively in amplitude during the course of life (Figs. 14–2B–D and Fig. 14–4). Parallel to the increase in notch amplitude is a corresponding decrease in phase 1 amplitude (the difference between resting potential and the minimum voltage during phase 1) (14,15). Our data indicate that notch amplitude does not reach a plateau in the canine heart but continues to increase until old age.

The duration of the epicardial action potential also shortens during postnatal development in the dog. Pacioretty and Gilmour (15) reported a biphasic change in APD with increasing age. At basic cycle lengths (BCL) of 500 or 2000 msec, APD_{90} (APD at 90% repolarization) increased gradually from 2 to 20 weeks of age and then decreased slightly thereafter until 60 weeks of age. In contrast, Jeck and Boyden (14) found only a monotonic decline in APD_{90} from 2 to more than 40 weeks of age in epicardium paced at a BCL of 1300 msec. The differing results may reflect the fact that the former study used epicardium from right ventricle and

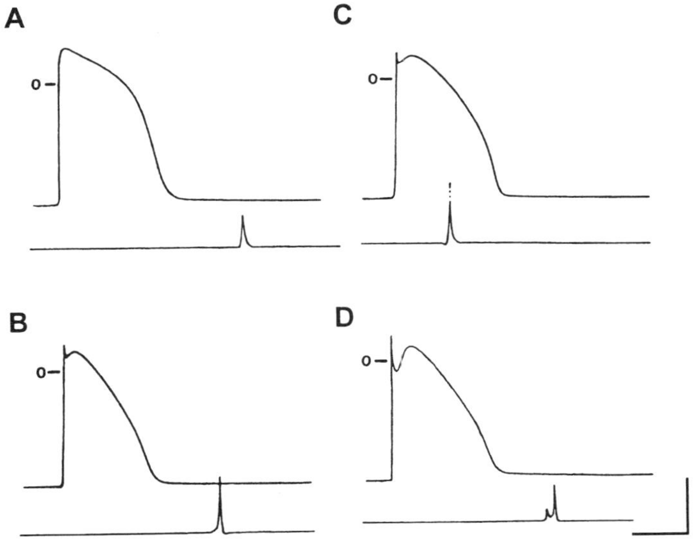

FIG. 14–2. Typical action potentials (upper traces) and *dV/dt* (lower traces) recorded from canine ventricular epicardium at (**A**) 2 months gestation, fetal; (**B**) 2 weeks; (**C**) 10 weeks; and (**D**) 60 weeks of age. Vertical and horizontal calibrations are 40 mV and 100 msec for action potentials. For *dV/dt,* the vertical calibrations are 200 V/sec (A–C) or 400 V/sec (D). Horizontal calibration for all *dV/dt* records is 10 msec. Basic cycle length (BCL) is 500 msec for A–D. (Reprinted with permission from ref. 15.)

the latter used it from left ventricle. A preliminary study suggests that action potential characteristics in epicardium may differ in the right versus left ventricle of the adult canine heart (16). The two groups also found differing effects on APA. Pacioretty and Gilmour (15) saw no change in APA from 2 to 60 weeks of age, whereas Jeck and Boyden (14) found a significant decrease in APA (11 mV) over this age range.

Resting membrane potential does not change significantly from the neonatal to adult stage of development in the dog. Indeed, resting membrane potential in fetal epicardium at 1–2 months of gestation is already polarized to the levels (~−85 mV) seen in neonatal and adult tissues and cells (14,15). Data are similar for upstroke velocity of phase 0 or *dV/dt* (14,15). However, Pacioretty and Gilmour (15) did find a large, though not significant, increase in dV/dt_{max} from 151.8 ± 22.6 to 250.7 ± 47.4 V/sec at 40 versus 60 weeks of age in canine epicardium.

Midmyocardium

It is now clear that the midmyocardial layer of the adult ventricle contains a distinct subtype of muscle cell, termed *M cells.* M cells differ from epicardial and endocardial cells in the manner in which they respond to heart rate. Deceleration of the stimulation rate results in an exaggerated prolongation of APD in M cells compared to epicardial or endocardial cells (9–11). To date, M cell behavior has been recorded in isolated canine midmyocardial tissue (9), single ventricular cells (2,17), and the canine heart in vivo (18,19). Cells displaying prolonged action potentials also exist in the deep myocardial layers of adult rat (20) and guinea pig hearts (21). Recently, M cells were demonstrated in the human heart using transmural slices obtained from normal donor hearts (22) or single cells isolated from ventricular biopsies (23). The functional significance of M cells in the heart remains unresolved. These cells may represent the true working myocardial cells of the heart. Some evidence indicates that prolonged repolarization in the M region is responsible for the U wave on the ECG (1,22,24). M cells are typically present in the deep subepicardial to midmyocardial layers of the ventricular wall. The M region constitutes ~40% of the cellular mass of the left ventricle in the adult canine heart (11) and ~30% in human (22). Estimates are not yet available for other species.

Very little is known about the development of the electrophysiologic characteristics of the midmyocardium. We examined the rate dependence of APD in midmyocardial myocytes obtained from 3-month-old puppies and adult (>2 years) dogs (Fig. 14–3). These age groups were selected for two reasons: (a) The major changes in development of the sympathetic innervation of the heart occur at 8–10 weeks of age in the dog (25–27). Thus, the sympathetic nervous system should be fully functional by 3 months of age. (b) The action potential notch is quite prominent by 3 months of age (Fig. 14–2), suggesting that features of the adult ventricle are present at this stage of postnatal development. As seen in Fig. 14–3, very little

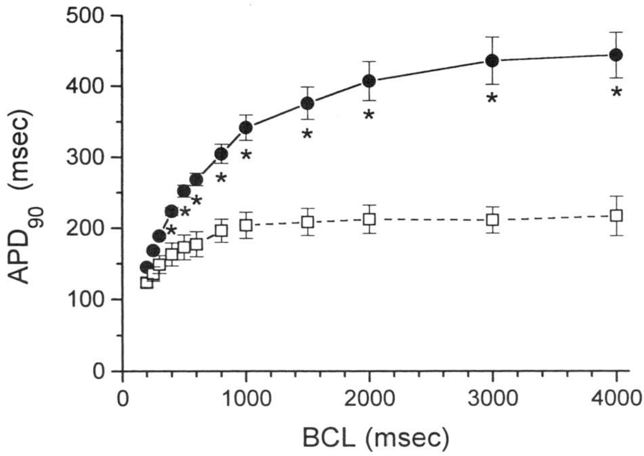

FIG. 14–3. Summary of the APD_{90}–rate relationships obtained in midmyocardial cells isolated from juvenile (3 months old; open squares) and adult dogs (>2 years old; filled circles). The APD_{90} was measured from action potentials recorded with glass microelectrodes in single cells dispersed from the midmyocardium of the left ventricular free wall (2–4 mm from epicardial surface). Cells were stimulated at each BCL (300–4000 msec) for 2 min before action potentials were recorded. The values are means ± S.E. for 18 (adult) or 8 (3-month) cells. $^*p <$ 0.05.

rate dependence of APD_{90} is present in midmyocardial myocytes at 3 months of age. In fact, the APD-rate relation is relatively flat when compared to that of cells from the adult. Similar results were seen in syncytial tissue preparations excised from these hearts. We did not observe M cell behavior in cells or tissues from hearts that ranged in age from 3 weeks to 3 months. The data suggest that maturation of the sympathetic nervous system does not play a role in expression of M cell behavior. Also, appearance of the action potential notch appears to precede the development of M cell behavior in the canine heart.

Endocardium

Perhaps the most dramatic changes in action potential characteristics occur in rat ventricular endocardium (Fig. 14–4). In this species, APD shortens by some threefold from birth to adulthood (12). The marked abbreviation of APD results primarily from loss of the plateau phase (phase 2) in the action potential during postnatal development (12,28,29). This is evident in Fig. 14–4, which depicts action potentials recorded at neonatal days 1–26 and in the adult rat heart. By about 21 days of age, the ventricular action potential resembles the spikelike configuration seen in the adult rat. Repolarization of the plateau in the adult ventricle consists of two phases, referred to as the early and late phases (Fig. 14–4). The early phase is relatively brief and followed by a more prolonged late phase that develops

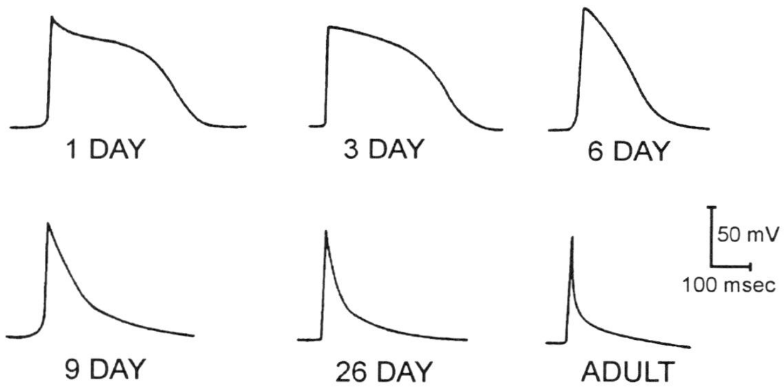

FIG. 14–4. Postnatal changes in the action potential configuration of the rat ventricle from 1 day to adult. Action potentials were recorded using glass microelectrodes in left ventricular papillary muscles at 24–26°C. Note that the progressive shortening of the action potential is attributable to abbreviation of the plateau. Also, two phases of repolarization (early and late phases) are clearly evident from day 9 onward. (Modified from ref. 28.)

at more negative potentials. Ironically, the action potential configuration seen in the neonatal rat ventricle at 1–3 days old is very similar to that recorded in the adult ventricle of most mammalian species (12,28,29). After maturation, APD prolongs steadily as the rat ages from a young adult, through middle age, and into senescence (30). Both the early and late phases of the action potential are prolonged in the ventricles of senescent rats (31,32).

In contrast to rat, the changes in action potential characteristics with age are far less striking in other mammals. In the guinea pig, resting membrane potential, action potential overshoot (OS), and dV/dt_{max} remain unchanged from birth until adulthood in papillary muscle or endocardial free wall preparations (33,34). The resting membrane potential averaged -86.0 ± 0.7 mV on neonatal day 1 versus -87.0 ± 0.5 mV in the adult. The values for OS and dV/dt_{max} in neonates (32.4 ± 0.8 mV and 164.9 ± 12.3 V/sec, respectively) are also similar to adult values (35.5 ± 0.6 mV and 182.4 ± 8.9 V/sec). However, a biphasic change in APD occurs with age in the guinea pig. Both APD_{50} and APD_{90} decrease progressively on neonatal days 1–5 and then increase from day 5 to adult (33,34). APD increases with age in the endocardium of only two species, guinea pig and rabbit. In all others, APD decreases progressively during postnatal development.

Conflicting data exist regarding the changes in electrophysiology of rabbit endocardium with age. Sanchez-Chapula et al. (13) compared action potential characteristics in papillary muscles isolated from neonatal (1–3-day) and adult rabbits at two stimulation frequencies (0.1 and 1.0 Hz). Resting membrane potential in neonatal papillary muscle was not significantly different from that in the adult, but the neonatal values were somewhat more negative. Similarly, APA did not differ in neonatal versus adult papillary muscles, but APA was slightly higher in the neonates. Osaka et al. (35) also examined action potentials in papillary muscles from neonatal (1–3-day) and adult rabbits. However, the neonatal papillary muscles had a significantly higher resting potential (-83.6 ± 1.2 versus -80.0 ± 1.5 mV) and *dV/dt* (134 ± 5 versus 120 ± 5 V/sec) than the adult muscles in this study. Both groups found that APD_{90} was significantly longer in the adult muscles than the neonates, but only at moderate (0.5 – 1.0 Hz) stimulation rates (13,35). At slow rates (0.1 Hz), APD_{90} was longer in the neonatal papillary muscles. The contrasting results obtained at different stimulation rates were due primarily to a blunted frequency response in neonatal muscles. APD_{90} shortens significantly following an increase in stimulation rate in adult papillary, whereas APD_{90} is relatively unaffected by rate changes in neonatal papillary muscles (13). In this respect, the APD-rate relation in endocardial tissues from neonatal rabbit hearts is very similar to that in epicardium (see earlier, under the section entitled "Epicardium").

Although the age-related changes in the epicardial action potential of the canine ventricle are well characterized, little data exist about the changes in endocardium. One microelectrode study found no difference in action potential parameters (resting membrane potential, APA, dV/dt_{max} or APD_{90}) in papillary muscles from neonatal (1–10-day) compared with adult dogs (36). A second study examined endocardial monophasic action potentials in open-chest puppies (4–6 months) and adults (37). This study found that APD_{70} was longer in puppies (204 ± 27 msec) than in adults (174 ± 22 msec). However, the difference was not statistically significant because of a large variation in the puppies. Thus, it is not clear whether the APD changes that occur in endocardium with age are biphasic, as is the case for epicardium.

Current data suggest that the canine heart is homogeneous with respect to electrophysiology during fetal development. Epicardial and endocardial action potentials in the fetal canine heart do not differ with respect to resting membrane potential, APA, *dV/dt,* and APD (15,38). Thus, it appears that the epicardial and endocardial layers become divergent in their electrophysiological characteristics after birth during the neonatal or juvenile stages of development.

IONIC BASIS FOR POSTNATAL CHANGES IN ELECTROPHYSIOLOGY OF THE HEART

Unless otherwise indicated, the following studies employed ventricular cells of transmural origin to investigate developmental changes in ionic currents. Thus, the results reflect the changes in a mixed population of cells derived from different ventricular layers.

The Inward Calcium Current (I_{Ca})

Action potential morphology in the neonatal and adult heart is determined via the interaction of several ionic currents. Of particular importance is the inward Ca^{2+} current. Two types of Ca^{2+} currents exist in the ventricular myocardium; the T-type (transient, $I_{Ca\text{-}T}$) and L-type (long-lasting, $I_{Ca\text{-}L}$). In the rat, $I_{Ca\text{-}L}$ is larger in amplitude and the time constant of decay of the current is slower in neonatal (2–7-day-old) versus adult rat ventricular cells (39,40). The changes in $I_{Ca\text{-}L}$ help explain the marked shortening of the action potential plateau that occurs in the rat ventricle during postnatal growth (Fig. 14–4). The development of the sarcoplasmic reticulum and its connection to the T-tubules may contribute to some of the differences in $I_{Ca\text{-}L}$ observed in neonatal versus adult rat ventricular cells (39). The immature ventricle may be more dependent on transsarcolemmal Ca^{2+} influx to generate tension because of the underdeveloped sarcoplasmic reticulum and deficient T-tubules. On the other hand, the adult ventricle relies largely on Ca^{2+} release from the sarcoplasmic reticulum to achieve the increased $[Ca^{2+}]_i$ needed for tension development. Currently, there is no evidence that $I_{Ca\text{-}T}$ is present in either the neonatal or adult rat ventricle (29,41).

The developmental changes in $I_{Ca\text{-}L}$ are well characterized in the rabbit ventricle. In the fetal heart, the amplitude and current density of $I_{Ca\text{-}L}$ (normalized from cell size) increase during gestation, whereas the voltage dependence for activation of $I_{Ca\text{-}L}$ remains essentially unchanged (42,43). However, the largest changes in $I_{Ca\text{-}L}$ occur after birth in the rabbit. The current density of $I_{Ca\text{-}L}$ in ventricular cells from adult rabbits is two to three times greater than that in neonates (2–5-day-old) (42–47). In contrast, the kinetic properties of $I_{Ca\text{-}L}$ (i.e., current–voltage relation and time course of inactivation) are similar in neonates and adults (43,46). There are two exceptions. First, the membrane potential for half-maximal inactivation of $I_{Ca\text{-}L}$ becomes less negative with age (-19 ± 2 mV in neonates versus -11 ± 2 mV in adults, $p < 0.05$) (43). Second, the time constant for recovery of $I_{Ca\text{-}L}$ from inactivation is prolonged in neonatal versus adult cells at test potentials from -80 to -40 mV (43). The latter result could explain the greater frequency dependence of $I_{Ca\text{-}L}$ seen in neonatal cells. Acceleration of the stimulation rate markedly decreases peak $I_{Ca\text{-}L}$ (elicited by a test pulse to +10 mV from a holding potential of -80 mV) in neonatal cells but has little effect on $I_{Ca\text{-}L}$ in the adult cells (43). At a holding potential of -40 mV, stimulation at faster rates inhibited peak $I_{Ca\text{-}L}$ in both neonatal and adult cells, but the effects of rate continued to be more pronounced in the neonatal cells.

Both $I_{Ca\text{-}L}$ and $I_{Ca\text{-}T}$ are present in adult rabbit ventricular cells. However, this is not the case in neonate cells. Wetzel et al. (44) found evidence of $I_{Ca\text{-}T}$ in only 39% of neonatal ventricular cells, whereas $I_{Ca\text{-}T}$ was present in 91% of the adult cells. The functional significance of a greater prevalence of $I_{Ca\text{-}T}$ in adult cells is not clear, since the exact roles of $I_{Ca\text{-}T}$ and $I_{Ca\text{-}L}$ in generation of the action potential and tension are not fully defined. Data are not yet available for developmental changes in $I_{Ca\text{-}L}$ or $I_{Ca\text{-}L}$ in the guinea pig or dog ventricle, although both $I_{Ca\text{-}T}$ and $I_{Ca\text{-}L}$ are present in the adult myocardium of these two species.

The Transient Outward Current (I_{to})

Postnatal development is associated with alterations in several K^+ currents that contribute to repolarization of the cardiac action potential. They include the transient outward current (I_{to}), the delayed rectifier current (I_K), and the inward rectifier current (I_{K1}). Of the K^+ currents, the greatest data are available for I_{to}. I_{to} consists of two components in most species; a slow component that is abolished by 4-aminopyridine (4-AP) and a fast component that is abolished by agents that inhibit Ca^{2+} release from the sarcoplasmic reticulum. The two components are termed the 4-AP-sensitive (I_{to1}) and Ca^{2+}-activated (I_{to2}) components.

Levels of I_{to1} increase significantly during postnatal development in rat ventricular myocytes (12,48). Wahler et al. (12) found a slight increase in I_{to1} amplitude between day 1 and days 8–10, but the largest increase occurred between days 8–10 and the adult. In contrast, Kilborn and Fedida (48) reported a dramatic increase in I_{to1} between days 1 and 10. However, the former study used freshly isolated rat ventricular cells, whereas the latter used cultured cells. Also, both studies used cells of transmural origin. Marked regional variations in I_{to} exist in the adult rat ventricle as in most species (i.e., I_{to} is larger in epicardium than in endocardium) (49). Thus, the increase in I_{to} amplitude that occurs after birth in the rat heart may be even greater in epicardium.

Postnatal development is also associated with an increase in I_{to} density in the rabbit ventricle. In the adult rabbit ventricle, I_{to} density is significantly greater in epicardial versus endocardial cells (4,13). One study has specifically measured I_{to} changes in rabbit epicardium versus endocardium with development (13). That study found that I_{to} densities in neonatal cells (1–3 days old) from the epicardium and endocardium were about one-half the current density in adults cells from the same layer. Also, the regional differences in I_{to} density seen in the adult rabbit ventricle were preserved in the neonatal heart cells. At +50 mV, I_{to} density averaged 7.9 ± 1.4 pA/pF in neonatal epicardial cells versus 6.1 ± 1.3 pA/pF in endocardial cells ($p < 0.05$). In adult cells, the corresponding values for I_{to} densities were 14.3 ± 2.0 pA/pF in epicardial cells and 11.1 ± 2.1 pA/pF in endocardial cells ($p < 0.05$) (13). The study also found differences in the kinetic behavior of I_{to} in the neonatal versus adult cells. Both the rate of inactivation of I_{to} and its recovery from inactivation were significantly faster in neonatal versus adult cells. The authors suggest that the marked differences in recovery kinetics of I_{to} could explain the blunted APD-rate relation recorded in neonatal versus adult rabbit ventricular preparations or cells (13).

The ventricular myocardium of the adult guinea pig is one of the few tissues in which an I_{to} current is not present (50). Also, there are no reports in the literature of an I_{to} in the ventricle of neonatal guinea pigs.

Changes in I_{to} with age are probably best characterized in the dog heart. A 4-aminopyridine-sensitive transient outward current (I_{to1}) begins to appear in canine epicardial cells by 2 weeks of age (15). Current density then progressively increases with age, but reaches a plateau at 20–40 weeks of age. The increase in I_{to1} is independent of the increase in cell size during this phase (15). At 20 weeks of age, the density of I_{to1} (14,15) is similar to that recorded in epicardium of adult dogs (17,51). The time constants of I_{to1} decay tend to increase significantly from 2 weeks (18.1 ± 1.6 msec) to 60 weeks (29.9 ± 2.2 msec) (15). In contrast, the

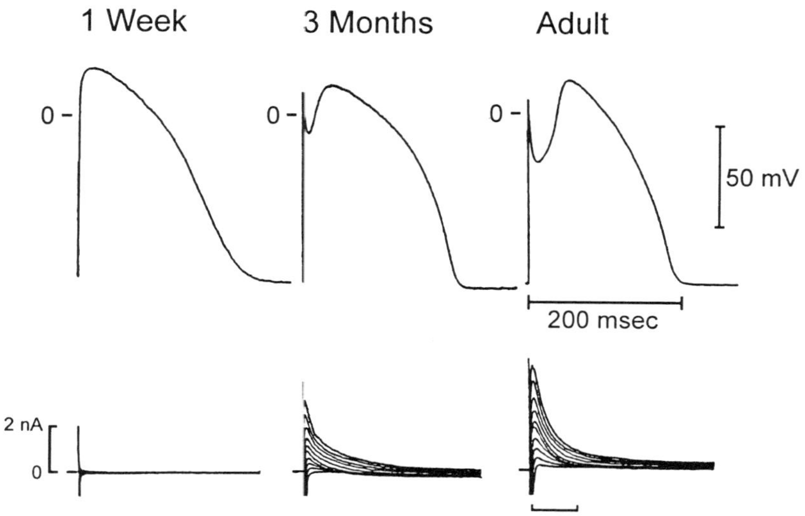

FIG. 14–5. Postnatal changes in action potential morphology and transient outward current (I_{to}) in canine ventricular epicardium. Top panels depict action potentials recorded at BCL of 2000 msec in epicardial tissues isolated at 1 week (left), 3 months (middle), and 1 year of age (right). Lower panels show typical I_{to} currents recorded using whole-cell patch-clamp in single cells isolated from the corresponding hearts. (Reprinted with permission from ref. 3.)

voltage dependence for steady-state inactivation of I_{to1} is unchanged over this age range. Thus, the major changes in I_{to1} with age include a large increase in amplitude and a slowing in its rate of decay.

The amplitude of I_{to1} varies markedly from epicardium to endocardium in most species. The density of I_{to1} is significantly greater in epicardial versus endocardial myocytes from the rat (49), rabbit (4), feline (52), canine (17), and human heart (8,53). The functional significance of a larger I_{to1} in epicardium than endocardium is unknown. It is clear that activation of I_{to1} underlies the action potential notch in the epicardium of several species, since inhibition of I_{to1} by 4-AP or rapid pacing abolishes the notch. In canine epicardium, the progressive development of the action potential notch with age is paralleled by an increase in I_{to1} amplitude to generate the characteristic "spike and dome" configuration of the adult (Fig. 14–5).

The Delayed Rectifier Current (I_K)

The delayed rectifier (I_K) plays a key role in the plateau phase and initiation of repolarization of the action potential. The delayed rectifier consists of a rapidly activating component (I_{Kr}) and a slowly activating component (I_{Ks}) that can be distin-

guished based on activation kinetics, threshold potential, sensitivity to benzenesulfonamide class III agents (E-4031 and dofetilide) and sensitivity to β-adrenergic stimulation (for reviews, see refs. 54,55). Both components of I_K are present in guinea pig (56), rabbit (57,58), and canine (59,60) ventricular cells, whereas only I_{Kr} exists in the feline (61,62) and possibly rat ventricle (63). A recent study of I_K in the human ventricle indicates that it also contains an I_{Kr} and I_{Ks} component (64). At present, the changes in I_K during development have not been investigated in the rat or rabbit ventricle.

Data are also limited about the developmental changes in I_K in the guinea pig ventricle. Wu et al. (65) studied postnatal changes in I_K in neonatal versus adult guinea pig ventricular cells. These authors found a larger slope conductance for I_K in neonatal cells (<1 day old) than in adult cells (702 ± 80 pS/pF versus 194 ± 23 pS/pF, $p < 0.01$). A decrease in the slope conductance of I_K is consistent with the age-related prolongation of APD seen in this species (33,34).

The distinctive APD-rate relation in canine midmyocardial or M cells is due, in large part, to a lesser contribution of I_K to repolarization. Specifically, the I_{Ks} tail current density is significantly smaller in M cells compared to epicardial and endocardial cells (59,60). In contrast, I_{Kr} tail current density is similar in the three cell types. At present, it is unclear at what age the postnatal changes in I_K density occur in the canine ventricle. Data presented in Fig. 14–3 suggest that M-cell behavior is not yet present in midmyocardial cells at 3 months of age. Paradoxically, β-adrenergic stimulation markedly increases I_{Ks} amplitude, yet M-cell expression occurs after maturation of the sympathetic nervous system in the canine ventricle (25–27,66). Thus, the event that triggers expression of M-cell behavior during postnatal development remains to be identified.

The Inward Rectifier Current (I_{K1})

The inward rectifier (I_{K1}) contributes to phase 3 repolarization of the cardiac action potential and to resting membrane potential. The inward rectification properties of I_{K1} allow K^+ efflux from cells at potentials near the resting membrane potential but limit K^+ loss at less polarized potentials. The current density of I_{K1} increases during fetal and neonatal development in most species. In the rat, I_{K1} density increases by a factor of 2–3 during early postnatal development (between days 3 and 10) and then remains constant (67,68) or decreases slightly (48). Age-dependent differences in single channel activity of I_{K1} were also observed in the rat ventricle. Wahler (67) reported that I_{K1} channels in adult myocytes consisted of two populations (30 and 42 pS conductances), whereas neonatal cells (<9 days old) exhibited only a 30-pS channel. Masuda and Sperelakis (68) also found only a 31 pS I_{K1} channel in neonatal (1–10-day-old) rat ventricular cells. The increase in I_{K1} amplitude with age may contribute to the dramatic shortening of the ventricular action potential in the rat (see Fig. 14–4). I_{K1} also contributes to maintenance of the resting potential, yet RMP remains virtually unchanged during postnatal development of the rat ventricle (67).

The developmental changes in I_{K1} in the rabbit heart are similar to those in rat. The increase in I_{K1} density in rabbit ventricular cells is most rapid during late fetal development but continues to increase from the neonate to adult (13,42). I_{K1} amplitude increases about sixfold from neonatal day 5 to the adult (475 ± 35 pA versus 2632 ± 310 pA, $p < 0.05$). Correspondingly, I_{K1} density increases from 27 ± 2 $\mu A/cm^2$ to 37 ± 35 $\mu A/cm^2$. Ironically, the increase in I_{K1} with age occurs when there is little change in APD_{90} in epicardium or endocardium. The resting membrane potential also does not change during postnatal development in epicardium (13) or endocardium (13,35), as might be expected with a large increase in I_{K1}.

Data are currently unavailable for the age-related changes in I_{K1} in the canine. However, I_{K1} levels do not differ among the epicardial, midmyocardial, and endocardial layers of the adult canine ventricle (17). In contrast, transmural differences in I_{K1} do exist in the ventricles of other species, such as the adult feline (69).

ELECTROCARDIOGRAPHIC CHANGES

The complex electrophysiologic changes that occur in the ventricles with age also register on the body surface ECG. ECGs in the neonate differ significantly from those in adult dogs with respect to every interval except the P wave (Table 14–1). In neonates, heart rate is significantly faster than in adult dogs (14,66). Once corrected for heart rate, the major age-related changes in the ECG correspond to differences in ventricular repolarization (Table 14–1). Neonates (0–14 days) and young dogs (57–58 days) require more time to complete repolarization than do adults (14). This is reflected by the significant decrease in QT_C and JT_C intervals in adult dogs versus neonates and juvenile animals.

TABLE 14–1. *Age-related changes in electrocardiographic intervals and durations in dogs*

	Intervals					
Age	RR (msec)	P (msec)	PR (msec)	QRS (msec)	QT_C	JT_C
Adult	582 ± 53	44 ± 3	148 ± 4	41 ± 2	273 ± 3	219 ± 3
64–68 days	357 ± 32	40 ± 0	117 ± 3*	37 ± 3	273 ± 8	212 ± 9
60–61 days	350 ± 23	35 ± 5	100 ± 6*	28 ± 3	283 ± 8	238 ± 8
57–58 days	280 ± 10	35 ± 5	102 ± 8*	35 ± 5	321 ± 6*	255 ± 10*
Neonate	269 ± 4*	36 ± 2	96 ± 3*	28 ± 2*	324 ± 2*	269 ± 3*

Modified from ref. 14, with permission.

Adult, >10 months of age; neonate, 0–14 days old; QT_C, rate-corrected QT interval using Bazzett's formula; JT_C, rate-corrected JT interval calculated as QT duration minus QRS duration and includes ST interval and T wave. Values are mean ± SEM.

*$p < 0.05$ versus adult.

SUMMARY

The mammalian heart evolves from a relatively homogeneous muscle at birth into a complex organ with diverse electrical properties in the adult. This evolution takes place over days to years, depending on the species. Postnatal development is associated with a shortening of the APD in all species (except guinea pig and rabbit) and an increase or decrease in inward and/or outward ionic currents. At present, large gaps still exist in our knowledge about the developmental changes that occur in the various ventricular layers of most species. The ionic basis for electrical heterogeneity in the heart must be identified in order to understand its response to aging, pharmacological interventions, and pathophysiologic conditions.

ACKNOWLEDGMENT

This work was supported by an NIH First Award (Grant HL43148). Dr. Lukas is the Myles Robinson Scholar.

REFERENCES

1. Antzelevitch C, Sicouri S. Clinical relevance of cardiac arrhythmias generated by afterdepolarizations: role of M cells in the generation of U waves, triggered activity and torsade de pointes. *J Am Coll Cardiol* 1994;23:259–277.
2. Lukas A, Antzelevitch C. The contribution of K^+ currents to electrical heterogeneity in the canine ventricular wall under normal and ischemic conditions. In: Dhalla NS, Singal PK, Takeda N, Beamish RE, eds. *Pathophysiology of heart failure.* Boston: Kluwer Academic Publishers, 1996: 439–456.
3. Antzelevitch C, Sicouri S, Lukas A, Nesterenko VV, Liu DW, Di Diego JM. Regional differences in the electrophysiology of ventricular cells: physiological and clinical implications. In: Zipes DP, Jalife J, eds. *Cardiac electrophysiology: from cell to bedside.* Philadelphia: WB Saunders; 1995: 228–245.
4. Fedida D, Giles WR. Regional variations in action potentials and transient outward current in myocytes isolated from rabbit left ventricle. *J Physiol (Lond)* 1991;442:191–209.
5. Kimura S, Bassett AL, Furukawa T, Cuevas J, Myerburg RJ. Electrophysiological properties and responses to simulated ischemia in cat ventricular myocytes of endocardial and epicardial origin. *Circ Res* 1990;66:469–477.
6. Kimura S, Bassett AL, Kohya T, Kozlovskis PL, Myerburg RJ. Simultaneous recording of action potentials from endocardium and epicardium during ischemia in the isolated cat ventricle: relation of temporal electrophysiologic heterogeneities to arrhythmias. *Circulation* 1986;74:401–409.
7. Litovsky SH, Antzelevitch C. Transient outward current prominent in canine ventricular epicardium but not endocardium. *Circ Res* 1988;62:116–126.
8. Nabauer M, Beuckelmann DJ, Uberfuhr P, Steinbeck G. Regional differences in current density and rate-dependent properties of the transient outward current in subepicardial and subendocardial myocytes of human left ventricle. *Circulation* 1996;93:168–177.
9. Sicouri S, Antzelevitch C. A subpopulation of cells with unique electrophysiological properties in the deep subepicardium of the canine ventricle: the M cell. *Circ Res* 1991;68:1729–1741.
10. Antzelevitch C, Sicouri S, Litovsky SH, Lukas A, Krishnan SC, Di Diego JM, Gintant GA, Liu DW. Heterogeneity within the ventricular wall: electrophysiology and pharmacology of epicardial, endocardial, and M cells. *Circ Res* 1991;69:1427–1449.
11. Sicouri S, Fish J, Antzelevitch C. Distribution of M cells in the canine ventricle. *J Cardiovasc Electrophysiol* 1994;5:824–837.

12. Wahler GM, Dollinger SJ, Smith JM, Flemal KL. Time course of postnatal changes in rat heart action potential and in transient outward current is different. *Am J Physiol* 1994;267:H1157–H1166.
13. Sanchez-Chapula J, Elizalde A, Navarro Polanco R, Barajas H. Differences in outward currents between neonatal and adult rabbit ventricular cells. *Am J Physiol* 1994;266:H1184–H1194.
14. Jeck CD, Boyden PA. Age-related appearance of outward currents may contribute to developmental differences in ventricular repolarization. *Circ Res* 1992;71:1390–1403.
15. Pacioretty LM, Gilmour RF, Jr. Developmental changes of action potential configuration and I_{to} in canine epicardium. *Am J Physiol* 1995;268:H2513–H2521.
16. Di Diego JM, Sicouri S, Litovsky SH, Antzelevitch C. Two components of the transient outward current in canine ventricular epicardium: right versus left. *Circulation* 1991;84:II-179. Abstract.
17. Liu DW, Gintant GA, Antzelevitch C. Ionic bases for electrophysiological distinctions among epicardial, midmyocardial, and endocardial myocytes from the free wall of the canine left ventricle. *Circ Res* 1993;72:671–687.
18. Wang Y, Hariman RJ, Gintant GA, Louie EK, Hwang MH, Loeb HS. A method for recording of intramyocardial monophasic action potential in intact dogs: in vivo evidence of M cells. *PACE* 1992;15:II–559. Abstract.
19. Hariman RJ, Wang Y, Sharif MA, Louie EK, Hwang MH, Loeb HS, Scanlon PJ. Early afterdepolarizations arising from M cells in intact dogs. *Circulation* 1992;86:I-301. Abstract.
20. Watanabe T, Delbridge LM, Bustamante JO, McDonald TF. Heterogeneity of the action potential in isolated rat ventricular myocytes and tissue. *Circ Res* 1983;52:280–290.
21. Watanabe T, Rautaharju PM, McDonald TF. Ventricular action potentials, ventricular extracellular potentials, and the ECG of guinea pig. *Circ Res* 1985;57:362–373.
22. Drouin E, Charpentier F, Gauthier C, Laurent K, Le Marec H. Electrophysiologic characteristics of cells spanning the left ventricular wall of human heart: evidence for presence of M cells. *J Am Coll Cardiol* 1995;26:185–192.
23. Peeters GA, Sanguinetti MC, Eki Y, Konarzewska H, Renlund DG, Karwande SV, Barry WH. Method for isolation of human ventricular myocytes from single endocardial and epicardial biopsies. *Am J Physiol* 1995;268:H1757–H1764.
24. Nesterenko VV, Antzelevitch C. M cells as the basis for the electrocardiographic U wave. *Circulation* 1992;86:I-302. Abstract.
25. Gauthier P, Nadeau RA, de Champlain J. The development of sympathetic innervation and the functional state of the cardiovascular system in newborn dogs. *Can J Physiol Pharmacol* 1975; 53:763–776.
26. Kralios FA, Millar CK. Functional development of cardiac sympathetic nerves in newborn dogs: evidence for asymmetrical development. *Cardiovasc Res* 1978;12:547–554.
27. Ursell PC, Ren CL, Danilo P, Jr. Anatomic distribution of autonomic neural tissue in the developing dog heart: I. Sympathetic innervation. *Anat Rec* 1990;226:71–80.
28. Langer GA, Brady AJ, Tan ST, Serena SD. Correlation of the glycoside response, the force staircase, and the action potential configuration in the neonatal rat heart. *Circ Res* 1975;36:744–752.
29. Fermini B, Schanne OF. Determinants of action potential duration in neonatal rat ventricle cells. *Cardiovasc Res* 1991;25:235–243.
30. Walker KE, Lakatta EG, Houser SR. Age associated changes in membrane currents in rat ventricular myocytes. *Cardiovasc Res* 1993;27:1968–1977.
31. Capasso JM, Malhotra A, Remily RM, Scheuer J, Sonnenblick EH. Effects of age on mechanical and electrical performance of rat myocardium. *Am J Physiol* 1983;245:H72–H81.
32. Wei JY, Spurgeon HA, Lakatta EG. Excitation-contraction in rat myocardium: alterations with adult aging. *Am J Physiol* 1984;246:H784–H791.
33. Agata N, Tanaka H, Shigenobu K. Developmental changes in action potential properties of the guinea-pig myocardium. *Acta Physiol Scand* 1993;149:331–337.
34. Pucelik P. Do differences develop in the electrogenesis of action potentials of the right and left ventricle of the guinea-pig heart during postnatal development. *Physiol Bohemoslov* 1983;32:193–202.
35. Osaka T, Ramza BM, Tan RC, Joyner RW. Developmental changes in the electrophysiologic properties of rabbit papillary muscles. *Pediatr Res* 1989;26:543–547.
36. Yabek SM, Kato R, Singh BN. Effects of hypoxia on the cellular electrical activity of adult and neonatal canine ventricular myocardium. *Pediatr Res* 1985;19:1263–1267.
37. Bosker H, Drake Holland AJ, ter Keurs HE, Noble MI, Passingham JE, Pepper JR, Main MJ, Wanless RB. On the change of the cardiac action potential with age: a study in dogs. *Cardiovasc Res* 1985;19:674–678.

38. Robinson RB, Reder RF, Danilo P Jr. Preparation and electrophysiological characterization of cardiac cell cultures derived from the fetal canine ventricle. *Dev Pharmacol Ther* 1984;7:307–318.
39. Cohen NM, Lederer WJ. Changes in the calcium current of rat heart ventricular myocytes during development. *J Physiol (Lond)* 1988;406:115–146.
40. Kojima M, Ishima T, Taniguchi N, Kimura K, Sada H, Sperelakis N. Developmental changes in beta-adrenoceptors, muscarinic cholinoceptors and Ca^{2+} channels in rat ventricular muscles. *Br J Pharmacol* 1990;99:334–339.
41. Cohen NM, Lederer WJ. Calcium current in isolated neonatal rat ventricular myocytes. *J Physiol (Lond)* 1987;391:169–191.
42. Huynh TV, Chen F, Wetzel GT, Friedman WF, Klitzner TS. Developmental changes in membrane Ca^{2+} and K^+ currents in fetal, neonatal, and adult rabbit ventricular myocytes. *Circ Res* 1992;70:508–515.
43. Wetzel GT, Chen F, Klitzner TS. Ca^{2+} channel kinetics in acutely isolated fetal, neonatal, and adult rabbit cardiac myocytes. *Circ Res* 1993;72:1065–1074.
44. Wetzel GT, Chen F, Klitzner TS. L- and T-type calcium channels in acutely isolated neonatal and adult cardiac myocytes. *Pediatr Res* 1991;30:89–94.
45. Wetzel GT, Chen F, Friedman WF, Klitzner TS. Calcium current measurements in acutely isolated neonatal cardiac myocytes. *Pediatr Res* 1991;30:83–88.
46. Osaka T, Joyner RW. Developmental changes in calcium currents of rabbit ventricular cells. *Circ Res* 1991;68:788–796.
47. Osaka T, Joyner RW. Developmental changes in the beta-adrenergic modulation of calcium currents in rabbit ventricular cells. *Circ Res* 1992;70:104–115.
48. Kilborn MJ, Fedida D. A study of the developmental changes in outward currents of rat ventricular myocytes. *J Physiol (Lond)* 1990;430:37–60.
49. Clark RB, Bouchard RA, Salinas Stefanon E, Sanchez Chapula J, Giles WR. Heterogeneity of action potential waveforms and potassium currents in rat ventricle. *Cardiovasc Res* 1993;27:1795–1799.
50. Hume JR, Uehara A. Ionic basis of the different action potential configurations of single guinea-pig atrial and ventricular myocytes. *J Physiol (Lond)* 1985;368:525–544.
51. Tseng GN, Hoffman BF. Two components of transient outward current in canine ventricular myocytes. *Circ Res* 1989;64:633–647.
52. Furukawa T, Myerburg RJ, Furukawa N, Bassett AL, Kimura S. Differences in transient outward currents of feline endocardial and epicardial myocytes. *Circ Res* 1990;67:1287–1291.
53. Wettwer E, Amos GJ, Posival H, Ravens U. Transient outward current in human ventricular myocytes of subepicardial and subendocardial origin. *Circ Res* 1994;75:473–482.
54. Tseng GN. Potassium channels: their modulation by drugs. In: Zipes DP, Jalife J, eds. *Cardiac electrophysiology: from cell to bedside.* Philadelphia: WB Saunders; 1995:260–269.
55. Colatsky TJ. Outward plateau currents and cardiac repolarization. In: Podrid PJ, Kowey PR, eds. *Cardiac arrhythmia: mechanisms, diagnosis, and management.* Baltimore: Williams & Wilkins; 1995:48–59.
56. Sanguinetti MC, Jurkiewicz NK. Two components of cardiac delayed rectifier K^+ current. Differential sensitivity to block by class III antiarrhythmic agents. *J Gen Physiol* 1990;96:195–215.
57. Carmeliet E. Voltage- and time-dependent block of the delayed K^+ current in cardiac myocytes by dofetilide. *J Pharmacol Exp Ther* 1992;262:809–817.
58. Salata J, Jurkiewicz NK, Jow B, Guinosso PJJ, Fermini B. Evidence for the slowly-activating component of the delayed rectifier K^+ current (I_{Ks}) in rabbit ventricular myocytes. *Biophys J* 1995; 68:A147. Abstract.
59. Gintant GA. Regional differences in I_K density in canine left ventricle: role of $I_{K,s}$ in electrical heterogeneity. *Am J Physiol* 1995;268:H604–H613.
60. Liu DW, Antzelevitch C. Characteristics of the delayed rectifier current (I_{Kr} and I_{Ks}) in canine ventricular epicardial, midmyocardial, and endocardial myocytes. A weaker I_{Ks} contributes to the longer action potential of the M cell. *Circ Res* 1995;76:351–365.
61. Follmer CH, Colatsky TJ. Block of delayed rectifier potassium current, I_K by flecainide and E-4031 in cat ventricular myocytes. *Circulation* 1990;82:289–293.
62. Follmer CH, Lodge NJ, Cullinan CA, Colatsky TJ. Modulation of the delayed rectifier, I_K, by cadmium in cat ventricular myocytes. *Am J Physiol* 1992;262:C75–C83.
63. Apkon M, Nerbonne JM. Characterization of two distinct depolarization-activated K^+ currents in isolated adult rat ventricular myocytes. *J Gen Physiol* 1991;97:973–1011.
64. Li GR, Feng J, Yue L, Carrier M, Nattel S. Two components of delayed rectifier potassium current in human ventricular myocytes. *Circ Res* 1996;78:689–696.

65. Wu MH, Su MJ, Lue HC. Inward rectifier and delayed outward potassium currents in isolated guinea-pig ventricular myocytes: maturation and its role in repolarization. *Acta Paediatr Sin* 1992;33:363–371.
66. Mace SE, Levy MN. Neural control of heart rate: a comparison between puppies and adult animals. *Pediatr Res* 1983;17:491–495.
67. Wahler GM. Developmental increases in the inwardly rectifying potassium current of rat ventricular myocytes. *Am J Physiol* 1992;262:C1266–C1272.
68. Masuda H, Sperelakis N. Inwardly rectifying potassium current in rat fetal and neonatal ventricular cardiomyocytes. *Am J Physiol* 1993;265:H1107–H1111.
69. Furukawa T, Kimura S, Furukawa N, Bassett AL, Myerburg RJ. Potassium rectifier currents differ in myocytes of endocardial and epicardial origin. *Circ Res* 1992;70:91–103.

The Developing Heart,
edited by Bohuslav Ošťádal et al.
Lippincott-Raven Publishers,
Philadelphia © 1997.

15

Biochemical Basis of Calcium Handling in Developing Myocardium

Mohinder S. Nijjar and Naranjan S. Dhalla

Institute of Cardiovascular Sciences, St. Boniface General Hospital Research Centre, and Department of Physiology, University of Manitoba, Faculty of Medicine, Winnipeg, Manitoba R2H 2A6, Canada

GENERAL BACKGROUND

An individual acquires different functions at different stages of development, that is, from fetus to adulthood (1); acquisition of these functions is achieved by alterations in tissue growth (cell division) and development (cell differentiation) (2). These developmental changes are accompanied by alterations in cellular events and organelles that are significant in the acquired heart function. For example, the developmental alterations in electrophysiologic properties such as the pacemaker activity and conduction as well as cardiac contractility reflect changes in heart function (3). These functions are associated with transfer of ions between different cellular compartments. In resting myocardial cell, the intracellular concentrations of cations are Na^+ (5 mM), K^+ (145 mM), and Ca^{2+} (0.1 μM) versus extracellular concentrations of Na^+ (140 mM), K^+ (4 mM), and Ca^{2+} (1.25 mM). Apparently there is a large concentration gradient of cations across the sarcolemmal (SL) membranes (4). On stimulation, the myocyte undergoes depolarization because of rapid influx of Na^+ from the extracellular compartment, followed by continuing slow inward movements of Na^+ and Ca^{2+} via slow channels during the plateau phase of an action potential. The cell is then repolarized by the efflux of K^+ to the resting state (5).

It is now well established that intracellular Ca^{2+} is involved in the excitation–contraction coupling process, regulation of cell metabolism, and cardiac function (4), and undergoes dynamic oscillations in response to electrical or chemical stimulus (6). During the plateau phase of an action potential, Ca^{2+} enters myocyte and stimulates Ca^{2+} release from the sarcoplasmic reticulum (SR), resulting in an elevation of intracellular Ca^{2+} that initiates muscle contraction (3). Ca^{2+} is then extruded from the cell by the SL Ca^{2+}-stimulated ATPase and Na^+–Ca^{2+} exchanger

(7) and is sequestered by the SR Ca^{2+}-stimulated ATPase to produce muscle relaxation (6). Calcium bound to SL may also modulate muscle contraction, since it regulates Ca^{2+} influx by modulating Ca^{2+} channels activity (8,9). To understand the molecular basis of changes in heart function during development, it is essential to consider the regulation of Ca^{2+} homeostasis in developing heart. A review of cellular events correlating the acquisition of heart function with changes in intracellular Ca^{2+} during development may provide some insight into regulatory mechanisms controlling heart function and may lead to the formulation of clinical strategies for treatment and prevention of heart disease. Because various neurotransmitters and

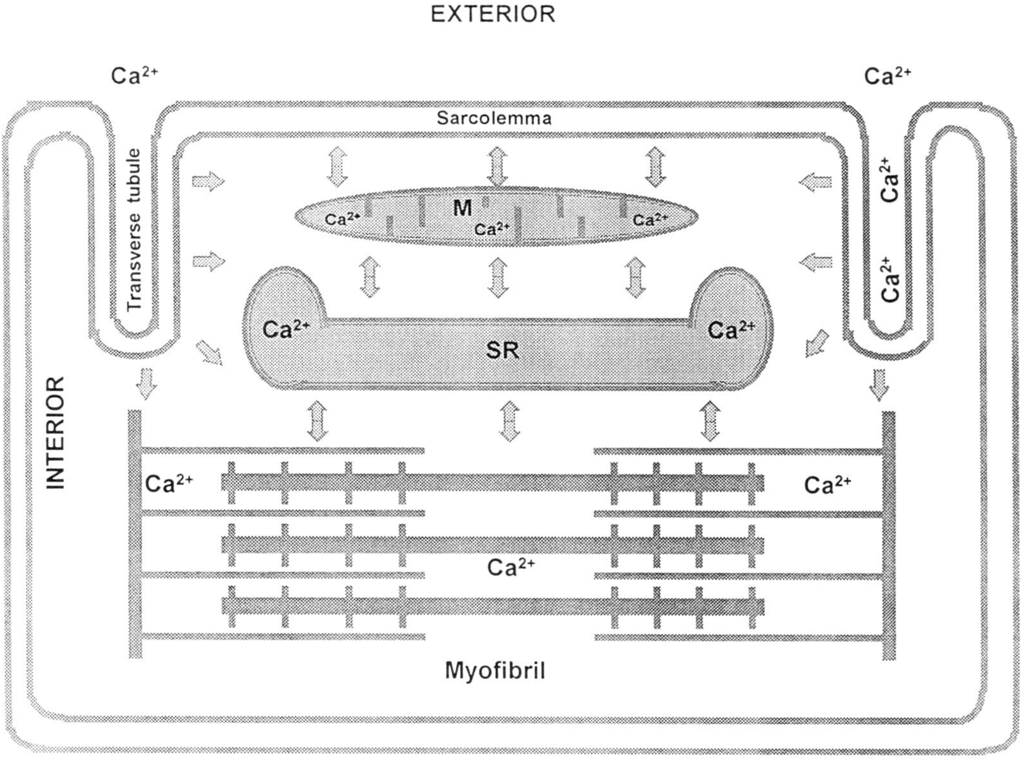

FIG. 15–1. A schematic representation of different components of cardiac muscle involved in heart function. The transfer of Ca^{2+} between different compartments is shown by arrows to indicate its significance and participation in excitation–contraction coupling process. Calcium enters myocyte via Ca^{2+} channels in sarcolemma in response to an electrical or a chemical stimulus. The resulting rise in intracellular Ca^{2+} induces Ca^{2+} release from the sarcoplasmic reticulum, and these together initiate full-strength muscle contraction. Calcium interacts with troponin C in myofilaments and causes dissociation of troponin T-I complex, and facilitates an interaction between myosin and actin to produce muscle contraction. Calcium is then taken up by the sarcoplasmic reticulum and is removed by sarcolemma to produce muscle relaxation. M, mitochondrion; SR, sarcoplasmic reticulum.

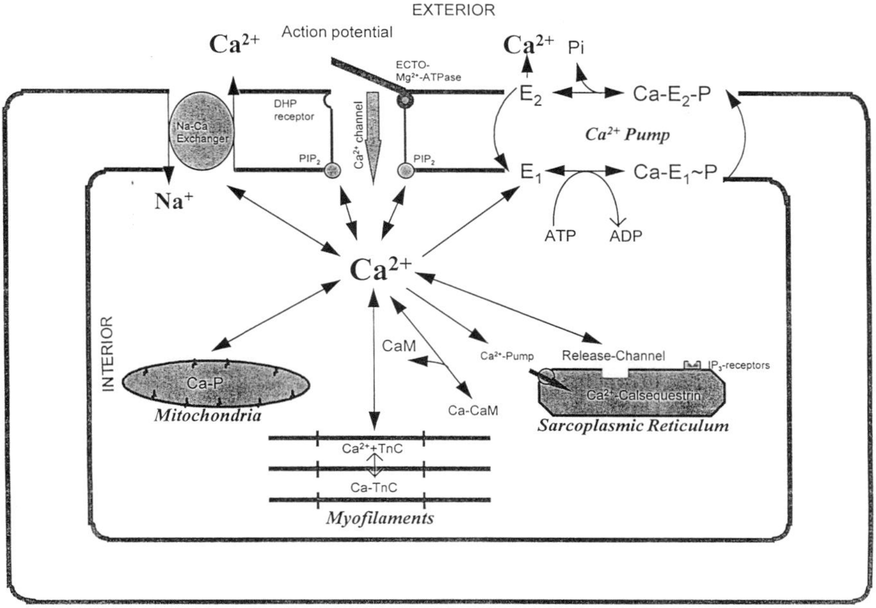

FIG. 15–2. A schematic diagram illustrates different transport systems that regulate intracellular calcium homeostasis. Calcium enters the cell via L-type Ca^{2+} channels that are blocked by dihydropyridine (DHP) analogs, and modulated by acidic phospholipids, particularly phosphatidylinositolmonophosphate and phosphatidylinositol-bisphosphate, and ecto-Mg^{2+}-ATPase. Calcium binding to low-affinity binding sites possibly to polyphosphoinositides at the inner side of sarcolemma also influence Ca^{2+} current through voltage-gated channels. Once Ca^{2+} enters the myocyte, it interacts with the sarcoplasmic reticulum to release Ca^{2+}. Calcium is extruded from the cell by Ca^{2+}–ATPase (pump) in sarcolemma. This enzyme exists in two forms E_1 and E_2. In the E_1 form the enzyme is located at the interior of sarcolemma, has a high affinity for Ca^{2+}, binds to Ca^{2+}, and undergoes phosphorylation by utilizing one ATP to a high-energy state E_1-P. This induces a conformational change that results in translocation of the enzyme complex to the outer side of membranes (E_2-P form), where it undergoes dephosphorylation. As a result, affinity of the enzyme for Ca^{2+} is reduced and Ca^{2+} is released into the extracellular environment. The enzyme then translocates itself to the interior of membranes and converts into E_1 form to undergo another cycle of Ca^{2+} binding and transfer. In addition, Ca^{2+} extrusion from the cell is primarily achieved by the reverse Na^+–Ca^{2+} exchanger, where Na^+ enters the cell because of its manyfold concentration gradient, and Ca^{2+} is transported extracellularly in exchange of Na^+ entry into myocyte. The cytoplasmic Ca^{2+} is also exchanged with that present in mitochondria. Calcium in myocytoplasm can bind reversibly with calmodulin (CaM) and other membrane proteins to provide Ca^{2+} buffering inside the myocyte. Some Ca^{2+} is bound to the myofibrillar protein such as troponin C (TnC) to facilitate interaction between myosin and actin to produce muscle contraction.

signal transduction pathways are involved in the control of heart function, an understanding of different membrane components of the signal transduction pathway can be seen to be a valuable piece of information. Although this subject has been reviewed by other investigators (3,10), we have focused primarily on literature concerning Ca^{2+} handling in the developing heart and/or isolated myocytes.

Ca^{2+} mediates the excitation–contraction coupling process in myocardium that involves Ca^{2+} influx during depolarization of cardiomyocytes and binding of Ca^{2+} to contractile proteins (6). Extracellular Ca^{2+} is critical for contraction of cardiac muscle during perinatal life from late fetal to early neonatal period of development (3,11), whereas Ca^{2+} from the intracellular sources is also required to induce muscle contraction in adult myocardium (12). The contraction of cardiac muscle involves different membrane systems, including the SL, transverse-tubules, SR, and mitochondria as well as the contractile proteins (Fig. 15–1). Calcium induces an interaction between myosin and actin to initiate muscle contraction. This involves formation of crossbridges with actin, hydrolysis of ATP, and myofilament shortening (13,14). A schematic representation of the excitation–contraction events is shown in Figure 15–2. The myocardial contraction occurs in three stages. The first stage is where Ca^{2+} interaction with actin is prevented by troponin (Tn)–tropomyosin (Tm) complex and thus no muscle contraction takes place. In the second stage, Ca^{2+} binds weakly to thin filaments, and cross-bridges react with thin filaments in a rapid "on–off steady state" but do not generate force. In the third and final stage, Ca^{2+} binds strongly with troponin C to induce rapid transition between different states to initiate muscle contraction (13,14). Accordingly, it is believed that when the intracellular concentration of Ca^{2+} is low, troponin T (TnT) complexes with Tm and the complex inhibits the interaction between actin and myosin filaments. When the intracellular concentration of Ca^{2+} is elevated in the myofilament space, Ca^{2+} binds to a regulatory site on troponin C. This relieves the inhibitory action of Tn–Tm complex on thin and thick filaments, thereby allowing an interaction between actin and myosin to produce muscle contraction. Thus, a clear insight into the mechanisms controlling Ca^{2+} homeostasis would assist in understanding cardiac muscle function in both developing and adult hearts.

DEVELOPMENT OF HEART FUNCTION

The contractile force in both the atrial and ventricular muscles increases with an increase in extracellular Ca^{2+} (3), but the sensitivity to Ca^{2+} appears to be higher in the fetus than in the neonate and adult hearts (15). The resting heart rate of awake unrestrained rats is low in newborn, reaches maximum at the age of 2.5 weeks, and declines thereafter to the adult level. The duration of isometric contraction correlates negatively with heart rate. Time to peak tension drops rapidly in the first few days postnatally, reaching a minimum at the age of 2.5 weeks, followed by slight prolongation toward adulthood. Recirculating fraction of activator Ca^{2+} increases in parallel with the heart rate. It seems that the postnatal increase in heart rate and duration of contraction shortening are closely associated with a shift in the activator Ca^{2+} from the extracellular to intracellular compartment (16). There is a slow decrease in the developed force from day 1 to 4, followed by an increase up to day 7. This is accompanied by a similar biphasic time course of the inotropic effect of Ca^{2+}. A reciprocal biphasic response is also observed during perfusion with verapamil, a well-known Ca^{2+} antagonist. The sensitivity to verapamil to induce negative inotropic effect rises from day 1 to 4 and then decreases at day 7 (17). The developmental alterations in chick heart muscle contraction show strong similarities with those of mammalian myocardium. Normalized twitch force of the intact trabeculae from chick left ventricle increases most markedly during the 3-day period around the time of hatching. Twitch force increases with an increase in extracellular Ca^{2+} concentration, and developmental increase in twitch force is accompanied by an increase in the maximal contractile capability of the muscle, which may be related to the maturation of contractile apparatus (i.e., proliferation of contractile proteins in myocardium). Ca^{2+} sensitivity of contractile apparatus in chick heart decreases with development in parallel with isoform switching in troponin T (18).

SOURCE OF INTRACELLULAR Ca^{2+} AND CONTRACTILE FORCE GENERATION

The source of intracellular Ca^{2+} to initiate contraction primarily in the cardiac muscle could be from the extracellular compartment and its entry via channels in SL and/or from the SR (3). It would appear that during the fetal/neonatal stages of development, muscle contraction is initiated by Ca^{2+} imported mainly from the extracellular compartment via Ca^{2+} channels in SL, whereas in the adult stage, Ca^{2+} released from the SR is also critical to produce muscle contraction (3). However, some evidence indicates that on depolarization Ca^{2+} bound to the inner leaflet of SL is released to interact with the contractile proteins to initiate muscle contraction directly (9). Ca^{2+} is then taken up by the SR and is removed by SL during relaxation of the cardiac muscle (9). These issues have been investigated by use of different Ca^{2+} inhibitors that are considered to block different Ca^{2+} channels and Ca^{2+} transport systems in the SL and SR membranes.

The contractile force in both atria and ventricular muscles of developing guinea pig was shown to increase with increasing extracellular Ca^{2+} concentration, and the sensitivity to Ca^{2+} was higher in fetus than in the neonate and adult hearts (15). Nicardipine, a blocker of voltage-gated Ca^{2+} channels in the outer membrane, abolished the contractile force in guinea pig atrial and ventricular muscle. Ryanodine, which blocks Ca^{2+} release from the SR, abolished the contractile force in atrial muscles from all age groups, but partially blocked the ventricular contractile force in neonate and adult, and increased the contractile force in fetus (15). Apparently, the SR function to release Ca^{2+} for myocardial contraction is less developed in fetal guinea pig than in neonatal and adult hearts (3), and the atrial contraction is more dependent on Ca^{2+} released from the SR than on that released by the ventricular contraction (15). Caffeine stimulated Ca^{2+} release from the SR and produced a positive inotropic effect on (isometric contractions) the ventricular strips from 3–15–day-old rats, but it had a negative inotropic effect on the cardiac muscle in adult rats (19). Such differential effects of caffeine on muscle twitch may be related to a shift from extracellular to intracellular source of Ca^{2+} (19). Ryanodine caused a depression of the caffeine- or Ca^{2+}-induced muscle tension in skinned muscle fibers (20). The depression of Ca^{2+}-induced contraction in fetus fibers caused by ryanodine was less affected than tension in adult fibers. These results show that SR Ca^{2+} release channels are modulated by extracellular Ca^{2+} and caffeine, and their relative insensitivity to ryanodine in the fetal fibers could contribute to resistance of the fetal heart to ryanodine (20). It is clear from the preceding evidence that the SR in fetal heart is not fully developed to store and release Ca^{2+} as well as to induce muscle contraction, whereas it is fully mature and functional in adult hearts (3). Some of the changes in Ca^{2+} handling mechanisms during development of the heart are shown in Table 15–1.

The sensitivity of atrial and ventricle muscle to contract in response to Ca^{2+} is dependent on the maturation of contractile apparatus that includes synthesis of myofibrillar proteins and their interaction with each other during contraction. The force of contraction in rat heart was decreased from day 1 to 4, followed by a steep increase up to day 12 (17). The development in cardiac contractile apparatus was accompanied by similar biphasic changes in the inotropic effect of Ca^{2+} (17). However, the sensitivity of contractile apparatus to Ca^{2+} was not changed. The sensitivity to negative inotropic agent, verapamil, showed reciprocal changes in that it was enhanced from day 1 to 4, and then decreased at day 7. These results show that the contractile function and inotropic responsiveness of rat heart change dramatically during the first week of life, and may be due to maturation of contractile apparatus in rat heart (17). The contractile force of chick left ventricle increased markedly during perinatal life (3 days around hatching) (18). These developmental changes in twitch force were accompanied by parallel changes in contractile capability of muscle (i.e., proliferation of contractile proteins) (18). The force of muscle contraction in response to Ca^{2+} depends on contractile capability of muscle (i.e., the presence of myofibrillar proteins). Ca^{2+} sensitivity of the contractile apparatus in chick heart decreased with development in parallel with isoform switching in troponin T (18). Calcium sensitivity of myofibrillar ATPase and fiber force in mam-

TABLE 15–1. *Developmental changes in heart components and functions*

Function/components	Fetal/newborn	Adult
Staircase phenomenon	Positive	Negative
Sarcoplasmic reticulum	Immature	Mature
Transverse tubules	Scarce	Many
Ca^{2+}-induced SR Ca^{2+} release	Absent	Functional
Number of myofilaments	Few	Numerous
Organization of myofilaments	Not aligned	Aligned

malian heart was higher in the newborn than in the adult; this change in Ca^{2+} sensitivity also correlated with switching in troponin T isoforms, which begins just before birth and is completed postnatally (13,20,21). The regulation of contraction in vertebrate heart muscle depends on Ca^{2+} binding to troponin C. Ca^{2+} binding to troponin C is modulated by troponin subunits (i.e., tropinin T and troponin I). In chick ventricle Ca^{2+} sensitivity is greater in early heart, where embryonic TnT predominates (22), and these changes in Ca^{2+} sensitivity cannot be attributed to troponin C, which is invariant during development (23). Calmidazolium is a calmodulin antagonist that binds to troponin C and alters Ca^{2+} troponin C–dependent activation of cardiac myofibrillar contractile activity (18). Mg^{2+}-dependent ATPase activity, which reflects myofibrillar function, was less stimulated by calmidazolium in neonatal than in adult rat hearts, indicating that the developmental changes in myofibrillar function are accompanied by transitions in thin filament proteins in response to calmidazolium. It would appear that developmentally related changes in troponin I isoforms contribute to the differential effects of calmidazolium on neonatal and adult cardiac myofibrils and the force of muscle contraction (24). The biomechanical changes indicating myofibrillar development and function in developing heart were consistent with histogenic findings in that there was a paucity in myofibrils in chick muscle, and lack of their alignment before embryonic day 5. There was a marked increase in myofibrils and their alignment in parallel to each other after 5 embryonic days (3,13,25).

Both acidosis and inorganic phosphate were observed to depress force generation by the contractile machinery of the chick heart (18). Protons compete with Ca^{2+} for the regulatory sites on TnC, and reduce Ca^{2+} binding to TnC (18,26). The depressant effect of acidosis, and inorganic phosphate on Ca^{2+} sensitivity increased with development in parallel with switch in tropinin I isoforms (18,27). Others have reported that Ca^{2+} sensitivity of myofibrillar ATPase or skinned fiber force is less affected by acidosis in the newborn than by that in the adult (28–30). The differential sensitivity is ascribed to switching in isoforms of troponin I, which begins in late fetal period and is complete in early neonatal life (22,28–30). Further studies have revealed that the decrease in maximum force generated by skinned fibers from mammalian skeletal muscle in response to acidosis was due to a decrease in the force per cross-bridge attachment, as well as a possible decrease in the number of attached cross-bridges (30).

GROWTH OF HEART

The pig heart grows at a maximal rate in the first 2–3 days of life because of volume overload imposed on the heart at birth (31). The growth of heart in vivo can be restrained by treatment with an angiotensin-converting enzyme inhibitor, enalapril maleate, or an angiotensin II receptor antagonist, DuP 753. Agonists stimulating β- and α-adrenergic receptors or angiotensin II receptors did not accelerate growth during in vitro perfusion of heart (31). It would appear that the rapid growth of the left ventricle of pig heart during the first 10 days of life is due largely to eccentric hypertrophy (31). During early neonatal myocardial growth, cardiac myocytes undergo a terminal differentiation (i.e., the cellular proliferation ceases). The growth of myocardium thereafter results from enlargement/hypertrophy of existing cells (2). Stimulation of α-adrenergic receptors in the neonatal rat heart muscle cells results in an increase in cell size, total protein, and mRNA encoding for fetal/neonatal contractile proteins isoforms. Similar changes in gene expression occur in pressure-load hypertrophy *in vivo* (2). Recent evidence indicates the production of peptide growth factors by mammalian myocardium, suggesting their role in cardiac growth and development. Another growth factor that is produced by nonmyocyte cells in culture was shown to induce hypertrophy of cardiac cells in culture (2). These findings suggest a role for cell–cell interaction in myocyte growth and differentiation.

The consumption of carbohydrate- or calorie-restricted diet during pregnancy causes ventricular arrhythmias, in addition to reduced fetal growth, and postnatal survival (32). The myocardial cell cultures from offsprings of mothers on restricted glucose and calorie diet showed no effect on the morphology, beating activity, and glucose utilization. ATP level was depressed in cultures exposed to amitriptyline (β-adrenergic receptor agonist), and the binding affinity of β-adrenergic receptors was increased in calorie-deficient diet (32). These results indicate that the maternal consumption of calorie-restricted diet during pregnancy may affect the myocardial functional capacity and integrity of the offspring. Hypocaloric feeding depresses heart function, causing cardiac atrophy, bradycardia, and decreased cardiac output (33). This appears to be due to compensatory, reversible, and asymmetric down-regulation of Ca^{2+} channels, and inhibition of the Ca^{2+} cycling process (33).

ROLE OF ADRENOCEPTORS IN HEART DEVELOPMENT

Maternal exposure to nicotine delayed the development of β-adrenergic receptor binding capabilities (pindolol binding to membranes) in cardiac membranes (34). The deficits in receptor binding were associated with marked subsensitivity of chronotropic responses to isoproterenol. The diminished binding to β-adrenergic receptor in response to isoproterenol or to preganglionic electrical stimulation of sympathetic nerves was evident after weaning and persisted into adulthood (34). These data demonstrate that the prenatal exposure to nicotine produces long-term alterations in adrenergic responsiveness of sympathetic target tissue (34). The electrophysiologic changes in developing heart are influenced by the sympathetic and parasympathetic innervation of heart (3). The neurotransmitter released regulates the intensity of the ventricular Ca^{2+} current (I_{Ca}) and is closely linked to contractile activation (5). The transmitter from sympathetic nerves stimulates the beta-adrenergic receptors–adenylyl cyclase–cyclic AMP system. This is mediated by the stimulatory GTP binding proteins (Gs), resulting in an increase in cyclic AMP, which activates protein kinase A to enhance phosphorylation of Ca^{2+} channels and thus regulate Ca^{2+} influx (3). The stimulation of muscarinic cholinergic receptors by acetylcholine inhibits adenylyl cyclase via an inhibitory guanine nucleotide binding (Gi) protein, resulting in reduced cyclic AMP production, which thereby antagonizes the effect of stimulation of adenylyl cyclase and cyclic AMP production by the activation of beta-adrenergic receptors (3). Both β-adrenergic receptor and cholinergic–muscarinic receptor linked signal transduction mechanisms are represented in Fig. 15–3. The development of different components of membrane signal transduction pathways in cardiac muscle function has been recently reviewed (3).

The number of α-1-adrenergic receptors was 60–120% higher in membranes from fetal or immature rats up to 25 days of age as compared to adult rats (35). The increased expression of α-1-adrenergic receptors in the developing heart relative to the adult heart is consistent with the hypothesis that α-1-adrenergic receptor stimulation may modulate protein synthesis and growth of mammalian myocardium (35). Treatment of neonatal rats with nerve growth factor modifies the receptor–effector coupling such that the innervated hearts at day 10 show high levels of a 41-kDa GTP regulatory protein that links the α-1-adrenergic receptors to the SL Na^+–K^+ pump (36). The receptor-effector pathway results in α-adrenergic-induced decrease in automaticity of heart. In contrast, noninnervated hearts at day 10 show lower levels of G protein and increases in automaticity induced by α-agonists (36). These results indicate that the development of sympathetic innervation is a determinant more of α- than of β-adrenergic modulation of ventricular rhythm (36). The coupling between α-1-adrenergic receptors to Ca^{2+} channels appears to change during heart development (37) and may explain the differential role of α- and β-adrenergic control of ventricle function. The α-adrenergic, angiotensin II, and endothelin signaling pathways modulate contraction of cardiac muscle (38); stimulation of PI turnover is involved in all three types of receptor stimulation. The genes expressing for phospholipase C isoforms change during development (38).

ROLE OF Ca^{2+} IN CARDIAC AND CELL FUNCTION

Ca^{2+} plays a central role in excitation–contraction coupling in muscle (4–7); some of the events associated with the entry and removal of Ca^{2+} as well as the regulation of intracellular Ca^{2+} are given in Fig. 15–2. In resting state, the intracellular level of Ca^{2+} in cardiac myocyte is low (μM) as compared with the extracellular concentration of Ca^{2+} (mM) (4). Indeed, $[Ca^{2+}]_i$ is precisely regulated by different mechanisms present in plasma and intracellular membranes (4,39). Calcium enters the cell via voltage-dependent and/or agonist-stimulated calcium channels (40) and by an electrogenic Na^+–Ca^{2+} exchanger driven by Na^+ gradient and membrane potential (41). Ca^{2+} is extruded from cardiac myocyte by the Ca^{2+}-stimulated ATPase (pump) in SL and is stored in the SR and/or mitochondria by another energy-dependent mechanism (39,42). Intracellular Ca^{2+} may also be sequestered by binding to cytosolic (calmodulin) and SR protein (calsequestrin), and membrane proteins such as channels, Ca^{2+}-ATPase, and Na^+–Ca^{2+} exchanger (39). The dynamic equilibrium between the free and membrane-bound Ca^{2+} provides the cell with Ca^{2+} buffering capacity (39) and is important for muscle contraction (9). The binding of Ca^{2+} to high-affinity proteins involves expression of hydrophobic sites upon complexation with Ca^{2+}. The association of high-affinity binding proteins with membranes is regulated by Ca^{2+} (43). These proteins could play an important role in mediating the transduction of Ca^{2+} signal from plasma membrane to the cell interior, and in mediating the interaction between the cytoskeletal and membrane components (39). Some agonists in the extracellular milieu interact with receptors (α-adrenergic and muscarinic-cholinergic) on the cell surface, resulting in the activation of phospholipase C to produce IP_3 and diacylglycerol (3,39). IP_3 mobilizes Ca^{2+} from the SR (44), and diacylglycerol stimulates protein kinase C to catalyze the phosphorylation of voltage-dependent Ca^{2+} channels (45,46), resulting in enhanced Ca^{2+} influx. Apparently, any derangements in one or more of the mechanisms discussed earlier would have serious metabolic and functional consequences.

During depolarization the cation permeability of SL membrane is enhanced (5); as a result, Ca^{2+} enters the cell along a concentration gradient (4). The depolarization of SL releases Ca^{2+} bound to the inner leaflet that diffuses to the contractile proteins to control muscle contraction. This Ca^{2+} is reaccumulated by SL and the SR during muscle relaxation (9). The contractility of any given beat was found to be a function of the preceding beat and of the duration of the preceding action potential. It has been proposed that Ca^{2+} entry via channels is inhibited by Ca^{2+} bound to the inner leaflet of the SL. The channel opens when this Ca^{2+} is released upon depolarization (9).

The function of Ca^{2+} pump in SR of myocardium in rats decreases with age, whereas the activity of SL Ca^{2+} pump increases (47). The rates of ATP-dependent Ca^{2+} accumulation by SR were similar in 3- and 6-month-old rat, whereas the rates of Ca^{2+} accumulation in membranes from 12-, 18-, and 24-month-old rats were significantly lower. The SL membranes from 18- and 24-month-old animals displayed substantially higher rates of ATP-dependent Ca^{2+} accumulation than membranes from 3-, 6-, and 12-month-old rat myocardium (47). The kinetic analysis revealed that maximum velocity had undergone age-related changes without any effect on the apparent affinity of Ca^{2+} accumulation. The combined Ca^{2+} transport activity (ATP-driven membrane Ca^{2+} pumps) of SL and SR declined with age. The effect of age on Ca^{2+} accumulation was minimal in young animals but became much pronounced with advancing age. It was suggested that the age-associated decline in Ca^{2+} transport of SR may involve uncoupling of energy transduction and ion translocation functions of membrane Ca^{2+} pump (47).

CALCIUM CHANNELS IN SARCOLEMMA

Voltage-Dependent Ca^{2+} Channels

The electrophysiological evidence indicates the opening of Ca^{2+} channels in a voltage- and time-dependent manner during membrane depolarization (4). The mechanism by which Ca^{2+} channels are opened on electrical stimulation is not defined, although this may be achieved by conformational changes in the integral SL proteins involving the phosphorylation of proteins and/or lipid components (3). It has been proposed that Ca^{2+}-Mg^{2+} ecto-ATPase may be involved in opening Ca^{2+} gates in the SL membranes (4). The slow inward movement of Ca^{2+} during the plateau phase of action potential appears to occur via slow Ca^{2+} channels whose function is dependent on energy (i.e., ATP) (4). Two types of Ca^{2+} channels are involved in excitation–contraction coupling in striated muscle: voltage-gated L-type Ca^{2+} channels on the transverse tubule that are blocked by dihydropyridines (DHP) and Ca^{2+} release channels in the SR that are inhibited by ryanodine (48). The expression of different components of the excitation–contraction coupling including Ca^{2+} channels is up-regulated during myogenic development in the rabbit (48). cDNA for different subunits (α-1, α-2, β-, and γ-subunits) of DHP receptors, and mRNA for α-1 subunit of cardiac DHP receptors were low in fetus, increased at birth, and reached adult levels thereafter. Ryanodine binding sites increase with age in both skeletal and cardiac muscle (48). These data reflect the molecular basis for functional maturation of the excitation–contraction coupling apparatus at birth, and during early postnatal development. Low levels of Ca^{2+} channel expression in fetal cardiac tissue make this tissue more sensitive to pharmacologic therapy with Ca^{2+} channel blockers (48). Some differences in the fetal/newborn and adult hearts with respect to the sensitivity of some pharmacologic agents are shown in Table 15–2.

Whole cell peak I_{Ca}, which reflects Ca^{2+} transfer across membrane in the plateau phase closely linked to muscle contraction and cell size, increased with age in rabbit ventricular myocytes (2,49). The most significant increase in I_{Ca} occurred after birth (50). Peak I_{Ca} density (I_{Ca}/unit cell surface area) also increased from day 21 of gestation to birth and then increased again from the neonatal to adult periods of development (50). The increase in I_{Ca} density may result from increased channel expression (50–52). The development of myofiber tension (early peak and phasic tension) is supported largely by Ca^{2+} influx across SL in immature myocardium. The density of atrial T-type Ca^{2+} channels was maximum at 5 weeks of age (53); the Ca^{2+}-channel density in isolated myocytes from 3.5-week-old rats was about 80% of maximum receptor density in myocytes from adult rat. In contrast, the density of L-type Ca^{2+} channels remained unchanged in rats from 3 to 14 weeks of age (53). Both T- and L-type Ca^{2+} channels were present after 2 days of culture of

TABLE 15–2. *Differential sensitivity of developing heart to drugs*

Drugs	Fetal/newborn	Adult
Nitrendipine	Enhanced	Diminished
Verapamil	High	Low
Ryanodine	Diminished	Enhanced
Ouabain	Low	High
Caffeine	Low	High

neonatal ventricular cardiomyocytes; however, after 7 days in culture, only L-types of Ca^{2+} channels were present (53).

Nitrendipine binding to intact ventricle and cultured myocytes was antagonized by nitrendipine analogs (nimodipine>nifedipine>nisoldipine), and dissociation constant for nitrendipine binding was between 0.4 and 0.5 nM (54). The binding of nitrendipine was inhibited by other antiarrhythmic agents, such as amiodarone, F13004, and bepridil. Half-maximal inhibition for verapamil and D600 was 0.23 and 0.26 μM, respectively (54). It appears that the plateau phase of action potential in cardiac myocyte was due to Ca^{2+} transfer via slow Ca^{2+} channels that were insensitive to nitrendipine at earlier stages of development. In the adult myocytes nitrendipine (50 nM) abolished the slow action potential due to slow Ca^{2+} transport via Ca^{2+} channels, and myocyte contraction (54). The density of Ca^{2+} channels that were sensitive to nitrendipine increased from embryonic chick heart from 40 fmol/mg protein at day 3 to 100 fmol/mg protein at day 14, and remained stable up to day 18. The number of binding sites then increased very rapidly to 210 fmol/mg protein on day 4 after hatching (54). The treatment with 6-hydroxydopamine resulted in a 35% increase in nitrendipine binding, whereas reserpine treatment had no effect. Apparently, nitrendipine binding sites or receptors exist at a very early stage of development (i.e., 3-day-old hearts) but do not correspond to functional slow Ca^{2+} channels. The nitrendipine-sensitive Ca^{2+} channels in myocytes may be regulated by innervation (54).

It is generally agreed that the SR is not fully developed during late gestation (fetal) and early neonatal period, and most of the Ca^{2+} for muscle contraction comes from the extracellular environment via L-type Ca^{2+} channels in SL. However, some recent evidence indicates significant contribution by SR to intracellular Ca^{2+}, which initiates muscle contraction at a much earlier stage of development (17,55). This evidence is based on the effectiveness of ryanodine to inhibit muscle contraction in developing heart (17). When Ca^{2+} transient was measured in a single isolated ventricular myocyte from day 11 embryonic chick heart, a positive staircase phenomenon was observed; nifedipine abolished the Ca^{2+} transient. Isoproterenol-induced rise in peak of Ca^{2+} transient was 70% inhibited by nifedipine, suggesting that most of the Ca^{2+} transient was associated with L-type Ca^{2+} channels, but a portion of the transient may be due to T-type Ca^{2+} channels and/or reverse Na^{+}/Ca^{2+} exchanger. Ryanodine inhibited the transient by 30%, indicating that SR was functional in embryonic chick heart well before Ca^{2+} transient via SL Ca^{2+} channels (55).

Agonist-Stimulated Ca^{2+} Channels

The events for signal transduction pathway depicted in Figs. 15–3 and 15–4 indicate that an integration of agonists such as hormones, neurotransmitters, or drugs with receptors on the outer cell surface leads to the activation of Ca^{2+} channels in membranes, resulting in enhanced Ca^{2+} influx, an elevation of intracellular Ca^{2+}, and muscle contraction (3). The stimulation of α-1-adrenoceptors by phenyl-

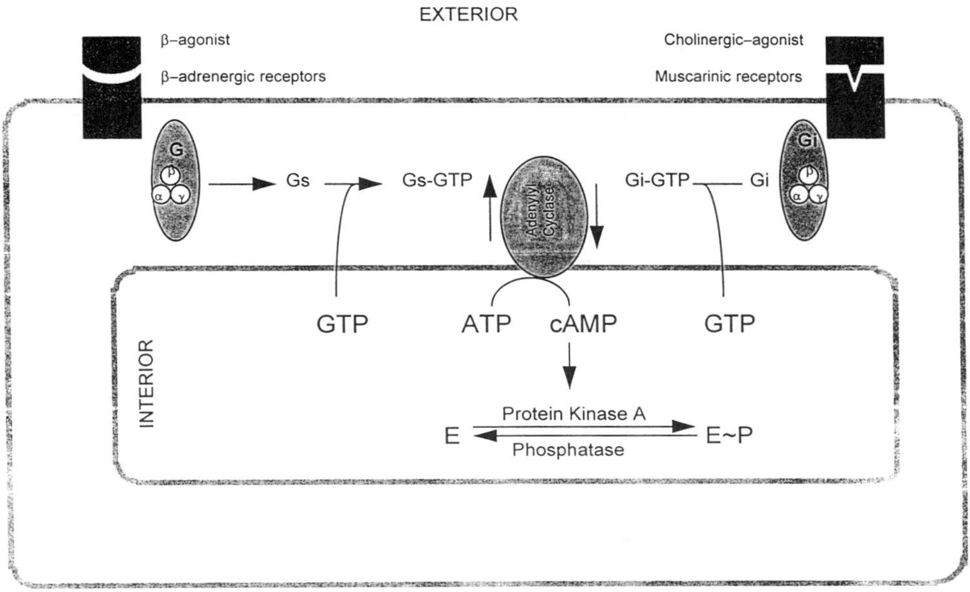

FIG. 15–3. Control of heart function by neurotransmitters released from sympathetic and parasympathetic nerve endings. These neurotransmitters interact with their specific receptors on sarcolemma, and the signal is transmitted via G protein to adenylyl cyclase enzyme located at the inside of membrane. Adenylyl cyclase catalyzes the formation of cyclic AMP. Norepinephrine interacts with β-adrenergic receptors in sarcolemma to induce dissociation of stimulatory guanine nucleotide binding protein (Gs) into its α-, β-, and γ-subunits. Gs-alpha combines with GTP, and the resulting complex activates adenylyl cyclase to produce more cyclic AMP. On the other hand, acetylcholine activates muscarinic cholinergic receptors to induce dissociation of inhibitory guanine nucleotide binding protein (Gi), and Gi-alpha combines with GTP. The Gi-alpha-GTP complex interacts with adenylyl cyclase, resulting in diminished enzyme activity and cyclic AMP production. Cyclic AMP then binds to the regulatory subunit of protein kinase A, causing its dissociation from active subunit of protein kinase A. Protein kinase A catalyzes phosphorylation of proteins (enzymes), including Ca^{2+} channels, resulting in enhanced Ca^{2+} influx and muscle contraction.

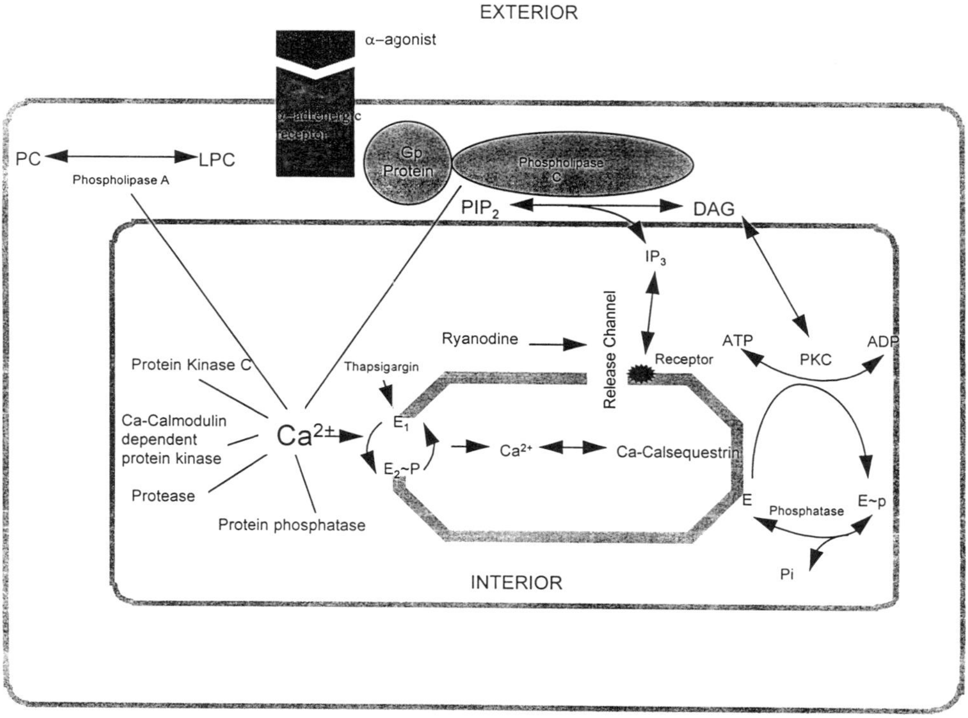

FIG. 15–4. A schematic diagram showing a membrane signal transduction pathway where stimulation of α-adrenergic receptors results in the activation of phospholipase C and production of inositol-1,4,5-triphosphate (IP_3) and diacylglycerol (DAG) from phosphatidylinositol-bisphosphate. IP_3 interacts with receptors on the sarcoplasmic reticulum, resulting in activation of Ca^{2+} release channels, and release of Ca^{2+} from the sarcoplasmic reticulum. Ryanodine inhibits Ca^{2+} release channels, preventing mobilization of Ca^{2+} from the sarcoplasmic reticulum in response to IP_3 and other agonists. Thapsigargin depletes the sarcoplasmic reticulum of Ca^{2+} by acting on Ca^{2+} pump ATPase. DAG activates protein kinase C such that the sensitivity of enzyme activation by Ca^{2+} is enhanced. Protein kinase C catalyzes the phosphorylation of numerous proteins, including Ca^{2+} channels. Intracellular Ca^{2+}, either directly or in combination with calmodulin, modulates the activities of a variety of enzymes to influence cell metabolism and is therefore an important regulator of cell function.

ephrine, when β-adrenoceptors were blocked by propranolol resulted in increased I_{Ca}. This action was prevented by prazosin (a blocker of α-adrenergic receptors) in myocytes from the neonatal heart but not in myocytes from young rat hearts (56). These results suggest that there may be a switch in coupling of α-1-adrenoceptor to Ca^{2+} channels during development of the cardiac tissue. The inotropic response to phenylephrine decreased significantly after 2 weeks of age and was blocked by prazosin, but not by propranolol (57). The inotropic potency of noradrenaline was highest neonatally and lower at all other ages up to 10-week-old rats. There were no significant differences in α-1- or β-1-adrenoceptor densities or affinities in ventricular membranes from 7-day-old and adult rats (57). Evidently, there was a decline in the positive inotropic response to sympathomimetic amines with age, and this decline was most pronounced for the α-1-adrenoceptor-mediated effects (57).

The maximum tension developed in response to isoproterenol in isolated left ventricular papillary muscles increased from 37 ± 7% at 3 days to 175 ± 33% at 21 days postnatally in rabbits, followed by a decrease to 68 ± 12% in young adult (58); this was due to increased sensitivity of the muscle to isoproterenol. The number of specific [^{3}H] dihydroalprenolol binding sites also increased from 3 to 21 days, which a subsequent decline to 32 ± 4.5% in young adult rats. The rise in cardiac contractility was related to an increase in the density of beta-adrenoceptors (58). Adenylyl cyclase activation by isoproterenol increased with age from 15 days fetal up to 7 days postnatally. However, the sensitivity of adenylyl cyclase to isoproterenol decreased from fetal to neonatal period in atria, and from the first day to the seventh day in ventricle (58). In contrast, the activation of adenylyl cyclase by forskolin did not change during the same period of development. A decrease in adenylyl cyclase response to isoproterenol accompanies the developmental decrease in chronotropic and inotropic sensitivity to β-adrenoceptor agonists. This decrease in sensitivity may be partly due to reduction in β-adrenoceptor density as well as to decreased coupling of receptors to adenylyl cyclase through G proteins (3,58).

The basal, isoproterenol-stimulated, and forskolin-stimulated adenylyl cyclase showed distinct developmental spikes of activity that were unrelated to changes in receptor binding sites but corresponded temporally to periods of sympathetic neuronal activation (59). The treatment of pregnant rats in late gestation with terbutaline (β-adrenergic receptor agonist), and dexamethasone enhanced immediately after birth the adenylyl cyclase activity and β-receptor binding in cardiac membranes, and delayed the appearance but exaggerated the magnitude of subsequent peaks in adenylyl cyclase activity (59). These results suggest that beta-adrenergic stimulation serves as a trophic factor controlling the ontogenetic rise of the adenylyl cyclase activity, and this regulation appears to involve the enzyme itself rather than changes in receptor binding capabilities or receptor-specific linkages. Consequently, administration of β-agonist and dexamethasone in late gestation can cause long-term alterations in enzyme activity and cardiac tissue responsiveness. Ca^{2+} entry into the cell may also be regulated by the sympathetic nervous system via release of norepinephrine, and β-adrenergic receptor activation (60,61). The stimulation of sympathetic nervous system also results in the release of ATP (62), which potentiates the contractile force of myocardium (63,64). The effects of ATP on myocardium are independent of cyclic AMP but appear to be mediated by specific receptors on SL (65,66). An interaction between ATP and its receptors at the cell surface enhances Ca^{2+} transport intracellularly and potentiates contractile force of myocardium (4). ATP-induced muscle contraction may be mediated by the enhanced turnover of inositol-containing lipids (67,68). Whether ATP-receptors are altered during the development of heart requires further studies.

SARCOLEMMAL Na^+–Ca^{2+} EXCHANGER AND Na^+–K^+-STIMULATED ATPase

As a consequence of underdeveloped SR, Na^+–Ca^{2+} exchange in SL assumes relatively greater importance in modulating Ca^{2+} fluxes in developing heart (69,70). Calcium uptake by Na^+-loaded SL vesicles isolated from fetal (28-day gestation), neonatal (24–48 hours), immature (14–16 days), and adult white rabbit hearts was stimulated by valinomycin, and inhibited by amiloride, reflecting the characteristics of Na^+–Ca^{2+} exchange (39). Initial velocity of Ca^{2+} uptake was significantly higher in fetal and newborn SL vesicles than in adult heart SL vesicles (69). Use of polyclonal antibody against the exchanger protein showed 2.5 times more exchanger content in fetal/newborn than in adult heart SL vesicles. Parallel changes in the Na^+–Ca^{2+} exchanger activity were noted during the same period of development (69). These data demonstrate that Na^+–Ca^{2+} exchanger was abundant and functionally active in late fetal and early neonatal periods of rabbit heart development, declining thereafter postnatally (69). Although Na^+–H^+ exchange system is also known to influence Ca^{2+}-movements in the myocardium indirectly, no studies regarding the behavior of this system have yet appeared in the literature.

The Na^+–K^+ ATPase and Na^+–Ca^{2+} exchange systems are considered important in excitation–contraction coupling in the heart (70,71). The sodium pump (Na^+–K^+ ATPase) activity and specific ouabain binding were higher in adult canine heart SL than during the neonatal period (1–5 postnatal days). The association–dissociation constants for ouabain binding were similar, but the maximal binding (Bmax) for ouabain was high in adult heart membranes (71). The Na^+–Ca^{2+} exchanger activity and its sensitivity to extracellular Ca^{2+} were not significantly different at two stages of development. Since Na^+–K^+ ATPase activity and ouabain binding were low in neonatal heart SL, Ca^{2+} flux via Na^+–Ca^{2+} exchanger may be important for canine heart function in the neonatal period (71). An inhibition of cardiac Na^+–K^+ ATPase activity decreases the driving force for Na^+–Ca^{2+} exchanger that increases cellular Ca^{2+} stores and contractility (72). Conditions that alter Na^+–K^+ ATPase abundance would change the Na^+–Ca^{2+} exchanger in a reciprocal fashion (72). In experimentally induced renovascular hypertension in rats, the expression (mRNA) of α-2 isoform of the Na^+–K^+ ATPase decreased in ventricles, whereas that for the Na^+–Ca^{2+} exchanger protein increased. During transition from hypo- to hyperthyroid state, the cardiac Na^+–K^+ ATPase alpha-1 isoform was increased twofold, with a concomitant reduction in Na^+–Ca^{2+} exchanger protein. The treatment of animals with antiarrhythmic amiodarone decreased α-2 Na^+–K^+ ATPase expression, and increased exchanger expression by a factor of 1.4 (72). The abundance of α-2 isoform of Na^+–K^+ ATPase in rat ventricle increased between 8 and 15 days of age, whereas the abundance of Na^+–Ca^{2+} exchanger protein decreased during the same period of heart development. The reciprocal changes in expression of Na^+–K^+ ATPase isoforms and Na^+–Ca^{2+} exchanger protein provide evidence for a homeostatic mechanism that would oppose changes in cellular Ca^{2+} stores driven by changes in Na^+–K^+ ATPAse activity (72). α-Adrenergic receptors on the cell surface appear to be coupled to Na^+–K^+ ATPase via GTP-binding protein (73). The treatment of neonatal rats with nerve growth factor (NGF) or its antibody modifies the receptor–effector coupling such that innervated hearts at day 10 show high levels of a 41-kDa GTP regulatory protein that links the α-1 receptors to the Na^+–K^+ pump. The receptor–effector pathway results in α-adrenergic-induced decreases in automaticity (73). In contrast, noninnervated hearts at day 10 show lower levels of the pertussis toxin–sensitive G protein and an increase in automaticity induced by α-agonists (73). These results are consistent with the view that the development of sympathetic innervation is a more determinant of α- than of β-adrenergic modulation of ventricular rhythm (73).

CALCIUM PUMP IN SARCOLEMMA

Ca^{2+} is extruded from cell by Ca^{2+}-pump (Ca^{2+}-stimulated ATPase) and by Na^+–Ca^{2+} exchanger in the SL membrane. The Ca^{2+}-pump utilizes Mg-ATP as a substrate with an apparent K_m of 0.2 μM, and its activity is stimulated by calmodulin (74). Since calmodulin content has been shown to undergo developmental alterations (75), one would expect changes in the modulation of Ca^{2+}-stimulated ATPase during heart development. It should be mentioned that the Ca^{2+}-pump is located on the inside of the membrane and exists in E_1 form, with a high affinity for Ca^{2+} (Fig. 15–2). On binding with Ca^{2+}, the pump protein undergoes phosphorylation (E_1-P), and this induces a conformational change in the enzyme to the E_2-P form such that the enzyme complex is translocated to the outside of the membrane. The enzyme then undergoes dephosphorylation to the E_2 form, which has low affinity for Ca^{2+} and releases Ca^{2+} extracellularly. The enzyme is then translocated to the inside of the cell membrane, where its affinity for Ca^{2+} is enhanced to promote Ca^{2+} binding (39). The enzyme transfers one Ca^{2+} from inside to outside of the cell and utilizes one ATP in each cycle (76). The transfer of Ca^{2+} from inside to outside is accompanied with transfer of H^+ from outside to inside of cardiac myocyte (77), and the resulting acidosis has a profound effect on cardiac muscle contraction (28–32).

Ca^{2+}-stimulated ATPase activity in SL was not altered significantly with age from 3 to 24 months in rat heart (47); the ATP-dependent Ca^{2+} accumulation by SL vesicles up to 12 months of age was also not significantly different, but increased in preparations from rats older than 12 months (47). In contrast, ATP-dependent Ca^{2+} accumulation by the SR vesicles decreased after 6 months of age. The Ca^{2+} pump activities in SL and SR did not change up to 12 months of age (47). Relative lack of information concerning the development of Ca^{2+} pump in heart SL may be relevant in that very little of the intracellular Ca^{2+} is pumped out by Ca^{2+}-stimulated ATPase, and most is achieved by Na^{+}–Ca^{2+} exchanger (39).

CALCIUM UPTAKE AND STORAGE IN THE SARCOPLASMIC RETICULUM

The SR accumulates Ca^{2+} from the cytoplasm via Ca^{2+} pump, which is the major protein in the SR membrane. Ca^{2+}–ATPase has a high affinity for Ca^{2+} (Ka 0.5 μM) and requires Mg-ATP as a substrate (39). It is well established that Ca^{2+} uptake by SR cisternae is dependent on ATP (movement of two Ca^{2+} per one ATP hydrolyzed) and reduces cytosol Ca^{2+} to a level that induces dissociation between Ca^{2+} and troponin C (39). Depolarization of the cell membrane is transmitted via transverse tubules to the interior of muscle cell, causing Ca^{2+} efflux from neighboring cisternae of the SR (78). The flow of charges in the tubular system would open Ca^{2+} channels in the terminal cisternae of SR to release Ca^{2+} to induce muscle contraction (39). Ca^{2+} uptake and Ca^{2+}-ATPase activity were significantly lower in the fetal and newborn SR membranes as compared with the adult (79). The protein content and mRNA expressing Ca^{2+} pump were 52–63% lower in the fetus than in the adult. The relationship between lower rates of Ca^{2+} uptake and Ca^{2+}–ATPase activity in fetal rabbit heart indicate genetic regulation of the SR Ca^{2+} pump and may be partly responsible for perinatal change in mammalian cardiac relaxation (79).

Shortening (muscle contraction) and intracellular Ca^{2+} transients of electrically paced, isolated adult rat myocytes were dependent on the presence of functional SR and were completely abolished by inhibitors of the Ca^{2+}–ATPase (i.e., cyclipiazonic acid and thapsigargin) or by the Ca^{2+} release inhibitor, ryanodine (80). Cardiomyocytes from neonatal rat elicited consistent intracellular Ca^{2+} transients even after complete inhibition of the SR function. These data show the significance of SR in regulating Ca^{2+} transients and shortening of cardiomyocytes during development (80). It should be mentioned that Ca^{2+}–ATPase exists in different isoforms that are expressed variably in different tissues during differentiation. However, Ca^{2+}–ATPase isoforms 1c, 1d, and 4a were expressed only in myocytes and neuronal cell lines and may be specific for excitable tissues (81). In particular, mRNA for isoform 1d was expressed specifically in heart and skeletal muscle. Myogenin is expressed in rat fibroblasts and converts myocytes to multinucleated myotubes that displayed plasma membrane Ca^{2+}-stimulated ATPase (PMCA) isoform-specific mRNAs 1c, 1d, and 4a, typical of differentiated muscle cells (81). It appears that the distribution of various PMCA isoform-specific mRNAs and their splicing variants is cell type and development specific, and that PMCA isoforms may play a role in determining functions of terminally differentiated muscle and neuronal cells (81).

Phospholamban is present in mature hearts and is phosphorylated by cyclic AMP-dependent protein kinase, but not in the presence of Ca^{2+} and calmodulin (82). Calcium uptake and Ca^{2+}-ATPase were low in fetal SR compared to adult control membranes, although affinity of enzyme for Ca^{2+} was similar (82). Both Ca^{2+}–ATPase and calsequestrin in SR membranes were low in fetal hearts compared to mature hearts. It appears that the age-related changes in Ca^{2+} transport and amounts of Ca^{2+}–ATPase and calsequestrin are related to changes in the regulation of intracellular Ca^{2+} concentration in fetal heart muscle, and its function (82). mRNA encoding for SR Ca^{2+}–ATPase (SERCA2) was present in cardiogenic plate on the 9-day-old presomite embryo before the first contraction (83). The expression (mRNA) encoding for SERCA2 was not differentially spliced during rat heart ontogenetic development, that is, from 14 fetal days to 24 months of age (84). When specific mRNA was measured relative to either 18 s RNA or myosin heavy chain mRNA, the amount of Ca^{2+}–ATPase mRNA increased substantially at the end of fetal life and 4 days postnatally, with a stable high level in adulthood (84).

In contrast to the Ca^{2+}–ATPase in the SR membranes, but like the one in SL membrane, the myofibrillar Ca^{2+}–ATPase is sensitive to calmodulin. The Ca^{2+}–ATPase activity in neonatal myofibrils was significantly less stimulated by calmidazolium, an antagonist of calmodulin, than by the enzyme from adult hearts (24). Variable concentration of calmodulin (75) or its inhibition by calmidazolium at different ages (24) would alter intracellular concentration of Ca^{2+} by modulating Ca^{2+}–ATPase activities in SL and myofibrils rather than the SR (85). Phospholamban is another protein present in SR (86), which modulates Ca^{2+}–ATPase activity by undergoing phosphorylation by cyclic AMP- and Ca^{2+}-phospholipid-dependent protein kinases (87,88). It has been suggested that phospholamban in its nonphosphorylated form is permanently attached to Ca^{2+}–ATPase and inhibits its activity. The phosphorylation of phospholamban induces a conformational change in the molecule so that it dissociates from Ca^{2+}–ATPase, resulting in the activation of the SR Ca^{2+} pump (87,88). The expression of phospholamban (mRNA) was present in 12-day-old embryos, but its distribution in heart tissue was opposite to that of SERCA2 mRNA and did not undergo developmental changes (83). Calsequestrin is an extrinsic, hydrophobic protein that binds large amounts of Ca^{2+} (40 mol/mol) with low affinity and acts as a Ca^{2+} storage protein in the SR lumen (84). This protein is found in the terminal cisternae of SR, which contain Ca^{2+} that is mobilized in response to depolarization (89). A single calsequestrin mRNA isoform was detected in rat heart that was not influenced by different stages of heart development (84).

Ca^{2+} RELEASE FROM THE SARCOPLASMIC RETICULUM

The activation of ICa in isolated myocytes elicited a sizable increase in intracellular Ca^{2+} released from the intracellular stores, as it was blocked by ryanodine.

The rate of Ca^{2+} release increased with age, indicating increased efficiency of Ca^{2+} signaling in mature myocytes (90). It would appear that I_{Ca}-gated release of Ca^{2+} from SR is the primary mechanism regulating Ca^{2+} signaling for contraction in mature human atrial myocytes (90). Extracellular calcium-induced Ca^{2+} release from SR is absent before birth, starts at about 2 days postnatally, and continues to increase to an adult level by the thirtieth day (91). This process develops in parallel to the development of SR and is accompanied by a decrease in Ca^{2+} entry through SL in rat ventricle (91). In early stages of development, a spanning protein that links SL or T-tubule to SR is lacking, and the principal source of Ca^{2+} for activation of contraction is *trans*-SL flux via Na^{+}–Ca^{2+} exchanger. In the adult stage, where the functional SR is linked to the surface membrane via the spanning protein, depolarization results in the opening of both SL voltage-dependent Ca^{2+} channels and SR Ca^{2+}-release channels, both contributing to the rise in intracellular Ca^{2+} (39,91). The release of Ca^{2+} from the SR is mediated by receptors that are activated by IP_3 (92–94), and inhibited by ryanodine (95–97). Receptors for Ca^{2+} release from SR appear to change in developing heart. Ryanodine produced a concentration-dependent depression of caffeine-induced transient tension in skinned muscle fibers of the rat. The fetal fibers were 26 times less sensitive to ryanodine than those of the adult (20). It would appear that SR receptors for release of Ca^{2+} in fetal and adult myocardium are modulated by Ca^{2+}, caffeine, and Mg^{2+} and that the SR is intimately involved in the delivery of Ca^{2+} to the contractile apparatus of cardiac cell on excitation (20).

An interaction of muscarinic and α-adrenergic agonists with cell surface receptors results in the activation of membrane phospholipase C to produce IP_3 (98), which mobilizes Ca^{2+} from the SR (99,100). Diacylglycerol stimulates protein kinase C to catalyze the phosphorylation of voltage-dependent Ca^{2+} channels (3). As a result, Ca^{2+} influx is enhanced, elevating intracellular Ca^{2+} to initiate muscle contraction; this signal transduction pathway involves receptors, G proteins, phospholipase C, and the second messenger IP_3. Different components of this signal transduction pathway undergo variations in developing tissues, variably affecting the heart function (i.e., cardiac muscle contraction) (3). Thus, this signal transduction pathway may constitute an important regulatory mechanism for the maintenance of Ca^{2+} homeostasis and muscle contraction. The release of Ca^{2+} from SR induced by IP_3 is quite rapid, and the amount of Ca^{2+} released is adequate to initiate muscle contraction. Because the IP_3-induced Ca^{2+} release has not been studied in developing heart, detailed investigation on IP_3 production, and IP_3-induced Ca^{2+} release from SR in developing heart is warranted.

STORAGE AND RELEASE OF CALCIUM BY MITOCHONDRIA

Both ATP and Ca^{2+} are required for many cellular processes and mediate physiologic responses such as the excitation–contraction in muscle (4–6) as well as stimulus-secretion coupling in brain and other tissues (101), whereas the intracellular concentration of Ca^{2+} is regulated precisely by different transport mechanisms (4,39). Any derangement in either one or all of these mechanisms (Fig. 15–5) would impair the Ca^{2+} homeostasis and cell metabolism, resulting in tissue dysfunction and necrosis. Excess intracellular Ca^{2+} is known to be toxic in different tissues, particularly cardiac muscle, since it induces changes in membrane permeability, impairs cell metabolism, and produces electrophysiologic abnormalities and heart dysfunction (4). This failure of cell function is believed to be due to depletion of high-energy intermediates that are rapidly utilized by active cation pumps in an attempt to restore the cation homeostasis (4,42,102). Excess intracel-

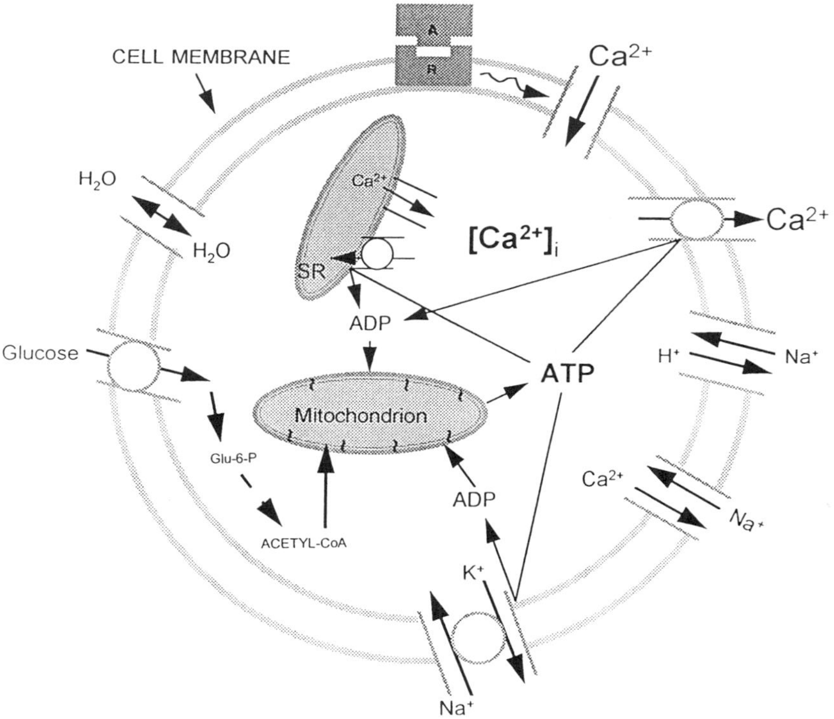

FIG. 15–5. A schematic diagram illustrating a possible relationship between high-energy phosphate (i.e., ATP) and different Ca^{2+} transport mechanisms regulating intracellular Ca^{2+} homeostasis. Ca^{2+} enters the cell via agonist-stimulated or voltage-dependent Ca^{2+} channels in response to a chemical or an electrical stimulus. Intracellular Ca^{2+} is actively taken up by the sarcoplasmic reticulum via Ca^{2+}–ATPase and extruded from the cell via another Ca^{2+} pump, and/or Na^{+}–Ca^{2+} exchanger. Ca^{2+} transfer across sarcolemma is influenced by the activity of Na^{+}–K^{+} pump and Na^{+}–H^{+} exchanger. The functions of these pumps and other transport mechanisms are influenced by high-energy compounds such as ATP and creatine phosphate. The metabolic conditions such as ischemia, anoxia, and impaired glucose metabolism in diabetes mellitus result in diminished levels of ATP and have a profoundly detrimental effect on the functions of different pumps.

lular Ca^{2+} is stored in SR (high-affinity, low-capacity system) and mitochondria (low-affinity but high-capacity system). Although SR is involved in dynamic changes in intracellular Ca^{2+} (Ca^{2+} transients), mitochondria store excess Ca^{2+} and may protect the cell from Ca^{2+} toxicity (39). Accumulation of Ca^{2+} may occur in other conditions where production of high-energy intermediates is diminished (i.e., ischemia, anoxia, hypoglycemia, and impaired glucose metabolism in diabetes mellitus) (42). Also, Ca^{2+} overload in mitochondria impairs oxidative phosphorylation, resulting in diminished production of ATP (4). According to chemiosmotic theory, Ca^{2+} uptake by mitochondria occurs as a result of negative membrane potential across inner membrane established by the activity of respiratory chain (103). The mitochondrial Ca^{2+} uptake is stimulated by inorganic phosphate because of the formation of insoluble calcium phosphates (104). It has been suggested that the mitochondrial matrix loading of Ca^{2+} in presence of phosphate seems to function as a safety device that enables mitochondria to buffer large amounts of Ca^{2+} when its concentration in the cytosol increases to levels sufficient to activate their low-affinity uptake system. This allows time for the cell to survive until the noxious agent that has elevated cytosolic Ca^{2+} is removed (39).

The newborn mammalian heart has less functional capacity than that of the adult, yet newborn myocardial mitochondrial respiratory activity is the same or exceeds that of the adult. The substrate-supported Ca^{2+} uptake in newborn heart mitochondria is twice that of adult and declines toward adult rates during the first 14 days (105). Both NADH- and succinate-linked respiration are equivalent to adult values at birth, increase transiently during the first 7 days, and then decline toward adult level. Creatine kinase activity is very low in 1–7-day-old newborn heart mitochondria and increases rapidly toward adult values after 10 days of age. The decreasing rates of Ca^{2+} uptake in development appear to be related not to respiratory activity, membrane potential, or increased cycling of Ca^{2+} but to a direct effect on the mitochondrial Ca^{2+} uniporter. It is significant to note that the developmental alterations in mitochondrial membrane phospholipids may be related to the increasing creatine kinase activity and decreasing Ca^{2+} uptake and respiration (105). The predominant role of mitochondria in comparison to SR for the regulation of intracellular Ca^{2+} in developing heart was described in earlier studies (106).

CALCIUM-BINDING PROTEINS

Some of the cytosolic Ca^{2+} binds reversibly to SL and other cell proteins such as troponin C, calmodulin, calcineurin, and calsequestrin; these proteins provide Ca^{2+} buffering in cells (39). Abnormalities in intracellular Ca^{2+} handling constitute the basis of heart dysfunction in essential hypertension and cardiac hypertrophy. Tropomyosin is elevated in hypertensive patients with ventricular hypertrophy (107). There appears to be an association between enhanced expression of tropomyosin in platelets and the development of cardiac hypertrophy, which may involve Ca^{2+} overload (107). It has been suggested that the age-related changes in

Ca^{2+} transport and the amount of Ca^{2+}-ATPase and calsequestrin may be related to changes in the regulation of intracellular Ca^{2+} concentration in fetal heart muscle and its function (82). Other investigators have reported that the rate of Ca^{2+} accumulation in the SR of rat heart myocytes grown in culture increased in a linear fashion as a function of culture age, whereas mRNA encoding for calsequestrin did not change in myocytes from 14-day fetal rat heart to 24 months of age (84). Calmodulin undergoes developmental alterations (83) and may be partly responsible for developmental changes in intracellular Ca^{2+}. In late gestation, calmodulin decreased while binding of [^{3}H]-quinuclidinyl benzilate (QNB) increased in developing rat hearts. After the second postnatal day, both calmodulin and QNB binding increased in parallel up to 10 days postnatally. It may well be that calmodulin regulates cholinergic functions in older rats via its ability to modulate intracellular Ca^{2+} in heart. However, relatively high levels of calmodulin during embryonic development may reflect other regulatory functions, such as cell growth and differentiation (73). Parallel changes in ontogenic profiles of two parameters do not conclusively demonstrate the cause-and-effect relationship between the two phenomena, unless it is subjected to more rigorous investigation. It is essential to either delay or expedite the appearance of one parameter and to see if the other parameter follows a similar profile. Further work is needed to determine the role of calmodulin in Ca^{2+} handling in developing heart.

SIGNAL TRANSDUCTION AND CALCIUM HANDLING

The positive force frequency response observed in fetal rat heart reverted to a highly negative response by the twelfth to fourteenth day postnatally. The biphasic mechanical responses directly paralleled reported changes in circulating glucocorticoid levels in developing rat (108). The force frequency response was maximally negative when the level of circulating glucocorticoids was low; the reversion of the negative force frequency response coincided with a gradual increase in the circulating level of glucocorticoids (108). The negative force frequency response was absent in the cortisol-treated developing rat heart, and a definite position pattern developed as the age of rat progressed. A high sensitivity to free Ca^{2+} seen in control fetal and newborn hearts diminished after the second postnatal week, and significantly reduced after the third postnatal week. Cortisol treatment prolonged the sensitivity to Ca^{2+} during the 3 weeks, and the hearts were more responsive to epinephrine. Apparently, the level of circulating cortisol influences force frequency response in developing rat heart (109), and this may, in part, be mediated by an increased number of β-adrenergic receptors in heart (108).

The stimulation of either α-adrenergic or muscarinic cholinergic receptors by appropriate agonists (neurotransmitter) results in the activation of phospholipase C, which hydrolyzes phosphatidylinositol bisphosphate to IP_3 and diacylglycerol. While IP_3 mobilizes Ca^{2+} from the SR, diacylglycerol stimulates protein kinase C, such that sensitivity of the enzyme to Ca^{2+} activation is enhanced. Consequently, phosphorylation of enzymes and/or other cellular proteins would occur, resulting in the modulation of cell metabolism and function. Protein kinase C appears to exist in different isoforms, which undergo differential alterations during development (110). Protein kinase C-alpha was present in fetal and 2-day-old neonatal heart extracts as well as in cultured neonatal rat ventricular myocytes. This isoform was essentially absent from adult heart extracts and ventricular myocytes. Protein kinase C-delta isoform was more abundant in fetal and neonatal heart than in adult myocardial extracts (110). The expression of PKC-alpha and PKC-delta isoforms declined during the first 2 postnatal weeks. Protein kinase C-zeta isoform was abundant in fetal heart and declined rapidly by the second postnatal day, and was essentially absent from adult heart extracts. Protein kinase C-epsilon was present at all developmental stages but was abundantly high in neonatal hearts. Protein kinase C-alpha isoform partitioned to the soluble fraction of unstimulated myocytes and was selectively translocated to the particulate fraction by Ca^{2+} (110). Thus, it can be appreciated that developmental changes in different components of the signal transduction system may yield valuable information on the biochemical basis of heart function during development.

SUMMARY AND CONCLUSIONS

It is clear from the evidence presented in this article that intracellular Ca^{2+} is critically involved in heart muscle contraction. The intracellular level of Ca^{2+} is regulated by a variety of cellular mechanisms such as Ca^{2+} influx via Ca^{2+} channels and Na^+–Ca^{2+} exchanger, its uptake, storage, and release by the SR and/or mitochondria, and Ca^{2+} binding to cytosolic and membrane proteins. Apparently, all these mechanisms undergo alterations during heart development, resulting in changes of intracellular Ca^{2+}, which modulates heart function (i.e., contraction either directly or indirectly) by influencing the cellular processes that are important for heart function. The developmental alterations in intracellular Ca^{2+} or associated changes in cellular processes may constitute the biochemical basis of heart function (i.e., muscle contraction at different stages of development). Ca^{2+} handling by the SR in the fetal/neonatal period is not fully developed, and the cardiac muscle relies primarily on the extracellular Ca^{2+} for contraction. The reliance of cardiac muscle on extracellular Ca^{2+} declines as the SR matures with age. In adult myocardium, SR is fully developed and provides sufficient Ca^{2+} to initiate full-strength muscle contraction. The sensitivity of contractile apparatus to Ca^{2+} also undergoes developmental alterations that are consistent with the acquisition of heart function. Differences in the sensitivities of heart during development to various drugs can be seen to highlight caution for the treatment of children during the early periods of their life. During the fetal/neonatal period of heart development, the myofilaments are scarce and not aligned to perform muscle contraction as in the adult stage, where adequate numbers of myofibrillar and associated proteins are present to produce full-strength contraction in cardiac muscle. It is also evident from the discussion that adequate numbers of mitochondria as well as the level of high-energy intermediates such as ATP and creatine phosphate are required to maintain Ca^{2+} homeostasis in cardiac muscle during development. Although some work concerning developmental changes in calmodulin and protein kinase C has appeared in the literature, a great deal of work on various other components of the signal transduction system in this regard remains to be carried out. In particular, mechanisms involved in the regulation of heart function during development need to be clarified before making any meaningful conclusions.

ACKNOWLEDGMENTS

This work was supported by the Medical Research Council of Canada (MRC Group in Experimental Cardiology). Dr. M. S. Nijjar was a visiting professor from the University of Prince Edward Island, Charlottetown, Canada.

REFERENCES

1. Greengard O. Hormonal regulation of enzyme synthesis differentiating mammalian tissues. In: Hommes FA, Van den Berg CJ, eds. *Normal and pathological development of energy metabolism.* London: Academic Press; 1975:55–61.
2. Long CS, Kariya K, Kams L, Simpson PC. Trophic factors for cardiac myocytes. *J Hypertens* 1990;8:S219–S224.
3. Kojima M, Sperelakis N, Sada H. Ontogenesis of transmembrane signaling systems for control of cardiac Ca^{2+} channels. *J Dev Physiol* 1990;14:181–219.
4. Dhalla NS, Elimban V, Rupp H, Takeda N, Nagano M. Role of calcium in cardiac cell damage and dysfunction. In: Sperelakis N, ed. *Physiology and pathophysiology of the heart.* 3rd ed. Boston: Kluwer Academic Publishers; 1995:605–623.
5. Klitzner TS. Maturational changes in excitation-contraction coupling in mammalian myocardium. *J Am Coll Cardiol* 1991;17:218–225.
6. Wier WG. Intracellular calcium during excitation-contraction coupling in mammalian ventricle. *Med Sci Sports Exerc* 1991;23:149–156.
7. Chapman RA, Coray A, McGuigan JAS. Sodium-calcium exchange in mammalian heart: the maintenance of low intracellular calcium concentration. In: Drake-Holland AJ, Noble MIM, eds. *Cardiac metabolism.* New York: John Wiley; 1983:117–150.
8. Lullmann H, Peters T. Plasmalemmal calcium in cardiac excitation-contraction coupling in heart muscle. *Prog Pharmacol* 1979;2:1–57.
9. Noble MIM, Drake-Holland AJ. Contractility of the heart as a function of sarcolemmal calcium handling. *J Cardiovasc Pharmacol* 1987;10(suppl 1):S107–S111.
10. Katz AM. Maturational changes in excitation-contraction coupling in mammalian myocardium. *J Am Coll Cardiol* 1991;17:218–225.
11. Jarmakani JM, Nakanishi T, George BL, Bers DM. The effect of extracellular calcium on myocardial mechanical function in the neonatal rabbit. *Dev Pharmacol Ther* 1982;5:1–52.
12. Chapman RA. Excitation-contraction coupling in cardiac muscle. *Prog Biophys Mol Biol* 1979; 35:1–52.
13. McAuliffe JJ, Gao L, Solaro RJ. Changes in myofibrillar activation and troponin C Ca^{2+} binding associated with troponin T isoform switching in developing rabbit heart. *Circ Res* 1990;66:1204–1216.
14. Solaro RJ. Molecular signaling in cardiac myofilaments. In: Dhalla NS, Beamish RE, Takeda N, Nagano M, eds. *The failing heart.* Philadelphia: Lippincott-Raven; 1995:109–114.
15. Agata N, Tanaka H, Shigenobu K. Inotropic effects of ryanodine and nicardipine on fetal, neonatal and adult guinea-pig myocardium. *Eur J Pharmacol* 1994;260:47–55.
16. Vornanen M. Force-frequency relationship, contraction duration and recirculating fraction of calcium in postnatally developing rat heart ventricles. *Acta Physiol Scand* 1992;145:311–321.

17. Ostadalova I, Kolar F, Ostadal B, Rohlicek J, Prochazka J. Early postnatal development of contractile performance and responsiveness to calcium, verapamil and ryanodine in the isolated rat heart. *J Mol Cell Cardiol* 1993;25:733–740.
18. Godt RE, Fogaca RT, Silva IK, Nosek TM. Contraction of developing avian heart muscle. *Comp Biochem Physiol* 1993;105:213–218.
19. Vornanen M. Effects of caffeine on the mechanical properties of developing rat heart ventricles. *Comp Biochem Physiol* 1984;78:329–334.
20. Su JY, Chang YI. Modulation of sarcoplasmic reticulum Ca^{2+} release channels by caffeine, Ca^{2+}, and Mg^{2+} in skinned myocardial fibres of fetal and adult rats. *Pflugers Arch* 1993;423:300–306.
21. Jin J-P, Lin JLC, Lin JJC. Troponin T isoform switching during heart development. *Ann NY Acad Sci* 1990;588:393–396.
22. Godt RE, Fogaca RTH, Nosek TM. Changes in force and calcium sensitivity in the developing avian heart. *Can J Physiol Pharmacol* 1991;69:1692–1697.
23. Roy RK, Sreter FA, Sarkar S. Changes in tropomyosin subunits and myosin light chains during development of chicken and rabbit striated muscles. *Dev Biol* 1979;69:15–30.
24. Murphy AM, Solaro RJ. Developmental differences in the stimulation of cardiac myofibrillar Mg^{2+}-ATPase activity by calmidazolium. *Pediatr Res* 1990;28:46–49.
25. Manasek FJ. Histogenesis of the embryonic myocardium. *Am J Cardiol* 1970;25:149–168.
26. El-Saleh SC, Solaro RJ. Troponin I enhances acidic pH-induced depression of calcium binding to the regulatory sites in skeletal troponin C. *J Biol Chem* 1988;263:3274–3278.
27. L'Ecuyer TJ, Schulte D, Lin JJC. Thin filament changes during in vivo rat heart development. *Pediatr Res* 1991;30:232–238.
28. Solaro RJ, El-Saleh SC, Kentish JC. Calcium, pH and the regulation of cardiac myofilament force and ATPase activity. *Mol Cell Biochem* 1989;89:163–167.
29. Martin AF, Ball K, Gao LZ, Kumar P, Solaro RJ. Identification and functional significance of troponin I isoforms in neonatal rat heart myofibril. *Circ Res* 1991;69:1244–1252.
30. Metzger JM, Moss RL. Effects on tension and stiffness due to reduced pH in mammalian fast-twitch and slow-twitch skinned skeletal muscle fibres. *J Physiol* 1990;428:737–750.
31. Beinlich CJ, Morgan HE. Control of growth in neonatal pig hearts. *Mol Cell Biochem* 1993;119:3–9.
32. Welder AA, Grant R, Kutschke RL, Anthony M, Bradlaw J, Acosta D. Effects of maternal calorie-restricted diet on development of the foetal heart, as evaluated in primary cultures of rat myocardial cells. *Food Chem Toxicol* 1991;29:445–452.
33. O'Brien PJ, Shen H, Bissonette D, Jeejeebhoy KN. Effects of hypocaloric feeding and refeeding on myocardial Ca and ATP cycling in the rat. *Mol Cell Biochem* 1995;142:151–161.
34. Navarro HA, Mills E, Seidler FE, Baker FE, Lappi SE, Tayyeb MI, Spencer JR, Slotkin TA. Prenatal nicotine exposure impairs beta-adrenergic function: persistent chronotropic subsensitivity despite recovery from deficits in receptor binding. *Brain Res Bull* 1990;25:233–237.
35. Schaffer W, Williams RS. Age-dependent changes in expression of alpha-1-adrenergic receptors in rat myocardium. *Biochem Biophys Res Commun* 1986;138:387–391.
36. Steinberg SF, Rosen TS, Malfatto G, Rosen MR. Beta-adrenergic modulation of cardiac rhythm in a rat model of altered sympathetic neural development. *J Mol Cell Cardiol* 1991;23(suppl 1):47–52.
37. Liu QY, Karpinski E, Pang PK. Changes in alpha-1-adrenoceptor coupling to calcium channels during development in rat heart. *FEBS Lett* 1994;338:234–238.
38. Hansen CA, Schroering AG, Robishaw JD. Subunit expression of signal transducing G proteins in cardiac tissue: implications for phospholipase C–beta regulation. *J Mol Cell Cardiol* 1995; 27:471–484.
39. Carafoli E. Intracellular calcium homeostasis. *Annu Rev Biochem* 1987;56:395–433.
40. Siesjo BK, Bengtsson F, Grampp W, Theander S. Calcium, excitotoxins, and neuronal death in the brain. *Ann NY Acad Sci* 1989;568:234–251.
41. Verity MA. Ca^{2+}-dependent processes as mediators of neurotoxicity. *Neurotoxicology* 1992;13: 139–148.
42. Xu KY, Zweier JL, Becker LC. Functional coupling between glycolysis and sarcoplasmic reticulum Ca^{2+} transport. *Circ Res* 1995;77:88–97.
43. Owens RJ, Crumpton MJ. Isolation and characterization of a novel 68,000-Mr Ca^{2+}-binding protein of lymphocyte plasma membrane. *Biochem J* 1984;219:309–316.
44. Streb H, Irvine RF, Berridge MJ, Schulz I. Release of Ca^{2+} from nonmitochondrial intracellular store in pancreatic acinar cells by inositol-1,4,5-triphosphate. *Nature* 1983;306:67–69.

45. Kikawa U, Kishimoto A, Nishzuka Y. The protein kinase C family: heterogeneity and its implications. *Ann Rev Biochem* 1989;58:31–44.
46. Baudry M, Evans J, Lynch G. Excitatory amino acids inhibit stimulation phosphatidylinositol metabolism by aminergic agonists in hippocampus. *Nature* 1986;319:329–331.
47. Narayanan N. Comparison of ATP-dependent calcium transport and calcium activated ATPase activities of cardiac sarcoplasmic reticulum and sarcolemma from rats of various ages. *Mech Ageing Dev* 1987;38:127–143.
48. Brillantes AM, Bezprozvannaya S, Marks AR. Developmental and tissue specific regulation of rabbit skeletal and cardiac muscle calcium channels involved in excitation-contraction coupling. *Circ Res* 1994;75:503–510.
49. Gomez JP, Potreau D, Branka JE, Raymond G. Development changes in Ca^{2+} currents from newborn rat cardiomyocytes in primary culture. *Pflugers Arch* 1994;428:241–249.
50. Wetzel GT, Chen F, Klitzner TS. Ca^{2+} channel kinetics in acutely isolated fetal, neonatal, and adult rabbit cardiac myocytes. *Circ Res* 1993;72:1065–1074.
51. Huynh TV, Chen F, Wetzel GT, Friedman WF, Klitzner TS. Developmental changes in membrane Ca^{2+} and K^+ currents in fetal, neonatal, and adult rabbit ventricular myocytes. *Circ Res* 1992; 70:508–515.
52. Kawano S, Dehaan RL. Developmental changes in the calcium currents in embryonic chick ventricular myocytes. *J Membr Biol* 1991;120:17–28.
53. Xu X, Best PM. Postnatal changes in T-type calcium current density in rat atrial myocytes. *J Physiol* 1192;454:657–672.
54. Renaud JF, Kazazoglou T, Schmid R, Romey G, Lazdunski M. Differentiation of receptor sites for [3H] nitrendipine in chick hearts and physiological relation to the slow Ca^{2+} channel and to excitation-contraction coupling. *Eur J Biochem* 1984;139:673–681.
55. DePaula Brotto MA, Creazzo TL. Ca^{2+} transients in embryonic chick heart: contributions from Ca^{2+} channels and the sarcoplasmic reticulum. *Am J Physiol* 270;39:H518–H525.
56. Liu QY, Karpinski E, Pang PK. Changes in alpha-1-adrenoceptor coupling to Ca^{2+} channels during development in rat heart. *FEBS Lett* 1994;338:234–238.
57. Inayatulla A, Li DY, Chemtob S, Varma DR. Ontogeny of positive inotropic responses to sympathomimetic agents and of myocardial adrenoceptors in rats. *Can J Physiol Pharmacol* 1994;72: 361–367.
58. Tanaka H, Shigenobu K. Role of beta-adrenoceptors–adenylate cyclase system in the developmental decrease in sensitivity to isoprenaline in foetal and neonatal rat heart. *Br J Pharmacol* 1990;100:138–142.
59. Navarro HA, Kudlacz EM, Slotkin TA. Control of adenylate cyclase activity in developing rat heart and liver: effects of prenatal exposure to terbutaline or dexamethasone. *Biol Neonate* 1991;60:127–136.
60. Reuter H. Calcium movements through cardiac cell membranes. *Med Res Rev* 1985;5:427–440.
61. Tsien RW. Calcium channels in excitable cell membranes. *Ann Rev Physiol* 1983;45:341–358.
62. Burnstock G. Purinergic nerves. *Pharmacol Rev* 1972;24:509–581.
63. DeYoung MB, Scarpa A. Extracellular ATP induces Ca^{2+} transients in cardiac myocytes which are potentiated by norepinephrine. *FEBS Lett* 1987;223:53–58.
64. Danziger RS, Raffaeli S, Moreno-Sanchez R, Sakai M, Capagrossi MC, Spurgeon HA, Hanford RG, Lakatta EG. Extracellular ATP has a potent effect to enhance cytosolic calcium and contractility in single ventricular myocytes. *Cell Calcium* 1988;9:193–199.
65. Williams M. Purine receptors in mammalian tissue: pharmacology and functional significance. *Ann Rev Pharmacol Toxicol* 1987;27:315–345.
66. Zhao D, Dhalla NS. [^{35}S] ATP gamma S binding sites in purified heart sarcolemma membrane. *Am J Physiol* 1990;258:C185–C188.
67. Scamps F, Maejoux E, Charlemagne D, Vassort G. Calcium current in single cells isolated from neonatal and hypertrophied rat heart. Effect of beta-adrenergic stimulation. *Circ Res* 1990; 67:1007–1016.
68. Legssyer A, Poggioli J, Renard D, Vassort G. ATP and other adenine compounds increase mechanical activity and inositol triphosphate production in rat heart. *J Physiol* 1988;401:185–199.
69. Artman M. Sarcolemmal Na^+–Ca^{2+} exchange activity and exchanger immunoreactivity in developing rabbit hearts. *Am J Physiol* 1992;263:H1506–H1513.
70. Sperelakis N. (Na^+–K^+)-ATPase activity of embryonic chick heart and skeletal muscles as a function of age. *Biochim Biophys Acta* 1972;266:230–237.

71. Hanson GL, Schilling WP, Michael LH. Sodium-potassium pump and sodium-calcium exchange in adult and neonatal canine cardiac sarcolemma. *Am J Physiol* 1993;264:H320–H326.
72. Maygar CE, Wang J, Azuma KK, McDonough AA. Reciprocal regulation of cardiac Na-K-ATPase and Na/Ca exchanger: hypertension, thyroid hormone, development. *Am J Physiol* 1995; 269:C675–C682.
73. Steinberg SF, Rose TS, Malfatto G, Rosen MR. Beta-adrenergic modulation of cardiac rhythm in a rat model of altered sympathetic neural development. *J Mol Cell Cardiol* 1991;23(suppl 1): 47–52.
74. Caroni P, Carafoli E. The Ca^{2+}-pumping ATPase of heart sarcolemma: characterization, calmodulin-dependence, and partial purification. *J Biol Chem* 1981;256:3263–3270.
75. Ho AKS, Shang K, Dufield R. Calmodulin regulation of the cholinergic receptor in the rat heart during ontogeny and senescence. *Mech Aging Dev* 1986;36:143–154.
76. Carafoi E, Chiesi M. Calcium pumps in the plasma and intracellular membranes. *Curr Top Cell Regul* 1992;32:209–241.
77. Niggli V, Sigel E, Carafoli E. The purified Ca^{2+} pump of human erythrocyte membrane catalyzes an electroneutral Ca^{2+}-H^{+} exchange in reconstituted lysosomal systems. *J Biol Chem* 1982;257: 2350–2356.
78. Franzini-Armstrong C. Structure of sarcoplasmic reticulum. *Fed Proc* 1980;39:2403–2409.
79. Fisher DJ, Tate CA, Phillips S. Developmental regulation of the sarcoplasmic reticulum calcium pump in the rabbit heart. *Pediatr Res* 1992;31:474–479.
80. Chiest M, Wrzosek A, Grueninger S. The role of the sarcoplasmic reticulum in various types of cardiomyocytes. *Mol Cell Biochem* 1994;130:159–171.
81. Hammes A, Oberdorf S, Strehler EE, Stauffer T, Carafoli E, Vetter H, Neyses L. Differentiation specific isoform mRNA expression of the calmodulin-dependent plasma membrane Ca^{2+}-ATPase. *FASEB J* 1994;8:428–435.
82. Michalak M. Sarcoplasmic reticulum membranes and heart development. *Can J Cardiol* 1987;3: 251–260.
83. Moorman AF, Vermeulen JL, Koban MU, Schwartz K, Lamers WH, Boheler KR. Patterns of expression of sarcoplasmic reticulum Ca^{2+}-ATPase and phospholamban mRNAs during rat heart development. *Circ Res* 1995;76:616–625.
84. Lompre AM, Lambert F, Lakatta EG, Schwartz K. Expression of sarcoplasmic reticulum Ca^{2+}-ATPase and calsequestrin genes in rat heart during ontogenic development and aging. *Circ Res* 1991;69:1390–1388.
85. Schulman H, Lou LL. Multifunctional Ca^{2+}/calmodulin dependent protein kinase: domain structure and regulation. *Trends Biochem Sci* 1989;14:62–66.
86. Le Peuch CJ, Demaille JG, Pechere JF. Radioelectrophoresis: a specific microassay of parvalbumins: application to muscle biopsies from men and other vertebrates. *Biochim Biophys Acta* 1978;537:153–159.
87. Movsesian MA, Nishikawa M, Adelstein RS. Phosphorylation of phospholamban by calcium-activated, phospholipid dependent protein kinase: stimulation of cardiac sarcoplasmic reticulum calcium uptake. *J Biol Chem* 1984;259:8029–8032.
88. Inui M, Saito A, Fleischer S. Purification of the ryanodine receptor and identity with feet structures of junctional terminal cisternae of sarcoplasmic reticulum from fast skeletal muscle. *J Biol Chem* 1987;262:1740–1747.
89. Yano K, Zarain-Herzberg A. Sarcoplasmic reticulum calsequestrins: structural and functional properties. *Mol Cell Biochem* 1994;135:61–70.
90. Hatem SN, Sweeten T, Vetter V, Morad M. Evidence for presence of Ca^{2+} channel-gated Ca^{2+} stores in neonatal human atrial myocytes. *Am J Physiol* 1995;268:H1195–H1201.
91. Fabiato A. Calcium release in skinned cardiac cells: variations with species, tissues, and development. *Fed Proc* 1982;41:2238–2244.
92. Streb H, Bayerdorffer E, Haase W, Irvine RF, Schulz I. Effect of inositol-1,4,5-triphosphate on isolated subcellular fractions of rat pancreas. *J Membr Biol* 1984;81:241–253.
93. Dawson AP, Irvine RF. Inositol-1,4,5-triphosphate-promoted Ca^{2+} release from microsomal fractions of rat liver. *Biochem Biophys Res Commun* 1984;120:858–864.
94. Prentki M, Biden TJ, Janjic D, Irvine RF, Berridge MJ, Wollheim CB. Rapid mobilization of Ca^{2+} from rat insulinoma microsomes by inositol-1,4,5-triphosphate. *Nature* 1984;309:562–564.
95. Sutko JL, Thompson LJ, Kort AA, Lakatta EG. Comparison of effects of ryanodine and caffeine on rat ventricular myocardium. *Am J Physiol* 1986;250:H786–H795.

96. Hansford RG, Lakkata EG. Relationship between cytosolic free Ca^{2+} concentration and the control of pyruvate dehydrogenase in isolated cardiac myocytes. *Biochem J* 1987;24:145–151.
97. Imagawa T, Smith JS, Coronado R, Campbell KP. Purified ryanodine receptor from skeletal muscle sarcoplasmic reticulum is the Ca^{2+}-permeable pore of the calcium release channel. *J Biol Chem* 1987;262:16636–16643.
98. Berridge MJ, Irvine RF. Inositol phosphates and cell signaling. *Nature* 1989;341:197–205.
99. Nicoletti F, Wroblewski JT, Novelli A, Alho H, Guyidotti A, Costa E. The activation of inositol phospholipid metabolism as a signal-transducing system for excitatory amino acids in primary cultures of cerebellar granule cells. *J Neurosci* 1986;6:1905–1911.
100. Giuramand J, Vines M, Recasens M. A specific transduction mechanism for the glutamate action on phosphoinositide metabolism via the quisqualte metabotropic receptor in rat brain synaptoneurosomes. II. Calcium dependency, cadmium inhibition. *J Neurochem* 1991;57:1501–1507.
101. Nicholls DG, Sihra TS. Synaptosomes possess an exocytotic pool glutamate. *Nature* 1986; 321:772–773.
102. Nayler WG, Daly MJ. Calcium and the injured cardiac myocytes. In: Sperelakis N, ed. *Physiology and pathophysiology of the heart.* 2nd ed. Boston: Kluwer Academic Publishers; 1989:527–540.
103. Rottenberg H, Scarpa A. Calcium uptake and membrane potential in mitochondria. *Biochemistry* 1974;13:4811–4819.
104. Rossi CS, Lehninger AL. Stoichiometric relationship between mitochondrial ion accumulation and oxidative phosphorylation. *Biochem Biophys Res Commun* 1963;11:441–446.
105. Wolf WJ, Rex KA, Geshi E, Sordahl LA. Postnatal changes in heart mitochondrial calcium and energy metabolism. *Am J Physiol* 1991;261:H1–H8.
106. Sulakhe PV, Dhalla NS. Excitation-contraction in heart. IV. Energy dependent calcium transport in the myocardium in developing rat. *Life Sci* 1970;9:1363–1370.
107. Crabos M, Yamakado T, Heizmann CW, Cerletti N, Buhler FR, Erne P. The calcium binding protein tropomyosin in human platelets and cardiac tissue: elevation in hypertensive cardiac hypertrophy. *Eur J Clin Invest* 1991;21:472–478.
108. Penefsky ZJ. Effects of glucocorticoids and catecholamines on maturing rat heart. *Comp Biochem Physiol* 1988;90:133–144.
109. Penefsky ZJ, Wolfe J, Greengard O, Bernstein J. Mechanical responses of developing Fisher rat heart: effects of steroid hormone. *J Dev Physiol* 1986;333–345.
110. Rybin VO, Steinberg SF. Protein kinase C isoform expression and regulation in the developing rat heart. *Circ Res* 1994;74:299–309.

The Developing Heart,
edited by Bohuslav Ošťádal et al.
Lippincott-Raven Publishers,
Philadelphia © 1997.

16

Postnatal Changes in Cardiac Calcium Regulation

Matti Vornanen

Department of Biology, University of Joensuu, 80101 Joensuu, Finland

Circulation pattern changes dramatically at birth and the reorganized blood flow exerts increasing demands on pump function of the heart. Therefore, it is not surprising that contractility of mammalian heart changes prominently during postnatal ontogeny. Maturational changes in cardiac performance are partially due to the increasing heart mass (1) but also result from age-dependent alterations in the contractile function of individual cells (2). Electrophysiologic properties (3–5), size and fine structure of ventricular myocytes (1,6), and isoform composition of contractile and regulatory proteins (7–9) go through a series of changes during postnatal maturation, which have profound influence on the pattern of contractile activation. In this article current knowledge on the developmental changes of excitation–contraction coupling (e–c coupling) in the rat heart is briefly reviewed.

ADULT TYPE OF EXCITATION–CONTRACTION COUPLING

Contraction of cardiac muscle cell is activated when cytoplasmic free Ca concentration rapidly rises from approximately 100 nM to 1 μM (10). Since cardiac muscle cell contains large amounts of molecules that efficiently buffer Ca, only 1% of the released Ca may be available for myofilament activation. To override the high buffering capacity of intracellular milieu the total Ca increase must be at least 50 μM to reach the free Ca concentration of 1 μM (11). The major source of contractile Ca in the adult mammals is the sarcoplasmic reticulum (SR), where the release is triggered by transsarcolemmal Ca influx (Ca-induced Ca release, CICR) (12). Recent evidence suggests that the e–c coupling mechanism is composed of thousands of independent release units. Each unit is composed of a cluster of SR Ca release channels in the subsarcolemmal cleft (13) and is triggered to open by local Ca currents through L-type Ca channels (14–19). The number of Ca-release channels/ryanodine receptors (RyR) is 4–10 times higher than the number of L-type Ca channels/dihydropyridine (DHP) receptors (20), suggesting that one Ca channel controls the opening of several SR Ca-release channels and that some Ca-release channels, because of their large size (~30 nm), are rather distant from the nearest DHP receptor.

The triggering efficiency of incoming Ca is strictly dependent on SR Ca load (12,21). Under experimental conditions that do not favor SR Ca loading or SR Ca release (room temperature, Na-free intracellular solution, intracellular Cs), the gain of CICR may be relatively low and Ca release within the RyR cluster seems to be under strict control of single Ca channel currents. In more physiologic conditions (body temperature, normal intracellular Na and K) the gain of CICR mechanism is probably several times higher (22), which may favor reverse Na–Ca exchange as an additional trigger for Ca release (23–26). Interestingly, the Na–Ca exchange protein has been located within the T-tubules (27–29), possibly in the same diffusionally restricted space between junctional SR and SL, where RyR and DHP receptors are localized (30). The importance of L-type Ca current as a trigger is well established, but further research is needed to elucidate the relative significance of L-type Ca current, reverse Na–Ca exchange, and other possible triggers (31) under physiologically relevant conditions.

SR FUNCTION DURING DEVELOPMENT

The SR of the newborn rat heart is morphologically deficient (6,32,33); consequently, the e–c coupling mechanism must be significantly different from the one described for adult heart. Although the SR is clearly rudimentary at the moment of birth, mRNA of SR Ca-ATPase is expressed in early fetal life, even before the heart tube has formed. Ca-ATPase mRNA is present already in 9-day-old rat embryo (34). In 12–15-day-old fetuses the mRNA concentration is still low but increases rapidly around the birth, so that adult level is reached at the fourth or fifth postnatal day (35,36). The density of cardiac SR Ca-release channels is relatively low at the end of gestation (0.22 pmol/mg protein) in comparison to the level in the adult rat heart (0.59 pmol/mg) (37), suggesting a prominent postnatal increase in SR participation in contractile activation. In accordance with this, CICR is totally absent in fetal rat heart but appears soon after birth (38,39). Progressive maturation of CICR occurs during several postnatal weeks, so that the sensitivity of adult rat is reached at the age of 30 days (39).

The increasing importance of SR Ca stores to contractile activation is evident from the pharmacologic blockade of SR function. Ryanodine binds specifically to Ca release channel and impairs the function of SR. In right ventricular strips of 3–4-day-old rats ryanodine (1 μM) causes approximately a 27% reduction in contractile force, while in the adult heart the reduction is about 83% (40) (their Fig. 7, corrected for the time-dependent deterioration). These numbers almost exactly correspond to the values of recirculating Ca for 6-day-old (27%) and adult rats (85%), with similar preparation and under very similar conditions (41). Experiments with perfused hearts show somewhat stronger negative inotropic effect of ryanodine on newborn rat heart. In 1-day-old rat, reduction of contractile force by 1 μM ryanodine was 53%, and in 7-day-old rat it was already 65% (42). In perfused heart contractile response represents mainly left ventricular function. Therefore, the stronger ryanodine response in perfused hearts could be due to faster development of SR in the left ventricle (6).

Minor contribution of SR Ca stores to contractile activation in newborn rat heart is also evident from the in vivo inhibition of SR Ca–ATPase. Cyclopiazonic acid (CPA), a specific blocker of SR Ca–ATPase (43), causes more than 80% inhibition of contractile force in right ventricular strips of adult rat heart but only 10% inhibition in 1-day-old rat (44).

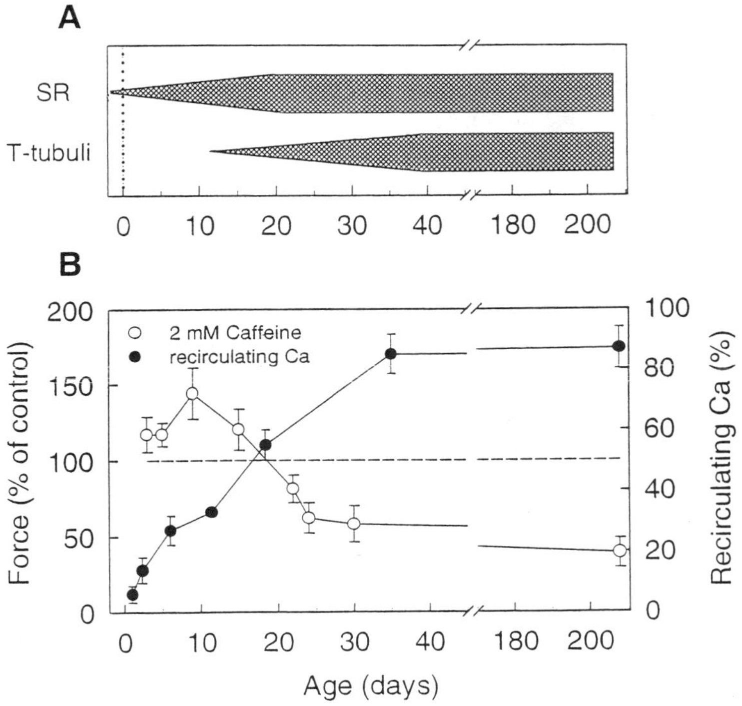

FIG. 16–1. Developmental changes in recirculating Ca and contractile response to caffeine (2 mM) in right ventricular strips of the rat heart. Postnatal maturation of SR and T-tubuli are schematically presented for comparison (**A**). The vertical dashed line in part **B** shows the transition from positive to negative inotropic effect in caffeine response and the 50% level of recirculating Ca. Recirculating fraction of activator Ca was determined from the decay of rest potentiation. Experimental temperature was 30°C and $[Ca]_0$ = 2.0 mM. (Data modified from refs. 41 and 46.)

The contribution of SR to contractile activation can be indirectly determined by calculating the recirculating fraction of activator Ca from the decay of potentiated contractile state (45). Analysis on right ventricular strips shows that in 1-day-old rat recirculating Ca corresponds to only 6% of the contractile force, but in 35-day-old rat it is already at the level of adult rat heart (85%) (41). This is well in line with the maturation of the CICR mechanism and ryanodine inhibition of contraction. Caffeine, although having other effects, such as myofilament Ca sensitization, releases SR Ca and inhibits its reuptake. The depletion of SR Ca by caffeine causes negative inotropic effect, which can be used as an indication of SR Ca stores in contractile activation. In the neonatal rat heart caffeine has prominent positive inotropic effect until day 15, but the response turns into a negative one before day 22 (46). Developmental changes in recirculating Ca and caffeine response occur parallel with the morphologic maturation of SR and T-tubuli (Fig. 16–1). When recirculating fraction of activator Ca and the effect of caffeine on contractile force are plotted as a function of age, the caffeine curve intersects the line for negative inotropic effect at the age of about 18 days, and the curve of recirculating Ca cuts the line of 50% at the age of 17 days. These two independent experiments suggest that control of contractile activation shifts from predominantly transsarcolemmal Ca influx to the one dominated by SR Ca release during the third postnatal week in rat.

EFFECT OF Ca CHANNEL BLOCKERS

The paucity of SR in newborn rat heart necessitates that Ca influx through sarcolemma (SL) from extracellular space is the main source of contractile Ca. In the light of current knowledge two putative routes for Ca influx exist, Ca channels and reverse Na–Ca exchange. Both L- and T-channel currents are present in neonatal rat ventricular cells but L-channel currents dominate (47,48). Blockade of L-type Ca channels will decrease contractile Ca directly by reducing sarcolemmal Ca influx to myofilaments and indirectly by reducing the trigger Ca. If Ca channel antagonist binding affinity does not change developmentally (40,49), the differences in contractile response to Ca antagonists should be due to developmental changes in e–c coupling. In cardiac preparations, which are directly dependent on sarcolemmal Ca influx, force decline should closely follow the occupation of Ca channels by the blocker. In preparations, which are predominantly dependent on CICR and where a relatively small fraction of the whole cell Ca current is sufficient to trigger full contraction (10), an appreciable number of channels could be blocked before the contractile force begins to decline. Therefore, the decreasing sensitivity of the isolated rat heart to the negative inotropic effect of calcium antagonists during postnatal ontogeny is an indication of a higher functional dependence of the immature heart on transsarcolemmal Ca influx (40,50,51). In 3–4-day-old rat heart 1 μM nifedipine practically abolishes contraction (suggesting a complete block of Ca channels), while the same dose reduces contraction force only 40% in the adults (40). Similarly, verapamil (0.5 mg l^{-1}) blocks contraction in 3-day-old rat but causes only about 20% reduction of contractile force in the adult rat (50). Even complete block of Ca current is unable to totally abolish the fast twitch in enzymatically isolated myocytes of the adult rat (23,52), suggesting that L-type Ca current is not the sole trigger for Ca release.

The relative insensitivity to ryanodine and complete inhibition of contraction by Ca channel blockers in newborn rat heart suggest that sarcolemmal Ca influx through L-type Ca channels directly activates contraction in newborn rats. Only a small portion of contraction seems to be dependent on SR Ca stores at this developmental stage. It should be noted, however, that block of Ca channels curtails the action potential duration and thereby inhibits possible Ca influx through reverse Na–Ca exchange (53).

POSTNATAL CHANGES IN Ca CURRENT

Several kinds of indirect evidence suggest that in the newborn rat heart sarcolemmal Ca transport mechanisms predominate and that during the early postnatal maturation SR Ca stores become increasingly important in the activation of contraction. However, it is not well understood whether both Ca channels and reverse Na–Ca exchange are involved, and to what extent these two putative influx routes contribute to the activation of contraction at different developmental stages of the rat heart. We have measured the contribution of sarcolemmal Ca current to total cellular Ca in six different developmental stages of postnatally developing rat heart (54). The peak amplitude of L-type Ca current increases about sevenfold from day 1 to the adult rat (Fig. 16–2A,E). This increase is, however, mainly due to the increase in cell size; accordingly, the Ca current density remains practically unaltered during the whole postnatal period (Fig. 16–2B,F). In fact, the contribution of Ca current to total cellular Ca is bigger in neonates than in adults because of slower inactivation of Ca current (Fig. 16–2C,G) and higher surface-to-volume ratio of neonatal rat myocytes (Fig. 16–2D,H). Our analysis suggests that the contribution of L-type Ca current to total cellular Ca is approximately sixfold in newborn rat (54 μmol L^{-1}) with comparison to the adults (8 μmol L^{-1}) (54). The total amount of Ca that is needed for maximal activation of myofilaments may approximate 50 μM in the adult rat (11). L-type Ca current produces an increment in total cytosolic Ca of approximately 10 μmol L^{-1} (11,54,55), which is probably able to activate less than 20% of the maximal twitch force in this age group. The Ca buffering capacity of newborn rat heart cells is not known but is probably not higher than in the adults, since the concentration of Ca buffers like SR Ca-ATPase and phospholamban is lower in newborn than in adult heart (36,56). Furthermore, Ca sensitivity of myofibrils is higher in newborn than in adult rats (38). Therefore, 54 μM of Ca, which flows through the L-type Ca channels, may be sufficient for almost full activation of myofilaments in the newborn rat heart.

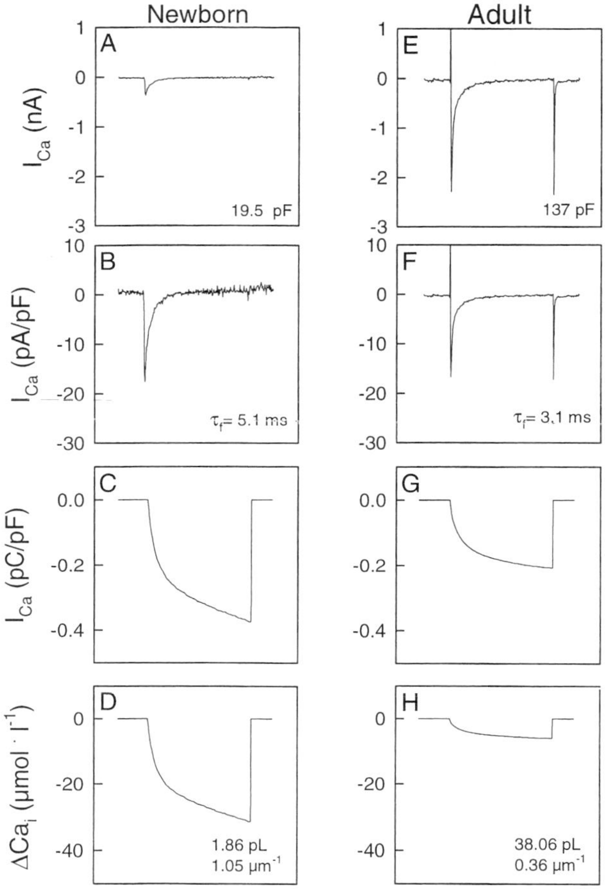

FIG. 16–2. A summary of factors that contribute to the higher transsarcolemmal Ca influx through L-type Ca channels in newborn rat myocytes in comparison to the adult cells. The top panels (**A,E**) show that the peak amplitude of Ca current is several times bigger in adult than in newborn (1-day-old) rat myocytes. In **B,F** the same Ca currents are normalized to capacitive surface area of the cells (19.5 and 137 pF) and show that the density of L-type Ca current is approximately the same in both age groups. Parts **C** and **G** show time integrals of the currents. Because of slower inactivation of the current in the newborn, the charge transfer through Ca channels is bigger in 1-day-old than in adult rat (τ_f, inactivation time constant of fast component of Ca current). The total increment in intracellular Ca due to Ca influx through L-type Ca current is shown in the lowest panels (**D,H**). The contribution of Ca current to total cellular Ca is approximately six times higher in newborn than in adult rat, largely because of the higher surface-to-volume ratio of the newborn myocytes (1.05 vs. 0.36/µm^{-1} for newborn and adult cells, respectively). The currents were elicited from the holding potential of −45 mV to pulse potential of 0 mV for 200 ms. Potassium was replaced with cesium both in extra- and intracellular solutions. Experimental temperature 36°C and $[Ca]_0$ = 1.8 mM.

Na–Ca EXCHANGER LEVELS AND ACTIVITY

Contribution of reverse mode of Na–Ca exchange to contractile Ca is suggested to be important in neonatal rabbit heart (53,57), since Ca influx through sarcolemmal Ca channels is considered to be insufficient for full activation of contraction (58–61). Exchanger mRNA level of the rat heart is maximal near the time of birth, 4–5 days before the peak expression of SR Ca-ATPase mRNA, and then declines postnatally (35,62). In accordance with this Na-dependent Ca uptake is higher in newborn cardiac tissue than in adult preparations (63).Whether the high Na–Ca exchange activity of the newborn rat heart is only involved in the removal of activator Ca or is also responsible for Ca influx is still undetermined. The relatively great Ca influx through the Ca channels, however, suggests that the reverse Na–Ca exchange may not be as important in the rat heart as it is suggested to be in the rabbit.

POSTNATAL DEVELOPMENT OF E–C COUPLING IN THE RAT HEART

It is evident that the contribution of SR to contractile Ca increases relatively rapidly during the postnatal maturation in rat. In Fig. 16–3 excitation–contraction coupling of the rat heart is divided into three different phases on the basis of physiologic, pharmacologic, and morphologic evidence. In the newborn rat heart major part of contractile Ca seems to come from extracellular space; this influx is thought to be mediated largely by L-type Ca channels. During the first postnatal week morphologic maturation of SR occurs, and dyadic couplings at the level of peripheral sarcolemma differentiate (6,32). The developmental phase from birth to the age of approximately 11 days is associated with increasing contribution of Ca release from dyadic SR at the level of peripheral SL. The development of T-tubules begins at the age of approximately 10 days (32) and leads to the differentiation of internal couplings of SR at the level of T-tubules (64). The development of the T-tubules, which coincides with the prominent increase in cell size, is associated with the change of SL-dominated Ca regulation to predominantly SR-based contractile activation during the third postnatal week (Fig. 16–3). This presentation is very general (e.g., neglecting the small but definite contribution of SR to contractile activation in the newborn animal). Furthermore, significant developmental differences may occur between different compartments of the heart (right vs. left ventricle; atria vs. ventricles), which have not yet been studied.

Although information on electrophysiologic and contractile properties of postnatally developing heart has increased substantially during the last decade, our understanding of contractile activation is in many respects fragmentary and based often on indirect evidence. Direct measurement of intracellular Ca transients (65) and quantification of different Ca transport systems of the cardiac myocyte are needed to elucidate quantitatively the contribution of intracellular and extracellular Ca pools to contractile activation in different phases of postnatal maturation.

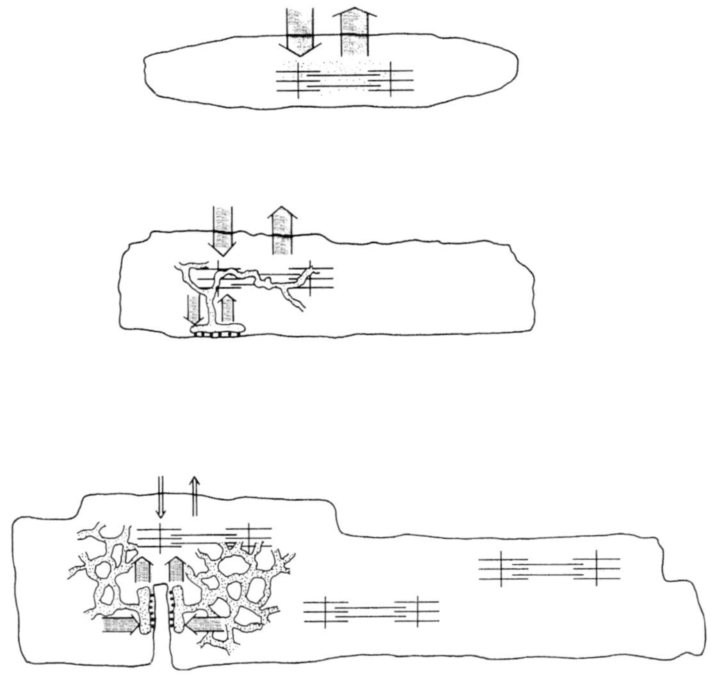

FIG. 16–3. Contribution of sarcolemmal Ca influx and Ca release from SR to contractile activation at different developmental stages of the rat heart ventricles. The postnatal development of contractile activation was divided in three different phases on the basis of morphologic differentiation of major ultrastructural features. In 1-day-old rat SR is sparsely developed and extracellular space is considered to be the major source of activator Ca. However, even at this phase a small contribution by SR is evident; approximately 10% according to the recirculating Ca (41) and CPA inhibition of contraction (44). From 2 days to approximately to 11 days of age is a period of rapid proliferation of SR, and the contribution of peripheral junctional SR to contractile activation increases. From 11 days on, T-tubules begin to develop and internal couplings at the level of T-tubules differentiate from the SR so that adult-type of e–c coupling is evident at the age of approximately 30 days. The cell contours are drawn to correspond to natural size differences. The thickness of the arrows describes the relative contribution of intra- and extracellular Ca to activation of contraction. (From ref. 41 with permission.)

SUMMARY

Subcellular structures and molecular mechanisms that are necessary for adult type of excitation–contraction coupling are absent or weakly developed in the heart of the newborn mammal. In the newborn rat ventricles T-tubuli are absent, sarcoplasmic reticulum (SR) is morphologically poorly developed, and its Ca-ATPase and Ca release channel content are lower than in the adult heart. Selective blocking of sarcolemmal Ca channels (verapamil, nifedipine) or SR function (ryanodine, cyclopiazonic acid) indicate that in newborn rat heart influx of extracellular Ca is the predominant route for contractile Ca, with relatively little contribution by SR Ca release. The major part of sarcolemmal Ca influx occurs probably through L-type Ca channels, which can bring approximately 50 μM of Ca in the newborn rat myocytes but only 10 μM in the adult cells. The larger contribution of sarcolemmal Ca influx in newborn rat heart is partly due to large sarcolemmal surface-to-volume ratio of newborn myocytes, partly affected by slow inactivation of Ca current in newborn ventricular cells. With advancing age Ca stores of SR become increasingly important for activation of contraction, so that adult–type excitation–contraction coupling is reached at the age of about 4 weeks in the rat heart.

ACKNOWLEDGMENT

This work was supported by the Academy of Finland.

REFERENCES

1. Clubb FJ, Bishop SP. Formation of binucleated myocardial cells in the neonatal rat. An index for growth hypertrophy. *Lab Invest* 1984;50:571–577.
2. Nassar R, Reedy M, Anderson PAW. Developmental changes in the ultrastructure and sarcomere shortening of the isolated rabbit ventricular myocyte. *Circ Res* 1987;61:465–483.
3. Wahler GM. Developmental increases in the inwardly rectifying potassium current of rat ventricular myocytes. *Am J Physiol* 1992;262:C1266–C1272.
4. Wahler GM, Dollinger S, Smith JM, Flemal KL. Time course of postnatal changes in rat heart action potential and in transient outward current is different. *Am J Physiol* 1994;267:H1157–H1166.
5. Gomez J-P, Potreau D, Branka J-E, Raymond G. Developmental changes in Ca^{2+} currents from newborn rat cardiomyocytes in primary culture. *Pflugers Arch* 1994;428:241–249.
6. Olivetti G, Anversa P, Loud AV. Morphometric study of early postnatal development in the left and right ventricular myocardium of the rat. II. Tissue composition, capillary growth, and sarcoplasmic alterations. *Circ Res* 1980;46:503–512.
7. Swynghedauw B. Developmental and functional adaptation of contractile proteins in cardiac and skeletal muscle. *Physiol Rev* 1986;66:710–771.
8. Reiser PJ, Westfall MV, Schiaffino S, Solaro RJ. Tension production and thin-filament protein isoforms in developing rat myocardium. *Am J Physiol* 1994;267:H1589–H1596.
9. Jin J-P, Lin JJ-C. Rapid purification of mammalian cardiac troponin T and its isoform switching in rat hearts during development. *J Biol Chem* 1988;263:7309–7315.
10. Cannell MB, Berlin JR, Lederer WJ. Effect of membrane potential changes on the calcium transient in single rat cardiac muscle cells. *Science* 1987;238:1419–1423.
11. Berlin JR, Bassani JWM, Bers DM. Intrinsic cytosolic calcium buffering properties of single rat cardiac myocytes. *Biophys J* 1994;67:1775–1787.
12. Fabiato A, Fabiato F. Contractions induced by a calcium-triggered release of calcium from the sarcoplasmic reticulum of single skinned cardiac cells. *J Physiol* 1975;249:469–495.
13. Stern MD. Theory of excitation–contraction coupling in cardiac muscle. *Biophys J* 1992; 63:497–517.
14. Lopez-Lopez JR, Shacklock PS, Balke CW, Wier WG. Local calcium transients triggered by single L-type calcium channel currents in cardiac cells. *Science* 1995;268:1042–1045.
15. Cannell MB, Cheng H, Lederer WJ. The control of calcium release in heart muscle. *Science* 1995;268:1045–1049.
16. Cheng H, Lederer WJ, Cannell MB. Calcium sparks: elementary events underlying excitation–contraction coupling in heart muscle. *Science* 1993;262:740–744.
17. Wier WG, Egan TM, Lopez-Lopez JR, Balke CW. Local control of excitation–contraction coupling in rat heart cells. *J Physiol* 1994;474.3:463–471.

18. Sham JSK, Cleeman L, Morad M. Functional coupling of Ca^{2+} channels and ryanodine receptors in cardiac myocytes. *Proc Natl Acad Sci USA* 1995;92:121–125.
19. Isenberg G, Han S. Gradation of Ca^{2+}-induced Ca^{2+} release by voltage-clamp pulse duration in potentiated guinea-pig ventricular myocytes. *J Physiol* 1994;480(3):423–438.
20. Bers DM, Stiffel VM. Ratio of ryanodine to dihydropyridine receptors in cardiac and skeletal muscle and implications for E–C coupling. *Am J Physiol* 1993;264:C1587–C1593.
21. Bassani JWM, Yuan W, Bers DM. Fractional SR Ca release is regulated by trigger Ca and SR Ca content in cardiac myocytes. *Am J Physiol* 1995;268:C1313–C1329.
22. Han S, Schiefer A, Isenberg G. Ca^{2+} load of guinea-pig ventricular myocytes determines efficacy of brief Ca^{2+} currents as trigger for Ca^{2+} release. *J Physiol* 1994;480.3:411–421.
23. Levi AJ, Brooksby P, Hancox JC. A role for depolarization induced calcium entry on the Na–Ca exchange in triggering intracellular calcium release and contraction in rat ventricular myocytes. *Cardiovasc Res* 1993;27:1677–1690.
24. Vornanen M, Shepherd N, Isenberg G. Tension–voltage relations of single myocytes reflect Ca release triggered by Na/Ca exchange at 35°C but not 23°C. *Am J Physiol* 1994;267:C623–C632.
25. Kohmoto O, Levi AJ, Bridge JHB. Relation between reverse sodium–calcium exchange and sarcoplasmic reticulum calcium release in guinea pig ventricular cells. *Circ Res* 1994;74:550–554.
26. Levi AJ, Spitzer KW, Kohmoto O, Bridge JHB. Depolarization-induced Ca entry via Na–Ca exchange triggers SR release in guinea pig cardiac myocytes. *Am J Physiol* 1994;266:H1422–H1433.
27. Porzig H, Li Z, Nicoll A, Philipson KD. Mapping of the cardiac sodium–calcium exchanger with monoclonal antibodies. *Am J Physiol* 1993;265:C748–C756.
28. Frank JS, Mottino G, Reid D, Molday RS, Philipson KD. Distribution of the Na^+–Ca^{2+} exchange protein in mammalian cardiac myocytes: an immunofluorescence and immunocolloidal gold-labeling study. *J Cell Biol* 1992;117:337–345.
29. Chen F. Mottino G, Klizner TS, Philipson KD, Frank JS. Distribution of the Na^+/Ca^{2+} exchange protein in developing rabbit myocytes. *Am J Physiol* 1995;268:C1126–C1132.
30. Langer GA, Wang SY, Rich TL. Localization of the Na/Ca exchange-dependent Ca compartment in cultured neonatal rat heart cells. *Am J Physiol* 1995;268:C119–C126.
31. Ferrier HR, Howlett SE. Contractions in guinea-pig ventricular myocytes triggered by a calcium-release mechanism separate from Na^+ and L-currents. *J Physiol* 1995;484.1:107–122.
32. Schiebler TH, Wolf HH. Elektronenmikroskopische Untersuchungen am Herzmuskel der Ratte während der Entwicklung. *Z Zellforsch* 1966;69:22–40.
33. Hirakow R, Gotoh T, Watanabe T. Quantitative studies on the ultrastructural differentiation and growth of mammalian cardiac muscle cells. *Acta Anat* 1980;108:144–152.
34. Moorman FM, Vermeulen JLM, Koban MU, Schwartz K, Lamers WH, Boheler KR. Patterns of expression of sarcoplasmic reticulum Ca^{2+}–ATPase and phospholamban mRNAs during rat heart development. *Circ Res* 1995;76:616–625.
35. Komuro I, Kurabayashi M, Shibazaki Y, Takaku F, Yazaki Y. Molecular cloning and characterization of a Ca^{2+} + Mg^{2+}–dependent adenosine triphosphatase from rat cardiac sarcoplasmic reticulum. *J Clin Invest* 1989;83:1102–1108.
36. Lompre AM, Lambert F, Lakatta EG, Schwartz K. Expression of sarcoplasmic reticulum Ca^{2+}-ATPase and calsequestrin genes in rat heart during ontogenetic development and aging. *Circ Res* 1991;69:1380–1388.
37. Ramesch V, Kresch MJ, Katz AM, Kim DH. Characterization of Ca^{2+}-release channels in fetal and adult rat heart. *Am J Physiol* 1995;269:H778–H782.
38. Fabiato A, Fabiato F. Calcium-induced release of calcium from the sarcoplasmic reticulum of skinned cells from adult human, dog, cat, rabbit, rat and frog hearts and from fetal and new-born rat ventricles. *Ann NY Acad Sci* 1978;307:491–522.
39. Fabiato A. Calcium release in skinned cardiac cells: variation with species, tissues, and development. *Fed Proc* 1982;41:2238–2244.
40. Wibo M, Bravo G, Godfraind T. Postnatal maturation of excitation–contraction coupling in rat ventricle in relation to the subcellular localization and surface density of 1,4-dihydropyridine and ryanodine receptors. *Circ Res* 1991;68:662–673.
41. Vornanen M. Force-frequency relationship, contraction duration and recirculating fraction of calcium in postnatally developing rat heart ventricle: correlation with heart rate. *Acta Physiol Scand* 1992;145:311–321.
42. Ostadalova I, Kolar F, Ostadal B. Inotropic effect of low extracellular sodium on perfused perinatal rat heart. *Can J Physiol Pharmacol* 1995;73:50–54.

43. Goeger DE, Rieley RT, Dorner JW, Cole RJ. Cyclopiazonic acid inhibition of the Ca^{2+} transport ATPase in rat skeletal muscle sarcoplasmic vesicles. *Biochem Pharmacol* 1988;37:978–981.
44. Agata N, Tanaka H, Shigenobu K. Possible action of cyclopiazonic acid on myocardial sarcoplasmic reticulum: inotropic effects on neonatal and adult rat heart. *Br J Pharmacol* 1993;108:571–572.
45. Kojima S, Wu ST, Wikman-Coeffelt J, Parmley WW. Contractile and intracellular Ca^{2+} decay in potentiated contractions following multiple extrasystolic beats. *Cell Calcium* 1995;18:155–164.
46. Vornanen M. Effects of caffeine on the mechanical properties of developing rat heart ventricles. *Comp Biochem Physiol* 1984;78C:239–334.
47. Wang R, Karpinski E, Pang PKT. Two types of voltage-dependent calcium channel currents and their modulation by parathyroid hormone in neonatal rat ventricular cells. *J Cardiovasc Pharmacol* 1991;17:990–998.
48. Rampe D, Skattebol A, Triggle DJ, Brown AM. Effects of McN-6186 on voltage-dependent Ca^{2+} channels in heart and pituitary cells. *J Pharmacol Exp Ther* 1989;248:164–170.
49. Boucek RJ Jr, Shelton ME, Artman M, Landon E. Myocellular calcium regulation by the sarcolemmal membrane in the adult and immature rabbit heart. *Basic Res Cardiol* 1985;80:316–325.
50. Skovranek J, Ostadal B, Pelouch V, Prochazka J. Ontogenetic differences in cardiac sensitivity to verapamil in rats. *Pediatr Cardiol* 1986;7:25–29.
51. Kolar F, Ostadal B, Papousek F. Effect of verapamil on contractile function of the isolated perfused rat heart during postnatal ontogeny. *Basic Res Cardiol* 1990;85:429–434.
52. Mitchell MR, Powell T, Terrar DA, Twist VW. Calcium-activated inward current and contraction in rat and guinea-pig ventricular myocytes. *J Physiol* 1987;391:545–560.
53. Klizner TS, Chen F, Raven RR, Wetzel GT, Friedman WF. Calcium current and tension generation in immature mammalian myocardium: effects of diltiazem. *J Mol Cell Cardiol* 1991;23:807–815.
54. Vornanen M. Contribution of Ca current to total cellular Ca in postnatally developing rat heart. *Cardiovasc Res* 1996;32:400–410.
55. Negretti N, Varro A, Eisner DA. Estimate of net calcium fluxes and sarcoplasmic reticulum calcium content during systole in rat ventricular myocytes. *J Physiol* 1995;486.3:581–591.
56. Harrer JM, Kiss E, Kranias EG. Application of the immunoblot technique for quantitation of protein levels in cardiac homogenates. *BioTechniques* 1995;18:995–997.
57. Artman M. Sarcolemmal Na^{+}–Ca^{2+} exchange activity and exchanger immunoreactivity in developing rabbit hearts. *Am J Physiol* 1992;263:H1506–H1513.
58. Wetzel GT, Chen F, Klizner TS. L- and T-type calcium channels in acutely isolated neonatal and adult cardiac myocytes. *Pediatr Res* 1991;30:89–94.
59. Osaka T, Joyner RW. Developmental changes in calcium currents of rabbit ventricular cells. *Circ Res* 1991;68:788–796.
60. Huynh TV, Chen F, Wetzel GT, Friedman WF, Klizner T. Developmental changes in membrane Ca^{2+} and K^{+} currents in fetal, neonatal, and adult rabbit ventricular myocytes. *Circ Res* 1992; 70:508–515.
61. Wetzel GT, Chen F, Klizner TS. Ca^{2+} channel kinetics in acutely isolated fetal, neonatal, and adult rabbit cardiac myocytes. *Circ Res* 1993;72:1065–1074.
62. Boerth SR, Zimmer DB, Artman M. Steady-state mRNA levels of the sarcolemmal Na^{+}–Ca^{2+} exchanger peak near birth in developing rabbit and rat hearts. *Circ Res* 1994;74:354–359.
63. Vetter R, Kemsies C, Schulze W. Sarcolemmal Na^{+}–Ca^{2+} exchange and sarcoplasmic reticulum Ca^{2+} uptake in several cardiac preparations. *Biomed Biochim Acta* 1987;46:375–381.
64. Nakamura S, Asai J, Hama K. The transverse tubular system of rat myocardium: its morphology and morphometry in the developing and adult animal. *Anat Embryol* 1986;173:307–315.
65. Hatem SN, Sweeten T, Vetter V, Morad M. Evidence for the presence of Ca^{2+} channel-gated Ca^{2+} stores in neonatal human atrial myocytes. *Am J Physiol* 1995;268:H1195–H1201.

The Developing Heart,
edited by Bohuslav Ošťádal et al.
Lippincott-Raven Publishers,
Philadelphia © 1997.

17

Perinatal Maturation of Myocardial Contraction: The Role of Na^{+}–Ca^{2+} Exchange

Peter S. Haddock, William A. Coetzee, Tomoe Y. Nakamura, Durisamy Balaguru, *Scott R. Boerth, and Michael Artman

**Department of Pediatrics and Neuroscience, NYU Medical Center, 560 Fifth Ave., New York, NY 10016, Department of Pharmacology, 3130 Medical Sciences Building, University of South Alabama College of Medicine, Mobile, AL 36688*

Contraction and relaxation of the mammalian heart result from a complex array of regulatory systems. These have evolved to precisely control the concentration of intracellular calcium bathing the contractile proteins throughout the cardiac cycle while working in harmony to produce a coordinated rhythm of contraction and relaxation. In the mature heart these systems must also be able to respond to changes in demand for cardiac output and changes in loading conditions to maintain a normal circulation. The same, of course, is true in the fetus and neonate. However, in this setting there are a range of differences in the functional maturity of the calcium regulatory systems that contribute to the age-related changes in the response of the neonate to inotropic interventions.

EXCITATION–CONTRACTION COUPLING IN DEVELOPING MYOCARDIUM

In contrast to the adult heart, the developing heart is less responsive to many physiologic and pharmacologic stimuli and exhibits major differences in the mechanisms underlying contraction and relaxation (1). The reasons for these differences are complex and undoubtedly include additional uncharacterized structural and biochemical factors. What is more clear, however, is that in many mammalian species the sarcoplasmic reticulum (SR) is either absent or significantly diminished at birth, relative to adult myocytes (2–4). For this reason, many of the contractile insufficiencies of the neonate have been attributed to an immature SR. Consequently, it has been proposed that the role of the sarcolemma in the regulation of intracellular calcium at the contractile proteins is significantly altered in the neonate to compensate for its reduced SR content and function (5–8).

DEVELOPMENTAL CHANGES IN SARCOPLASMIC RETICULUM FUNCTION

During the early phases of systole in the adult heart, membrane depolarization triggers the opening of L-type calcium channels and results in an influx of calcium from the extracellular space (9). It is thought that the relatively small amount of calcium entering the cells via this route is insufficient in itself to initiate contraction. However, this pool of calcium is believed to propagate a large release of calcium from the SR (via the SR calcium release channel) that is subsequently responsible for contraction, a process that has been termed calcium-induced calcium release (10). Relaxation occurs by a subsequent reduction in cytosolic Ca^{2+} from a high systolic level to a low resting level via (a) Ca^{2+}–ATPase-mediated calcium sequestration into the SR, (b) the sarcolemmal Na^{+}– Ca^{2+} exchanger, and (c) a sarcolemmal Ca^{2+}–ATPase. During normal relaxation the sarcolemmal mechanisms are believed to extrude an amount of calcium equivalent to that which entered via the calcium entry pathways.

Studies to investigate the altered contractile activity in mature and developing hearts have pointed to striking morphologic and functional differences in the SR of mammalian hearts (2,11–16). Both the process of SR calcium release and subsequent calcium uptake are significantly underdeveloped in the neonate compared to the adult. This reduction in SR function has been demonstrated, for example, in ryanodine binding studies that have shown that SR calcium release channel numbers are significantly reduced in SR vesicles prepared from fetal sheep ventricle (13). While a decrease in channel numbers does not necessarily equate with a change in contractile function, it has also been shown that ryanodine exerts little effect on contracting preparations of fetal and newborn myocardium. This is in direct contrast to adult hearts, in which a negative iontropic response to ryanodine is observed. Additional supportive data for a diminished SR function in neonatal heart have also been provided by studies in which a lower level of mRNA encoding for SR Ca^{2+}–ATPase in developing heart compared to the adult has been quantified (17). All these data are consistent with the concept that fetal and newborn hearts are more dependent upon transsarcolemmal calcium fluxes to initiate contraction and relaxation. This is in contrast to the mature myocardium, in which the SR plays the predominant role in cycling calcium to and from the contractile proteins.

CALCIUM TRANSPORT IN IMMATURE MYOCYTES

It has been suggested that the sarcolemma may be the major avenue for calcium delivery to the contractile proteins in the immature heart, which may account for an increased sensitivity to dihydropyridine-type calcium channel antagonists (18–20). While a number of studies have been carried out to address this hypothesis, the data are difficult to reconcile with subsequent studies in which perinatal changes in calcium current have been characterized. Wetzel et al. obtained convincing data that L-type calcium current density (pA/unitary area of membrane) is significantly lower in neonatal rabbit myocytes (1–5 days of age), concluding that calcium current increases during cardiac development (21). What processes, therefore, are responsible for calcium influx in the neonatal heart in the face of an increased dependency on transsarcolemmal calcium flux and a decreased calcium current density? These disparate observations can be reconciled if calcium influx were to occur in the newborn heart via an alternative sarcolemmal ion transport mechanism. Subsequently, it has been proposed that the sarcolemmal Na^+–Ca^{2+} exchanger may provide a plausible mechanism by which calcium influx may occur in the developing heart. Na^+–Ca^{2+} exchange activity is itself indirectly sensitive to calcium channel antagonists through temporal changes in intracellular calcium concentration (22,23). Therefore, the negative iontropic response of neonatal myocytes to calcium channel blockers (24,25) may be of a combined effect on both Ca^{2+} channels and the Na^+–Ca^{2+} exchanger. Electrophysiologic experiments, employing the whole-cell voltage-clamp technique, have provided an additional tool to address this question. In this setting, diltiazem blocked the inward calcium current (26). Furthermore, Klitzner et al. have mapped the correlation between twitch length and action potential duration in response to diltiazem and demonstrated that the reduction in action potential duration contributes (at least in part) to a reduction in twitch tension (27). It is proposed that, in the developing heart, L-type calcium channels are not the only route for calcium entry to initiate contraction.

Na^+–Ca^{2+} EXCHANGE IN THE IMMATURE HEART

By virtue of its stoichiometry (3 Na^+ transported in return for each Ca^{2+} ion), the Na^+–Ca^{2+} exchanger is an electrogenic sarcolemmal ion transporter. While the physiologic role of the Na^+–Ca^{2+} exchanger has been extensively studied in the mature myocardium (9,28–35), this level of information does not extend to the ontogeny of Na^+–Ca^{2+} exchange. Nakanishi and Jarmakani were among the first to speculate an enhanced role for Na^+–Ca^{2+} exchange in the contractile function of neonatal rabbit hearts based upon functional responses to rapid changes in extracellular sodium concentration (36). Similarly, Hoerter et al. quantified the contractile response of isolated neonatal papillary muscles in response to rapid reduction in extracellular sodium concentration and inferred from this and additional morphologic data that Na^+–Ca^{2+} exchange was relatively more important in regulating relaxation in immature rabbit hearts (6,37).

EXPRESSION AND FUNCTIONAL DEVELOPMENT OF Na^+–Ca^{2+} EXCHANGE ACTIVITY

A number of studies—using sodium-loaded sarcolemmal vesicles prepared from the hearts of fetal, neonatal, immature, and adult animals—have been carried out to characterize developmental changes in Na^+–Ca^{2+} exchange activity during car-

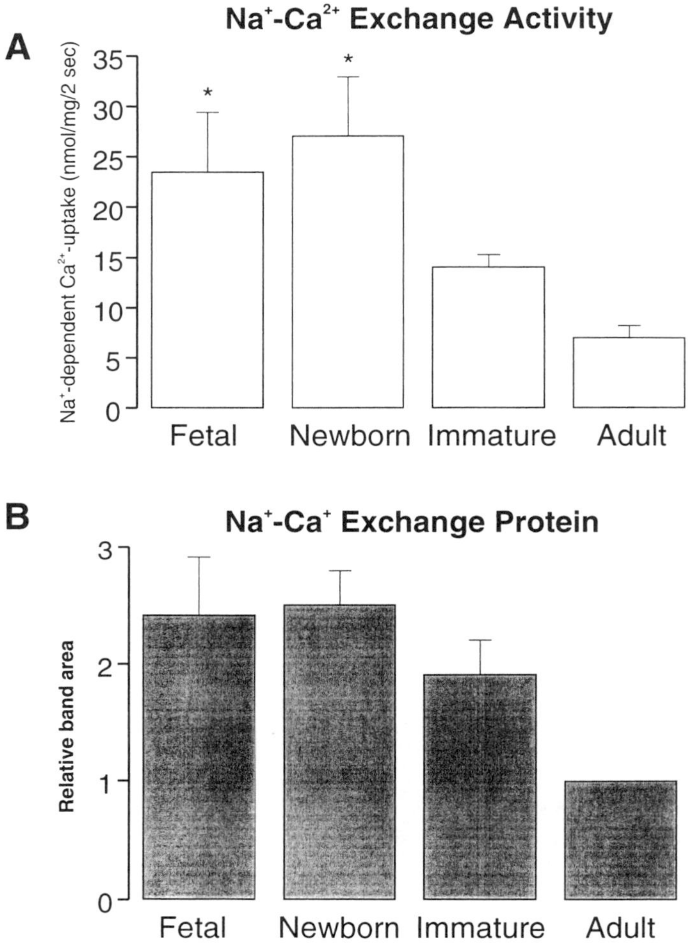

FIG. 17–1. Na^+–Ca^{2+} exchange activity and protein levels during postnatal development. (**A**) A comparison of the initial velocity of Na^+–Ca^{2+} exchange in sarcolemmal vesicles prepared from the hearts of different-aged rabbits. Data are normalized for the fraction of competent vesicles in each age group. (*Different from adult, $p = 0.03$. $n = 4 - 7$ hearts per age group.) (**B**) Relative immunoreactivity quantified using video densitometric scanning of protein slot blots. Band areas were normalized against the appropriate adult value on an individual nitrocellulose membrane. $n = 5$ separate preparations per group. (Redrawn with permission from ref. 39.)

diac development. In one such study, Vetter and Will established that Na^+–Ca^{2+} exchange activity in the chicken increased linearly prior to and early after hatching, followed by a subsequent fall in activity at approximately 10 days posthatching (38). Studies in our laboratory were performed to characterize Na^+–Ca^{2+} exchange in late fetal (28 days gestation), newborn (1–2 days old), immature (14–16 days old) and adult rabbit myocardium (39). We quantified both Na^+–Ca^{2+} exchanger activity (in terms of the initial rate of Na^+-dependent Ca^{2+} uptake) and the relative amount of exchanger protein (using Western analysis). Data from these studies are summarized in Fig. 17–1. Both exchanger activity and protein levels in vesicles from fetal and newborn hearts were significantly raised during gestation and immediately following birth compared to immature and adult preparations.

STEADY-STATE Na^+–Ca^{2+} EXCHANGER mRNA LEVELS

The correlation between Na^+–Ca^{2+} exchange activity and protein levels suggests that the postnatal decrease in exchanger activity is a consequence of increased ex-

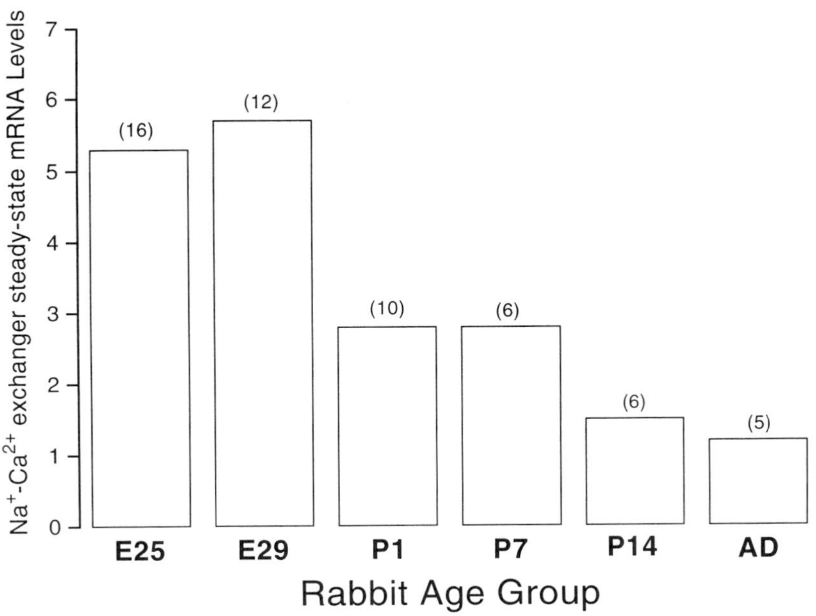

FIG. 17–2. Na^+–Ca^{2+} exchanger mRNA levels during cardiac development. Steady-state Na^+–Ca^{2+} exchanger mRNA levels in fetal (25 days [E25] and 29 days [E29]), newborn (1 day [P1]), immature (7 days [P7] and 14 days [P14]), and adult (AD) rabbit hearts. Densitometric quantitation of hybridized exchanger cDNA was normalized to the hybrid oligo(dT) and expressed relative to the adult levels. There were two determinations per age group. The number of hearts pooled for each age group is shown in parentheses. (Redrawn with permission from ref. 40.)

changer expression rather than functional alterations of existing protein. One danger in the evaluation of data from sarcolemmal vesicle experiments is that the enrichment of sarcolemmal preparations may vary between different age groups. To address this concern we measured steady-state Na^+–Ca^{2+} exchange mRNA levels in hearts from both developing rabbits and rats (40). These changes were quantified by Northern blot and slot blot analyses using poly(A^+) RNA isolated from ventricular tissue and normalized by reprobing with [^{32}P] 5′-end-labeled oligo(dT). From these experiments we established that mRNA levels peak at or around birth and subsequently decline during development. Maximal levels were approximately sixfold greater in the late fetal rabbit and eightfold greater in the early newborn rat. These data are summarized in Fig. 17–2 and support the concept that a feature of normal mammalian cardiac development is a maximal expression of Na^+–Ca^{2+} exchange protein at the time of birth. As the sarcoplasmic reticulum subsequently develops there is a parallel decline in exchanger expression. These observations suggest that the developmental regulation of cardiac Na^+–Ca^{2+} exchanger expression involves pretranslational control mechanisms.

DISTRIBUTION OF Na^+–Ca^{2+} EXCHANGER IN DEVELOPING MYOCARDIUM

Na^+–Ca^{2+} exchange activity is associated with a series of 70-, 120-, and 160-kDa proteins (41) and has been cloned and sequenced in canine myocardium (42). Frank et al. and Kieval have also localized the Na^+–Ca^{2+} exchanger to the sarcolemma using elegant immunocytochemical techniques (43,44). There is still, however, some dispute as to whether the exchanger is homogeneously distributed throughout the sarcolemma or whether it may be more abundant in T-tubules. Chen et al. recently studied the distribution of the exchanger in the developing rabbit heart using a high-affinity monoclonal antibody (R3F1) that recognizes two neighboring, nonoverlapping sequences localized to the hydrophilic region of the Na^+–Ca^{2+} exchanger (45). In adult rabbit myocytes the Na^+–Ca^{2+} exchanger was localized in the peripheral sarcolemma and especially in the T-tubules. In contrast, Na^+–Ca^{2+} exchanger protein was predominantly located in the peripheral sarcolemma in 5-day-old myocytes. By 11 days of age, labeling paralleled development of the T-tubules such that Na^+–Ca^{2+} exchange protein appeared in the tubules as soon as they formed.

Na^+–Ca^{2+} EXCHANGE CURRENT DENSITY DURING POSTNATAL DEVELOPMENT

Many of the data obtained to evaluate developmental changes in Na^+–Ca^{2+} exchange activity have been derived from experiments utilizing enriched sarcolemmal preparations. However, one disadvantage of this type of experiment is that it is difficult to interpret whether the exchanger is functionally more active in *intact* myocytes isolated from newborn hearts. To address this issue we undertook a series of electrophysiologic experiments in which Na^+–Ca^{2+} exchange activity was quantified in terms of Na^+–Ca^{2+} exchange current density in ventricular myocytes isolated from different-aged animals (46). Experiments were performed using both rabbit myocytes (which have a sparse SR at birth) and guinea pigs (which, in contrast to the rabbit, exhibit a more developed and extensive sarcoplasmic reticulum at birth). Voltage-clamp techniques were used to characterize Na^+–Ca^{2+} exchange current, which was defined as the Ni^{2+}-sensitive current (when all other known electrogenic currents were blocked). In addition, Na^+–Ca^{2+} exchange current records were normalized against cell capacitance (an index of cell size and functional membrane surface area). Figure 17–3 shows results of normalized Ni^{2+}-sensitive currents grouped according to age. From these experiments we were able to establish that in the rabbit, Na^+–Ca^{2+} exchange current was relatively well devel-

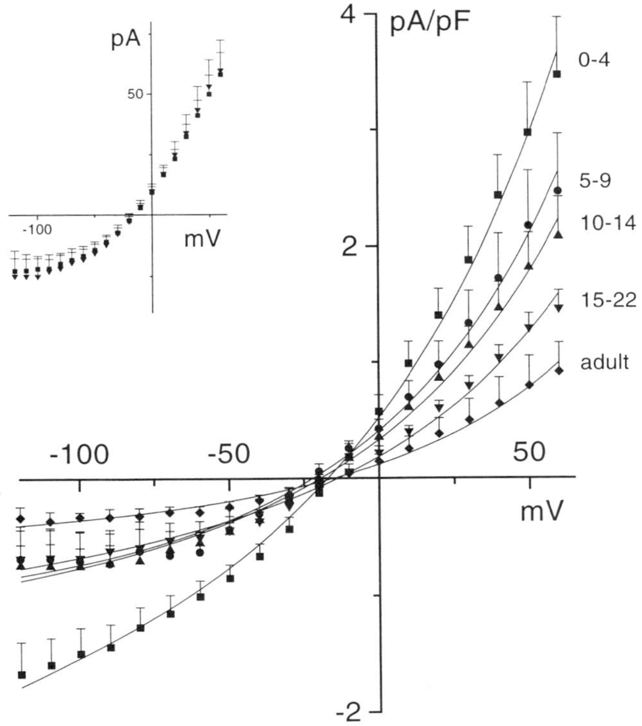

FIG. 17–3. Postnatal reduction in Na^+–Ca^{2+} exchange current. Summary of Ni^{2+}-sensitive membrane currents of myocytes from different-age rabbits. Results were pooled as follows: 0–4 days (■; *n* = 24), 5–9 days (●; *n* = 8), 10–14 days (▲; *n* = 17), 15–22 days (▼; *n* = 16), and adult (◆; *n* = 3). Current was normalized against cell capacitance (an index of cell surface area). The inset compares uncorrected current from 0–4-days group with that from 15–22-days group. (Redrawn with permission from ref. 46.)

oped at birth, after which time it declined (with a time constant of approximately 10 days) to reach adult levels by 2–3 weeks of age. Na^+–Ca^{2+} exchange current decreased at both positive and negative membrane potentials. Interestingly, these electrophysiologic data correlated with (a) Na^+-dependent Ca^{2+} uptake data obtained in sarcolemmal vesicle studies, (b) the postnatal decrease in Na^+–Ca^{2+} exchange mRNA levels, and (c) the age-related changes in Na^+–Ca^{2+} exchange protein content. Together these data support the concept that Na^+–Ca^{2+} exchange is a dominant mechanism for regulating intracellular calcium concentration in the immature myocardium.

Relaxation in newborn myocytes may occur predominantly through calcium extrusion by the Na^+–Ca^{2+} exchanger as opposed to Ca^{2+} uptake by the SR. In the mature myocardium, the Na^+–Ca^{2+} exchanger is also thought to contribute to relaxation by promoting Ca^{2+} efflux. Importantly, the Na^+–Ca^{2+} exchanger is reversible and can theoretically operate in a reverse mode in intact tissues under conditions such as an elevated intracellular sodium concentration. During the action potential in immature myocytes, the absence of a large inward Ca^{2+} current and the diminished calcium-induced calcium release from the SR may favor Ca^{2+} entry via the Na^+–Ca^{2+} exchange mechanism and provide the necessary rise in intracellular calcium to propagate contraction. This is supported by data from nonmammalian species that lack intracellular calcium stores, such as the shark, in which the Na^+–Ca^{2+} exchange has been shown to contribute to contraction and relaxation of cardiac myocytes (47).

Data regarding the density of functional Na^+–Ca^{2+} exchange protein molecules can also be derived from these electrophysiologic experiments. The absolute magnitude of Na^+–Ca^{2+} exchange current remained unchanged during the first 22 days after birth in the face of a decreasing Na^+–Ca^{2+} exchange current density. This paradigm requires additional experiments to resolve but may reflect the influence of additional mechanism(s) that modulate Na^+–Ca^{2+} exchange activity during development.

DOES THE Na^+–Ca^{2+} EXCHANGE CONTRIBUTE TO Ca^{2+} INFLUX IN THE IMMATURE MYOCARDIUM?

When compared to the adult, the newborn heart appears to be relatively more dependent upon Na^+-dependent Ca^{2+} influx during the action potential. While theoretically the Na^+–Ca^{2+} exchanger can operate in a reverse mode, the contribution of Na^+–Ca^{2+} exchange in the adult heart to Ca^{2+} influx under normal conditions is a matter of contention. In the mature heart, Na^+–Ca^{2+} exchange normally operates to extrude calcium from the cell during relaxation (9). However, a significant number of studies have recently pointed to a reversal of Na^+–Ca^{2+} exchange during systole in a variety of species and under selected conditions (including an elevated intracellular sodium concentration) (48,52). Levi et al. have shown that calcium influx via Na^+–Ca^{2+} exchange is insufficient to elicit contraction when L-type calcium current is blocked in the mature myocardium. However, in the immature heart there is a diminished level of Ca^{2+} release from the SR that may consequently enhance calcium influx via Na^+–Ca^{2+} exchange. In addition, Conforti et al. have demonstrated that the plateau of the action potential is prolonged in the fetal rat heart (53), which they attributed to replacement of the fast sodium current with a sustained slow-inactivating sodium current. The possibility arises that the Na^+–Ca^{2+} exchanger brings calcium into the cell during the action potential to provide calcium for contraction in the fetal and newborn heart. During relaxation, calcium would be removed by Na^+–Ca^{2+} exchange, possibly enhanced in the immature myocardium because of the decreased Ca^{2+} sequestration by the underdeveloped SR. This concept is illustrated in Fig. 17–4.

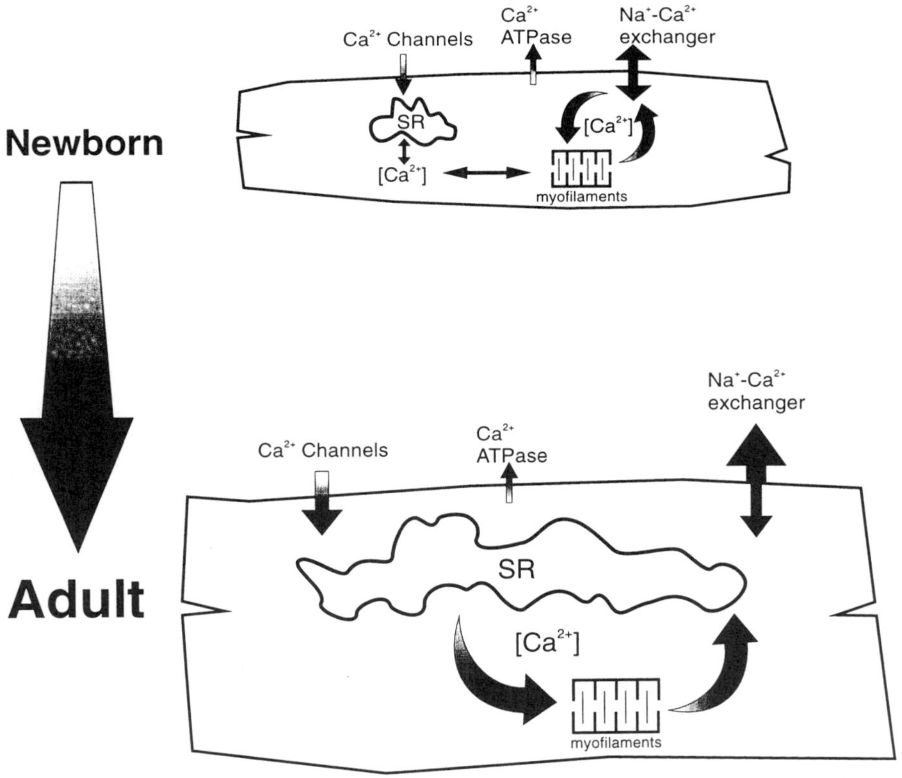

FIG. 17–4. Schematic illustration of a proposed role for Na^+–Ca^{2+} exchange in contraction and relaxation during cardiac development. The sizes of the various components reflect their relative magnitude and function. The Na^+–Ca^{2+} exchange may play a significantly greater role in the regulation of contraction and relaxation in the immature heart that has a functionally immature SR.

OTHER FACTORS REGULATING Na^+–Ca^{2+} EXCHANGE ACTIVITY DURING POSTNATAL DEVELOPMENT

Factors that influence the postnatal down-regulation of Na^+–Ca^{2+} exchange expression remain largely uncharacterized. Circulating thyroid hormone levels have been described as a classical modulator of cardiac gene expression, providing, for example, a stimulus for a postnatal isoform switch in myosin heavy chain (MHC) isozymes that peaks 3 weeks after birth (54,55). Furthermore, thyroid hormone status affects expression of the genes encoding β-adrenergic receptors (56), atrial natriuretic factor (57), the ryanodine receptor (58), phospholamban (59), the Na^+–K^+–ATPase (60), and the sarcoplasmic reticulum Ca^{2+}–ATPase (SERCA2) (58,61). The time course of changes in thyroid hormone status and an up-regulation of SERCA2 mirror the temporal down-regulation of Na^+–Ca^{2+} exchange expression, suggesting that thyroid hormone status may be related to the modulation of Na^+–Ca^{2+} exchange expression during the first 3 weeks after birth. Further supportive data have been provided in a series of experiments in which Kolar et al. measured contractile function of hearts isolated from euthyroid, hyperthyroid, and hypothyroid newborn rats (62). They elegantly demonstrated that hyperthyroid animals were less dependent, whereas the hypothyroid animals were more dependent on transsarcolemmal calcium flux for contraction. These findings also correlated with their data regarding an increased SR function in hyperthyroid animals compared to hypothyroid animals. A surge in circulating thyroid hormone upon birth may contribute to the maturation of SR function and thereby contribute to the postnatal transition from sarcolemmal dependency in the neonate to SR dependency in the adult.

We recently quantified steady-state mRNA levels encoding cardiac Na^+–Ca^{2+} exchange and SERCA2 proteins in euthyroid, hypothyroid, and hyperthyroid rabbit pups (63). We also included an additional group of animals whose induced hypothyroid state was subsequently reversed using *l*-thyroxine. Northern analysis demonstrated that in hypothyroid (propylthiouracil-treated) animals, expression of Na^+–Ca^{2+} exchange mRNA increased while that of SERCA2 decreased. The converse was true in the hyperthyroid (*l*-thyroxine-treated) animals. Blocking the postnatal surge of thyroid hormone (by administering propylthiouracil from gestational day 25 through 21 days after birth) prevented the normal postnatal down-regulation of cardiac Na^+–Ca^{2+} exchange expression. These data are summarized in Fig. 17–5 and support the hypothesis that thyroid hormone status reciprocally regulates cardiac Na^+–Ca^{2+} exchange and SERCA2 expression. Vetter et al. have also recently examined the relationship between Na^+–Ca^{2+} exchange activity and sarcoplasmic reticulum Ca^{2+}–ATPase (64) and found an inverse relationship between their function and postnatal expression, suggesting that there is a coordinated pretranslational level of control of the cellular mechanisms that regulate calcium. The reciprocal effect on Na^+–Ca^{2+} exchange and SERCA2 may contribute to the effects of thyroid status on myocardial contractile function. Interestingly, Magyar et al. have also published data from a study in which they demonstrated

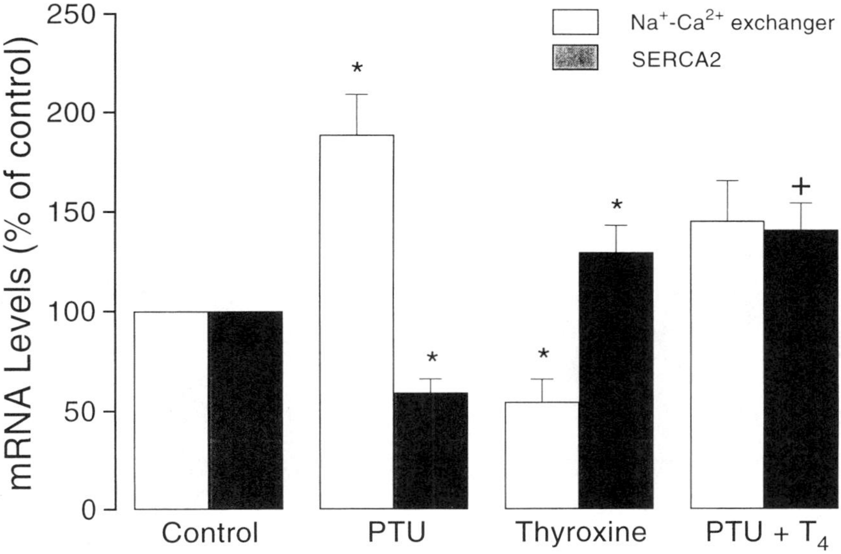

FIG. 17–5. Thyroid hormone status regulates Na^+–Ca^{2+} exchange mRNA levels. Poly(A^+) RNA was isolated from the ventricles of adult rabbit hearts that were either euthyroid, hypothyroid, hyperthyroid, or hypothyroid reversed control and analyzed on Northern slot-blots. Densitometric measurements of hybridized Na^+–Ca^{2+} exchange and SERCA2 cDNA were normalized to the amount of hybridized oligo(dT) and expressed as a percentage of the euthyroid control. (*Different from control ($p < 0.05$). +Different from PTU alone. [PTU = propylthiouracil; T_4 = thyroxine].) (Redrawn with permission from ref. 63.)

that Na^+–Ca^{2+} exchange abundance is reciprocally regulated to the levels of Na^+–K^+ ATPase, including during perinatal development. These data provide evidence for a homeostatic mechanism by which changes in calcium stores are minimized by changes in the activity of ion transporters.

IMPLICATIONS FOR EXCITATION–CONTRACTION COUPLING AND FUTURE GOALS

Many of the fundamental processes that control excitation–contraction coupling are modulated during the transition from birth to adulthood, and these changes are summarized in Fig. 17–6. However, a thorough characterization of both normal and abnormal expression, functional activity, and the processes controlling the concentration of calcium bathing the contractile elements during perinatal development of the heart is still required. A future challenge must be to establish whether, in the face of a diminished SR, the Na^+–Ca^{2+} exchange operates in a reverse mode to allow calcium entry and direct propagation of contraction of the im-

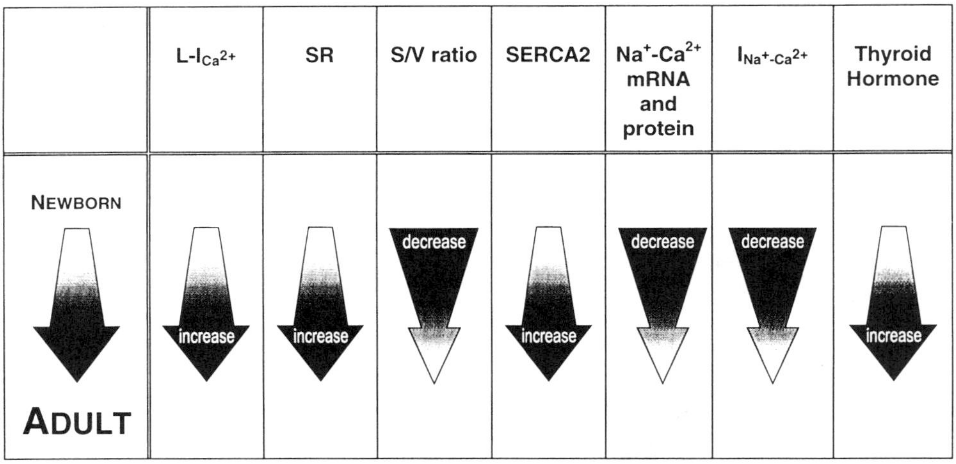

FIG. 17–6. Summary of changes in myocardial ion exchange and channel function, in addition to additional physiologic parameters during perinatal development. Thyroid hormone levels do not control excitation–contraction coupling but may control levels of elements involved in e–c coupling. (L-$I_{Ca^{2+}}$ = l-type calcium current; SR = sarcoplasmic reticulum; S/V = surface to volume; SERCA2 = sarcoplasmic reticulum Ca^{2+} – ATPase.)

mature heart. If such a mechanism is confirmed there may be many physiologic and pharmacologic implications.

SUMMARY

Despite the relative functional immaturity of many calcium regulatory systems, the neonatal heart is able to respond to changing demands for cardiac output. However, compared to the adult, the developing heart exhibits major differences in the processes underlying contraction and relaxation and in its response to many physiologic and pharmacologic stimuli. One major difference between the adult and neonatal heart is the relative immaturity of the sarcoplasmic reticulum (SR) at birth and, as a consequence, the increased dependence upon transsarcolemmal calcium flux to propagate contraction and relaxation in the neonate. However, in the rabbit, for example, the density of L-type (dihydropyridine-sensitive) calcium channels is low at birth, increasing subsequently during development. What processes, therefore, are primarily responsible for calcium influx and efflux in the neonatal heart in the face of both a decrease in calcium channel density and an underdeveloped SR? In this chapter we have described in detail many of the differences between the adult and neonatal hearts' regulation of intracellular calcium levels during the cardiac cycle. In particular, we have highlighted developmental changes in the expression and function of one particular sarcolemmal calcium transport mechanism—the Na^+–Ca^{2+} exchanger—that is thought to have an enhanced role in e–c coupling in the neonatal heart. A better understanding of the cellular basis for age-related changes of the processes controlling calcium handling will allow the development of new strategies for altering the inotropic state of the neonatal heart.

REFERENCES

1. Bassani RA, Bassani JWM, Bers DM. Mitochondrial and sarcolemmal Ca^{2+} transport reduce $[Ca^{2+}]_i$ during caffeine contractures in rabbit cardiac myocytes. *J Physiol (Lond)* 1992;453:591–608.
2. Nakanishi T, Jarmakani JM. Developmental changes in myocardial mechanical function and subcellular organelles. *Am J Physiol* 1984;246:H615–H625.
3. Pegg W, Michalak M. Differentiation of sarcoplasmic reticulum during cardiac myogenesis. *Am J Physiol* 1987;252:H22–H31.
4. Arai M, Otsu K, Maclennan DH, Periasamy M. Regulation of sarcoplasmic reticulum gene expression during cardiac and skeletal muscle development. *Am J Physiol* 1992;262:C614–C620.
5. Nakanishi T, Seguchi M, Takao A. Development of the myocardial contractile system. *Experientia* 1988;44:936–944.
6. Hoerter J, Mazet F, Vassort G. Perinatal growth of the rabbit cardiac cell: possible implications for the mechanism of relaxation. *J Mol Cell Cardiol* 1981;13:725–740.
7. Klitzner T, Friedman WF. Excitation–contraction coupling in developing mammalian myocardium: evidence from voltage clamp studies. *Pediatr Res* 1988;23:428–432.
8. Chin TK, Friedman WF, Klitzner TS. Developmental changes in cardiac myocyte calcium regulation. *Circ Res* 1990;67:574–579.
9. Barry WH, Bridge JHB. Intracellular calcium homeostasis in cardiac myocytes. *Circulation* 1993;87:1806–1815.
10. Fabiato A. Appraisal of the physiological relevance of two hypotheses for the mechanism of calcium release from the mammalian cardiac sarcoplasmic reticulum: calcium-induced release versus charge-coupled release. *Mol Cell Biochem* 1989;89:135–140.
11. Riva E, Hearse DJ. *The developing myocardium.* Mt. Kisco, NY: Futura, 1991.
12. Kaufman TM, Horton JW, White DJ, Mahony L. Age-related changes in myocardial relaxation and sarcoplasmic reticulum function. *Am J Physiol* 1990;259:H309–H316.
13. Mahony L, Jones LR. Developmental changes in cardiac sarcoplasmic reticulum in sheep. *J Biol Chem* 1986;261:15257–15265.
14. Penefsky ZJ. Studies on mechanism of inhibition of cardiac muscle contractile tension by ryanodine. *Pflugers Arch–Eur J Physiol* 1974;347:173–184.
15. Seguchi M, Harding JA, Jarmakani JM. Developmental change in the function of sarcoplasmic reticulum. *J Mol Cell Cardiol* 1986;18:189–195.
16. Tanaka H, Shigenobu K. Effect of ryanodine on neonatal and adult rat heart: developmental increase in sarcoplasmic reticulum function. *J Mol Cell Cardiol* 1989;21:1305–1313.
17. Fisher DJ, Tate CA, Phillips S. Developmental regulation of the sarcoplasmic reticulum calcium pump in the rabbit heart. *Pediatr Res* 1993;31:474–479.
18. Artman M, Graham TP, Boucek RJ. Effects of postnatal maturation on myocardial contractile responses to calcium antagonists and changes in contraction frequency. *J Cardiovasc Pharmacol* 1985;7:850–855.
19. Seguchi M, Jarmakani JM, George BL, Harding JA. Effects of Ca^{2+} antagonists on mechanical function in the neonatal heart. *Pediatr Res* 1986;20:838–842.
20. Boucek RJ Jr., Shelton M, Artman M, Mushlin PS, Starnes VA, Olson RD. Comparative effects of verapamil, nifedipine, and diltiazem on contractile function in the isolated immature and adult rabbit heart. *Pediatr Res* 1984;18:948–952.
21. Wetzel GT, Chen FH, Klitzner TS. L- and T-type calcium channels in acutely isolated neonatal and adult cardiac myocytes. *Pediatr Res* 1991;30:89–94.
22. Haworth RA, Goknur AB, Hunter DR. Control of the Na^+–Ca^{2+} exchanger in isolated heart cells. I. Introduction of Na–Na exchange in sodium-loaded cells by intracellular calcium. *Circ Res* 1991;69:1506–1513.
23. Haworth RA, Goknur AB. Control of the Na^+–Ca^{2+} exchanger in isolated heart cells. II. Beat-dependent activation in normal cells by intracellular calcium. *Circ Res* 1991;69:1514–1524.

24. Zheng JS, Christie A, De Young MB, Levy MN, Scarpa A. Synergism between cAMP and ATP in signal transduction in cardiac myocytes. *Am J Physiol* 1992;262:C128–C135.
25. Boachieansah G, Kane KA, Rankinn AC. Effects of a combination of acidosis, lactate, and lysophosphatidylcholine on action potentials and ionic currents in guinea pig ventricular myocytes. *J Cardiovasc Pharmacol* 1992;20:538–546.
26. Klitzner TS, Chen F, Raven RR, Wetzel GT, Friedman WF. Calcium current and tension generation in immature mammalian myocardium: effects of diltiazem. *J Mol Cell Cardiol* 1991;23:807–815.
27. Dagnino L, Larigne J-P, Nemer M. Increased transcripts for B-type natriuretic peptide in spontaneously hypertensive rats: quantitative polymerase chain reaction for atrial and brain natriuretic peptide transcripts. *Hypertension* 1992;20:690–700.
28. Katz AM. *Physiology of the heart.* New York: Raven Press, 1992.
29. Beuckelmann DJ, Wier WG. Mechanism of release of calcium from sarcoplasmic reticulum of guinea pig cardiac cells. *J Physiol (Lond)* 1988;405:233–255.
30. Ellis D. Na–Ca exchange in cardiac tissue. In: Harris P, Poole-Wilson PA, eds. *Advances in myocardiology.* New York: Plenum Medical; 1985:295–312.
31. Sheu S-S, Blaustein MP. Sodium/calcium exchange and control of cell calcium and contractility in cardiac and vascular smooth muscles. In: Fozzard HA, Haber G, Jennings RB, Katz AM, Morgan HE, eds. *The heart and cardiovascular system.* New York: Raven Press; 1991:903–943.
32. Blaustein MP, Dipolo R, Reeves JP. *Sodium–calcium exchange: proceedings of the Second International Conference.* New York: New York Academy of Sciences, 1991.
33. Philipson KD. The cardiac Na^+–Ca^{2+} exchanger. In: Langer GA, ed. *Calcium and the heart.* New York: Raven Press; 1990:85–108.
34. Reeves JP. Sodium-calcium exchange. In: Bronner F, ed. *Intracellular calcium regulation.* New York: Liss; 1990:305–347.
35. Philipson KD, Nicoll DA. Molecular and kinetic aspects of sodium–calcium exchange. *Int Rev Cytol* 1993;137C:199–227.
36. Nakanishi T, Jarmakani JM. Effect of extracellular sodium on mechanical function in the newborn rabbit. *Dev Pharmacol Ther* 1981;2:188–200.
37. Hoerter J, Vassort G. Participation of the sarcolemma in the control of relaxation of the mammalian heart during perinatal development. In: Chazov E, Smirnov V, Dhalla NS, eds. *Advances in myocardiology.* New York: Plenum Medical; 1982:373–380.
38. Vetter R, Will H. Sarcolemmal Na^+–Ca^{2+} exchange and sarcoplasmic reticulum calcium uptake in developing chick heart. *J Mol Cell Cardiol* 1986;18:1267–1275.
39. Artman M. Sarcolemmal Na^+–Ca^{2+} exchange activity and exchanger immunoreactivity in developing rabbit hearts. *Am J Physiol* 1992;263:H1506–H1513.
40. Boerth SR, Zimmer DB, Artman M. Steady-state mRNA levels of the sarcolemmal Na^+–Ca^{2+} exchanger peak near birth in developing rabbit and rat hearts. *Circ Res* 1994;74:354–359.
41. Philipson KD, Longoni S, Ward R. Purification of the cardiac Na^+–Ca^{2+} exchange protein. *Biochim Biophys Acta* 1988;945:298–306.
42. Lompre AM, Lambert F, Lakatta EG, Schwartz K. Expression of sarcoplasmic reticulum Ca^{2+}–ATPase and calsequestrin genes in rat heart during ontogenic development and aging. *Circ Res* 1991;69:1380–1388.
43. Frank JS, Mottino G, Reid D, Molday RS, Philipson KD. Distribution of the Na^+–Ca^{2+} exchange protein in mammalian cardiac myocytes: an immunofluorescence and immunocolloidal gold-labelling study. *J Cell Biol* 1992;117:337–345.
44. Kieval RS, Bloch RJ, Lindenmayer GE, Ambesi A, Lederer WJ. Immunofluorescence localization of the Na–Ca exchanger in heart cells. *Am J Physiol* 1992;263:C545–C550.
45. Chen F, Mottino G, Klitzner TS, Philipson KD, Frank JS. Distribution of the Na^+–Ca^{2+} exchange protein in developing rabbit myocytes. *Am J Physiol* 1995;268:C1126–C1132.
46. Artman M, Ichikawa H, Avkiran M, Coetzee WA. Na^+–Ca^{2+} exchange current density in cardiac myocytes from rabbits and guinea pigs during postnatal development. *Am J Physiol* 1995;268: H1714–H1722.
47. Nabauer M, Morad M. Modulation of contraction by intracellular Na^+ via Na^+–Ca^{2+} exchange in single shark (*Squalus acanthias*) ventricular myocytes. *J Physiol (Lond)* 1992;457:627–637.
48. Bers DM, Christensen DM, Nguyen TX. Can Ca entry via Na–Ca exchange directly activate cardiac muscle contraction? *J Mol Cell Cardiol* 1988;20:405–414.
49. Leblanc N, Hume JR. Sodium current–induced release of calcium from cardiac sarcoplasmic reticulum. *Science* 1990;248:372–376.

50. Bers DM. Species differences and the role of sodium–calcium exchange in cardiac muscle relaxation. *Ann NY Acad Sci* 1991;639:375–385.
51. Nuss HB, Houser SR. Sodium–calcium exchange–mediated contractions in feline ventricular myocytes. *Am J Physiol* 1992;263:H1161–H1169.
52. Levi AJ, Brooksby P, Hancox JC. A role for depolarisation induced calcium entry on the Na^+–Ca^{2+} exchange in triggering intracellular calcium release and contraction in rat ventricular myocytes. *Cardiovasc Res* 1993;27:1677–1690.
53. Conforti L, Tohse N, Sperelakis N. Tetrodotoxin-sensitive sodium current in rat fetal ventricular myocytes: contribution to the plateau phase of action potential. *J Mol Cell Cardiol* 1993;25: 159–173.
54. Lompre AM, Mercadier JJ, Wisnewsky C, et al. Species and age-dependent changes in the relative amounts of cardiac myosin isoenzymes in mammals. *Dev Biol* 1981;84:286–290.
55. Watras J. Changes in rat cardiac myosin during development and in culture. *J Mol Cell Cardiol* 1981;13:1011–1021.
56. Birk E, Tyndall MR, Erickson LC, Rudolph AM, Roberts JM. Effects of thyroid hormone on myocardial adrenergic b-receptor responsiveness and function during late gestation. *Pediatr Res* 1992;31:468–473.
57. Zimmerman RS, Gharib H, Zimmerman D, Heublein D, Burnett JCJ. Atrial natriuretic peptide in hypothyroidism. *J Clin Endocrinol Metab* 1987;64:353–355.
58. Arai M, Otsu K, Maclennan DH, Alpert NR, Periasamy M. Effect of thyroid hormone on the expression of mRNA encoding sarcoplasmic reticulum proteins. *Circ Res* 1991;69:266–276.
59. Kiss E, Jakab G, Kranias EG, Istvan E. Thyroid hormone-induced alterations in phospholamban protein expression: regulatory effects on sarcoplasmic reticulum Ca^{2+} transport and myocardial relaxation. *Circ Res* 1994;75:245–251.
60. Horowitz B, Hensley CB, Quintero M, Azuma KK, Putnam D, McDonough AA. Differential regulation of Na^+–K^+–ATPase alpha 1, alpha 2 and beta subunit mRNA and protein levels by thyroid hormone. *J Biol Chem* 1990;265:14308–14314.
61. Rohrer D, Dillman WH. Thyroid hormone markedly increases mRNA encoding for sarcoplasmic reticulum calcium ATPase in the rat heart. *J Biol Chem* 1988;263:6941–6944.
62. Kolar F, Seppet EK, Vetter R, et al. Thyroid control of contractile function and calcium handling in neonatal rat heart. *Pflugers Arch–Eur J Physiol* 1992;421:26–31.
63. Boerth SR, Coetzee WA, Artman M. Ontogeny and hormonal regulation of cardiac Na–Ca exchange expression in rabbits. *Annals of the New York Academy of Sciences.* 1996;779:536–538.
64. O'Neill SC, Donoso P, Eisner DA. The role of $[Ca^{2+}]_i$ and $[Ca^{2+}]$sensitization in the caffeine contracture of rat myocytes: measurement of $[Ca^{2+}]_i$ and $[caffeine]_i$. *J Physiol (Lond)* 1990;425:55–70.

The Developing Heart,
edited by Bohuslav Ošťádal et al.
Lippincott-Raven Publishers,
Philadelphia © 1997.

18

The Role of the Sarcoplasmic Reticulum Calcium–ATPase and Its Regulatory Protein Phospholamban in the Developing Myocardium

Maren U. Koban, Samuel Y. Boateng, and Kenneth R. Boheler

Imperial College of Science, Technology and Medicine, National Heart and Lung Institute, Division of Cardiothoracic Surgery, Dovehouse Street, London SW3 6LY, United Kingdom

Regional and functional differences within the developing myocardium occur through the progressive diversification of cells and through the appropriate expression and interaction of proteins within cells. Vertebrate hearts are derived from the two sides of the developing embryo through movement of precardiac cells in the visceral mesoderm toward the midline. On meeting, these cells fuse in a time-dependent and in a craniocaudal (head-to-tail) direction to form the primitive heart tube. The primitive cardiac tube subsequently forms an S-shaped structure that loops to bring the more caudally (tail) located atrial regions to a position cranial and behind the ventricular regions. With further development, the ventricular regions form trabeculae, the atrial and ventricular regions septate to form four chambers, and valves develop (1). At birth, the myocardium undergoes a number of morphologic changes characterized especially by an increase in ventricular wall thickness. Fetal and, to some extent, neonatal cardiocytes retain the capacity to divide, whereas in the adult, cardiac myocytes do not normally divide (2). Therefore, just after birth, in response to aging or increased blood pressure, the myocardium increases its mass principally through hypertrophy of a preexisting and fixed population of myocytes.

As with the morphologic characteristics just described, the contractile and lusitropic characteristics of the developing heart change dramatically during development. The initial rate of pulsation in the primitive ventricle is very slow and insufficiently strong to set blood in motion through the developing blood vessels. Once fusion of the precardiac cells has extended far enough to establish the atrial regions, and subsequently the sinoatrial regions, the cardiac tube begins to pulsate more regularly and heart rate is increased. At this point, the efficiency of the pump is enhanced dramatically: instead of slow, nonpropagated, and ineffective contractions, a peristaltoid sweep starting in the more rapidly beating atrium is transmitted to the ventricle. The heart is now efficient enough to pump blood in motion. With further development, particularly of the conduction system, contraction becomes more rhythmic and efficient (3–5).

The application of molecular markers to the study of the spatial distribution of proteins involved in contraction (myosin heavy chain and actin) and relaxation (sarcoplasmic reticulum [SR] calcium–ATPase and phospholamban) have been useful in explaining some of the functional aspects of myocardial differentiation (4,6). Specifically, a model system has been proposed to explain how gradients of expression of these mRNAs and proteins along the tubular heart can explain, in conjunction with other molecular markers, how blood can be propelled unidirectionally by the evolving heart in the developing embryo and fetus (4,6). Although based partially on extrapolation of results from the adult myocardium, the regional expression of sarco(endo)plasmic reticulum calcium ATPase (SERCA) and phospholamban is hypothesized to be a critical factor in determining the rate of relaxation in various regions of the embryonic and fetal heart, and it is this aspect of development that will be the focus of this chapter.

THE SR Ca–ATPase AND PHOSPHOLAMBAN

The Ca^{2+}/Mg^{2+}-dependent ATPase of the sarcoplasmic reticulum is a mammalian ion transport enzyme whose function in heart is to move Ca^{2+} from the cytoplasm to the sarcoplasmic reticulum (7–9). The Ca–ATPase catalyzes the transport of Ca^{2+} from the cytoplasm to the SR lumen in an ATP-dependent process through transfer of the terminal phosphate group of ATP to an aspartate residue, formation of an enzyme–phosphate (E–P) intermediate, and translocation of two Ca^{2+} ions to the lumen of the SR (8,9). Cloning and sequencing of full-length complementary DNAs (cDNAs) have permitted the identification of three different mammalian genes for the SERCA: SERCA1, 2, and 3 (7–9). The SERCA1 gene is expressed almost exclusively in fast-twitch skeletal muscle, whereas SERCA3 is expressed in many cell types at relatively low levels. Alternative splicing of the SERCA2 gene transcript gives rise to two isoforms: the cardiac and slow-twitch SERCA2a, and the smooth muscle and nonmuscle SERCA2b. The difference between the SERCA2a and 2b proteins is confined to the extreme carboxy-terminal tail. The 2b isoform differs from the 2a isoform by replacement of the last four amino acids (SERCA2a) with a 49-amino-acid extension (SERCA2b). Comparison of rat cardiac Ca–ATPase messenger RNA (mRNA) with the slow isoform isolated from human kidney and rabbit slow skeletal muscle reveals a very strong nucleotide conservation. Only 8-, 7-, and 6-amino-acid substitutions are seen between rat and rabbit, rat and human, and rabbit and human, respectively. None of the substitutions occur in the proposed functional domains, apart from the nucleotide-binding domain of the rat clone whose sequence resembles more closely that of human and rabbit fast-twitch skeletal muscle isoform, which would concur functionally with the rapid contraction of the rat heart. The SERCA2 gene isoform SERCA2a is the predominant isoform in cardiac tissue.

Ca–ATPase activity is regulated by phospholamban, a small homopentameric phosphoprotein located like the Ca–ATPase mainly in the longitudinal sarcoplasmic reticulum (10). Phospholamban is encoded by a single gene and is expressed as a single protein with no isoform diversity. Each monomer of the homopentameric structure is 52 amino acids in length and can be separated into two functional domains (9). Domain 1 is a hydrophilic α-helical domain localized at the cytoplasmic surface of the SR. Domain 2 is a transmembrane hydrophobic domain of greater than 20 uncharged residues, where tightly interacting intramembraneous leucine residues are important for maintaining the stability of the pentameric structure. On each subunit of the homopentamer are found two serine residues and one threonine residue that can be phosphorylated. Phosphorylation of serine 16 and threonine 17 by protein kinase A and the Ca^{2+}/calmodulin-dependent protein kinase seems to be critical for phospholamban to function as a regulatory protein for SERCA2. In the nonphosphorylated form, phospholamban acts as an inhibitor of SERCA; when phosphorylated, this inhibition is removed.

Previously, we reported the presence of four phospholamban transcripts of different lengths that were generated by at least four signals for polyadenylation: one each at 2.3 kb and 2.0 kb and at least two between 0.6 and 1.0 kb (11). We speculated that a fifth transcript length might be present in rat myocardium at around 1.0 kb that could use a putative polyadenylation signal (ataaaaa) identified at nucleotides 944 to 950. To test this possibility, Northern blots were examined using a probe specific to the very 3′ end of our longest cDNA clone, pRCPLB1. For this purpose, a 280-bp PCR fragment was generated using as primers an oligonucleotide corresponding to nucleotides 883–899 and the T3 primer of the plasmid. The purified PCR fragment was labeled with ^{32}P using the specific SK primer and the Klenow fragment of DNA polymerase I. When hybridized, only the 2.3- and 2.0-kb phospholamban transcripts were detected (data not shown), indicating that at least in adult myocardium, there are only four major transcript lengths for phospholamban in rat.

A novel cDNA (pRCSER6) for the SR Ca–ATPase has also been isolated from a rat cardiac cDNA library (12) that contains two signals for polyadenylation. This clone arose from a transcript that was generated by alternative splicing of the 3′end of the gene. RNA processing had been proposed to give rise to four classes of SERCA2 transcripts: one for SERCA2a and three for SERCA2b (13) in muscle and brain. The second transcript in rat heart represents a second form of the SERCA2a mRNAs that is characterized by the addition of 128 nucleotides at the extreme 3′ end of the transcript (data not shown). As such, it contains two signals for polyadenylation. The coding region of this transcript is unchanged, however, and would give rise to a protein of the expected 997 amino acids when translated.

It is currently unclear what role in the cell, if any, is played by differences in the 3′ untranslated regions of the mRNAs coding for phospholamban and the SR Ca–ATPase. There is some evidence for the influence of the 3′ untranslated region toward stability and localization of the mRNA transcripts. Recent work by Rastinejan and Le Cam has shown that 3′ untranslated regions can be involved in growth and differentiation of the cells (NMU2) as well as in regulation of gene expression (14,15). The potential role of the different extensions in the 3′ untranslated regions of phospholamban and SERCA2a transcripts remains to be elucidated, particularly to see if they play any role during development and/or in disease states.

SR Ca–ATPASE AND PHOSPHOLAMBAN EXPRESSION IN THE EMBRYONIC AND FETAL RAT HEART

The spatial distribution of the SR Ca–ATPase and phospholamban were determined using in situ hybridization techniques in collaboration with A. F. M. Moorman in Amsterdam (11,16). Detection of SERCA2 was first seen at approximately

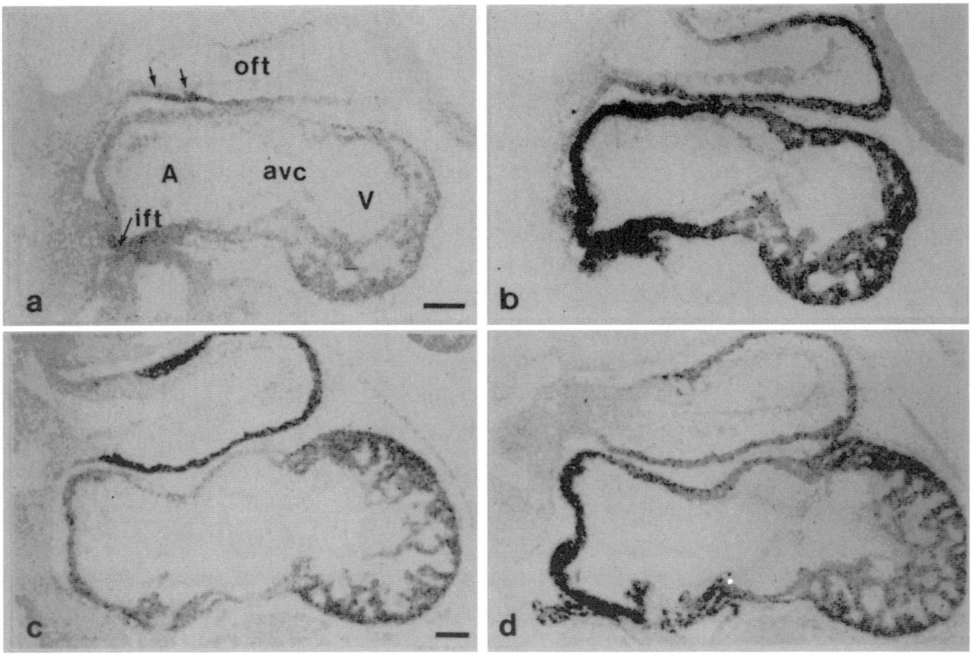

FIG. 18–1. Patterns of expression of phospholamban mRNA (a and c) and sarcoplasmic reticulum Ca–ATPase mRNA (b and d) in sagittal sections of the rat heart at embryonic days 12 (a and b) and 13 (c and d). Phospholamban mRNA can now be detected for the first time in the inflow tract (ift) and outflow tract (oft) of the rat heart at embryonic day 12. A = atrium; avc = atrioventricular canal; and v = ventricle. Bar = 100 μm. (Reproduced with permission from Patterns of expression of sarcoplasmic reticulum Ca^{2+}–ATPase and phospholamban mRNAs during rat heart development. American Heart Association, 1995.)

9 embryonic days (ED) throughout the horseshoe-shaped cardiogenic plate in the presomite embryo. At this time the heart tube has not yet formed. No transcripts for phospholamban were detected. One day later, SERCA2 mRNAs can be detected along the entire heart tube and are present as a weak gradient, with the highest amounts seen at the venous pole (inflow tract) and a relatively weaker expression seen at the arterial pole. At 12 ED of development (Fig. 18–1), SERCA2 transcripts are detectable as a gradient of expression throughout most of the myocardium, greater in the dorsal wall of the atrium and inflow tract, and lesser in the ventricle and outflow tract. The weakest signals for SERCA2 are apparently in the outflow tract. Phospholamban transcripts are also first seen at 12 ED. Although not detectable at this stage in most of the myocardium, phospholamban transcripts are present at low levels in the most distal regions of the outflow tract and to a lesser degree in the dorsal wall of the atrium and inflow tract. Ventricular expression of phospholamban is first seen at 13 ED (see Fig. 18–1). At this time, transcripts for phospholamban also appear as a gradient, with the greatest expression seen in the outflow tract, decreasing toward the atrial regions and inflow tract. The gradient of phospholamban expression is opposite to that seen for SERCA2 expression. This general pattern of SERCA2 mRNA expression and phospholamban expression is maintained throughout embryonic and early fetal development (13–16 ED) (Table 18–1). Both SERCA2 and phospholamban expression tend to be present at lower levels in the atrioventricular junction than in the adjacent atrium and ventricle. A four-chamber view of SERCA2 and phospholamban mRNA expression illustrates the relative expression of these mRNAs in fetal heart at 20 ED, and for comparison, α- and β-MHC expression are also

TABLE 18–1. *Expression of cardiac S Reticulum Ca–ATPase and phospholamban (PLB) mRNA in embryonic and fetal rat heart development*

Age	mRNA	IFT	Atrium	A-V	Ventricle	OFT
10 ED	Ca–ATPase	++++	++++	+++	+++	++
	PLB	–	–	–	–	–
11 ED	Ca–ATPase	++++	++++	+++	+++	++
	PLB	–	–	–	–	–
12 ED	Ca–ATPase	++++	++++	++	+++	++
	PLB	±	–	–	–	+
13 ED	Ca–ATPase	++++	++++	++	+++	++
	PLB	±	±	±	++	+++
16 ED	Ca–ATPase	++++	++++	++	+++	+
	PLB	±	±	++	+++	+++
20/22 ED	Ca–ATPase	*	++++	++	++++	*
	PLB	*	+	+	+++	**

*Incorporation into the atrium when the semilunar valves have evolved.

**The OFT at this time has either partially disappeared or been incorporated into the right ventricle.

A-V, atrioventricular junction; ED, days of embryonic development; IFT, inflow tract; OFT, outflow tract.

Reproduced with permission from Molecular aspects of myocardial differentiation. *Eur Heart J* 1995; (16) 3–7.

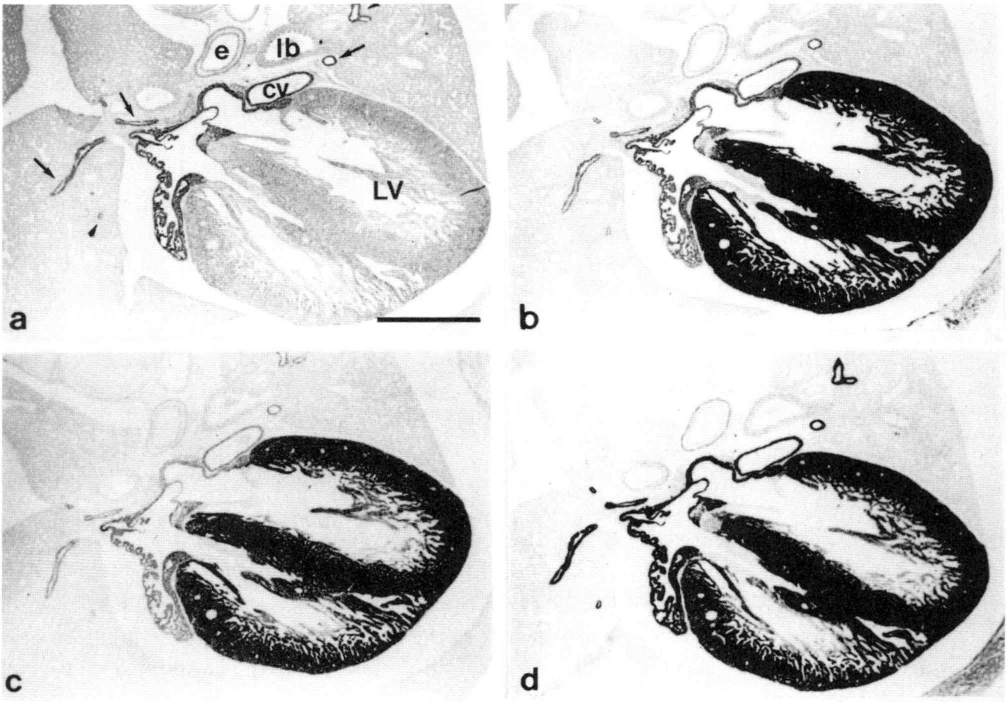

FIG. 18–2. Four-chamber view of a fetal rat heart at embryonic day 20. Overview demonstrates the myocardium surrounding the pulmonary (*arrows*) and caval veins (cv). Serial sections were hybridized to probes specific for α-myosin heavy chain (a), β-myosin heavy chain (b), phospholamban (c), and sarcoplasmic reticulum Ca–ATPase (d). At this stage of development, α-myosin heavy chain is largely confined to the atria; whereas β-myosin heavy chain is present mostly in ventricle. (e = esophagus; lb = left principal bronchus; cv = caval vein; and LV = left ventricle. Bar = 1 mm.) (Reproduced with permission from Patterns of expression of sarcoplasmic reticulum Ca^{2+}–ATPase and phospholamban mRNAs during rat heart development. American Heart Association, 1995.)

shown (Fig. 18–2). At this time the differences in atrial versus ventricular SERCA2 expression become less pronounced, but phospholamban expression remains greater in the ventricles than in atria.

SR Ca–ATPASE AND PHOSPHOLAMBAN EXPRESSION IN ADULT RAT HEART

RNA Expression

Total RNA was isolated from rat ventricles (left or right) and atria according to the methods of Chomczynski and Sacchi (17). Phospholamban mRNA expression was determined by slot blot hybridizations, and the data were normalized to 18S ribosomal RNA expression to control for any potential loading differences, as previously described (18,19). No significant difference in mRNA expression could be detected between the left and right ventricles, but a difference was demonstrated between ventricle and atria (11). The presence of phospholamban transcripts in atria was found to be 2.7 times less in atria (4.8 arbitrary units) than in ventricles (12.7 arbitrary units).

Protein Expression

The main question arising from the in situ hybridization work was whether or not differences in RNA expression would translate into differences in protein expression. To address this question, total protein was isolated from adult rat hearts by homogenizing frozen ventricular (left or right) and atrial tissue in 1.0% sodium dodecyl sulfate containing 1 mM phenyl methyl sulfonylfluoride. Protein concentrations were determined using the Bradford protein assay. Total protein (25 μg) was separated on the basis of size by SDS-polyacrylamide gel electrophoresis (PAGE) and transferred to nitrocellulose membranes (20). For phospholamban, proteins were separated on 12% gels; for the SR Ca–ATPase, total protein was separated on 7.5% PAGE gels (21). The membranes were probed with either a monoclonal antibody specific for phospholamban (kindly provided by J. Wang, Calgary, Canada) or a polyclonal antibody specific for the SR Ca–ATPase (kindly provided by F. Wuytack, Leuven Belgium). Signals were detected using the enhanced chemiluminescence system and exposed to ECL film (Amersham) according to the manufacturer's instructions. After probing, bound antibodies were removed by washing the membrane (1% SDS, 15 mM TRIS buffer pH 6.8, 0.02% β-mercaptoethanol) at 50°C for 30 minutes. The membranes were then stained with 0.15% amido black. The specific signals for the SR Ca–ATPase and phospholamban generated by the ECL system and the amido black staining of total protein were scanned using the Pdquest system and the ECL signals were expressed as a ratio of amido black staining (total protein transferred to the nitrocellulose membrane) (20,21).

SR Ca–ATPase levels and phospholamban levels were determined by Western blot analyses as just described. In the adult rat heart, SR Ca–ATPase levels were found to be greater in atria than in ventricle (Fig. 18–3a). Additionally, more SR Ca–ATPase was seen in the right ventricle than in the left ventricle. In contrast, phospholamban proteins were more prevalent in the left ventricle than in the right ventricle, and both ventricles had more phospholamban protein than the atria. (Fig. 18–3b). The protein data seen are reminiscent to those described earlier in the embryonic and fetal rat hearts examined by in situ mRNA hybridizations. For phospholamban, the data are also analogous to those seen at the mRNA level in adult. These data imply that for the most part in the adult rat, phospholamban expression is determined by the levels of mRNA expression. For Ca–ATPase there is some evidence to suggest a dissociation between mRNA levels and protein levels in certain

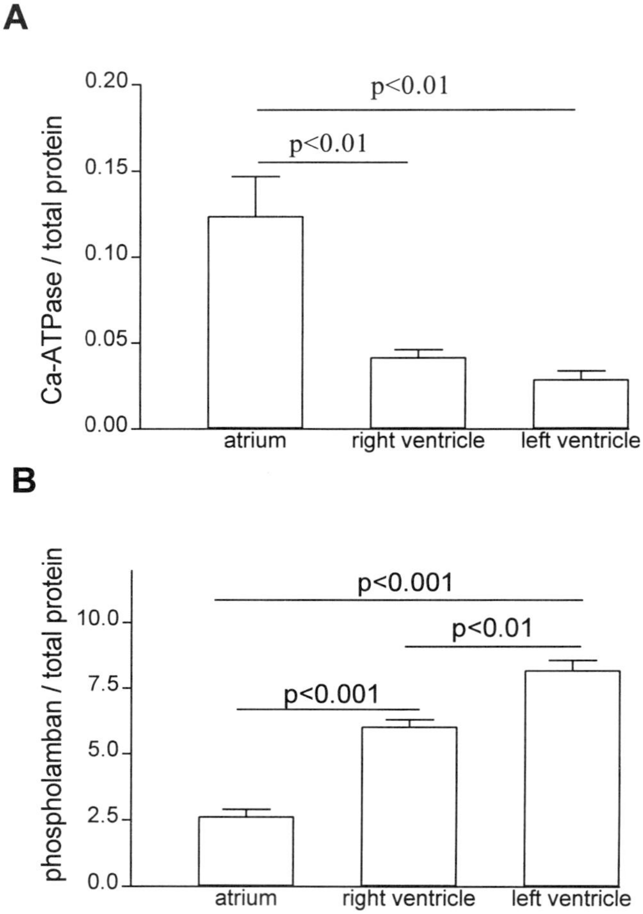

FIG. 18–3. Relative protein expression of the sarcoplasmic reticulum Ca+ATPase (a) and phospholamban (b) in adult rat heart. The data are expressed in arbitrary units and each graph represents the mean value of four samples analyzed simultaneously.

models of cardiac hypertrophy (21), but importantly for this study, the proteins levels are consistent with those described for the embryonic and fetal rat heart: greater expression in the atria than in the ventricles.

RATIO OF SR Ca–ATPASE TO PHOSPHOLAMBAN: FUNCTIONAL IMPLICATIONS

A change in the relative amounts of either the SR Ca–ATPase or phospholamban protein leads to a change in the ratio of Ca–ATPase to phospholamban (Fig. 18–4).

Any change in this ratio has functional consequences, and apparently, it is the quantity of phospholamban protein, and perhaps not so much the phosphorylation state of phospholamban in transgenic animals, that is most important for affecting contraction and relaxation. For example, the absence of phospholamban in a knockout mouse results in enhanced myocardial performance (22). In those mice lacking ventricular phospholamban and analyzed relative to controls, heart rate and blood pressure were unchanged; however, cardiac contraction and relaxation, measured in isolated heart preparations, were both significantly increased. The increased affinity of the SERCA pump for Ca^{2+} in the phospholamban-deficient mice was to the same extent as the removal of phospholamban inhibition by beta-adrenocepter stimulation in wild-type mice. Furthermore, perfusion of the isolated hearts from the phospholamban-deficient mice with an isoproterenol-containing perfusate produced no additional increases in the cardiac functional parameters. In contrast, transgenic mice that overexpress phospholamban about twice as much as controls, and for which there was no evidence of phosphorylation differences, showed an important decrease in myocardial performance (23). Isolated cardiac myocytes from these transgenic mice had a diminished shortening fraction and decreased rate of shortening. Additionally, the time it took for the myocytes to re-lengthen was increased. These differences could, however, all be abolished by isoproterenol stimulation and phosphorylation of phospholamban. Finally, and in normal mouse hearts, Koss et al. showed that an increased ratio of Ca–ATPase to phospholamban in atrium versus ventricle leads to significantly shorter times to half relaxation in isolated myocytes, and to shortened contraction times in atrial muscle relative to ventricles (24). Taken together, these data indicate that changes in the ratio of SR Ca–ATPase to phospholamban between compartments in rat heart lead to important differences in contractile parameters.

If the protein data are extrapolated from adult myocardium to the embryonic and fetal rat heart, then it would be expected that as in adult, differences in the relative

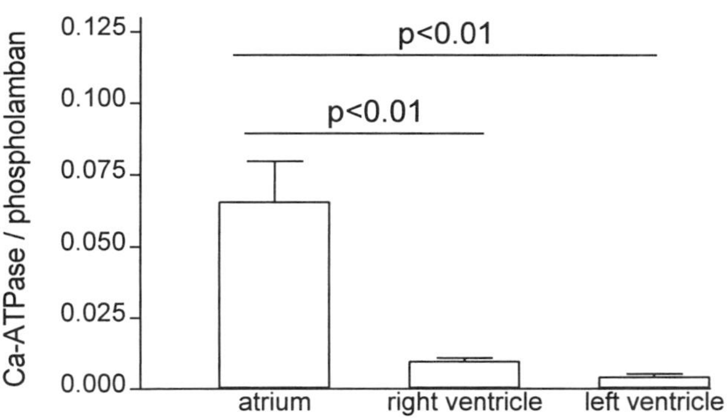

FIG. 18–4. The ratios of the sarcoplasmic reticulum Ca–ATPase to phospholamban protein in atria and right and left ventricles of adult rat heart. The ratios were determined from the data presented in Fig. 18–3.

protein proportions of SERCA to PLB in different regions of the embryonic heart would also have important functional consequences. In the adult, the protein expression of the SR Ca–ATPase is greater in atria than in ventricle, whereas the presence of PLB is greater in ventricle than in atria. These data are similar to the mRNA gradients seen in the embryonic and fetal rat heart (see Table 18–1). If the mRNA levels are indicative of the protein levels, then these data predict that the rate of relaxation would be faster where the ratio of SERCA to PLB is greater. In the atrial region of the embryonic heart, the amount of SR Ca–ATPase protein is predicted to be much greater than that of PLB; as such, the ratio should be large and relaxation times should be short. In fact, the inflow tract and atrial regions of the myocardium have been shown to have a more rapid contraction and a more rapid rate of relaxation than ventricular regions and the outflow tract of the developing heart (4–6). In the adult myocardium, rapid atrial relaxation allows for an increased time for venous return and as a consequence more atrial filling. During the next atrial contraction of the cardiac cycle, the atrial blood reservoir is pumped to the ventricle to improve cardiac output. In the embryonic heart, an analogous situation could be envisaged. Blood returning from the periphery should have adequate time to enter the inflow tract and atrial regions of the heart, so that on the next contraction, blood can be pumped swiftly into the ventricular region. Before relaxation begins in the atrial region, the ventricles contract, and with the help of the cardiac jelly, blood should continue its forward momentum toward the outflow tract without regurgitation into the atrial regions. Likewise, the outflow tract in the embryonic heart—with its relatively long action potential duration, peristaltoid contraction form, and slow propagation of impulse—functions to prevent regurgitation of blood (25). As the ratio of SERCA2 to PLB is low in this region of the developing heart, the relaxation rate should be very slow, and as a consequence, should permit prolonged contraction times. These results are consistent with the spatial distribution of the SR Ca–ATPase and PLB transcripts and are supportive of a model that can partially explain how blood can be moved unidirectionally in the absence of valves in the embryonic heart.

SUMMARY

The embryonic heart can pump blood in a single direction in the absence of one-way valves. Functionally, the unidirectional movement of blood can be partially explained through the use of molecular markers to determine the temporal and spatial distribution of cardiac proteins. In this study, the patterns of expression of the important cardiac sarcoplasmic reticulum calcium-adenosine triphosphatase (SERCA2) and phospholamban (PLB) were examined at both the mRNA and protein levels in the developing and adult heart. The mRNA expression of SERCA2 and PLB are seen as gradients in the developing heart; and in the adult, the relative protein expression of these proteins leads to a ratio of SERCA2 to PLB that is greater in atria than in ventricle. The results are consistent with a model where relaxation is more rapid in atria than in ventricle, and are supportive of a molecular model that can partially explain how blood can be moved unidirectionally in the absence of valves in the embryonic heart.

ACKNOWLEDGMENTS

This work was supported by project grants to KRB from the British Heart Foundation (PG/95093 and PG/93148). M. Koban was supported by Professor J. Holtz (Halle, Germany) and the Bundesministerium fur Forschung und Technik (01ZZ9105-1.23). The authors would especially like to thank JLM Vermeulen and AFM Moorman (Amsterdam, The Netherlands) for all their support both in data analysis and in the performance of the *in situ* hybridizations.

REFERENCES

1. Manasek FJ. Embryonic development of the heart. I. A light and electron microscopic study of myocardial development in the early chick embryo. *J Morphol* 1968;125:329–365.
2. Anversa P, Olivetti G, Loud AV. Morphometric study of the early post-natal development in the left and right ventricular myocardium of the rat. I. Hypertrophy, hyperplasia and binucleation of myocytes. *Circ Res* 1980;46:495–502.
3. Patten BM. Initiation and early changes in the character of the heartbeat in vertebrate embryos. *Physiol Rev* 1949;29:31–47.
4. Moorman AFM, Lamers WH. A molecular approach towards the understanding of early heart development: an emerging synthesis. In: El Hag A, ed. *The molecular biology of muscle.* Vol 46. Cambridge: Society for Experimental Biology; 1992:285–300.
5. Counch JR, West TC, Hoff HE. Development of the action potential of the prenatal rat heart. *Circ Res* 1969;24:19–31.
6. Moorman AFM, Lamers WH. Molecular anatomy of the developing heart. *Trends Cardiovasc Med* 1994;4:257–264.
7. Arai M, Matsui H, Periasamy M. Sarcoplasmic reticulum gene expression in cardiac hypertrophy and heart failure. *Circ Res* 1994;74:555–564.
8. Lompre AM, Anger M, Levitsky D. Sarco(endo)plasmic reticulum calcium pumps in the cardiovascular system: function and gene expression. *J Mol Cell Cardiol* 1994;26:1109–1121.
9. Wynne DG, Koban MU, Boheler KR. Molecular mechanisms of relaxation. In: Yacoub M, ed. *Annual of Cardiac Surgery.* 8th ed. Philadelphia: Current Science; 1995:29–37.
10. Colyer J. Control of the calcium pump of cardiac sarcoplasmic reticulum: a specific role for the pentameric structure of phospholamban: *Cardiovasc Res* 1993;27:1766–1771.
11. Moorman AFM, Vermeulen JLM, Koban MU, Schwartz K, Lamers WH, Boheler KR. Patterns of expression of sarcoplasmic reticulum Ca^{2+}-ATPase and phospholamban mRNAs during rat heart development. *Circ Res* 1995;76:616–625.
12. Martin XJ, Schwartz K, Boheler KR. Characterization of a novel transcript of retroviral origin expressed in rat heart and liver. *J Mol Cell Cardiol* 1995;27:589–597.
13. Wuytack F, Raeymaekers L, De Smedt H, Eggermont JA, Missiaen L, Van Den Bosch L, De Jaegere S, Verboomen H, Plessers L, Casteels R. Ca^{2+}-transport ATPases and their regulation in muscle and brain. *Ann NY Acad Sci* 1992;671:82–91.
14. Rastinejad F, Blau HM. Genetic complementation reveals a novel regulatory role for 3′ untranslated regions in growth and differentiation. *Cell* 1993;72:903–917.
15. Le Cam A, Legraverend C. Transcriptional repression, a novel function for 3′untranslated regions. *Eur J Biochem* 1995;231:620–627.
16. Boheler KR, Moorman AFM. Molecular aspects of myocardial differentiation. *Eur Heart J* 1995;16(suppl N):3–7.
17. Chomczynski P, Sacchi N. Single-step method of RNA isolation by acid guanidinium thiocyanate-phenol-chloroform extraction. *Anal Biochem* 1987;162:156–159.

18. Mendez RE, Pfeffer JM, Ortola FV, Bloch KD, Anderson S, Seidman JG, Brenner BM. Atrial natriuretic peptide transcription, storage and release in rats with myocardial infarction. *Am J Physiol* 1987;243:H1449–H1455.
19. Boheler KR, Carrier L, de la Bastie D, Allen PD, Komajda M, Mercadier JJ, Schwartz K. Skeletal actin mRNA increases in the human heart during ontogenic development and is the major isoform of control and failing adult hearts. *J Clin Invest* 1991;88:323–330.
20. Latif N, Baker CS, Dunn MJ, Rose ML, Brady P, Yacoub MH. Frequency and specificity of anti-heart antibodies in patients with dilated cardiomyopathy detected using SDS-PAGE and Western blotting. *J Am Coll Cardiol* 1993;22:1378–1384.
21. Boateng SY, Seymour AML, Bhutta NS, Dunn MJ, Yacoub MH, Boheler KR. Sub-antihypertensive doses of ramipril normalize calcium ATPase expression and function following cardiac hypertrophy in rats (submitted).
22. Luo W, Grupp IL, Harrer J, Ponniah S, Grupp G, Duffy JJ, Doetschman T, Kranias EG. Targeted ablation of the phospholamban gene is associated with markedly enhanced myocardial contractility and loss of β-agonist stimulation *Circ Res* 1994;75:401–409.
23. Kadambi VJ, Ponniah S, Harrer JM, Hoit BD, Dorn II GW, Walsh RA, Kranias EG. Cardiac-specific overexpression of phospholamban alters calcium kinetics and resultant cardiomyocyte mechanics in transgenic mice. *J Clin Invest* 1996;97:533–539.
24. Koss KL, Ponniah S, Keith Jones W, Grupp IL, Kranias EG. Differential phospholamban gene expression in murine cardiac compartments. *Circ Res* 1995;77:342–353.
25. de Jong F, Opthof T, Wilde AAM, Janse MJ, Charles R, Lamers WH, Moorman AFM. Persisting zones of slow impulse conduction in developing chicken hearts. *Circ Res* 1992;71:240–250.

The Developing Heart,
edited by Bohuslav Ošťádal et al.
Lippincott-Raven Publishers,
Philadelphia © 1997.

19

Calcium/Calmodulin-Dependent Protein Phosphorylation in Cardiac Sarcoplasmic Reticulum

Njanoor Narayanan, Ande Xu, and Thomas Netticadan

Department of Physiology, University of Western Ontario, London, Ontario, N6A 5C1, Canada

In the heart, the sarcoplasmic reticulum (SR) plays a central role in regulating cytosolic Ca^{2+} concentration, and therefore, muscle contraction and relaxation. Opening of voltage-gated L-type Ca^{2+} channels in response to depolarization permits the entry of a small amount of Ca^{2+} from the extracellular fluid (1–3). This Ca^{2+} influx into the cardiomyocyte triggers massive Ca^{2+} release from the SR through activation of the Ca^{2+} release channels (known as the ryanodine receptor, RYR), and the consequent increase in cytoplasmic Ca^{2+} produces myofilament activation and muscle contraction (1–6). Subsequently, active sequestration of Ca^{2+} back into the SR lumen by a Ca^{2+}-pumping ATPase (Ca^{2+}-ATPase) in the SR lowers the cytoplasmic Ca^{2+}, thus promoting muscle relaxation (3–5). Considerable evidence suggests that, physiologically, the Ca^{2+} uptake and release functions of the SR are subject to regulation by protein phosphorylation and dephosphorylation. Thus, the Ca^{2+} sequestering function of the SR Ca^{2+}–ATPase is well known to be regulated by the phosphorylation of an intrinsic SR protein, phospholamban (7–10). Current evidence suggests that interaction of nonphosphorylated phospholamban with the ATPase inhibits Ca^{2+} pumping and that phosphorylation of phospholamban by cAMP-dependent protein kinase (PKA) or Ca^{2+}/calmodulin-dependent protein kinase (CaM kinase) disrupts the ATPase–phospholamban interaction, leading to removal of inhibition and consequent stimulation of Ca^{2+} pumping (7–10). Recently, direct phosphorylation of the cardiac SR Ca^{2+}–ATPase by membrane-associated and exogenous CaM kinase has been demonstrated (11,12). This phosphorylation, occurring at a serine residue, resulted in stimulation of ATP hydrolysis and Ca^{2+} transport (11–13). Thus, direct phosphorylation of the Ca^{2+}–ATPase may provide an additional mechanism for the regulation of SR Ca^{2+} pump function. In cardiac SR, the RYR–Ca^{2+} release channel also undergoes phosphorylation by CaM kinase (11,12,14,15) as well as cAMP (15,16) and cGMP-dependent

(15) protein kinases. The functional consequence of RYR phosphorylation has not been clearly established, although stimulation of Ca^{2+} release upon RYR phosphorylation by CaM kinase has been observed under some conditions (14). In this chapter, we review the studies demonstrating phosphorylation of Ca^{2+}–ATPase in addition to RYR and phospholamban, by CaM kinase in cardiac SR, ontogenetic expression of this regulatory system, and the physiologic implications of the phosphorylation of multiple targets by CaM kinase in transmembrane Ca^{2+} cycling.

IDENTIFICATION OF Ca^{2+}–ATPase AS A SUBSTRATE FOR CAM KINASE IN CARDIAC SR

Observations, originally reported from this laboratory (17–20) and subsequently confirmed by others (21,22) have described the presence of two distinct cytosolic proteins in heart muscle capable of modulating the Ca^{2+} uptake and release functions of the SR. One of these proteins, with an apparent molecular mass of 43 kDa, inhibits ATP-dependent Ca^{2+} uptake by SR vesicles in vitro (17–22) and stimulates Ca^{2+} release from the SR (19,21,22); the other, with an apparent molecular mass 64 kDa, reverses the effects of 43-kDa protein (18,20,21). Recently, we found that calmodulin potentiated the action of 64-kDa protein in reversing the inhibition of SR Ca^{2+} uptake produced by the 43-kDa protein (23). In attempting to understand the mechanism of action of calmodulin, we examined calmodulin-dependent protein phosphorylation in cardiac SR. When SR vesicles isolated from rabbit heart ventricles were incubated in a phosphorylation assay medium, a protein of approximate molecular mass 105 kDa underwent strong Ca^{2+}/calmodulin-dependent phosphorylation, in addition to phospholamban (7–10,24) and RYR-Ca^{2+} release channel (14,15), the two previously characterized substrates for CaM kinase (Fig. 19–1). Western immunoblotting and immunoprecipitation experiments using a Ca^{2+}–ATPase-specific antibody led to the identification of the phosphorylated 105-kDa peptide band as the Ca^{2+}-pumping ATPase of SR. It was also established that the observed phosphorylation of the Ca^{2+}–ATPase is not due to the formation of the acylphosphate (aspartyl phosphate) intermediate of the Ca^{2+}–ATPase (25), because (a) phosphorylation was dependent on both Ca^{2+} and calmodulin (11,12); (b) acylphosphate does not survive the alkaline conditions of SDS-polyacrylamide gel electrophoresis (26); (c) phosphorylation is fully resistant to hydroxylamine treatment (27); and (d) the major amino acid undergoing phosphorylation was identified as serine (11).

CHARACTERISTICS OF Ca^{2+}/CALMODULIN-DEPENDENT PHOSPHORYLATION OF THE Ca^{2+}–ATPase AND IDENTIFICATION OF THE PHOSPHORYLATION SITE

The cardiac and slow-twitch skeletal muscle express the same Ca^{2+}–ATPase isoform (SERCA 2a) that is distinct from that expressed in fast-twitch skeletal muscle

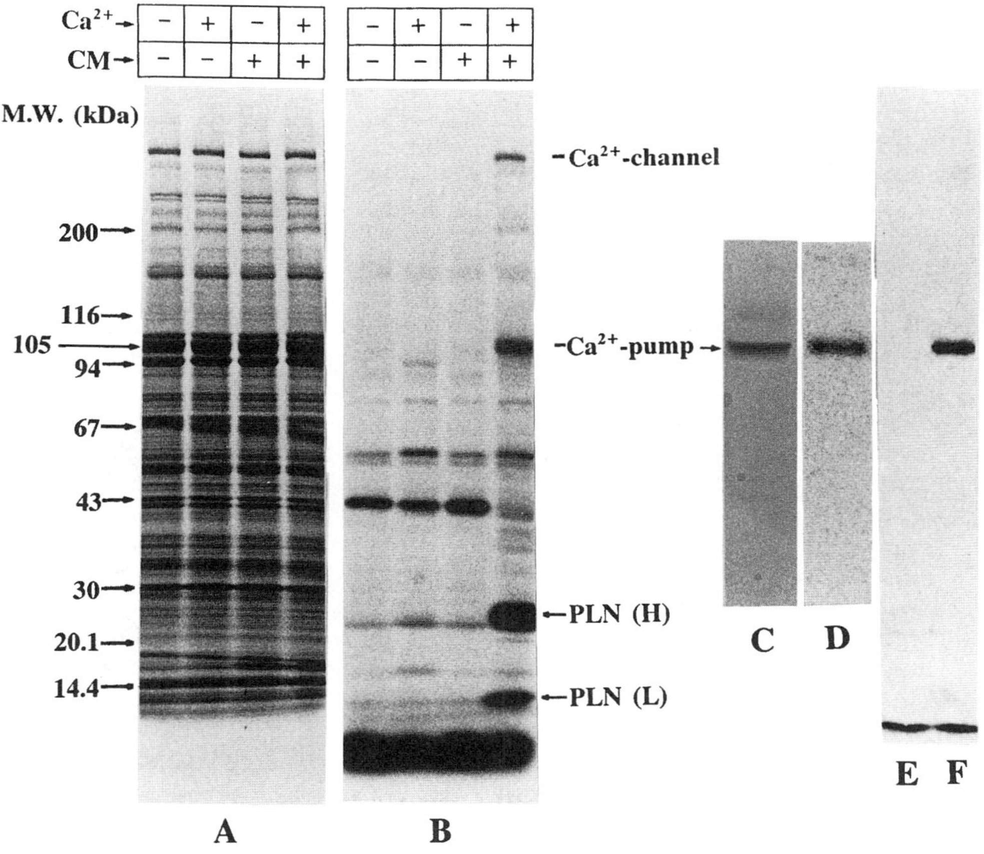

FIG. 19–1. Phosphorylation of Ca^{2+} pump (Ca^{2+}–ATPase), Ca^{2+}-release channel, and phospholamban (PLN; H, high-molecular-weight form; L, low-molecular-weight form) in rabbit cardiac SR by membrane-associated CaM kinase. (**A**) Coomassie blue-stained SDS-polyacrylamide gel showing SR protein profile. (**B**) Autoradiogram of the same gel. (**C**) Western immunoblot of the 105-kDa phosphorylated peptide band excised from the gel showing immunoreactivity with SR Ca^{2+}–ATPase-specific antibody. (**D**) Autoradiogram of the Western immunoblot. (**E,F**) Autoradiogram of proteins fractionated on SDS polyacrylamide gel after subjecting phosphorylated SR to immunoprecipitation protocol in the absence (E) and presence (F) of Ca^{2+}–ATPase-specific antibody. The phosphorylation reaction was carried out for 3 min in the presence or absence of Ca^{2+} and calmodulin (CM) as indicated. (From Xu et al., ref. 11. Reprinted with permission.)

(SERCA 1) (28–31). These two isoforms show about 84% sequence homology (29,30), similar transmembrane topologies and tertiary structures (32,33), and qualitatively similar enzymatic properties (34), all of which likely reflect the uniformity in their function, namely, active Ca^{2+} transport. On the other hand, the limited structural differences among the Ca^{2+}–ATPase isoforms may signify subtle variations in their intrinsic functional properties (35–37) and/or susceptibility to mechanisms of physiologic regulation. We examined whether the CaM kinase-mediated phosphorylation of the Ca^{2+}–ATPase is specific to the cardiac/slow-twitch muscle isoform. Studies using SR vesicles isolated from slow-twitch (*soleus*) and fast-twitch (*adductor magnus*) skeletal muscles of the rabbit showed Ca^{2+}/calmodulin-dependent phosphorylation of the Ca^{2+}–ATPase in slow-twitch muscle SR but not in fast-twitch muscle SR (Fig. 19–2). Thus, an endogenous CaM kinase capable of phosphorylating the Ca^{2+}–ATPase is present in cardiac and slow-twitch muscle SR. Exogenously added α-CaM kinase II stimulated the phosphorylation of the Ca^{2+}–ATPase in cardiac and slow-twitch muscle SR but failed to induce phosphorylation of the Ca^{2+}–ATPase in fast muscle SR (11,12,27). Therefore, the absence of an appropriate CaM kinase does not account for the inability of the fast-twitch muscle SR Ca^{2+}–ATPase isoform (SERCA 1) to undergo phosphorylation. The isoform specificity of CaM kinase phosphorylation of the Ca^{2+}–ATPase was confirmed in other studies that demonstrated phosphorylation of SERCA 2a but not SERCA 1 expressed in HEK-293 cells by α-CaM kinase II (13). The SERCA 2a isoform contains three serine residues in its primary structure (in positions 38, 167, and 531) that have minimal consensus sequence (R-X-X-S/T) for phosphorylation by CaM kinase (38). Site-directed mutagenesis studies have led to the identification of Ser^{38} as the residue undergoing phosphorylation by CaM kinase (13). The SERCA 1 isoform lacks phosphorylatable serine or threonine in position 38, and the amino acid sequence upstream of this site shows several substitutions, at least some of which are nonconservative (29). These structural differences may explain the inability of SERCA 1 to undergo phosphorylation by CaM kinase (13). Recently, we have found that the SERCA 2b isoform of the Ca^{2+}–ATPase expressed in coronary vascular smooth muscle also undergoes phosphorylation by CaM kinase (Fig. 19–3); except for having an extended carboxy terminus, SERCA 2b is structurally identical to SERCA 2a (39).

Phosphorylation of the Ca^{2+}–ATPase by endogenous, membrane-associated CaM kinase could be observed in cardiac SR isolated from several mammalian species, including rabbit, rat, guinea pig, dog (A. Xu and N. Narayanan, unpublished) and man (G. Hassenfus, W. Schillinger, A. Xu and N. Narayanan, unpublished). Detailed studies on the characteristics of Ca^{2+}–ATPase phosphorylation by CaM kinase have been performed using rabbit cardiac SR (11,12). Phosphorylation of the Ca^{2+}–ATPase by endogenous CaM kinase occurs rapidly, reaching a maximum within 2 min at 37°C (Fig. 19–4). The time course of phosphorylation of the Ca^{2+}–ATPase is similar to that seen for phospholamban and RYR–Ca^{2+} release channel. Phosphorylation is strongly pH-dependent, increasing about sixfold, with an increase in pH from 6.5 to 9 (12). The striking pH dependence of Ca^{2+}–ATPase

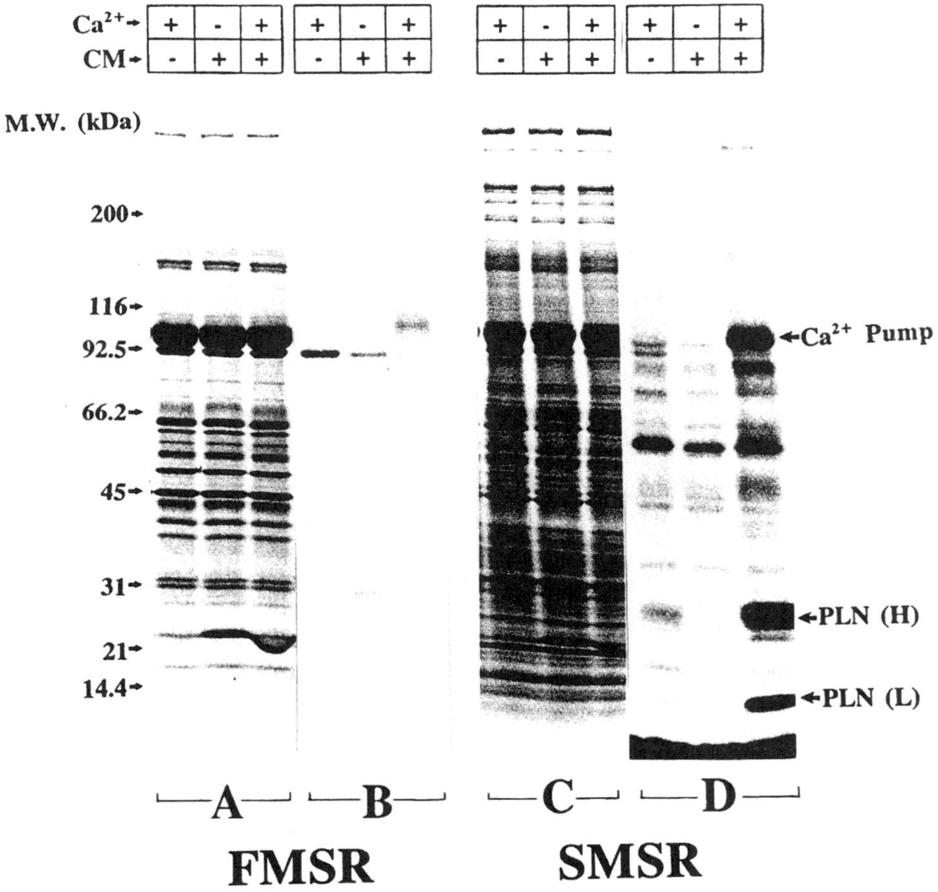

FIG. 19–2. Comparison of Ca^{2+}/calmodulin-dependent protein phosphorylation in rabbit fast-twitch skeletal muscle (*adductor magnus*) SR (FMSR) and rabbit slow-twitch skeletal muscle (*soleus*) SR (SMSR). Panels A and C show Coomassie blue-stained SDS-polyacrylamide gels showing SR protein profiles; panels B and D show the corresponding autoradiograms. The phosphorylation reaction was carried out for 3 min in the presence or absence of Ca^{2+} and calmodulin (CM) as indicated. (Modified from Hawkins et al., ref. 12.)

phosphorylation by CaM kinase correlates with the pH-dependent alterations in SR Ca^{2+}–ATPase function. For example, (a) in isolated SR vesicles, acidification results in depression of Ca^{2+}–ATPase activity and Ca^{2+} sequestration (40,41); (b) in cardiac cells, Ca^{2+} loading of the SR declines with decreasing (7.4–6.2) pH (42); and (c) intracellular acidosis is accompanied by a decrease in the rates of muscle relaxation (43). Phosphorylation has been found to result in increased turnover rates of the Ca^{2+}–ATPase (see later), and therefore, the observed pH-dependent

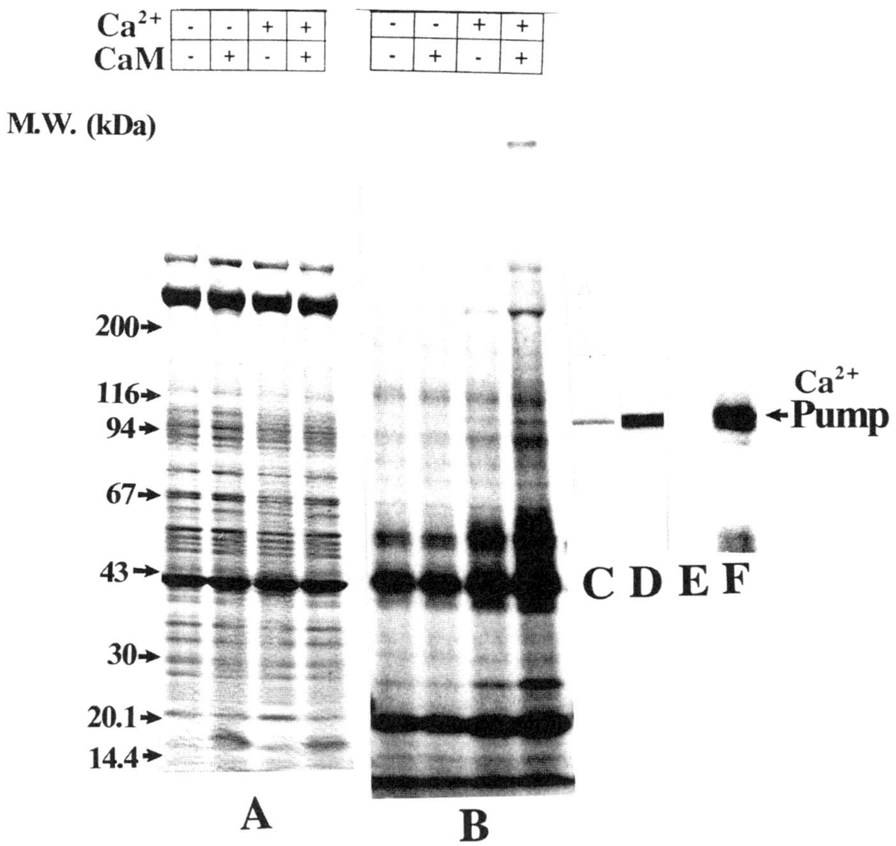

FIG. 19–3. Phosphorylation of the Ca^{2+}–ATPase (Ca^{2+}-pump) in coronary artery smooth muscle SR by endogenous CaM kinase. (**A**) Coomassie blue-stained SDS-polyacrylamide gel showing SR protein profile. (**B**) Autoradiogram of the same gel. (**C**) Western immunoblot of the peptide band corresponding to ~115 kDa excised from the gel showing immunoreactivity with the SERCA2-specific antibody. (**D**) Autoradiogram of the immunoblot. (**E,F**) Autoradiogram of proteins fractionated on SDS-polyacrylamide gel after subjecting the phosphorylated membranes to immunoprecipitation protocol in the absence (E) or presence (F) of SERCA2-specific antibody. The phosphorylation reaction was carried out for 2 min in the presence or absence of Ca^{2+} and calmodulin as indicated.

changes in Ca^{2+}–ATPase phosphorylation imply that the SR Ca^{2+} pump activity will be depressed at lower pH (due to low levels of Ca^{2+}–ATPase phosphorylation) and enhanced at higher pH (due to high levels of Ca^{2+}–ATPase phosphorylation).

Phosphorylation of the cardiac SR Ca^{2+}–ATPase by CaM kinase increases with increasing temperature up to 30°C with no further change at temperatures up to 40°C (12). Phosphorylation is maximal with 0.2 μM calmodulin and is half-maximal with ~50 nM calmodulin (27).

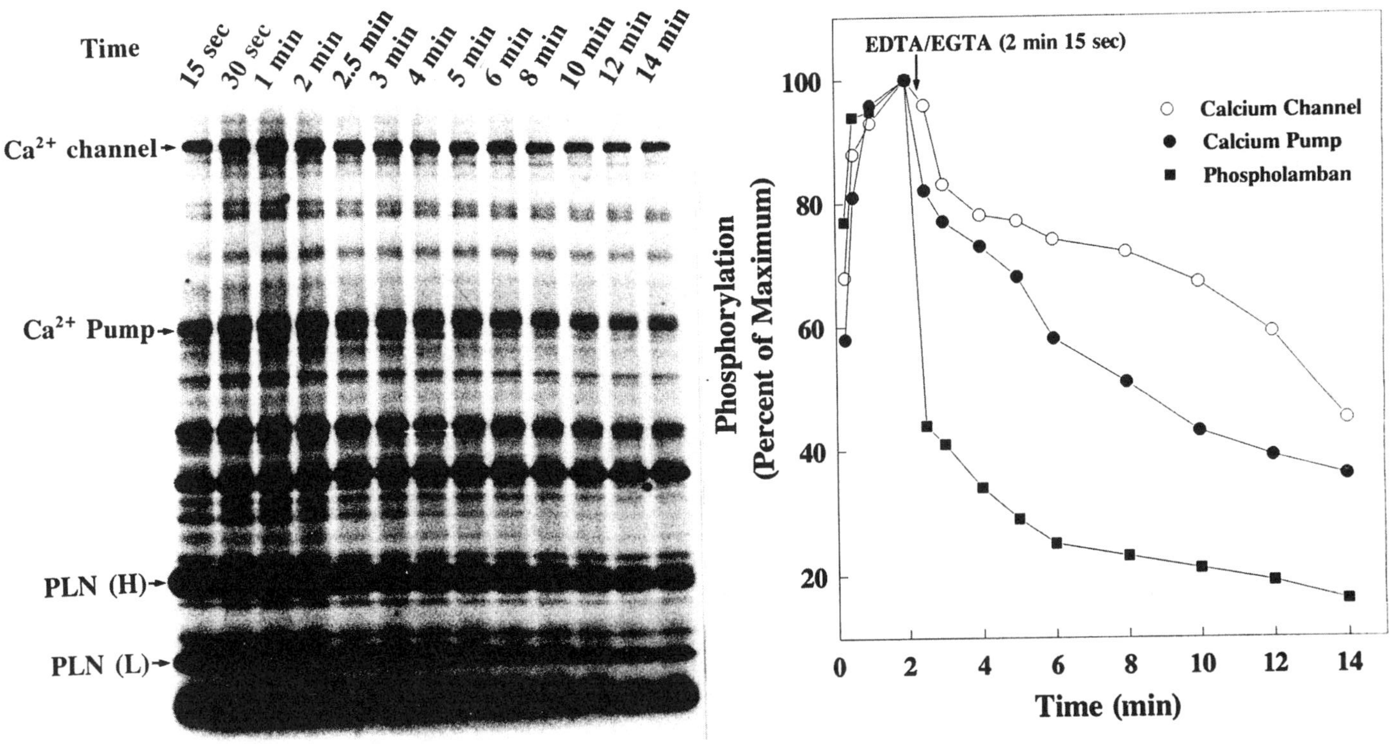

FIG. 19–4. Time course of phosphorylation and dephosphorylation of Ca^{2+} pump, Ca^{2+} channel, and phospholamban in rabbit cardiac SR. The SR membranes were incubated in a phosphorylation assay medium in the presence of Ca^{2+} and calmodulin, and the time course of phosphorylation was monitored by removing aliquots at the various time intervals indicated. The time course of dephosphorylation was monitored similarly after the addition (at 2 min 15 s) of a mixture of EDTA/EGTA to chelate Mg^{2+} and Ca^{2+}. The left panel shows an autoradiogram depicting the time-dependent changes in phosphorylation of SR proteins fractionated on SDS-polyacrylamide gel; the right panel shows quantification of phosphorylation in the peptide bands corresponding to Ca^{2+} pump, Ca^{2+} channel and phospholamban. (From ref. 11. Reprinted with permission.)

In isolated cardiac SR vesicles, the magnitude of Ca^{2+}–ATPase phosphorylation by CaM kinase was found to be intermediate between the Ca^{2+} release channel and phospholamban and the ratio of ^{32}P incorporation into Ca^{2+} channel: Ca^{2+}–ATPase: phospholamban has been estimated to be about 0.5:1:5. The molar ratio of phospholamban to Ca^{2+}–ATPase in cardiac SR membrane has not been clearly established (44), but a ratio of one mole of phospholamban per mole of Ca^{2+}–ATPase has been suggested (45). Since phospholamban is a homopentamer (46,47) with each monomer having one phosphorylation site (Thr^{17}) for CaM kinase (48), a fivefold higher phosphorylation of phospholamban relative to Ca^{2+}–ATPase (with a single phosphorylation site at Ser^{38}) (13) is to be expected. The findings with cardiac SR are in accordance with this and suggest that CaM kinase phosphorylates one mole of Ca^{2+}–ATPase and one mole of phospholamban pentamer concurrently in this membrane. However, quantification of ^{32}P incorporation into Ca^{2+}–ATPase protein suggested that only a small proportion (<20%) of the Ca^{2+} pump units in the SR membrane underwent phosphorylation by CaM kinase under the experimental conditions used (11,12). The reasons for the low level of phosphorylation are not clear, but potential contributing factors include preexisting endogenous phosphorylation, incomplete inhibition of protein phosphatase activity, and/or the influence of membrane constituents on Ca^{2+}–ATPase confrontation, which in turn may dictate accessibility of the phosphorylation site to CaM kinase.

Phosphorylation of the Ca^{2+}–ATPase and other CaM kinase substrates in cardiac SR was also found to be influenced markedly by factors other than pH, temperature, and preexisting endogenous phosphorylation. For example, inclusion of KCl (120 mM) in the phosphorylation assay medium was found to produce inhibition (~60%) of phospholamban phosphorylation while having no effect on Ca^{2+}–ATPase and Ca^{2+} channel phosphorylation (A. Xu and N. Narayanan, unpublished). On the other hand, addition of NaF (10 mM), a conventional protein phosphatase inhibitor, in the phosphorylation assay medium resulted in stimulation (~60%) of phospholamban phosphorylation and inhibition (~40–50%) of Ca^{2+}–ATPase and Ca^{2+} channel phosphorylation (49). Recently, fluoride has been shown to interact with and inhibit the Ca^{2+}–ATPase (36,37,50,51); therefore, the inhibitory effect of fluoride on Ca^{2+}–ATPase phosphorylation may be due to fluoride-induced alteration in the enzyme conformation. The critical dependence of Ca^{2+}–ATPase conformation on its ability to undergo phosphorylation by CaM kinase is demonstrated by the finding that creation of a CaM kinase phosphorylation site in SERCA 1, which mimicked the phosphorylation site (Ser^{38}) in SERCA 2, did not result in CaM kinase phosphorylation of SERCA 1 (13). The presence of fluoride in the assay medium may have contributed to the failure to detect substantial phosphorylation of the Ca^{2+}–ATPase in previous studies. Recently, we have observed that ruthenium red, a widely used RYR Ca^{2+}-release channel blocker, produces virtually complete inhibition of CaM kinase–mediated phosphorylation of the cardiac RYR Ca^{2+}-release channel (85% inhibition with 30 μM ruthenium red) while having no effect on phospholamban phosphorylation and only a modest effect (25% inhibition with 30 μM ruthenium red) on Ca^{2+}–ATPase phosphorylation (52). It seems likely that the interaction of physiologic and pharmacologic ligands with target proteins in the SR may produce conformational changes in CaM kinase substrates, which in turn may influence their phosphorylation by CaM kinase.

In cardiac SR, phosphorylation of Ca^{2+}–ATPase, RYR Ca^{2+}-release channel, and phospholamban could be readily stimulated by exogenously added α-CaM kinase II (11,12). Interestingly, we have found that KN-62, a specific inhibitor of CaM kinase II (53), did not inhibit protein phosphorylation by the endogenous, SR-associated CaM kinase under conditions in which phosphorylation by exogenous α-CaM kinase II was completely inhibited (54). Recently, novel isoforms of CaM kinase II have been identified in heart (55) and aorta (56); the SR-associated CaM kinase appears to be a δ-isoform of CaM kinase II (57).

EFFECT OF CaM KINASE–MEDIATED PHOSPHORYLATION ON Ca^{2+}–ATPase FUNCTION

The impact of Ser^{38} phosphorylation of the Ca^{2+}–ATPase by CaM kinase has been assessed by determining the effect of phosphorylation on the catalytic and ion transport functions of the ATPase. Purified Ca^{2+}–ATPase preparations (free of phospholamban and other membrane constituents) from cardiac SR (Fig. 19–5) and slow-twitch muscle SR (12) could be phosphorylated by CaM kinase II and phosphorylation resulted in nearly twice as much catalytic activity (rate of Ca^{2+}-stimulated ATP hydrolysis) of the enzyme without any appreciable change in $K_{0.5}$ for Ca^{2+}. Analysis of the effect of Ca^{2+}–ATPase phosphorylation on its Ca^{2+} transport function in native SR membranes is rendered difficult by the concurrent phosphorylation of phospholamban, which in turn stimulates Ca^{2+}-pump activity. However, some studies have suggested that, unlike in cardiac SR, Ca^{2+}–ATPase and phospholamban are poorly coupled in slow-twitch muscle SR (58,59). We have observed marked stimulation of Ca^{2+} uptake activity of slow-twitch muscle (rabbit soleus) SR following preincubation of the membranes in a phosphorylation assay medium containing Ca^{2+} and calmodulin (12). Under the experimental conditions employed, the magnitude of stimulation of Ca^{2+} uptake by SR could be correlated well with a corresponding increase in Ca^{2+}–ATPase phosphorylation by the endogenous CaM kinase. These findings suggest that CaM kinase–mediated phosphorylation of the Ca^{2+}–ATPase leads to stimulation of its enzymatic and ion transport functions, resulting in increased turnover rate of the Ca^{2+} pump. This view was further supported by the finding that when SERCA 2 isoform of the Ca^{2+}–ATPase is expressed in a heterologous system (HEK 293 cells) lacking phospholamban, phosphorylation of the enzyme by CaM kinase results in stimulation of V_{max} of Ca^{2+} transport without alteration in Ca^{2+} binding affinity of the ATPase (Fig. 19–6 and ref. 13). Our finding that phosphorylation of the Ca^{2+}–ATPase alters the V_{max} of ATP hydrolysis (11,12) and Ca^{2+} transport (13) without influencing the $K_{0.5}$ for Ca^{2+} is of particular interest. Phospholamban phosphorylation is

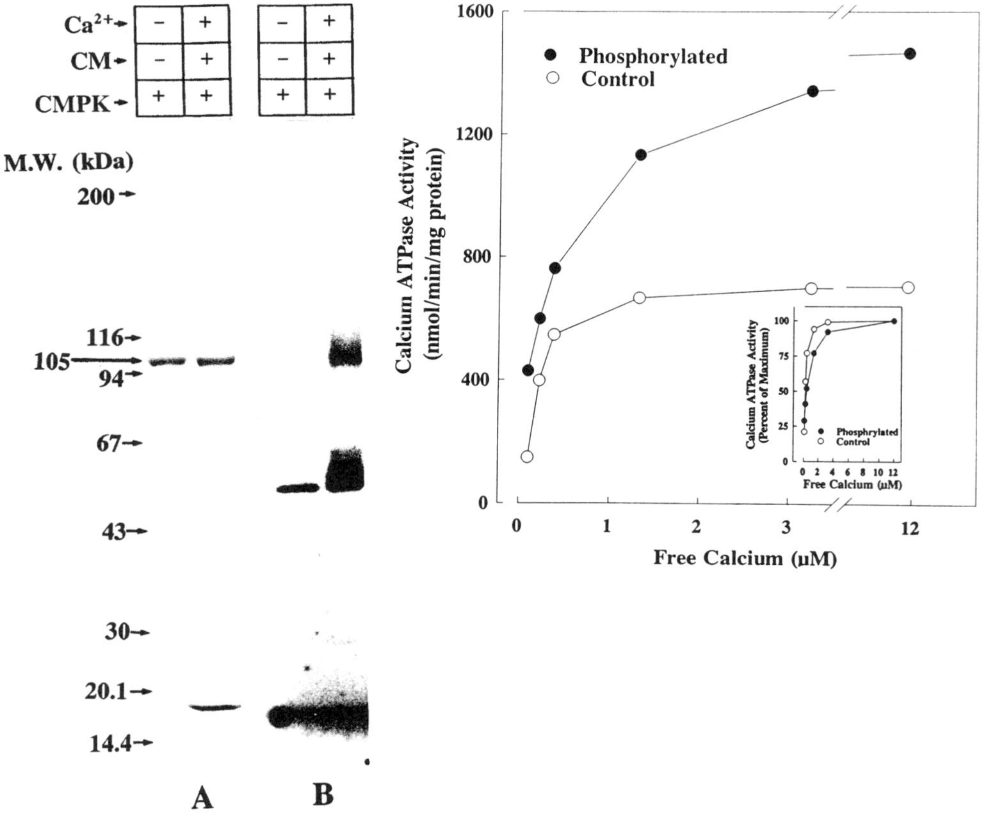

FIG. 19–5. Phosphorylation and stimulation of purified rabbit cardiac SR Ca^{2+}–ATPase by exogenous CAM kinase. Left panel: Phosphorylation of purified cardiac SR Ca^{2+}–ATPase (Ca^{2+} pump) by exogenous CaM kinase. (**A**) Coomassie Blue-stained polyacrylamide gel. (**B**) Autoradiogram of the same gel. Phosphorylation of the purified Ca^{2+}–ATPase was performed for 3 min in the presence of exogenous CaM kinase II (CMPK) at a concentration of 0.25 μM with or without Ca^{2+} and calmodulin (CM) as indicated. Following phosphorylation, the samples were subjected to SDS-polyacrylamide gel electrophoresis (A) and autoradiography (B). Right panel: Effect of CaM kinase-catalyzed phosphorylation of cardiac SR Ca^{2+}–ATPase on its enzymatic function. Ca^{2+}–ATPase purified from cardiac SR was allowed to undergo phosphorylation in the presence of exogenous CaM kinase, Ca^{2+}, and calmodulin (CM) with nonradioactive ATP (0.8 mM) (instead of [γ-^{32}P] ATP) as substrate. Ca^{2+}–ATPase subjected to the same incubation protocol in the absence of CaM kinase, Ca^{2+}, and calmodulin served as control (unphosphorylated enzyme) for this experiment. Aliquots of phosphorylated ATPase were transferred to an ATPase reaction medium to determine Ca^{2+}-stimulated ATPase activity. The assays were performed at varying concentrations of free Ca^{2+} as indicated. (From ref. 11. Reprinted with permission.)

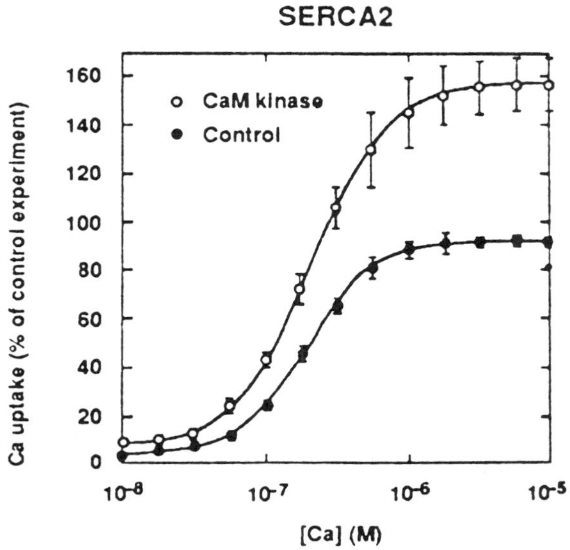

FIG. 19–6. Stimulation of Ca^{2+} uptake by SERCA 2 upon its phosphorylation by CaM kinase. SERCA 2 was expressed in HEK-293 cells. Microsomes containing the SERCA 2 enzyme were harvested from these cells and subjected to phosphorylation by exogenous α-CaM kinase II. The phosphorylated and unphosphorylated (control) microsomes were then assayed for Ca^{2+} uptake activity at varying free Ca^{2+} concentrations as indicated. The Ca^{2+} uptake rate (nmol/min/mg of microsomal protein) of phosphorylated microsomes was normalized to the activity of control microsomes and is shown as a percentage of the control Ca^{2+} uptake rate. In these experiments phosphorylation of SERCA 2 by CaM kinase was localized to Ser^{38}. (From ref. 13. Reprinted with permission.)

thought to activate the Ca^{2+}–ATPase mainly through a decrease in the enzyme's $K_{0.5}$ for Ca^{2+} (58,60,61), although an increase in V_{max} may also occur (44). Thus, the positive V_{max} effect of phosphorylation of the Ca^{2+}–ATPase and the positive $K_{0.5}$ effect of phosphorylation of phospholamban may provide a powerful, mutually complementary mechanism for the stimulation of Ca^{2+} pumping in cardiac muscle and slow-twitch skeletal muscle SR. Such a mechanism would be of particular physiologic significance in these slow-contracting muscle types, where myofilament activation and contraction result from binding of Ca^{2+} to a single Ca^{2+}-specific site on troponin C (6). This site has much lower affinity for Ca^{2+} than the Ca^{2+} binding sites on Ca^{2+}–ATPase (6). Given the higher intrinsic affinity of the Ca^{2+}–ATPase for Ca^{2+} (even when associated with phospholamban, the apparent affinity of the Ca^{2+}–ATPase for Ca^{2+} is at least 25 times higher than that of the Ca^{2+}-specific site on troponin C [cf. refs. 6, 34]), it is unlikely that an increase in Ca^{2+} affinity alone would be sufficient to cause a large increase in the rate of Ca^{2+} uptake (and therefore relaxation rate) in the presence of systolic levels of cytoplasmic Ca^{2+} concentration. It would, however, allow the SR to accumulate more Ca^{2+}

for future release. When complemented with an increase in V_{max}, the two would form a powerful mechanism for the cell to increase both the rate and amount of Ca^{2+} uptake into SR. This, in turn, would facilitate enhancement of both heart rate (because of faster mechanical restitution) and contractility (because of greater SR Ca^{2+} load available for release).

DEPHOSPHORYLATION OF THE Ser^{38}-PHOSPHORYLATED SR Ca^{2+}–ATPase

The presence of protein phosphatase activity has been demonstrated in cardiac SR, and some properties of the enzyme involved in the dephosphorylation of phospholamban have been described (62–64). We have observed that the SR-associated protein phosphatase(s) can also catalyze the dephosphorylation of Ca^{2+}–ATPase and Ca^{2+}-release channel (Fig. 19–4 and ref. 11). Under the experimental conditions used in our studies the rate of dephosphorylation of CaM kinase substrates differed in the order, phospholamban > Ca^{2+}–ATPase > Ca^{2+} channel. The identity of the protein phosphatase(s) involved in dephosphorylation of the Ca^{2+}–ATPase and the factors influencing protein dephosphorylation remain to be established.

DEVELOPMENTAL EXPRESSION OF Ca^{2+}/CALMODULIN-DEPENDENT PROTEIN PHOSPHORYLATION IN CARDIAC SR

Striking morphologic and functional changes occur during prenatal and postnatal development of the mammalian heart. In several species studied, the contractile force of the unit myocardium, ventricular compliance, and cardiac reserve increase with development (65–67). Ultrastructural studies suggest significant postnatal development of the SR (68,69), and there is evidence that the Ca^{2+}-pump activity (70–72) as well as Ca^{2+}-induced Ca^{2+}-release property (73) may develop after birth. Despite the growing recognition of CaM kinase in regulating SR Ca^{2+} cycling in the adult, little is known about the developmental expression of SR-associated CaM kinase and its role in the fetal and neonatal heart. Recently, we have examined the ontogenetic expression of CaM kinase and Ca^{2+}/calmodulin-dependent SR protein phosphorylation in the rabbit heart. These studies utilized SR-enriched membrane vesicles isolated from fetal (21 and 28–30 days gestation), newborn (2 days postnatal), and adult rabbits. Western immunoblotting analysis detected the presence of Ca^{2+}–ATPase, Ca^{2+}-release channel and phospholamban in SR of all ages tested (74). Phosphorylation studies revealed the presence of CaM kinase–dependent phosphorylation of Ca^{2+}–ATPase, Ca^{2+}-release channel, and phospholamban as early as 21 days gestation. An antibody specific for δ-CaM kinase II, detected a small amount of this CaM kinase isoform in SR at 21 days gestation; the amount of SR-associated δ-CaM kinase was maximal just prior to birth (28–30 days gestation) and declined to near adult levels by 2 days postnatal (74). Using antibodies against α- and β-isoforms of CaM kinase II, we could not detect these isoforms in the adult or developing rabbit heart. The δ-CaM kinase–mediated phosphorylation per unit of Ca^{2+} pump was greatest in the fetus and decreased toward adulthood; phospholamban phosphorylation was proportionately less than Ca^{2+}–ATPase phosphorylation in the fetal SR (74). Thus, Ca^{2+}–ATPase phosphorylation may serve as the main regulatory mechanism for Ca^{2+} uptake into SR during fetal life.

IMPLICATIONS OF THE PHOSPHORYLATION OF MULTIPLE SR SUBSTRATES BY CaM KINASE

By virtue of its ability to phosphorylate the Ca^{2+}–ATPase, RYR Ca^{2+}-release channel, and phospholamban, CaM kinase may play a key role in the regulation of transmembrane Ca^{2+} cycling in the SR, and therefore muscle contraction and relaxation. We have observed that, in contrast to the strong phosphorylation of the Ca^{2+}–ATPase by CaM kinase, PKA causes only weak phosphorylation of the Ca^{2+}–ATPase in cardiac and slow-twitch muscle SR (12). On the other hand, both kinases produce strong phosphorylation of phospholamban (12). These findings suggest that while PKA can produce stimulation of Ca^{2+}-pump activity via phosphorylation of phospholamban, CaM kinase can cause stimulation of SR Ca^{2+} pump activity via phospholamban phosphorylation as well as through direct phosphorylation of the Ca^{2+}–ATPase. In cardiac SR, phosphorylation of the RYR Ca^{2+}-release channel is about five times higher than that produced by PKA (12). Although the functional consequence of Ca^{2+} channel phosphorylation has not been clearly established (75), enhanced Ca^{2+} release upon Ca^{2+} channel phosphorylation by CaM kinase has been demonstrated in cardiac SR (14). Thus, it appears that the SR-associated CaM kinase has a unique capacity to regulate the Ca^{2+} uptake as well as the Ca^{2+} release functions of the SR because of its ability to phosphorylate Ca^{2+}–ATPase, phospholamban, and Ca^{2+}-release channel (see Fig. 19–7). However, to be physiologically effective, the function and activity of CaM kinase need to be coordinated with the events in muscle contraction and relaxation. For example, CaM kinase–mediated phosphorylation and activation of the Ca^{2+}-release channel would be fruitful if it were to occur coincident with or soon after the excitatory event involving membrane depolarization and the onset of muscle contraction. Likewise, CaM kinase–mediated phosphorylation of Ca^{2+}–ATPase and phospholamban would be meaningful if it were to occur coincident with or soon after the cessation of contraction and the onset of the relaxation phase. It is not known whether the cardiomyocytes possess mechanisms to orchestrate timely and sequential targeting of the SR-bound CaM kinase to its specific substrates. In this regard, it is of considerable interest that a recent study reported membrane depolarization-dependent modulation of CaM kinase activity and consequent changes in transmembrane Ca^{2+} fluxes in cardiac sarcolemma (76). Depolarization of the SR membrane may favor Ca^{2+}-release channel phosphorylation, and repolarization may favor Ca^{2+}–ATPase phosphorylation by the SR-bound (and cytosolic) CaM kinase. Consistent with this possibility, we have obtained evidence suggesting that the "open state" but not the "closed state" conformation of the cardiac SR Ca^{2+}-release channel is subject to phosphorylation by SR-associated (and exogenously added) CaM kinase (52). We have also observed that a 64-kDa cytosolic protein (P_{64}) from heart muscle, which is capable of modulating Ca^{2+} transport across the SR in vitro (23), stimulates Ca^{2+}–ATPase phosphorylation while producing concomitant inhibition of Ca^{2+}-release channel phosphorylation in cardiac SR by the membrane-associated CaM kinase (77). P_{64} may serve to target the SR-bound CaM kinase from the Ca^{2+} channel to the Ca^{2+}–ATPase, and this may be facilitated by membrane repolarization. Future studies should be aimed to investigate these conceptual possibilities and the functional roles of SR-associated CaM kinase in vivo.

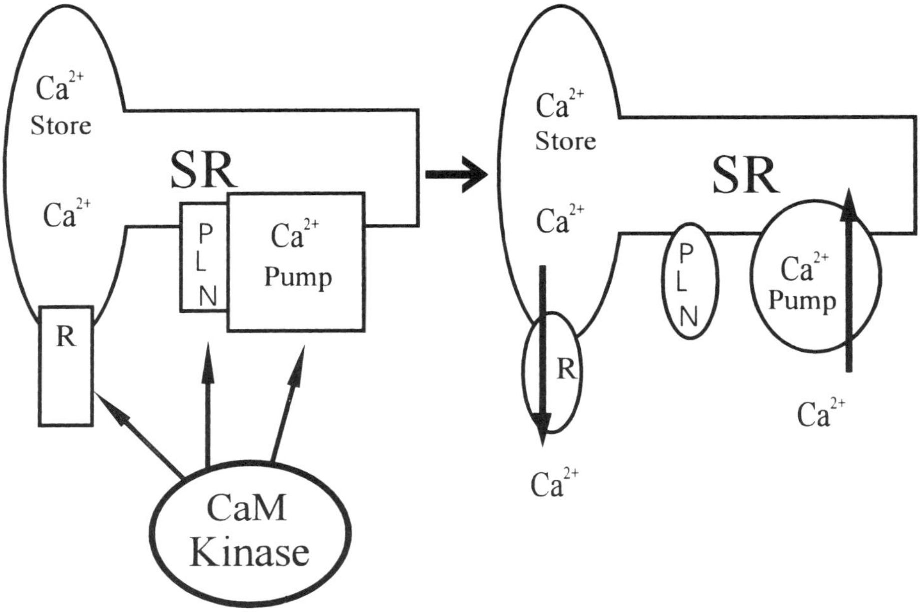

FIG. 19–7. Regulation of the Ca^{2+} uptake and release functions of cardiac SR through phosphorylation of multiple substrates by membrane-associated CaM kinase. In cardiac SR, membrane-bound CaM kinase phosphorylates three major proteins, namely, phospholamban (PLN) Ca^{2+}–ATPase (Ca^{2+} pump), and Ca^{2+}-release channel (R, ryanodine receptor). Phosphorylation is accompanied by changes in protein conformation and function. In its unphosphorylated state, phospholamban associates with the Ca^{2+} pump and inhibits Ca^{2+} pumping. Phosphorylation of phospholamban results in disruption of the physical interaction between the two proteins and the stimulation of Ca^{2+} pumping, mainly because of an increase in the affinity of the Ca^{2+}–ATPase for Ca^{2+}. Direct phosphorylation of the Ca^{2+}–ATPase and consequent changes in enzyme conformation results in stimulation of Ca^{2+} pumping due to an increase in V_{max} of ATP hydrolysis and Ca^{2+} transport. Phosphorylation of Ca^{2+} channel results in the activation of Ca^{2+} release, apparently due to an increase in the duration of the open state of the channel.

SUMMARY

In cardiac sarcoplasmic reticulum (SR), a membrane-associated Ca^{2+}/calmodulin-dependent protein kinase (CaM kinase) phosphorylates three major proteins, namely, phospholamban, Ca^{2+}-release channel (ryanodine receptor), and Ca^{2+}–ATPase (Ca^{2+} pump). Phosphorylation of phospholamban results in stimulation of SR Ca^{2+} pump activity, apparently because of the disruption of a preexisting inhibitory interaction between Ca^{2+}–ATPase and phospholamban. The functional consequence of ryanodine receptor phosphorylation has not been clearly established, but some evidence suggests that phosphorylation is associated with activation of Ca^{2+} release caused by an increase in the duration of the open state of the channel. Direct phosphorylation of the Ca^{2+}–ATPase by CaM kinase results in enhanced catalytic activity of the enzyme without alteration in its Ca^{2+} sensitivity. The phosphorylation of the Ca^{2+}–ATPase is isoform specific in that the cardiac and slow-twitch skeletal muscle isoform (SERCA 2), but not the fast-twitch skeletal muscle isoform (SERCA1), undergo phosphorylation by CaM kinase. Studies using SERCA 1 and SERCA 2 isoforms and their mutants expressed in a heterologous system have resulted in (a) confirmation of the isoform specificity of Ca^{2+}–ATPase phosphorylation by CaM kinase, (b) identification of Ser^{38} as the site in SERCA 2 phosphorylated by CaM kinase, and (c) demonstration of phosphorylation-induced increase in V_{max} of Ca^{2+} transport by the SERCA 2 enzyme. These observations suggest that in cardiac muscle, CaM kinase–mediated phosphorylation of Ca^{2+}–ATPase and phospholamban may serve mutually complementary roles in stimulating SR Ca^{2+} sequestration and therefore the speed of muscle relaxation. The SR-associated CaM kinase has been identified as a δ-isoform of CaM kinase II. Expression of this CaM kinase isoform and phosphorylation of Ca^{2+}–ATPase, phospholamban, and ryanodine receptor by the SR-associated δ-CaM kinase could be detected as early as 21 days of gestation in the rabbit. It appears that the CaM kinase regulatory system develops concurrently with the morphogenesis of the SR.

ACKNOWLEDGMENTS

We thank Susan Hunt for secretarial assistance and Bruce Arppe for preparing illustration photographs. The studies from the authors' laboratory reported here were supported by a grant from the Medical Research Council of Canada.

REFERENCES

1. Fabiato A. Time and calcium dependence of activation and inactivation of calcium-induced calcium release from the sarcoplasmic reticulum of a skinned canine cardiac purkinje cell. *J Gen Physiol* 1985;85:247–290.
2. Fleischer S, Inui M. Biochemistry and biophysics of excitation–contraction coupling. *Annu Rev Biophys Biophys Chem* 1989;18:333–364.

3. Bers DM. *Excitation–contraction coupling and cardiac contractile force.* Dordrecht: Kluwer Academic Press, 1991.
4. Lytton J, MacLennan DH. Sarcoplasmic reticulum: In: Fozzard HA, ed. *The heart and cardiovascular system.* New York: Raven Press; 1992:1203–1222.
5. Feher JJ, Fabiato A. Cardiac sarcoplasmic reticulum calcium uptake and release. In: Langer GA, ed. *Calcium and the heart.* New York: Raven Press; 1990:199–268.
6. Thompson RB, Warber KD, Potter JD. Calcium at the myofilaments. In: Langer GA, ed. *Calcium and the heart.* New York: Raven Press; 1990:127–165.
7. Tada M, Katz AM. Phosphorylation of sarcoplasmic reticulum and sarcolemma. *Annu Rev Physiol* 1982;44:401–423.
8. Davies BA, Edes I, Gupta RC, Young EF, Kim HW, Steenart NAE, Szymanska G, Kranias EG. The role of phospholamban in the regulation of calcium transport by cardiac sarcoplasmic reticulum. *Mol Cell Biochem* 1990;99:83–88.
9. Tada M, Kadoma M, Inui M, Fugi JI. Regulation of Ca^{2+} pump from cardiac sarcoplasmic reticulum. *Meth Enzymol* 1988;157:107–154.
10. Colyer J. Control of the calcium pump of cardiac sarcoplasmic reticulum: a specific role for the pentameric structure of phospholamban? *Cardiovasc Res* 1993;27:1766–1771.
11. Xu A, Hawkins C, Narayanan N. Phosphorylation and activation of the Ca^{2+}-pumping ATPase of cardiac sarcoplasmic reticulum by a Ca^{2+}/calmodulin-dependent protein kinase. *J Biol Chem* 1993;268:8394–8397.
12. Hawkins C, Xu A, Narayanan N. Sarcoplasmic reticulum calcium pump in cardiac and slow-twitch skeletal muscle but not fast-twitch skeletal muscle undergoes phosphorylation by endogenous and exogenous Ca^{2+}/calmodulin-dependent protein kinase: characterization of optimal conditions for calcium pump phosphorylation. *J Biol Chem* 1994;269:31198–31206.
13. Toyofuku T, Kurzydlowski K, Narayanan N, MacLennan DH. Identification of Ser^{38} as the site in cardiac sarcoplasmic reticulum Ca^{2+}–ATPase that is phosphorylated by Ca^{2+}/calmodulin-dependent protein kinase. *J Biol Chem* 1994;269:26492–26496.
14. Witcher DR, Kovacs RJ, Schulman H, Cefali DC, Jones LR. Unique phosphorylation site on the cardiac ryanodine receptor regulates Ca^{2+} channel activity. *J Biol Chem* 1991;266:11144–11152.
15. Takasago T, Imagawa T, Shigekawa M. Phosphorylation of the cardiac ryanodine receptor by cAMP-dependent protein kinase. *J Biochem (Tokyo)* 1989;106:872–877.
16. Takasago T, Imagawa T, Furukawa K, Ogurusu T, Shigekawa M. Regulation of the cardiac ryanodine receptor by protein kinase-dependent phosphorylation. *J Biochem (Tokyo)* 1991;109:163–170.
17. Narayanan N, Lee P, Newland M, Khandelwal RL. Evidence for an endogenous protein inhibitor of sarcoplasmic reticulum calcium pump in heart muscle. *Biochem Biophys Res Commun* 1982;108:1158–1164.
18. Narayanan N, Newland M, Neudorf D. Inhibition of sarcoplasmic reticulum calcium pump by cytosolic protein(s) endogenous to heart and slow skeletal muscle but not fast skeletal muscle. *Biochem Biophys Acta* 1983;735:53–66.
19. Narayanan N, Bedard P, Waraich T. Effects of endogenous calcium transport inhibitor from heart muscle on the active calcium uptake and passive calcium release properties of sarcoplasmic reticulum. *Can J Physiol Pharmacol* 1989;67:999–1006.
20. Donat ME, Su N, Narayanan N. Ontogeny of cytosolic proteins capable of modulating sarcoplasmic reticulum calcium transport in heart muscle. *Mol Cell Biochem* 1991;106:41–48.
21. Chiesi M, Geurini D. Characterization of heart cytosolic proteins capable of modulating calcium uptake by sarcoplasmic reticulum. 1. Isolation of a protein with protective activity and its identification as muscle albumin. *Eur J Biochem* 1987;162:365–370.
22. Chiesi M, Schwaller R. Characterization of heart cytosolic proteins capable of modulating calcium uptake by sarcoplasmic reticulum. 2. Identification of actin isoforms with inhibitory activity. *Eur J Biochem* 1987;162:371–377.
23. Xu A, Narayanan N. Purification, amino-terminal sequence and functional properties of a 64 kDa cytosolic protein from heart muscle capable of modulating calcium transport across the sarcoplasmic reticulum in vitro. *Mol Cell Biochem* 1994;132:7–14.
24. LePeuch CJ, Haiech J, Demaille JG. Concerted regulation of cardiac sarcoplasmic reticulum calcium transport by cyclic adenosine monophosphate-dependent and calcium/calmodulin-dependent phosphorylations. *Biochemistry* 1979;18:5150–5157.
25. Inesi G. Mechanisms of calcium transport. *Annu Rev Physiol* 1985;47:573–601.
26. Buss JE, Stull JT. Measurement of chemical phosphate in proteins. *Meth Enzymol* 1983;99:7–14.

27. Narayanan N. Multiple roles for the membrane-associated Ca^{2+}/calmodulin-dependent protein kinase in the regulation of sarcoplasmic reticulum function in heart muscle. In: Dhalla NS, Pierce GN, Panagia V, eds. *Pathophysiology of heart failure.* Norwell: Kluwer Academic Publishers; 1995:225–243.
28. MacLennan DH, Brandl CJ, Korezak B, Green NM. Amino acid sequence of a Ca^{2+}+Mg^{2+}-dependent ATPase from rabbit muscle sarcoplasmic reticulum, deduced from its complementary DNA sequence. *Nature* 1985;316:696–700.
29. Brandl CJ, Green NM, Korezak B, MacLennan DH. Two Ca^{2+}-ATPase genes: homologies and mechanistic implications of deduced amino acid sequences. *Cell* 1986;44:597–607.
30. Brandl CJ, deLeon S, Martin DR, MacLennan DH. Adult forms of the Ca^{2+}–ATPase of sarcoplasmic reticulum: expression in developing skeletal muscle. *J Biol Chem* 1987;262:3768–3774.
31. Zarain-Herzberg A, MacLennan DH, Periasamy M. Characterization of rabbit sarco(endo)plasmic reticulum Ca^{2+}–ATPase gene. *J Biol Chem* 1990;265:4670–4677.
32. MacLennan DH, Toyofuku T, Lytton J. Structure–function relationships of endoplasmic reticulum type Ca^{2+} pumps. In: Scarpa A, Carafoli E, Papa S, eds. *Ion-motive ATPases: structure, function and regulation.* New York: New York Academy of Sciences; 1992:1–10.
33. Inesi G, Kirtley ME. Structural features of cation transport ATPases. *J Bioenerg Biomembr* 1992; 24:271–283.
34. Lytton J, Westlin M, Burk SE, Shull GE, MacLennan DH. Functional comparisons between isoforms of the sarcoplasmic or endoplasmic reticulum family of calcium pumps. *J Biol Chem* 1992; 267:14483–14489.
35. VanWinkle WB, Tate CA, Blick RJ, Entman ML. Nucleotide triphosphate utilization by cardiac and skeletal muscle sarcoplasmic reticulum: evidence for hydrolysis cycle not coupled to intermediate acylphosphate formation and calcium translocation. *J Biol Chem* 1981;256:2268–2274.
36. Narayanan N, Su N, Bedard P. Inhibitory and stimulatory effects of fluoride on the calcium pump of cardiac sarcoplasmic reticulum. *Biochem Biophys Acta* 1991;1070:83–91.
37. Hawkins C, Xu A, Narayanan N. Comparison of the effects of fluoride on the calcium pumps of cardiac and fast-twitch skeletal muscle sarcoplasmic reticulum: evidence for tissue-specific qualitative difference in calcium-induced pump conformation. *Biochem Biophys Acta* 1994;1191:231–243.
38. Pearson RB, Woodgett JR, Cohen P, Kemp BE. Substrate specificity of a multifunctional calmodulin-dependent protein kinase. *J Biol Chem* 1985;260:14471–14476.
39. Gunteski-Hamblin AM, Grebb J, Shull GE. A novel calcium pump expressed in brain, kidney and stomach is encoded by an alternative transcript of the slow-twitch muscle sarcoplasmic reticulum Ca^{2+}-ATPase gene: identification of cDNAs encoding Ca^{2+} and other cation-transporting ATPases using an oligonucleotide probe derived from the ATP binding site. *J Biol Chem* 1988;263: 15032–15040.
40. Nakamura Y, Schwartz A. Possible role of intracellular calcium metabolism by [H^+] in sarcoplasmic reticulum of skeletal and cardiac muscle. *Biochem Biophys Res Commun* 1970;41:830–836.
41. Mandel F, Kranias EG, DeGende AG, Sumidar M, Schwartz A. The effect of pH on the transient state kinetics of Ca^{2+}–Mg^{2+}–ATPase of cardiac sarcoplasmic reticulum: a comparison with skeletal muscle sarcoplasmic reticulum. *Circ Res* 1982;50:310–317.
42. Fabiato A. Use of Aequorin for the appraisal of the hypothesis of the release of calcium from the sarcoplasmic reticulum induced by a change of pH in skinned cardiac cells. *Cell Calcium* 1985; 6:95–108.
43. Orchrad CH, Kentish JH. Effects of changes of pH on the contractile function of cardiac muscle. *Am J Physiol* 1990;258:C967–C981.
44. Sasaki T, Inui M, Kimura Y, Kimura T, Tada M. Molecular mechanism of regulation of Ca^{2+} pump ATPase by phospholamban in cardiac sarcoplasmic reticulum: effects of synthetic phospholamban peptides on Ca^{2+} pump ATPase. *J Biol Chem* 1992;267:1674–1679.
45. Tada M, Inui M, Yamada M, Kadoma M, Kuzuya T, Abe H, Kakiuchi S. Effects of phospholamban phosphorylation catalyzed by adenosine 3′ : 5′-monophosphate- and calmodulin-dependent protein kinases on calcium transport ATPase of cardiac sarcoplasmic reticulum. *J Mol Cell Cardiol* 1983; 15:335–346.
46. Wegener AD, Jones LR. Phosphorylation-induced mobility shift in phospholamban in sodium dodecyl sulfate-polyacrylamide gels. *J Biol Chem* 1984;259:1834–1841.
47. Fujii J, Kadoma M, Tada M, Toda H, Sakiyama F. Characterization of structural unit of phospholamban by amino acid sequencing and electrophoretic analysis. *Biochem Biophys Res Commun* 1986;138:1044–1050.

48. Simmemman HKB, Collins JH, Theibert JL, Wegener AD, Jones LR. Sequence analysis of phospholamban. *J Biol Chem* 1986;261:13333–13341.
49. Xu A, Narayanan N. Differential effects of fluoride on Ca^{2+}/calmodulin-dependent phosphorylation in cardiac sarcoplasmic reticulum. *FASEB* 1994;8:A162. Abstract.
50. Murphy AJ, Coll RJ. Fluoride is a slow, tight-binding inhibitor of the Ca^{2+}–ATPase of sarcoplasmic reticulum. *J Biol Chem* 1992;267:5229–5235.
51. Troullier A, Girardet JL, Dupont Y. Fluoraluminate complexes are bifunctional analogues of phosphate in sarcoplasmic reticulum Ca^{2+}–ATPase. *J Biol Chem* 1992;267:22821–22829.
52. Netticadan T, Xu A, Narayanan N. Ruthenium red inhibits Ca^{2+}/calmodulin-dependent phosphorylation of Ca^{2+}-release channel in cardiac sarcoplasmic reticulum. *Can J Cardiol* 1994;10:93A. Abstract.
53. Tokumitsu H, Chijwar T, Hagiwara M, Mitzutani A, Terasawa M, Hidaka H. KN-62, 1-[*N,O*-bis(1,5-isoquinolinesulfonyl)-*N*-methyl-*N*-methyl-L-tyrosyl]-4-phenylpiperazine, a specific inhibitor of Ca^{2+}/calmodulin-dependent protein kinase II. *J Biol Chem* 1990;265:4315–4320.
54. Hawkins CE, Xu A, Narayanan N. Evidence that the Ca^{2+}/calmodulin-dependent protein kinase intrinsic to cardiac sarcoplasmic reticulum is not CaM kinase II. *J Mol Cell Cardiol* 1994;26: CLXXXIX. Abstract.
55. Edman CF, Schulman H. Identification and characterization of δ_B-CaM kinase and δ_C-CaM kinase from rat heart, two new multifunctional Ca^{2+}/calmodulin-dependent protein kinase isoforms. *Biochem Biophys Acta* 1994;1221:89–101.
56. Schworer CM, Rothblum LI, Thekkumkara TJ, Singer HA. Identification of novel isoforms of δsubunit of Ca^{2+}/calmodulin-dependent protein kinase II: differential expression in rat brain and aorta. *J Biol Chem* 1993;268:14443–14449.
57. Baltas LG, Karczewski P, Krause EG. The cardiac sarcoplasmic reticulum phospholamban kinase is a distinct δ-CaM kinase isozyme. *FEBS Lett* 1995;373:71–75.
58. Briggs FN, Lee KF, Wechsler AW, Jones LR. Phospholamban expressed in slow-twitch and chronically stimulated fast-twitch muscles minimally affects calcium affinity of sarcoplasmic reticulum Ca^{2+}–ATPase. *J Biol Chem* 1992;267:26056–26061.
59. Kirchberger MA, Tada M. Effects of adenosine 3′,5′-monophosphate-dependent protein kinase on sarcoplasmic reticulum isolated form cardiac and slow and fast contracting skeletal muscles. *J Biol Chem* 1976;251:725–729.
60. Morris GL, Cheng HC, Colyer J, Wang JH. Phospholamban regulation of cardiac sarcoplasmic reticulum (Ca^{2+}–Mg^{2+})–ATPase: mechanism of regulation and site of monoclonal antibody interaction. *J Biol Chem* 1991;266:11270–11275.
61. Toyofuku T, Kurzydlowski K, Lytton J, MacLennan DH. Amino acids Glu^2 to Ile^{18} in the cytoplasmic domain of phospholamban are essential for functional association with the Ca^{2+}–ATPase of sarcoplasmic reticulum. *J Biol Chem* 1994;269:3088–3094.
62. MacDougall LK, Jones LR, Cohen P. Identification of the major protein phosphatases in mammalian cardiac muscle which dephosphorylate phospholamban. *Eur J Biochem* 1991;196:725–734.
63. Kranias EG. Regulation of calcium transport by protein phosphatase activity associated with cardiac sarcoplasmic reticulum. *J Biol Chem* 1985;260:11006–11010.
64. Steenaart NAE, Ganin JR, DiSalvo J, Kranias EG. The phospholamban phosphatase associated with cardiac sarcoplasmic reticulum is a type 1 enzyme. *Arch Biochem Biophys* 1992;293:17–24.
65. Davies P, Dewar J, Tynan M, Ward R. Postnatal changes in the length–tension relationship of cat papillary muscles. *J Physiol* 1975;253:95–102.
66. Nakanishi T, Seguchi M, Takao A. Development of the myocardial contractile system. *Experientia* 1988;44:936–944.
67. Anderson PAW, Glick KL, Marning A, Crenshaw C Jr. Developmental changes in cardiac contractility in fetal and postnatal sheep: in vitro and in vivo. *Am J Physiol* 1984;247:H371–H379.
68. Ishikawa H, Yamada F. Differentiation of the sarcoplasmic reticulum and T-system in developing mouse cardiac muscle. In: Lieberman M, Sano T, eds. *Developmental and physiological correlates of cardiac muscle.* New York: Raven Press; 1975;1:21–35.
69. Olivetti G, Anversa P, Loud AV. Morphometric study of early postnatal development in the left and right ventricular myocardium of the rat. II. Tissue comparison, capillary growth, and sarcoplasmic alterations. *Circ Res* 1980;46:503–512.
70. Maylie JG. Excitation–contraction coupling in neonatal and adult myocardium of cat. *Am J Physiol* 1982;242:H834–H843.
71. Nakanishi T, Jarmakani JM. Developmental changes in myocardial mechanical function and subcellular organelles. *Am J Physiol* 1984;246:H615–H625.

72. Nayler WG, Fassold E. Calcium accumulation and ATPase activity of cardiac sarcoplasmic reticulum before and after birth. *Cardiovasc Res* 1977;2:213–237.
73. Fabiato A. Calcium release in skinned cardiac cells: variations with species, tissues and development. *Fed Proc* 1982;41:2238–2244.
74. Hawkins C, Xu A, Narayanan N. Ontogeny of Ca^{2+}/calmodulin-dependent protein phosphorylation in cardiac sarcoplasmic reticulum. *Proc Can Fed Biol Soc* 1994;37:173. Abstract.
75. Hain J, Onoue H, Mayrleitner M, Fleischer S, Schindler H. Phosphorylation modulates the function of the calcium release channel of sarcoplasmic reticulum from cardiac muscle. *J Biol Chem* 1995; 270:2074–2081.
76. Xiao RP, Cheng H, Lederer WJ, Suzuki T, Lakatta EG. Dual regulation of Ca^{2+}/calmodulin-dependent protein kinase II activity by membrane voltage and by calcium influx. *Proc Natl Acad Sci USA* 1994;91:9659–9663.
77. Hawkins C, Xu A, Narayanan N. Divergent effects of a cytosolic protein on Ca^{2+}/calmodulin-dependent protein kinase (CaM kinase) mediated phosphorylation of calcium pump and calcium channel in cardiac sarcoplasmic reticulum (SR). *Proc Can Fed Biol Soc* 1993;38:81. Abstract.

The Developing Heart,
edited by Bohuslav Ošťádal et al.
Lippincott-Raven Publishers,
Philadelphia © 1997.

20

Inotropic Responsiveness of the Perinatal Rat Heart

Bohuslav Ošťádal, Ivana Ošťádalová, and Frontisek Kolář

Institute of Physiology, Academy of Sciences of the Czech Republic,
Vídeňská 1083, 142 20 Prague 4, Czech Republic

Developmental variations of the contractile response of the mammalian heart have been described for most of the positive and negative inotropic drugs (for review see refs. 1,2). It seems likely that, despite significant interspecies differences, developmental changes may exist in all mammals, depending on the degree of maturation of systems involved in the control of contractile functions. There are, however, many controversies concerning the mechanisms of developmental variations in cardiac responsiveness that may partly reflect the different animal species studied. Nevertheless, it is worth noting that the ontogenetic conclusions are often based on the comparison of the adult myocardium with one randomly selected and poorly defined "fetal" or "neonatal" stage. Such an approach, probably sufficient for the study of later stages of ontogenetic development, is not acceptable for the perinatal period because rapid changes may occur during this phase of life (for rev. see ref. 3). Detailed information on the development of the contractile performance and response to inotropic agents during the perinatal period has been lacking. Furthermore, the experimental data on the ontogenetic differences in cardiac contractile responsiveness were obtained exclusively on healthy individuals. This approach is, however, far from clinical situations where interventions acting in the critical developmental periods may have serious consequences for further maturation.

Therefore, we examined the development of contractile properties of the cardiac muscle during the perinatal period in rats. Particular attention was paid (a) to the normal development of basal contractile performance, (b) to the inotropic effect of Ca^{2+}, verapamil (a sarcolemmal [SL]–L-type Ca^{2+} channel blocker), ryanodine (an inhibitor of Ca^{2+} release channel of the sarcoplasmic reticulum [SR]) and low extracellular sodium; (c) to the inotropic responsiveness of chronically hypoxic and malformed perinatal hearts. For this purpose, isolated heart was perfused in the Langendorff mode under constant pressure, proportional to the mean blood pressure for the given developmental stages (4,5), and electrically stimulated. The contractile function of the heart (developed force [DF], g, and its first derivative +

$(dF/dt)_{max}$, g.s^{-1}), was measured using an isometric force transducer and evaluated automatically with an on-line computer (6). Studies included in this survey have been carried out on the rat; the term *perinatal* means from prenatal day 20 up to the first week of postnatal life (3).

NORMAL DEVELOPMENT

Basal Contractile Performance

Cardiac development during the perinatal period is, at least in rats, not linear. Three different phases can be distinguished, prenatal and two postnatal: before and after the fourth day. This feature is also reflected in the time course of cardiac growth: the relative heart weight decreases from prenatal day 20 to day 22 and then increases, attaining a maximum value on postnatal day 4 (Fig. 20–1). The faster rate of growth just after birth is obviously due to the fact that the heart has to cope with a suddenly increased workload. This adaptation is associated with a rapid, predominantly hyperplastic growth of rat cardiac cells that starts to decrease between days 4 and 5 of postnatal life (7–9). The decrease in the heart weight to body weight ratio, characteristic for further postnatal development (10), suggests that the heart is working more effectively.

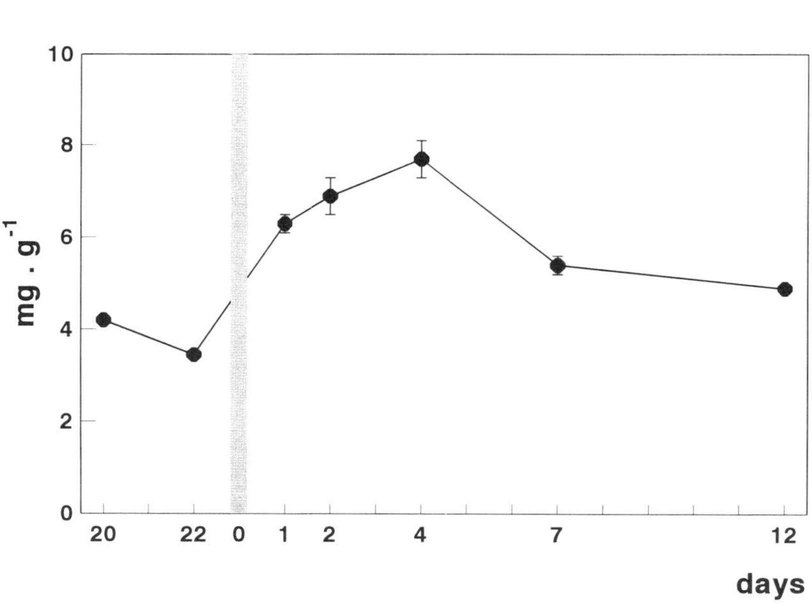

FIG. 20–1. Development of relative heart weight during the perinatal period of the rat. Values are means ± SEM. (Data partly from ref. 6.)

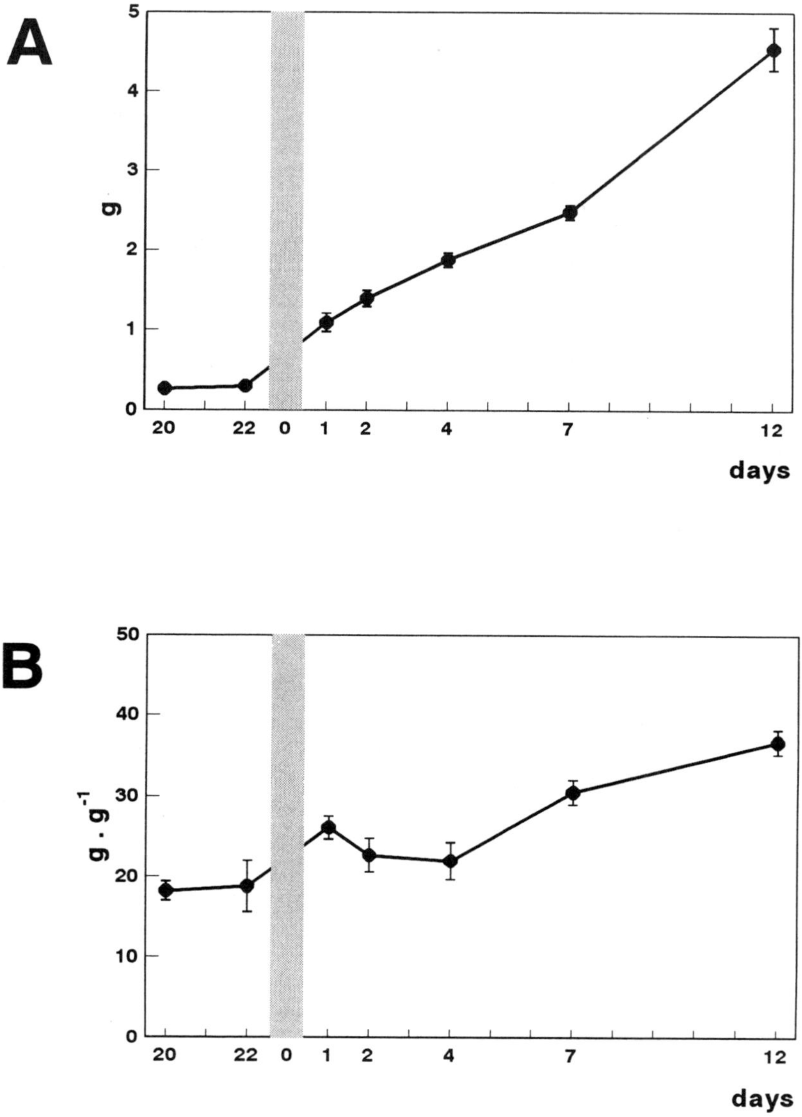

FIG. 20–2. Changes of DF (developed force) during the perinatal period of the rat. Values are means ± SEM. (**A**) absolute values of DF. (**B**) DF normalized to heart weight. (Data partly from ref. 6.)

The value of developed force DF increased throughout the whole investigated period (Fig. 20–2A); the maximum rate of contraction $+(dF/dt)_{max}$ exhibited a similar trend. The value of DF, normalized to heart weight, has a triphasic time course (Fig. 20–2B). The increase up to the day 1 of postnatal life is followed by a decrease until day 4 and a subsequent increase. This indicates that other factors than the simple growth of contractile units may also play a role. The increase of contractile performance of the mammalian hearts during the postnatal development (11) has been largely attributed (a) to an age-dependent change in α- and β-myosin heavy chain expression resulting in transition from low to high ATPase activity of myosin isoforms (for a review see ref. 12) and (b) to the maturation of the mechanisms controlling the intracellular calcium transients at the level of SR and SL. The contraction of perinatal myocardium depends to a large extent on the influx of Ca^{2+} across the SL via the calcium channels. During further development the ability of SR to accumulate calcium increases and there is a progressive maturation of calcium release from the SR. However, detailed day-by-day changes in the development of calcium transport and in myosin isoforms during the perinatal period are not known (13).

Inotropic Responsiveness

Ryanodine

The functional contribution of the SR to the control of myocardial contraction is believed to be reflected in the negative inotropic response to ryanodine. As follows from our data, a 40% decrease of contractile force due to ryanodine was already observed in 20-day-old fetuses, more than 50% drop being found in 1-day-old animals (Fig. 20–3). This is in good agreement with the results of Wibo et al. (14) which suggest that a substantial proportion of functional SR is already present in newborn rats. The same concentration of ryanodine (10^{-6} mol/L) almost completely inhibits the contractile activity of adult cardiac tissues (13–16).

Calcium and Calcium Antagonists

The sensitivity to the inotropic effect of Ca^{2+} (expressed as a percentage of the maximum value) increased significantly from prenatal day 20 to day 22 (Fig. 20–4); it did not change appreciably during the subsequent period, that is, up to day 7 of postnatal life. Except for 20-day-old fetuses, a maximum response in all experimental groups was attained at a concentration of 5.0–7.5 mmol/L. In the youngest fetal group the response to Ca^{2+} increased in the whole concentration range, that is, the maximum performance may be attained at an even higher concentration than 10 mmol/L (Fig. 20–4A). The absolute maximum value of DF increased during the whole period under study. On the other hand, DF normalized to

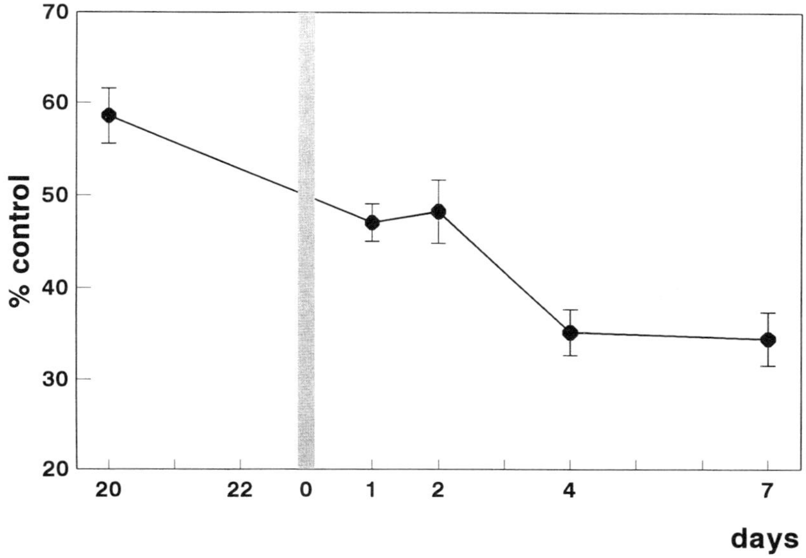

FIG. 20–3. Effect of ryanodine on DF (developed force) during the perinatal period of the rat. Values are means ± SEM. (Data partly from ref. 6.)

heart weight decreased from prenatal day 22 to day 4 of postnatal life and then increased again up to the end of the first postnatal week (Fig. 20–4B).

Postnatal day 4 appears to be critical also in the development of the contractile response to the calcium antagonist verapamil (Fig. 20–5). The highest sensitivity to the negative inotropic effect was observed not on day 1 of postnatal life, as expected, but on day 4. This means that the sensitivity to verapamil increases between day 1 and 4. Later, the sensitivity of the rat myocardium to the calcium antagonists starts to decrease, in accordance with our previously published results (16,17). The biphasic time-course may be hypothetically explained by a higher availability of intracellular calcium on day 1 than on day 4 because of the disproportionate development of different ways of Ca^{2+} entry during this period: a decreasing leakage of the immature cell membrane, insensitive to verapamil, and a slowly increasing number of functional calcium channels (18). Furthermore, shortly after birth (day 1–3) these channels (L-type) are localized at the SL surface only because T-tubules are not yet developed. During further ontogeny the number of sarcolemmal Ca^{2+} channels increases in newly occurring T-tubules in the close vicinity of terminal cisternae of SR. This favors the amplification mechanism of Ca^{2+}-induced Ca^{2+} release from the SR and makes myocardial function less dependent on the influx of extracellular Ca^{2+} (13).

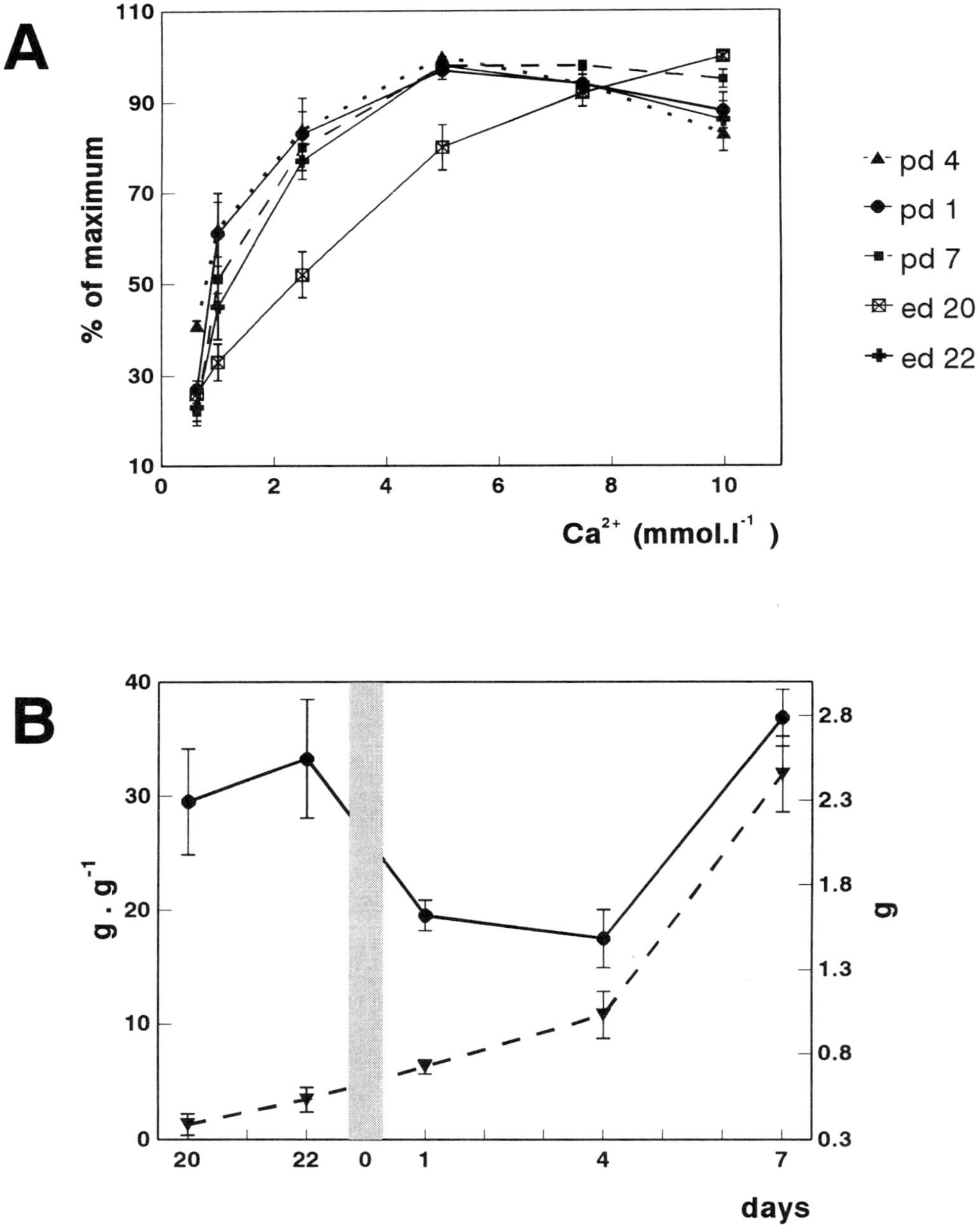

FIG. 20–4. (**A**) Sensitivity of the perinatal rat heart to Ca^{2+}. Effect of increasing concentration of extracellular Ca^{2+} on DF (developed force) expressed as a percentage of the maximum values. (**B**) Absolute values of maximum DF (developed force), dotted line; maximum DF normalized to heart weight, full line. Values are means ± SEM. (Data partly from ref. 6.)

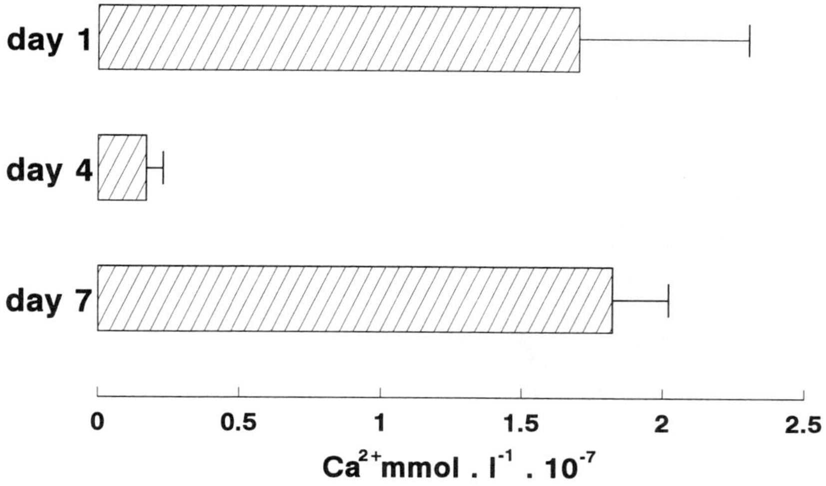

FIG. 20–5. Sensitivity of the perinatal rat heart to the calcium antagonist verapamil (expressed as IC_{50}, that is, the concentration of verapamil that decreased cardiac contractility by 50%). Values are means ± SEM. (Data partly from ref. 6.)

Low Extracellular Sodium

Low extracellular sodium (LES) induces Ca^{2+} loading of adult cardiomyocytes: the increase in intracellular Ca^{2+} concentration is caused by a change in the ratio of outward to inward Ca fluxes via the Na^{+}–Ca^{2+} exchanger (19). In the adult isolated perfused rat heart, the inotropic response to LES was described to consist of three phases: an initial increase of DF, followed by a depression of contractions together with an increase of resting tension, and finally a delayed increase of DF (20,21).

Our results have shown (22) that the pattern of inotropic response of the perfused immature heart to LES (35 mmol/L^{-1}) significantly differs from that described in adults, both qualitatively and quantitatively (Fig. 20–6). In fetal hearts (prenatal day 20) LES induced a persistent increase of contractions, whereas on postnatal days 1 and 2 this positive inotropic response was only transient. The LES-induced increase of the resting force was first observed on postnatal day 2, but in a limited numbers of animals. The first signs of the triphasic response appeared on the fourth day of postnatal life. The age-dependent quantitative difference was most pronounced in phase 3 (delayed increase of DF), which in immature heart (day 4) did not reach the starting control values. During further development, the magnitude of phase 3 increased in a stepwise manner, but even on day 7, the last day of our observation, it did not attain the adult level.

The absolute values of the initial increase of contractions were significantly higher up to postnatal day 2 compared with 4- and 7-day-old hearts. This supports

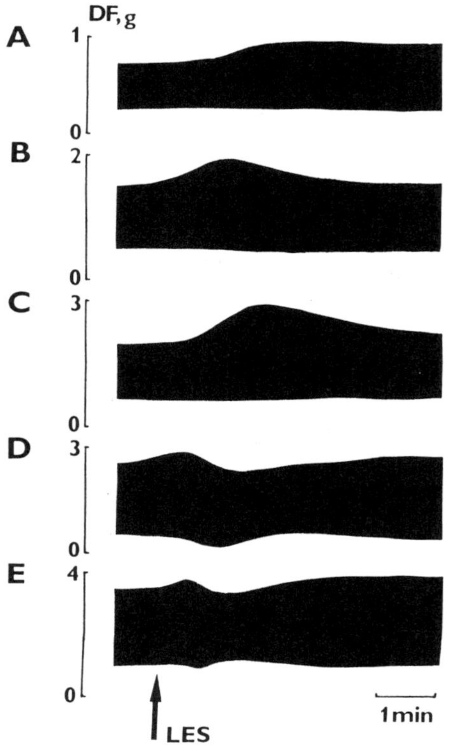

FIG. 20–6. Inotropic response to low extracellular sodium (LES). Actual records of developed force (DF) on prenatal day 20 (**A**) and postnatal days 1 (**B**), 2 (**C**), 4 (**D**), and 7 (**E**). *Arrow* indicates the onset of perfusion with LES (35 mmol.l^{-1} Na^+). (Reproduced with permission from ref. 22.)

the observation that the activity of Na^+–Ca^{2+} exchange decreases in rats during the early postnatal period (23). The secondary depression of contraction and the rise of the resting force appeared to be the consequence of the short intracellular Ca^{2+} overload. Furthermore, the recovery of contractions and the delayed positive inotropic response may be the result of the intracellular redistribution of excessive Ca^{2+} into the SR and mitochondria (21).

It is obvious that a satisfactory explanation of the rapid perinatal changes in cardiac inotropic responses to LES is hardly possible on the basis of the present incomplete information about cardiac development. A detailed analysis of the age-dependent mechanisms controlling the actual intracellular concentrations of Na^+ and Ca^{2+} is therefore highly desirable.

EFFECT OF PRENATAL PATHOLOGIC INTERVENTIONS

Prenatal Hypoxia

Pathogenetic factors acting during the prenatal period (e.g., stress, hypoxia, toxic effects of drugs) may have serious consequences for further maturation

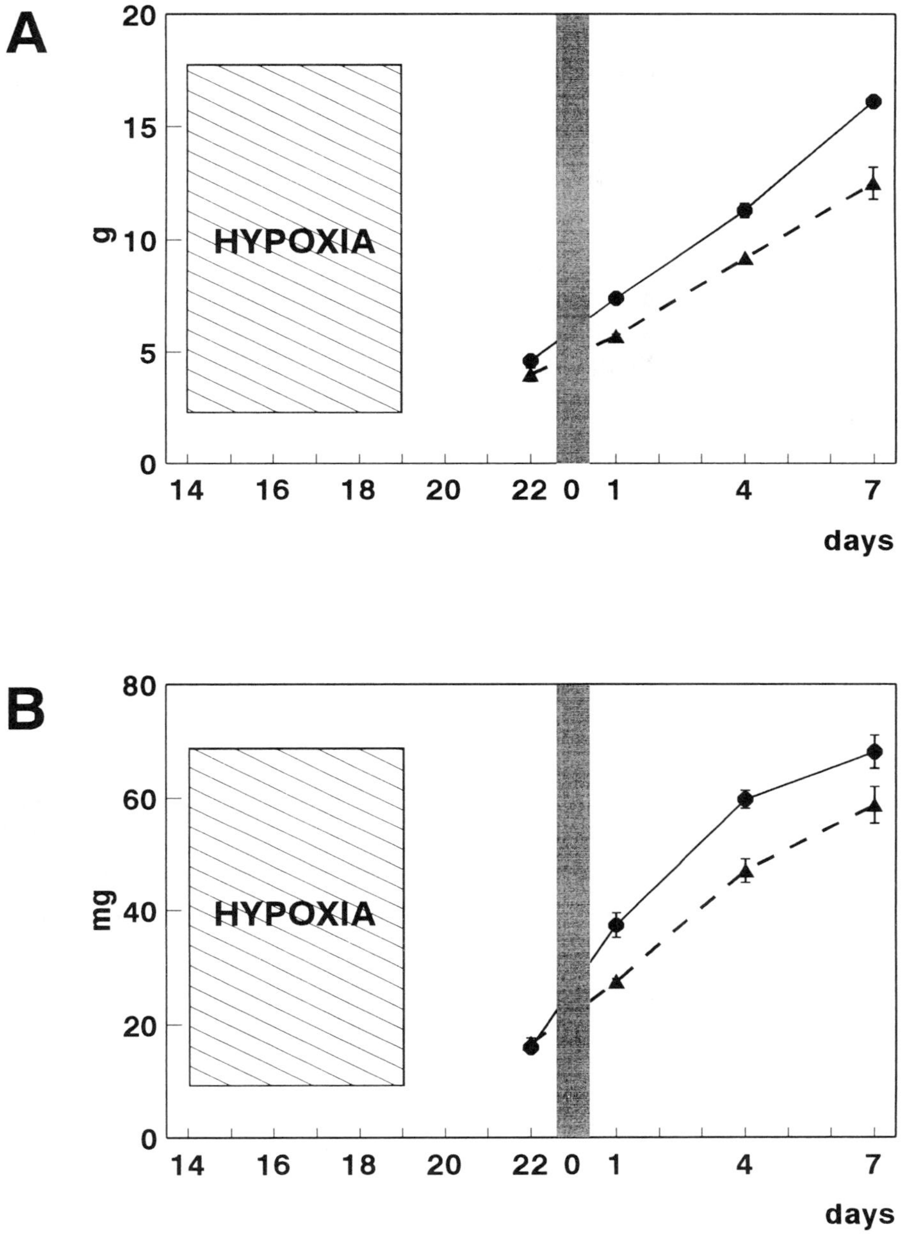

FIG. 20–7. The effect of prenatal intermittent high-altitude hypoxia (*dotted column*) on the (**A**) body weight and (**B**) heart weight during the perinatal period of the rat. Dotted line, experimental group; full line, controls. Values are means ± SEM. (Data from ref. 26.)

(24,25). The aim of our study was, therefore, to evaluate the cardiac contractile function in rats exposed prenatally to hypoxic stress. Experimental pregnant rats were exposed to intermittent high-altitude hypoxia simulated in a barochamber from day 14 to day 18 of pregnancy. The fetuses were investigated on day 22 of pregnancy and the offspring on days 1, 4, and 7 of postnatal life (26).

Body and heart weights were significantly lower in experimental rats as compared with the controls starting from day 1 of postnatal life (Fig. 20–7). The sensitivity to the inotropic effect of Ca^{2+} (expressed as a percentage of the maximum value of DF) was in experimental animals significantly decreased on prenatal day 22. This trend was apparent on postnatal day 1 and disappeared on days 4 and 7 (Fig. 20–8).

Our results have shown that prenatal maternal hypoxia influenced the body growth of the offspring as well as cardiac inotropic responsiveness to extracellular Ca^{2+}. The effect occurred with some delay but persisted even 12 days after the last

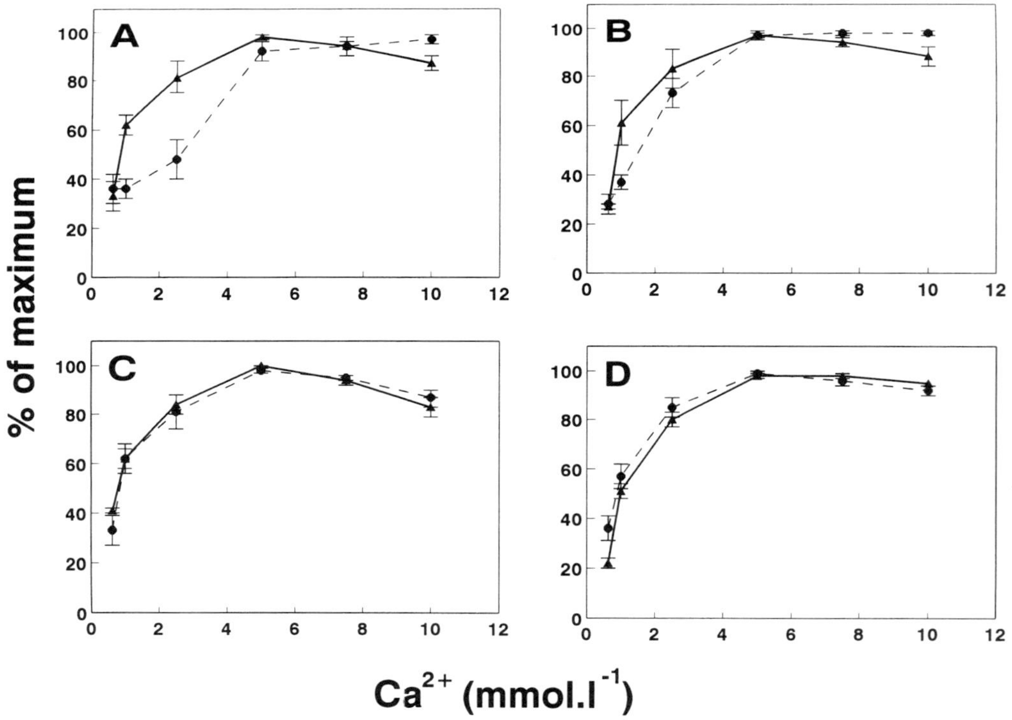

FIG. 20–8. The effect of prenatal intermittent high-altitude hypoxia on the sensitivity to increasing Ca^{2+} concentration expressed as percentage of maximum value of DF (developed force) in the control (*full dots*) and experimental hearts (*circles*) on prenatal day 22 (**A**) and postnatal days 1 (**B**), 4 (**C**), and 7 (**D**). Values are means ± SEM. (Data from ref. 26.)

exposure. This may suggest that the development of Ca^{2+} handling could be altered. The preceding changes may be induced by at least three different factors: undernutrition, stress-induced catecholamines and maternal hypoxia per se. Our results do not permit us to determine the most relevant cause. It seems interesting to mention that even a short period of perinatal hypoxia could induce permanent changes in the rat pulmonary vasculature (27,28). The possibility that prenatal hypoxia alters different physiologic processes that are activated by the lack of oxygen must also be taken into consideration.

Retinoic Acid–Induced Malformations

Congenital heart disease is the most frequent major malformation in the human population. It is due to chromosomal anomalies (8%) and to teratogenic agents in the environment (2%), but 90% of cases have a multifactorial origin (29). Most of the embryogenetic theories are still purely speculative; one reason is the absence of an adequate animal model for experimental analysis of the pathogenesis of congenital heart disease. It has been shown that administration of all-*trans* retinoic acid to pregnant dams induced cardiac malformations such as transposition of great arteries and double outlet right ventricle (30). Retinoic acid obviously interferes with cardiac development: it passes through the cell membrane, to be bound by a cellular retinoic acid-binding protein. Nuclear retinoic acid receptors are involved in the interactions with DNA and DNA transcription. This mechanism is responsible for the various biological effects known to influence almost every tissue in an organism (31). The aim of our study was to compare the inotropic effect of increasing concentrations of Ca^{2+} in the fetal rat heart with and without retinoic acid-induced malformations. For this purpose, pregnant Wistar rats were given 125 $mg.kg^{-1}$ of all-*trans* retinoic acid by gastric tubing on embryonic day 13 and 13.5 (32).

Our results have shown that the administration of retinoic acid influenced the growth of rat fetuses (2.52 $\pm$ 0.07 g and 3.30 $\pm$ 0.14 g, respectively), supporting the view that its effect is more complex and that heart is not the only target tissue. Retinoic acid negatively influenced the contractile parameters of fetal (20-day-old) rat hearts. The most pronounced was this effect on DF at most Ca^{2+} concentrations (Fig. 20–9A). The sensitivity to Ca^{2+}, expressed as the concentration at which 30% of maximum was attained, was significantly lower in malformed heart; but the sensitivity did not differ at higher Ca^{2+} concentrations (Fig. 20–9B). This implies that the malformed heart is significantly more dependent on the extracellular sources of Ca^{2+}.

From our data, however, it is difficult to distinguish whether the described changes are due to a retinoic acid effect on Ca^{2+} handling or to abnormal cardiac morphology. Detailed analysis of myocardial ultrastructure in retinoic acid–exposed hearts, with particular attention to the systems involved in Ca^{2+} handling, may be very helpful in this respect. Moreover, no data are yet available on the hemodynamic alterations in different types of retinoic acid–induced malformations.

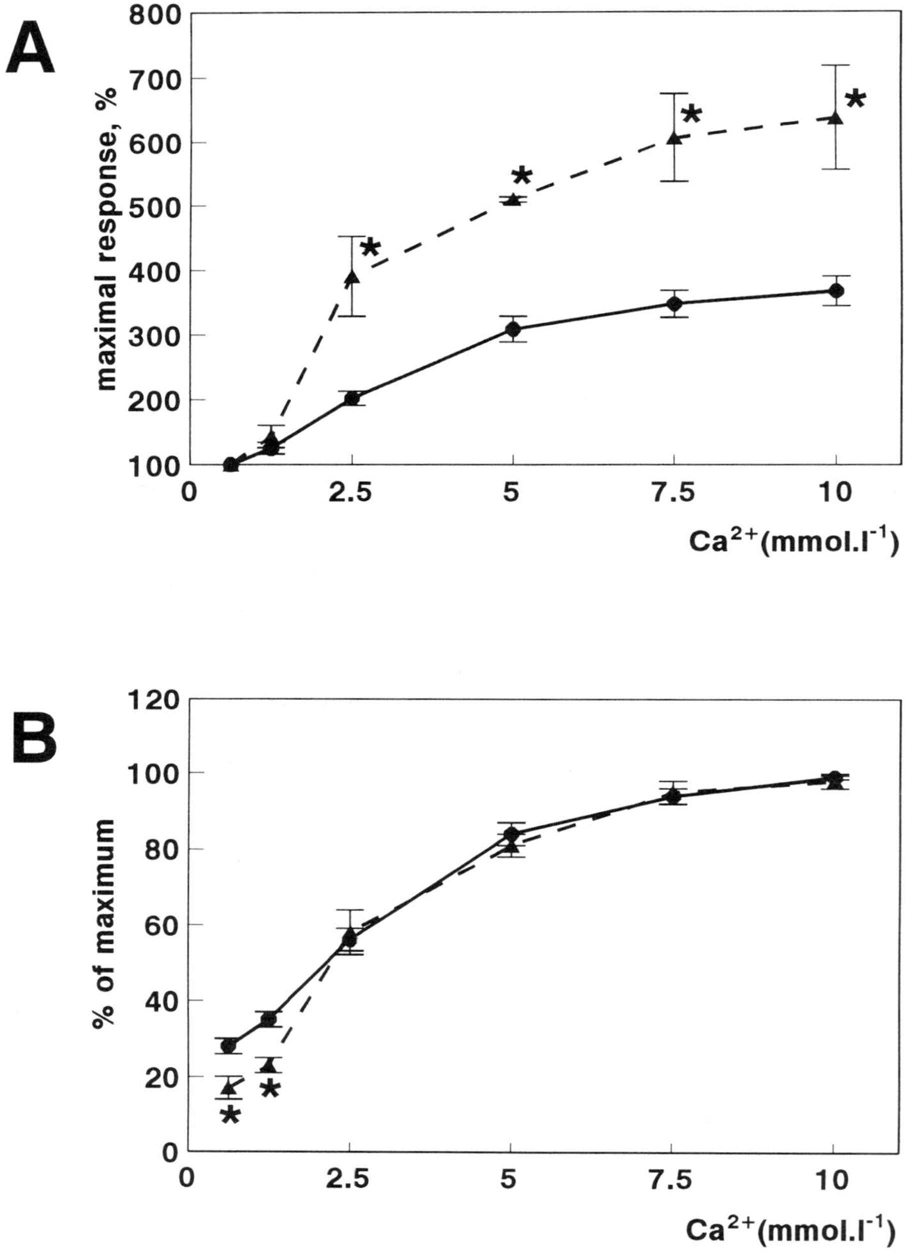

FIG. 20–9. The effect of retinoic acid on the inotropic response to increasing Ca^{2+} concentration expressed as a percentage of the lowest value of DF (developed force) (**A**) and as a percentage of the maximum value of DF (**B**) of control (*circles*) and malformed (*triangles*) hearts. Values are means ± SEM. (Reproduced with permission from ref. 32.)

SUMMARY

Our data show that the perinatal development of cardiac contractile function and its regulation at the level of Ca^{2+} transport is not linear and changes dramatically at least up to the end of the first week of life. The changes are obviously due to a disproportion between rapidly increasing functional demands and the structural and functional ability of the myocardium to fulfil these requirements. Prenatal interventions may significantly alter the cardiac function and inotropic responsiveness even postnatally. Our results suggest that rapidly changing inotropic responsiveness must be taken into account when inotropic drugs are used in clinical practice during early phases of ontogenetic development.

ACKNOWLEDGMENT

This study was supported by research grant 3508-3 from the Czech Ministry of Health.

REFERENCES

1. Artman M. Developmental changes in myocardial contractile responses to inotropic agents. *Cardiovasc Res* 1992;26:3–13.
2. Ošťádal B, Kolář F, Škovránek J, Ošťádalová I. Ontogenetic development of cardiac inotropic responsiveness. In: Ošťádal B, Dhalla NS, eds. *Heart function in health and disease.* Dordrecht: Kluwer Academic, 1993.
3. Riva E, Hearse DJ. *The developing myocardium.* Mount Kisco, NY: Futura, 1991.
4. Lichtfield JB. Blood pressure in infant rats. *Physiol Zool* 1958;31:1–6.
5. Zicha J, Kuneš J, Jelínek J. Experimental hypertension in young and adult animals. *Hypertension* 1986;8:1096–1104.
6. Ošťádalová I, Kolář F, Ošťádal B, Rohlíček V, Rohlíček J, Procházka J. Early postnatal development of contractile performance and responsiveness to Ca^{2+}, verapamil and ryanodine in the isolated rat heart. *J Mol Cell Cardiol* 1993;25:733–740.
7. Anversa P, Olivetti G, Loud AV. Morphometric study of early postnatal development in the left and right ventricular myocardium of the rat. I. Hypertrophy, hyperplasia, and binucleation of myocytes. *Circ Res* 1980;46:495–502.
8. Rakušan K, Jelínek J, Korecký B, Soukupová M, Poupa O. Postnatal development of muscle fibres and capillaries in the rat heart. *Physiol Bohemoslov* 1965;14:32–33.
9. Zak R. Development of proliferative capacity of cardiac muscle cells. *Circ Res* 1974;53:suppl II; 17–26.
10. Ošťádal B, Wachtlová M, Bílý J, Rakušan K, Poupa O. Weight of the heart in the rat before and after birth. *Physiol Bohemoslov* 1967;16:111–115.
11. Nakanishi T, Seguchi M, Takao A. Development of the myocardial contractile system. *Experientia* 1988;44:936–944.
12. Swynghedauw B. Developmental and functional adaptation of contractile proteins in cardiac and skeletal muscles. *Physiol Rev* 1986;66:710–771.
13. Tanaka H, Shigenobu K. Effect of ryanodine on neonatal and adult rat heart: developmental increase in sarcoplasmic reticulum function. *J Mol Cell Cardiol* 1989;21:1305–1313.
14. Wibo M, Bravo G, Godfraind T. Postnatal maturation of excitation–contraction coupling in rat ventricle in relation to the subcellular localization and surface density of 1,4-dihydropyridine and ryanodine receptors. *Circ Res* 1991;68:662–673.
15. Chin TK, Friedman WF, Klitzner TS. Developmental changes in cardiac myocyte calcium regulation. *Circ Res* 1990;67:574–579.

16. Kolář F, Ošt'ádal B, Papoušek F. Effect of verapamil on contractile function of the isolated perfused rat heart during postnatal ontogeny. *Basic Res Cardiol* 1990;85:429–434.
17. Škovránek J, Ošt'ádal B, Pelouch V, Procházka J. Ontogenetic differences in cardiac sensitivity to verapamil in rats. *Pediatr Cardiol* 1986;7:25–29.
18. Kazazoglou T, Schmid A, Renaud JF, Ladzunski M. Ontogenic appearance of Ca^{2+} channels characterized as binding sites for nitrendipine during development of nervous, skeletal and cardiac muscle systems in the rat. *FEBS Lett* 1983;164:75–79.
19. Bers DM. Early transient depletion of extracellular Ca during individual cardiac muscle contractions. *Am J Physiol* 1983;244:H462–H468.
20. Watanabe H, Ishide N, Takishima T. Twitch contractions during low Na^{+}-induced $[Ca^{2+}]_i$ overload in rat ventricular muscle. *Am J Physiol* 1987;253:H737–H744.
21. Kolář F, Cole WC, Ošt'ádal B, Dhalla NS. Transient inotropic effects of low extracellular sodium in perfused rat heart. *Am J Physiol* 1990;259:H712–H719.
22. Ošt'ádalová I, Kolář F, Ošt'ádal B. Inotropic effect of low extracellular sodium on perfused perinatal rat heart. *Can J Physiol Pharmacol* 1995;73:50–54.
23. Vetter R, Studer R, Reinecke H, Drexler H, Holm J. Postnatal expression changes of cardiac sarcolemmal Na^{+}/Ca^{2+} exchanger and sarcoplasmic reticulum Ca^{2+} ATPase are inversely related. *J Mol Cell Cardiol* 1993;25:S93.
24. Benedetti TJ. Life-threatening complications of betamimetic therapy for pre-term labor inhibition. *Clin Perinatol* 1986;13:843–852.
25. Ošt'ádal B, Beamish RE, Barwinski J, Dhalla NS. Ontogenetic development of cardiac sensitivity to catecholamines. *J Appl Cardiol* 1989;4:467–486.
26. Ošt'ádalová I, Ošt'ádal B, Kolář F. Effect of prenatal hypoxia on contractile performance and responsiveness to Ca^{2+} in the isolated perinatal rat heart. *Physiol Res* 1995;44:135–137.
27. Heymann MA, Hoffman JIE. Persistent pulmonary hypertension syndromes in the newborn. In: Weir EK, Reeves JT, eds. *Pulmonary hypertension.* Mount Kisco, NY: Futura; 1984:45–71.
28. Hampl V, Herget J. Perinatal hypoxia increases hypoxic pulmonary vasoconstriction in adult rats recovering from chronic exposure to hypoxia. *Am Rev Resp Dis* 1990;142:619–624.
29. Pexieder T, Bloch D, Beuret A. Eurocat collaborative study of congenital heart disease. *Eur J Epidemiol* 1989;5:254–262.
30. Pexieder T, Pfinzenmaier RM, Prados-Frutos JC. Prenatal pathogenesis of the transposition of the great arteries. *Teratology* 1990;41:584–596.
31. Pexieder T, Pfinzenmaier RM, Prados-Frutos JC. Prenatal pathogenesis of the transposition of great arteries. In: *Transposition of the great arteries 25 year after Rahskind balloon septosomy.* Darmstadt: Steinkopff Verlag; 1992:11–27.
32. Ošt'ádalová I, Pexieder T, Ošt'ádal B, Kolář F. Inotropic effect of increasing concentration of Ca^{2+} in the fetal rat heart with retinoic acid-induced malformations. *Pediatr Res* 1995;38:892–895.

The Developing Heart,
edited by Bohuslav Ošt'ádal et al.
Lippincott-Raven Publishers,
Philadelphia © 1997.

21

Digitalis Sensitivity in Developing Heart

*Jagdish C. Khatter and +Robert J. Hoeschen

Departments of Medicine (Cardiology) and Pharmacology and Therapeutics, Health Sciences Centre* and St. Boniface General Hospital+, 700 William Avenue, Winnipeg, Manitoba, R3E 0Z3 Canada*

It has been known for some time that newborn infants tolerate serum levels of digoxin almost twice as high as those of adults (1–3). This is equally true for most animal species (4–7). No substantial differences are found in absorption, distribution, or elimination of digoxin between infants and adults (8–11) or young and adult animals (12,13). Cardiac glycosides bind specifically to membrane-bound enzyme Na^+–K^+–ATPase and inhibit this enzyme in various tissues, including cardiac muscle. The enzyme is generally considered the receptor site for digitalis.

MEMBRANE-BOUND Na^+–K^+–ATPase ENZYME AND ITS FUNCTION

Na^+–K^+-activated adenosine triphosphatase (Na^+,K^+–ATPase) is a ubiquitous plasma membrane enzyme that plays a fundamental role in animal cells. By means of continuous function, transmembrane gradients of Na^+ and K^+, resting membrane potential and cell volume are maintained (14). It is believed that Na^+, K^+–ATPase changes its affinity for Na^+ and K^+ alternatively in the cycle of the ATP hydrolysis reaction coupled with the active transport of Na^+ and K^+. According to the postalbers scheme (15–18) deduced from kinetic studies on ATP hydrolysis by the enzyme, Na^+ binds to the intracellular Na^+ sites (5) on the E1 form of the enzyme and accelerates the phosphorylation from ATP. The formed Na^+ E1 ~ p.Mg^{2+} transforms to E2 p.Mg^{2+}, and this change is accompanied with the transport of Na^+ from the inside to the outside of the cell. Potassium then binds to the extracellular K^+ sites (5) on E2. p.Mg^{2+} and the formed K^+. E2-p.Mg^{2+} dephosphorylates to K.E2. Release of the K^+ E2 accompanied with the transport of K^+ from the outside to the inside of the cell is accelerated by the rebinding of Na^+ and ATP.

THE FUNCTIONAL Na^+,K^+–ATPase ISOFORMS IN THE MYOCARDIUM

Mammalian Na^+,K^+–ATPase is a noncovalent oligomer of equimolar amounts of α and β subunits that make up the mature functional enzyme (14). Three isoforms of the catalytic subunit have been identified, designated as α_1, α_2, and α_3 (19,20). Tissue-specific expression of αsubunit isoforms has been associated with the presence of various classes of Na^+,K^+–ATPase manifesting different sensitivities to inhibition by cardiac glycosides (21–24). The α_1 and α_3 mRNA isoforms are expressed in neonatal myocardium, whereas α_1 and α_2 mRNAs, but not the α_3 mRNA, are present in the adult atrial and ventricular muscle (20,25); α_2 mRNA comprises a minor component of α-mRNA isoforms in the normal adult rat heart (20,25). The developmental changes in the rat myocardium Na^+,K^+–ATPase have been shown by Orlowski and Lingrel (26), who demonstrated that, during the short interval between the second to the fifth postnatal days, the abundance of mRNAα_1, mRNAα_3, and mRNAβ remains relatively constant. However, the abundance of mRNAα_3 markedly decreases and that of mRNAα_2 increases between the fifth and fifteenth postnatal days. Guinea pig left ventricular muscle, on the other hand, contains two distinct molecular forms of the Na^+,K^+–ATPase catalytic α subunit (27), with high affinity contributing 55% and low affinity contributing 45%, respectively. The high-affinity molecular form is suggested to be involved in the positive inotropic effect of digitalis, whereas the low-affinity form may be involved in both inotropy and toxicity (27). The physiologic role of β subunit remains uncertain.

THYROIDAL ENHANCEMENT OF MYOCARDIAL Na^+,K^+–ATPase

Thyroid hormone (T3) stimulates the Na^+,K^+–ATPase of a variety of mammalian target tissues (28,29). The enhancement of Na^+,K^+–ATPase activity by T3 is associated with increased numbers of specific ouabain binding of Na^+-dependent phosphorylation sites of plasma membranes isolated from target tissues (30,31). Thyroid hormone induction of Na^+,K^+–ATPase in target tissues expressing more than one αisoform mRNAs, such as myocardium, raised the possibility of selective or preferential regulation of isoform-specific gene expression. In the developing rat neonatal brain, however, hypothyroidism reduced the expression of both the high and low ouabain sensitivity forms of the enzyme (32). These findings imply that differential regulation of the high-affinity form by T3 may be tissue specific. In hypothyroid rat myocardium, for example, the low-ouabain-sensitive Na^+,K^+–ATPase (K_i = 10^{-4} M) accounts for approximately 95% of the enzyme activity, while the high-ouabain-sensitive enzyme activity ($K_i = 3 \times 10^{-7}$ M) amounts to 5% of the total activity. Administration of T3 increased total Na^+,K^+ – ATPase activity by 1.6 times; the low-ouabain-sensitive activity increased 1.5 times, whereas high-ouabain-sensitive activity was stimulated by a factor of 3.2 (14). T3 thus enhances myocardial Na^+,K^+ – ATPase subunit mRNA abundance and Na^+,K^+–

ATPase activity and that the expression of the high- and low-ouabain-sensitive activities are probably a reflection of the abundance of the α_2 and α_1 isoforms, respectively. The thyroid hormone concentrations in the serum of neonatal rats are negligible at birth and increase dramatically during the first 2 weeks postnatally (33–35). The abundance of mRNAα_1, mRNAα_3, and mRNAβ, on the other hand, remains constant between the second and fifth postnatal days (32). The abundance of mRNAα_3, however, markedly decreases, and that of mRNAα_2 increases between the fifth and fifteenth postnatal days. The notion that T3 may act as a "molecular switch" has also been looked at by others (33) and in our laboratory. In the euthyroid neonates between the ages of 3 and 7 days, mRNAα_1, mRNAα_3, and mRNAβ_1 abundances are nearly constant, whereas mRNAα_2 is undetectable. During the intervals between postnatal days 7 and 21, mRNAα_3 decreases to negligible levels and mRNAα_2 becomes expressed and increased in abundance to account for 23.5% of the mRNAα pool by the twenty-first postnatal day. Although the decrease in mRNAα_3 occurs postnatally, while there is an increase in mRNAα_2, the percentage change is not the same, and it is unlikely that a "molecular switch" from one isoform to the other occurs in postnatal development. It is more likely that T3 augments the abundance of Na^+,K^+–ATPase subunit mRNAs for existing isoforms in the neonatal myocardium. It is, however, clear from the data published in the literature that the high-affinity isoenzyme (α_2 isoform) is involved in the inotropic effect of digitalis as found in rat (36), ferret (37), dog (38), and human (39).

DEVELOPMENTAL CHANGE IN THE MYOCARDIAL Na^+,K^+–ATPASE RECEPTOR BINDING CHARACTERISTICS OF CARDIAC GLYCOSIDES

Although the presence of high- and low-affinity isoenzymes in the myocardium may provide an explanation to the apparent differences of digitalis tolerance in human newborns or young and adult animals, the binding characteristics of the cardiac glycosides to the Na^+,K^+–ATPase enzyme receptor may ultimately reflect the differences in its sensitivity. Furthermore, the ultimate inotropic or toxic response of cardiac glycosides is determined by the amount of Ca^{2+} delivered to the contractile proteins at a given time (40), which may depend upon the developmental status of Na^+–Ca^{2+} exchanger.

Khatter and Hoeschen (41), using guinea pig heart, have earlier demonstrated that the number of digitalis receptor sites increases progressively in the fetus (45 days fetus, 2.2 pmol/mg potential and newborn (9.1 pmol/mg protein), and reaches adult level (13.3 pmol/mg protein) at 21–25 days of age. The affinity of the Na^+,K^+–ATPase receptor sites for ouabain (K_d, 8.68–9.22×10^{-9} mol/L) remain unchanged during development. Thus, there is a continuous developmental increase in Na^+,K^+–ATPase activity in fetal and newborn guinea pig hearts; maturity occurs at the age of 21–25 days (41). The ability of ouabain to inhibit the enzyme, however, remains the same throughout the development of guinea pig, with 50% inhibition occurring at 0.1 μmol/L concentration. Sperelakis (42) has also reported that the activity of Na^+,K^+–ATPase increases sharply during embryonic development in chick heart. Berman and Shortencarrier (43) have reported much higher Na^+,K^+–ATPase activity in adult sheep as compared to the fetus. The observations made by Atwood and Dunkley (44) that the newborn and adult sheep have the same myocardial Na^+,K^+–ATPase activity, however, remains unexplained.

DIGITALIS RESPONSE IN GUINEA PIG DURING DEVELOPMENT

In a whole animal model, ouabain (5 μg kg^{-1} min^{-1}) was infused in saline solution via the external jugular vein until fatal cardiac arrhythmias appeared (13). The fetal cardiac arrhythmias were characterized by 6–8 successive ventricular ectopics leading to sustained ventricular tachycardia and/or ventricular fibrillation. Figure 21–1 shows a typical recording of EKG, left ventricular pressure (LVP), and *dp/dt* before (basal) and after the infusion of ouabain in an adult (3 months old)

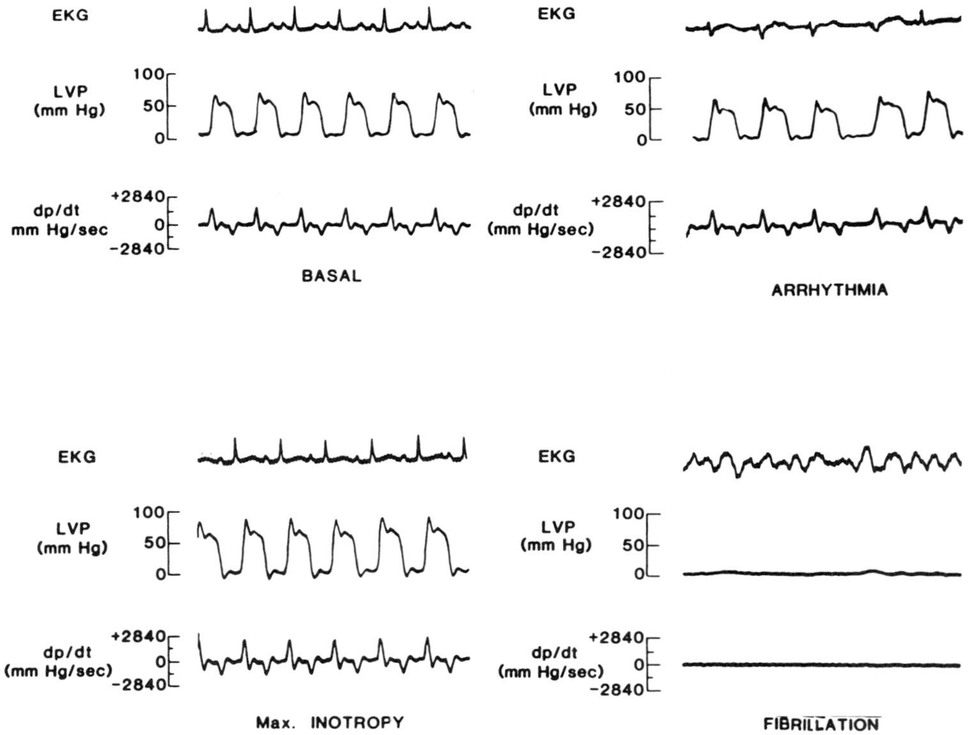

FIG. 21–1. Simultaneous recording of EKG, left ventricular pressure (LVP), and LV*dp/dt* before and during the infusion of 5 μg kg^{-1} min^{-1} ouabain, through external jugular vein in 3-month-old guinea pigs.

guinea pig. The basal LVP or its *dp/dt* of 3–5-day-old guinea pigs did not differ significantly from the values of 3-month-old guinea pig. The heart rate at 1–5 days old was, however, about 5% higher than that of 3-month-olds. Infusion of 0.04 ± 0.004 mg/kg ouabain in adult guinea pigs caused a maximal increase in + *dp/dt* of 43%. A total of 0.1 ± 0.004 mg/kg was necessary to initiate ventricular arrhythmias, whereas 0.14 ± 0.007 mg/kg ouabain was lethal. Guinea pigs of 1–5 days required 0.037 ± 0.007 mg/kg of ouabain for a maximum inotropic response of 37% increase over the basal *dp/dt*. The appearance of arrhythmias, on the other hand, was significantly delayed in 1–5-day-olds and required 75% more ouabain to initiate a toxic response. These developmental differences in tolerance of digitalis in guinea pig myocardium can be explained by lower density of receptor sites and reduced Na^+,K^+–ATPase activity in newborns and younger animals reported by us earlier (13).

DEVELOPMENTAL ALTERATIONS IN Na^+–Ca^{2+} EXCHANGE

It is now widely accepted that the effect of cardiac glycosides results from glycoside-induced inhibition of the membrane Na^+,K^+–ATPase, a rise in the intracellular Na^+ and subsequent increase in the intracellular Ca^{2+} through Na^+–Ca^{2+} exchange mechanisms. Tissue calcium has been reported to be lower in newborn rabbits than in the adult animals (45). In a recent study in our laboratory (13), using isolated sarcolemmal vesicles, it was demonstrated that the Na^+-dependent Ca^{2+} efflux activity is age dependent. The apparent rates of Ca^{2+} efflux seemed to be lower in the isolated myocardial sarcolemmal vesicles at 3 days of age than at 10 days of age, which in turn were lower than rates from adult animals. Similarly, substantial differences were observed in Na^+-dependent accumulated Ca^{2+}, both in initial period and in plateau phase, between the different age groups (13). The rate of Ca^{2+} uptake in myocardial sarcolemmal vesicles from 3-day-old guinea pig is significantly slower than that of 10-day-old guinea pigs, which in turn is significantly slower than that in vesicles from 3-month-old adult guinea pigs (13). Since digitalis sensitivity is a consequence of ultimate change in cellular Ca^{2+} metabolism, the observed developmental differences in Na^+–Ca^{2+} exchanger activity may be important.

SUMMARY

The apparent differences of digitalis tolerance in human newborns and adults or young and adult animals may be a consequence of several developmental changes. The initial binding interaction of digitalis to its receptor sites seems to be crucial to its ultimate response of inotropy or cardiotoxicity. The availability of high-affinity α_2 isoform of Na^+,K^+–ATPase receptor may thus be an important determinant for the positive inotropic response and the expression of both high-affinity α_2 and low-affinity α_3 isoforms for the differential cardiotoxicity during development. The developmental increase in the density of receptor sites observed by us (41) may thus represent an increase in both α_2 and α_3 isoforms. The inotropic dose of cardiac glycosides, which elicit a dose-dependent increase in the intracellular Na^+ activity (40, 46), may thus bind to high-affinity α_2 isoform of Na^+,K^+–ATPase and toxic concentration, which causes marked accumulation of intracellular Na^+ and intracellular Ca^{2+} (40,47,48), and may bind to both low-affinity α_3 and high-affinity α_2 isoform of the enzyme. The developmental changes in the thyroid hormone may play a role in the expression of these isoforms of the enzyme Na^+,K^+–ATPase. The activity of Na^+–Ca^{2+} exchanger is another important factor in determining the sensitivity of digitalis, as the exchanger is ultimately responsible for Na^+-related alteration in intracellular calcium and consequently sensitivity to digitalis (13,47,49). We have recently demonstrated a correlation between the developmental change in Na^+–Ca^{2+} exchanger activity and ouabain-induced inotropy and cardiotoxicity in guinea pig (13). Finally, toxic doses of ouabain have also been shown to release norepinephrine from the adrenergic nerve terminals (50). The extent to which this mechanism contributes to developmental sensitivity to digitalis is not clearly understood.

ACKNOWLEDGMENT

This work was supported by a grant to Dr. J. C. Khatter from the Heart and Stroke Foundation of Manitoba.

REFERENCES

1. Hayes C, Butler VP, Gersony VM. Serum digoxin studies in infants and children. *Pediatrics* 1975;52:561–568.
2. Gorodischer R, Jusko WT, Yaffo ST. Tissue and erythrocyte distribution of digoxin in infants. *Clin Pharmacol Ther* 1976;19:256–263.
3. Halkins H, Radomsky M, Bleiden L, et al. Steady state serum digoxin concentration in relation to digitalis toxicity in neonates and infants. *Pediatrics* 1978;61:184–188.
4. Wollenberger A, Jehl J, Karsh ML. Influence of age on the sensitivity of guinea-pig and its myocardium to ouabain. *J Pharmacol Exp Ther* 1953;108:52–60.
5. Halloran KH, Schimpff SC, Nicolas JG, Talner NS. Digitalis tolerance in young puppies. *Pediatrics* 1970;46:730–736.
6. Berman MA, Melmon KK, Rudolph AM. Differential effects of digoxin at comparable concentrations in tissue of fetal and adult sheep. *Circ Res* 1977;41:635–642.
7. Khatter JC, Agbanyo M, Hoeschen RJ, et al. Mitochondrial calcium overload in digitalis induced mechanical toxicity. In: Beamish R, Panagia V, Dhalla NS, eds. *Pharmacological aspects of heart disease*. Boston: Nijhof; 1987:313–327.
8. Dungan WT, Doherty JD, Harvey C, et al. Titrated digoxin XVIII studies in infants and children. *Circulation* 1973;46:983–988.
9. Hayes J, Butler VP, Gersony WM. Serum digoxin studies in infants and children. *Pediatrics* 1973;52:561–568.
10. Hernandez A, Burton RM, Patakhan et al. Pharmacodynamics of ^{3}H-digoxin in infants. *Pediatrics* 1969;44:418–428.
11. Wattrell G, Anderson KE. Clinical pharmacokinetics of digoxin in infants. *Clin Pharmacokinet* 1977;2:17–31.

12. Singh S, Gadgil S, Mirkin S. Age dependent factors influencing digoxin. Pharmacokinetics in the post-natal puppy. *Res Commun Chem Pathol Pharmacol* 1978;21:87–101.
13. Khatter JC, Agbanyo M, Navaratnam S, et al. Mechanisms of developmental increase in the sensitivity to ouabain. *Dev Pharmacol Ther* 1989;12:128–136.
14. Jorgenson PL. Mechanism of the Na^+,K^+–ATPase pump protein structure and confirmations of the pure Na^+,K^+–ATPase. *Biochem Biophys Acta* 1982;694:27–68.
15. Robinson JD, Flashner MS. The Na^+,K^+–ATPase enzymatic and transport properties. *Biochem Biophys Acta* 1979;549:145–176.
16. Post RL. Na^+,K^+–ATPase. In: Mukohata Y, Packer L, eds. *Cation flux across biomembranes.* New York: Academic Press; 1979:3–19.
17. Fukushima Y, Post RL. Binding of divalent cation to phosphoenzyme of Na^+,K^+–ATPase. *J Biol Chem* 1978;153:6853–6862.
18. Gicu GG, Melikian J, Faramarz I-B. Thyroidal enhancement of rat myocardial Na^+,K^+–ATPase; Preferential expression of α_2 activity mRNA abundance. *J Membrane Biol* 1990;115:273–282.
19. Shull GE, Greeb J, Lingrel JB. Molecular cloning of three distinct forms of the Na^+,K^+–ATPase α-subunit form from brain. *Biochemistry* 1986;25:8125–8132.
20. Young RM, Lingral JB. Tissue distribution of mRNA's encoding the α isoforms and β subunits of rat Na^+,K^+–ATPase. *Biochem Biophys Res Commun* 1987;145:52–58.
21. Charlemagne D, Moixent JM, Pretescille M, et al. Ouabain binding sites and Na^+,K^+–ATPase activity in rat cardiac hypertrophy. *J Biol Chem* 1986;261:185–189.
22. Swendner RJ, Farshi SK. Rat cardiac ventricle has two Na^+,K^+–ATPase with different affinities for ouabain: developmental changes in immunologically different catalytic subunits. *Proc Natl Acad Sci USA* 1987;84:8404–8407.
23. Takyasu K, Tamkun MM, Renaud KJ, et al. Ouabain sensitive Na^+,K^+–ATPase activity expressed in mouse L cells by transfection with DNA encoding the α-subunit of an avian Na^+ pump. *J Biol Chem* 1988;263:4347–4354.
24. Urayama O, Sweadner KJ. Ouabain sensitivity of α_3 isoenzyme of rat Na^+,K^+–ATPase. *Biochem Biophys Res Commun* 1988;156:796–800.
25. Orlowski J, Lingrel JB. Tissue-specific and developmental regulation of rat Na^+,K^+–ATPase catalytic α isoform and β subunit mRNAs. *J Biol Chem* 1988;263:10436–10442.
26. Orlowski J, Lingrel JB. Differential expression of the Na^+,K^+–ATPase α_1 and α_2 subunit genes in a murine myogenic cell line. Induction of the α_2 isozyme during myocyte differentiation. *J Biol Chem* 1988;263:17817–17821.
27. Bertrand IB, Maixent JM, Guede FG, et al. Two functional Na^+,K^+–ATPase isoforms in the left ventricle of guinea pig heart. *Eur J Biochem* 1991;196:129–133.
28. Curfman GD, Crowley TJ, Smith TW. Thyroid-induced alterations in myocardial Na^+,K^+–ATPase, monovalent cation active transport and cardiac glycoside binding. *J Clin Invest* 1977;59:586–590.
29. Philipson KD, Edelman IS. Thyroid hormone control of Na^+,K^+–ATPase and K^+-dependent phosphatase. *Am J Physiol* 1977;232:C196–C201.
30. Lo CS, August T, Liberman UA, et al. Dependence of renal Na^+,K^+–ATPase activity on thyroid status. *J Biol Chem* 1976;251:7826–7833.
31. Lin MH, Akera T. Increased Na^+,K^+–ATPase concentrations in various tissues of rats caused by thyroid hormone treatment. *J Biol Chem* 1978;253:723–726.
32. Schmitt CA, McDonough AA. Thyroid hormone regulates α and α_+ isoforms of Na^+,K^+–ATPase during development in neonatal rat brain. *J Biol Chem* 1988;26:17643–17649.
33. Dubois JD, Dussalt JH. Ontogenesis of thyroid function in the neonatal rat. Thyroxin (T4) and T3 production rates. *Endocrinology* 1977;101:435–441.
34. Dussault JH, Labrie F. Development of hypthalamic–pituitary–thyroid axis in the neonatal rat. *Endocrinology* 1975;97:1321–1324.
35. Young RA, Meyers B, Alex S, et al. Thyroxin binding to serum thyronine-binding globulin in thyroidectomized adult and normal-neonate rats. *Endocrinology* 1988;122:2318–2323.
36. Lelievee LG, Charlemagne D, Mouas C, et al. Respective involvement of high and low affinity digitalis receptors in the inotropic response of isolated rat heart to ouabain. *Biochem Pharmacol* 1986;35:3449–3455.
37. Ng YC, Akera T. Two classes of ouabain binding sites in ferret heart and two forms of Na^+,K^+–ATPase. *Am J Physiol* 1987;252:H1016–H1022.
38. Maxient JM, Charlemagne D, Chapelle B, et al. Two Na^+,K^+–ATPase isoenzymes in canine cardiac myocytes: molecular basis of inotropic and toxic effects of digitalis. *J Biol Chem* 1987;262: 6842–6848.

39. Rasmussen HH, Teneick RE, Okita GT, et al. Inhibition of electrogenic Na^+ pumping attributable to binding of cardiac steroids to high affinity pump sites in human atrium. *J Pharmacol Exp Ther* 1985;235:629–635.
40. Khatter JC, Agbanyo M, Navaratnam S, et al. Digitalis cardiotoxicity: cellular Ca^{2+} overload a possible mechanism. *Basic Res Cardiol* 1989;84:553–563.
41. Khatter JC, Hoeschen RJ. Developmental increase of digitalis receptors in guinea pig heart. *Cardiovasc Res* 1982;16:80–85.
42. Sperelakis N. Na^+,K^+–ATPase activity of embryonic heart and skeletal muscle as a function of age. *Biochem Biophys Acta* 1972;266:230–237.
43. Berman W, Shortencarrier W. Ouabain interaction with myocardial Na^+,K^+–ATPase from fetal and adult sheep. *Circulation* 1980;62(suppl III):24.
44. Atwood GF, Dunkley SP. Maturity of the ouabain sensitive Na^+,K^+–ATPase receptor in the newborn lamb heart. *Circulation* 1972;45/46(suppl II):36.
45. George BL, Nakaniski T, Jarmakani JM. The effect of developmental changes in membrane permeability to Ca^{2+} on cardiac function. *Pediatr Res* 1979;13:344–347.
46. Lee CO, Dagostino M. Effect of strophantidin on intracellular Na^+ ion activity and twitch tension of constantly driven canine cardiac Purkinje fibers. *Biophys J* 1982;40:185–198.
47. Goshima K, Wakabayashi S. Involvement of a Na^+, Ca^{2+} exchange system in the genesis of ouabain-induced arrhythmias of cultured myocardial cells. *J Mol Cell Cardiol* 1981;13:489–509.
48. Wier WG, Hess P. Excitation contraction coupling in cardiac Purkinje fibers: effects of cardiotonic steroids on the intracellular calcium transient, membrane potential and contraction. *J Gen Physiol* 1984;83:395–415.
49. Khatter JC, Navaratnam S, Hoeschen RJ. Protective effect of verapamil upon ouabain-induced arrhythmias. *Pharmacology* 1988;38:380–389.
50. Lathers CM, Roberts J. Digitalis cardiotoxicity revisited. *Life Sci* 1970;27:1713–1733.

The Developing Heart,
edited by Bohuslav Ošťádal et al.
Lippincott-Raven Publishers,
Philadelphia © 1997.

22

Age-Related Changes in the Contractile Response to Endothelin-1 and in Binding Characteristics of the Endothelin Receptor in Rat Ventricular Myocardium

Yumi Katano, *Akira Ishihata, and *Masao Endoh

*Division of Theoretical Nursing, Department of Nursing, Yamagata University School of Medicine, *Department of Pharmacology, Yamagata University School of Medicine, Yamagata 990-23, Japan*

Endothelin (ET) is an endogenous vasoactive peptide of 21 amino acids originally isolated from cultured medium of porcine aortic endothelial cells (1), which may be involved in the pathogenesis of various cardiovascular diseases. The incidence of cardiovascular disorders caused by coronary artery disease increases with advancing age, but the role of ET in this increase is unknown. We previously reported that the ET-1-induced coronary vasoconstriction increased with age in the isolated perfused rat heart (2).

It is now well established that a high density of ET receptors is found in mammalian myocardium (3–5), and these receptors mediate an increase in cardiac contractility in both experimental animals and humans (5–11). It has been reported that myocardial ET receptors are up-regulated in some pathologic states, such as ischemia and postischemic reperfusion (12), posthypoxic reoxygenation (13), and cyclosporine-induced cardiotoxicity (14), while the receptors are down-regulated in streptozotocin-induced diabetes (15) and hypertension (16).

Evans et al. (17) have found that unstimulated cultured endocardial endothelial cells express ET-1 mRNA and release ET-1 into superfusing effluent, and ET-1 released from this source could exert positive inotropic effect (PIE) in isolated cardiac myocytes with no intervention with coronary perfusion. Although ET-1 facilitates cardiac hypertrophy in experimental models (18), it remains unclear whether the PIE induced by ET is beneficial or detrimental to the heart under given pathophysiologic states.

Although the influence of senescence on cardiac β-adrenergic action has been addressed extensively, little is known about the influence of age on the inotropic response mediated by ET receptors. We reported previously that the PIE of ET-1 decreased with age in isolated perfused rat heart (2). In the present study we further examined mechanisms of the age-related changes in the ET-1-induced PIE in relation to the ET receptor binding in rat ventricular myocardium.

METHODS AND MATERIALS

Animals

For this study 2-, 6-, and 27-month-old male Fisher 344 rats were obtained from Charles River Japan (Atsugi, Japan).

Isolated Papillary Muscle Preparations

The rat was lightly anesthetized with ether, and papillary muscles were isolated from right ventricle. Muscles were mounted in 10-ml organ baths containing Krebs-Ringer bicarbonate solution (37 ± 0.1°C) of the following composition (in mM): NaCl 118, KCl 4.7, $NaHCO_3$ 24.9, $MgSO_4$ 1.18, KH_2PO_4 1.18, $CaCl_2$ 1.25, glucose 11, ascorbic acid 0.057. The buffer solution was aerated with a mixture of 95% O_2 and 5% CO_2 (pH 7.4). The muscles were electrically stimulated by square-wave pulses of 5-ms duration and a voltage about 20% above the threshold, at a frequency of 1 Hz. The force of isometric contraction was recorded on a thermal pen writing oscillograph (WR 3701, Graphic, Tokyo, Japan) by means of strain-gauge transducers (T7-15-240, Orientec, Tokyo, Japan). After an equilibration period of 1 hour, (±)-bupranolol (3×10^{-7} M) was added into the bath to eliminate the influence of endogenous norepinephrine on the direct effect of the test drugs. Bupranolol at this concentration did not affect the basal force of contraction. ET-1 was administered in a cumulative manner by stepwise increases (by log 0.5 units). When a steady level of contractile force was achieved at each concentration, peak force and time course of isometric contractions were measured. The contraction of mammalian myocardium is dependent on both Ca^{2+} flux across the plasma membrane and Ca^{2+} release from the sarcoplasmic reticulum (SR). Since Ca^{2+} release from SR plays an essential role in the development force in adult rat myocardium, and cyclopiazonic acid (CPA; 3×10^{-6} M) is a specific inhibitor of Ca^{2+}–ATPase in the SR (19), we used CPA to examine the role of SR in the age-related changes in ET-1 induced PIE in the rat ventricular muscle.

[^{125}I]-Labeled ET-1 Binding Assay

Details of the experimental procedure used to prepare the membrane fraction and of the binding assay were described previously (5). Briefly, pieces of ventricular muscle, including free walls and septum, were excised and homogenized in 10 volumes of ice-cold buffer (0.25 M sucrose containing 5 mM tris [hydroxymethyl] aminomethane [Tris] HCl and 1 mM $MgCl_2$, pH7.4) by means of a Polytron PT-10 (Kinematica, Lucerne, Switzerland) three times for 15 sec at a setting of 7. The homogenate was centrifuged at $500 \times g$ for 15 min at 4°C. The supernatant was filtered through a single layer of cheesecloth and centrifuged at $50{,}000 \times g$ for 20 min at 4°C. The resulting pellet was washed twice with ice-cold incubation buffer (50 mM Tris HCl, 10 mM $MgCl_2$, pH 7.5) by repeated resuspension and recentrifugation. The final pellet was resuspended in ice-cold incubation buffer, yielding a protein concentration of ~1 mg/ml.

The binding assay was carried out as follows: the incubation mixture contained 150 μl of membrane suspension (150–300 μg of protein), 50 μl of various concentrations of [^{125}I]-labeled ET-1, and 50 μl of incubation buffer containing 0.1% bovine serum albumin (BSA). The incubation began by adding [^{125}I]-labeled ET-1 and was carried out for 90 min at 25°C and terminated by adding 2 ml of ice-cold incubation buffer. Aliquots were taken and subjected to rapid filtration over a Whatman GF/C glass filter in an M-24R-type cell harvester (Brandel Biochemical Research & Development Labs, Gaithersburg, MD). The filters were washed rapidly with 12 ml (3×4 ml) of ice-cold incubation buffer. After drying for 1 hour at 90°C, the radioactivity bound to the membrane was counted by means of Gamma Counter (1470 Wallac Wizard, Turku, Finland) at an efficiency of 82%.

Nonspecific binding of [^{125}I]-labeled ET-1 was defined as the radioactivity bound to the membrane that was not displaced by a high concentration of unlabeled ET-1 (10^{-6} M). Specific binding of [^{125}I]-labeled ET-1 was defined as total binding minus nonspecific binding, which amounted to ~50% at 2.5 nM [^{125}I]-labeled ET-1. Protein was determined by the method of Lowry et al. (20).

Statistics

Experimental values are presented as means ± SEM. Differences between the groups were evaluated by one-way analysis of variance (ANOVA), including Dunnett's test and Duncan's multiple range test. A p value smaller than 0.05 was considered to be significant.

Drugs

Drugs used were ET-1 (Peptide Institute, Osaka, Japan), CPA (Sigma Chemical, St. Louis, MO, USA), (±)-bupranolol hydrochloride (Kaken Pharmaceutical Co., Osaka), and bovine serum albumin (BSA; Sigma Chemical, St. Louis, MO, USA). ET-1 was dissolved in redistillated water containing 0.01% BSA. CPA, which was dissolved in about 50% dimethyl sulfoxide as stock solution of 1.2 mM, was applied in a volume of 25 μl into the bath.

RESULTS

Influence of Aging on Myocardial Contractility

Basal force of contraction, total duration of contraction, time to peak tension, and half relaxation time ($RT_{1/2}$) were presented in Table 22–1. These parameters were measured at a steady-state level prior to the administration of (±)-bupranolol (3×10^{-7} M). There were no significant age-related changes in basal force of contraction. Total duration of contraction and time to peak tension tended to prolong with aging, but the difference was not significant. The $RT_{1/2}$ in 27-month-old rats was significantly longer than the value in 2- or 6-month-old rats.

Influence of Aging on the Inotropic Response to ET-1

Concentration–response curves for the inotropic effects of ET-1 at different ages are shown in Fig. 22–1. ET-1 elicited a concentration-dependent PIE in 2- and 6-month-old rats, but it scarcely affected the force of contraction in 27-month-old rats. In 2- and 6-month-old rats the PIE was induced at concentrations of 3×10^{-9} M and higher, the maximum response being achieved at 3×10^{-8} M. The maximum response to 3×10^{-8} M ET-1 was reached at 10–15 min after administration. The basal force of contraction and the maximal force in response to ET-1 (3×10^{-8} M) were 1.03 ± 0.14 and 1.52 ± 0.16 mN (n = 5) in 2-month-old, 0.99 ± 0. 13 and 1.28 ± 0.14 mN in 6-month-old (n = 5), and 1.05 ± 0.20 and 1.07 ± 0.22 mN in 27-month-old (n = 6), respectively. The maximum response to ET-1 amounted to 25.4 ± 7.2% of the maximum response to isoproterenol in 2-month-old and 14.9 ± 5.3% in 6-month-old rats, respectively. In aged rats, the positive inotropic response to isoproterenol also decreased in 27-month-old rats (data not shown).

Influence of CPA on the Inotropic Response to ET-1

CPA (3×10^{-6} M) was applied into the bath for 15–20 min before ET-1. The vehicle of CPA (3×10^{-6} M) did not affect the force of contraction in three age groups. CPA (3×10^{-6} M) alone produced a decrease in contractile force by 22.6 ± 4.0% in 2-month-old (n = 5), 23.6 ± 2.3% in 6-month-old (n = 6), and 14.4 ±

TABLE 22–1. *Basal force, total duration of contraction, time to peak force, and half relaxation time*[a]

Age (mo)	n	Basal force (mN)	Total duration of contraction (ms)	Time to peak force (ms)	Half relaxation time (ms)
2	5	0.83 ± 0.08	148.0 ± 6.04	51.0 ± 2.45	35.0 ± 0.95
6	5	0.88 ± 0.15	148.0 ± 3.74	52.6 ± 1.50	39.8 ± 2.75
27	6	0.99 ± 0.22	166.7 ± 8.43	61.3 ± 3.33	45.3 ± 2.39*

[a]Values are means ± SEM; n, numbers of experiments; *$P < 0.05$ vs 2-month-old rats.

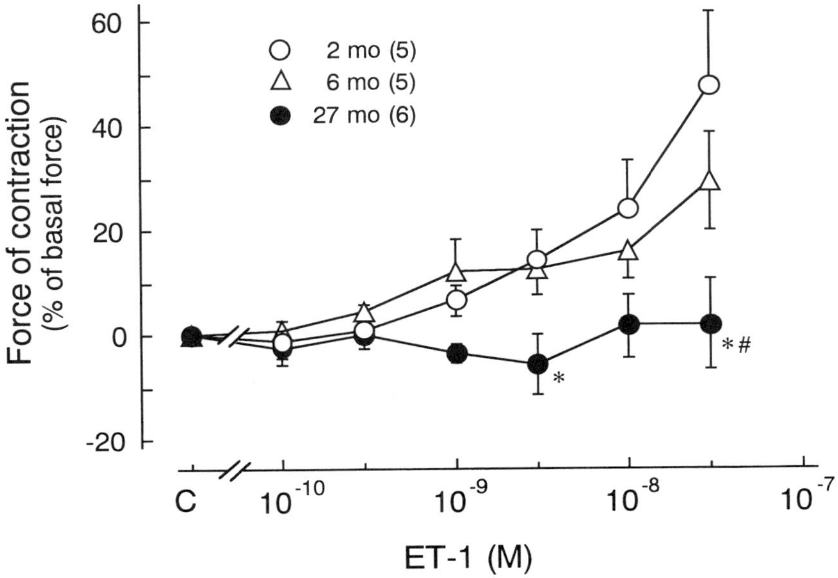

FIG. 22-1. Concentration–response curves for the positive inotropic effect of endothelin-1 in ventricular papillary muscles isolated from 2-, 6-, and 27-month-old rats. Papillary muscles were driven electrically at 1 Hz at 37°C in the presence of 3×10^{-7} M of (±)-bupranolol. *Ordinate,* force of contraction expressed as a percentage of the basal force of contraction. *Abscissa,* logarithmic concentration of endothelin-1. Figures in parentheses are numbers of experiments (n). Basal force of contraction, 1.03 ± 0.14 mN in 2-month-olds, 0.99 ± 0.13 mN in 6-month-olds, and 1.05 ± 0.20 mN in 27-month-old rats, respectively. All values presented are mean ± SEM. $^{*}P < 0.05$ (vs 2-month-old rats), $^{\#}P < 0.05$ (vs 6-month-old rats).

3.2% in 27-month-old rats (n = 6), respectively. The concentration–response curves for the inotropic response to ET-1 in the absence or the presence of CPA were shown in Fig. 22–2. Although $RT_{1/2}$ in 2- or 6-month-old rats was significantly briefer than that in 27-month rats (Table 22–1), CPA (3×10^{-6} M) diminished the difference among three age groups in $RT_{1/2}$ (data not shown). The PIE of ET-1 was markedly attenuated by CPA in 2-month-old rats. The PIE of ET-1 in 6-month-old rats was attenuated by the CPA, but the difference was not significant. CPA did not affect the effect of ET-1 in 27-month-old rats.

Influence of Age on ET-1 Binding Sites

Saturation binding isotherms for [^{125}I]-labeled ET-1 in the membrane fractions derived from rat ventricular muscles were determined. The membrane yields were not significantly different among three age groups. The values for maximal binding (B_{max}) of ET-1 and dissociation constant (K_D) determined by Scatchard analysis of the specific binding of [^{125}I]-labeled ET-1 to the membrane fraction derived from ventricles of different ages are shown in Table 22–2. The B_{max} in 27-month-

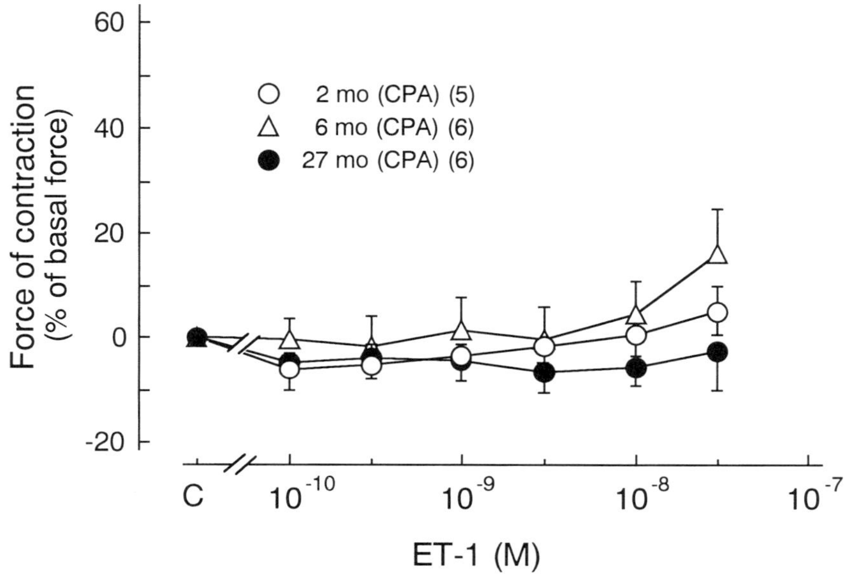

FIG. 22-2. Concentration–response curves for the positive inotropic effect of endothelin-1 in the presence of CPA (3×10^{-7} M) in ventricular papillary muscles isolated from 2-, 6-, and 27-month-old rats. Papillary muscles were driven electrically at 1 Hz at 37°C in presence of 3×10^{-7} M of (±)-bupranolol. *Ordinate,* force of contraction expressed as a percentage of the basal force of contraction. *Abscissa,* logarithmic concentration of endothelin-1. Figures in parentheses are numbers of experiments (*n*). Basal force of contraction, 1.17 ± 0.04 mN in 2-month-old, 1.46 ± 0.37 mN in 6-month-old, and 1.52 ± 0.43 mN in 27-month-old rats, respectively. All values presented are mean ± SEM.

TABLE 22–2. *B_{max} and K_D values for [^{125}I]-labeled ET-1 bindings to membrane fraction derived from 2-, 6-, and 27-month-old rat ventricular muscles[a]*

Age (mo)	[^{125}I]ET-1 Specific binding: B_{max} (fmol/mg protein)	K_D value (nM)
2	505.4 ± 29.4	0.16 ± 0.06
6	477.0 ± 43.8	0.24 ± 0.08
27	819.7 ± 80.8[*,#]	0.30 ± 0.02

[a]Values are means ± SE of four experiments. *$P < 0.05$ vs. 2-month-old rats, #$P < 0.05$ vs. 6-month-old rats.

old rats was significantly higher than those in 2- and 6-month-old rats, whereas the K_D values were not significantly different among three age groups.

DISCUSSION

In ventricular papillary muscles isolated from 2- and 6-month-old Fisher 344 rats, ET-1 elicited a PIE in concentration-dependent manner with no significant differences between both aged rats. By contrast, the PIE of ET-1 was markedly decreased in 27-month-old rats. These results are consistent with our previous findings that the ET-1 induced PIE decreased with age in isolated perfused rat heart (11).

α_1-Adrenoceptor agonists and angiotensin II activate protein kinase C in cardiac muscle cells, producing the second messengers diacylglycerol and 1,4,5-inositol trisphosphate, and elicit the PIE with closely resembling characteristics in respect to alteration of contractile parameters (5,21,22), which implies the involvement of identical intracellular signal transduction pathway. Since ET-1 stimulates phosphoinositide (PI) hydrolysis in cardiac muscle, it is highly likely that ET-1 shares an identical signal transduction process to α_1-agonists and angiotensin II (5).

Kimball et al. (23) reported that the inotropic efficacy of α_1-adrenoceptor stimulation was diminished during senescence in rat ventricular muscle and postulated that the age-related decline in α_1-adrenoceptor responsiveness is mediated in part by a decrease in cardiac α_1-adrenoceptor density. Although B_{max} values for α_1-adrenoceptors (23,24), β-adrenoceptors (25), and digitalis receptors (26) have been reported to decrease with age, the B_{max} of [^{125}I]-ET-1 binding in rat ventricular membrane was even higher in aged rats (27-month-old) than in younger rats (2- and 6-month-old). There was no significant difference in B_{max} between 2-month-old and 6-month-old rats. The affinity for ET-1 was unaltered with aging. Because the B_{max} value was expressed as fmoles per milligram protein, it is not known in the present study whether the receptor density per cell or per sarcolemmal surface area is altered with age. While ventricular wet weight increased between 2- and 6-month-old rats, no further increase was observed between 6- and 27-month-old rats. The protein yield of partially purified membrane preparations per tissue mass was not affected by aging (data not shown). Gu et al. (27) reported that the density of [^{125}I]ET-1 binding sites in cardiac membranes isolated from 5- to 7-day-old, 20-day-old and 8- to 9-week-old rats decreased with age without changes in the affinity for [^{125}I]ET-1 binding. However, in this study the influence of senescence beyond middle age was not investigated.

Although it has been shown that characteristics of myocardial ET receptors are modulated in certain pathologic conditions (12–16), little is known about the age-related changes in ET receptors in myocardium. Our results indicate that the diminished cardiac response to ET-1 in aged rats may be due to uncoupling of ET-1 receptors to subsequent signal transduction processes. Further experiments are required to elucidate the mechanism and pathophysiologic relevance of the up-regulation of ET-1 receptors with age.

Although the subcellular mechanism for the PIE of ET-1 is not yet fully clarified, stimulation of PI hydrolysis catalyzed by ET receptor activation (5) may play a crucial role, as is the case with α_1-adrenoceptor agonists (21) and angiotensin II (22). The PI hydrolysis is postulated to be coupled to multiple regulatory processes, including various types of ion channel, such as the Ca^{2+}, K^+, and Cl^- channels; ion transport systems that include Na^+–H^+ exchange; and the responsiveness of Ca^{2+} of contractile proteins (28–32). Damron et al. (32) reported that ET may elicit the PIE through protein kinase C–dependent inhibition of K^+ channels to result in a prolongation of action potential duration and an increase in Ca^{2+} influx across the sarcolemma.

It is considered that the Ca^{2+} release from the SR plays a central role in the excitation–contraction coupling in the adult rat myocardium. In the present study, the relaxation time of the isometric force of contraction was significantly prolonged in 27-month-old rats as compared with those 2- and 6-month-old. These findings suggest that the Ca^{2+} uptake and release function of SR may be deteriorated in the aged rats and support the view that the diminished SR Ca^{2+}–ATPase activity in aged rats may contribute to the age-related changes in relaxation and the ET-1-induced PIE. CPA could be an effective pharmacologic tool to dissect the role of SR because it has been demonstrated that CPA is a highly selective inhibitor of Ca^{2+}–ATPase in the SR (19). The PIE of ET-1 was markedly attenuated by CPA in 2- and 6-month-old rats. After treatment with CPA, the difference among three age groups in $RT_{1/2}$ and the PIE of ET-1 was diminished, indicating that the decrease in Ca^{2+}–ATPase activity in the SR may be crucial for the age-related changes in the ET-1-induced PIE. The diminished function of cardiac SR (33) and the lower content of the Ca^{2+}–ATPase protein in cardiac SR isolated from senescent rats have been reported previously (34). Thus, the diminished function of cardiac SR may contribute significantly to the blunted responsiveness to ET-1 of the senescent heart. Further study is required to elucidate whether the decrease in inotropic response to ET-1 occurs also in other signal transduction processes and which steps are most crucial for the age-related modulation.

SUMMARY

The PIE of ET-1 was markedly decreased in aged rats. The PIE of ET-1 in 2- and 6-month-old rats was markedly attenuated by CPA. After treatment with CPA, the difference among the three age groups in the inotropic response disappeared. These findings suggest that the decreased function of SR to uptake and release Ca^{2+} may contribute significantly to the age-related changes in the ET-1 induced PIE. The density of ET-1 binding sites was even higher in 27-month-old rats than in 2- and 6-month-old rats, indicating that the diminished cardiac response to ET-1 in aged rats may be largely due to uncoupling of ET-1 receptors to subsequent signal transduction processes and/or to the diminished function of cardiac Ca^{2+} pump in sarcoplasmic reticulum.

ACKNOWLEDGMENTS

This work was partly supported by a Grant-in-Aid for Scientific Research (C) (No. 05834003) from the Ministry of Education, Science, Sports, and Culture of Japan and a Grant-in-Aid for Aging Research from Yamagata Prefecture, Japan.

REFERENCES

1. Yanagisawa M, Kurihara H, Kimura S, Tomobe Y, Kobayashi M, Mitsui Y, Yazaki Y, Goto K, Masaki T. A novel potent vasoconstrictor peptide produced by vascular endothelial cells. *Nature* 1988;332:411–415.
2. Katano Y, Ishihata A, Morinobu S, Endoh M. Modulation by aging of the coronary vascular response to endothelin-1 in the rat isolated perfused heart. *Naunyn-Schmiedbergs Arch Pharmacol* 1993;348:82–87.
3. Davenport AP, Nunez DJ, Hall JA, Kaumann AK, Brown MJ. Autoradiographical localization of binding sites for porcine [^{125}I] endothelin-1 in humans, pigs and rats: functional relevance in humans. *J Cardiovasc Pharmacol* 1989;13:S166–S170.
4. Ishikawa T, Li LM, Shinmi O, Kimura S, Yanagisawa K, Goto K, Masaki T. Characteristics of binding of endothelin-1 and endothelin-3 to rat hearts. *Circ Res* 1991;69:918–926.
5. Takanashi M, Endoh M. Characterization of positive inotropic effect of endothelin on mammalian ventricular myocardium. *Am J Physiol* 1991;261:H611–H619.
6. Moravec CS, Reynolds EE, Stewart RW, Bond M. Endothelin is a positive inotropic agent in human and rat heart in vitro. *Biochem Biophys Res Commun* 1989;159:14–18.
7. Krämer BK, Smith TW, Kelly RA. Endothelin and increased contractility in adult rat ventricular myocytes. *Circ Res* 1991;68:269–279.
8. Li K, Stewart DJ, Rouleau JL. Myocardial contractile action of endothelin-1 in rat and rabbit papillary muscles. *Circ Res* 1991;69:301–312.
9. Wang JX, Paik G, Morgan JP. Endothelin-1 enhances myofilament Ca^{2+}-responsiveness in aequorin-loaded ferret myocardium. *Circ Res* 1991;69:582–589.
10. Qui ZH, Wang JX, Perreault CL, Meuse AJ, Grossman W, Morgan JP. Effects of endothelin on intracellular Ca^{2+} and contractility in single ventricular myocytes from the ferret and human. *Eur J Pharmacol* 1992;214:293–296.
11. Katano Y, Ishihata A, Endoh M. Detrimental adaptation of cardiovascular receptor-mediated regulation with age: changes in cardiac and coronary responses to endothelin-1 in isolated perfused rat heart. In: Nagano M, Takeda N, Dhalla NS, eds. *The adapted heart.* New York: Raven Press; 1994:477–490.
12. Liu J, Chen R, Casley DJ, Nayler WG. Ischemia and reperfusion increase ^{125}I-labeled endothelin-1 binding in rat cardiac membranes. *Am J Physiol* 1990;258:H829–H835.
13. Liu J, Gu XH, Casley DJ, Nayler WG. Reoxygenation, but neither hypoxia nor intermittent ischemia increases ^{125}I-labeled endothelin-1 binding to rat cardiac membranes. *J Cardiovasc Pharmacol* 1990;15:436–443.
14. Nayler WG, Gu XH, Casley DJ, Panagiotopoulos S, Liu J, Mottram PL. Cyclosporine increases endothelin-1 binding site density in cardiac cell membranes. *Biochem Biophys Res Commun* 1989; 163:1270–1273.
15. Nayler WG, Liu J, Panagiotopoulos S, Casley DJ. Streptozotocin-induced diabetes reduces the density of ^{125}I-labelled endothelin-1 binding sites in rat cardiac membranes. *Br J Pharmacol* 1989;97:993–995.
16. Gu XH, Casley DJ, Cincotta M, Nayler WG. ^{125}I-Labelled endothelin-1 binding to brain and cardiac membranes from normotensive and spontaneously hypertensive rats. *Eur J Pharmacol* 1990;177:205–209.
17. Evans HG, Lewis MJ, Shah AM. Modulation of myocardial relaxation by basal release of endothelin from endocardial endothelium. *Cardiovasc Res* 1994;28:1694–1699.
18. Ito H, Hirata Y, Hiroe M, Tsujino M, Adachi S, Takamoto T, Nitta M, Taniguchi K, Marumo F. Endothelin-1 induces hypertrophy with enhanced expression of muscle-specific genes in cultured neonatal rat cardiocytes. *Circ Res* 1991;69:209–215.

19. Goeger DE, Rieley RT, Dorner JW, Cole RJ. Cyclopiazonic acid inhibition of the Ca^{2+}-transport ATPase in rat skeletal muscle sarcoplasmic reticulum vesicles. *Biochem Pharmacol* 1988;37:978–981.
20. Lowry OH, Rosebrough NJ, Farr AL, Randall RJ. Protein measurement with the Folin phenol reagent. *J Biol Chem* 1951;193:265–275.
21. Endoh M, Hiramoto T, Ishihata A, Takanashi M, Inui J. Myocardial α_1-adrenoceptors mediate positive inotropic effect and changes in phosphatidylinositol metabolism: species differences in receptor distribution and the intracellular coupling process in mammalian ventricular myocardium. *Circ Res* 1991;68:1179–1190.
22. Ishihata A, Endoh M. Pharmacological characteristics of the positive inotropic effect of angiotensin II in the rabbit ventricular myocardium. *Br J Pharmacol* 1993;108:999–1005.
23. Kimball KA, Cornett LE, Seifen E, Kennedy RH. Aging: changes in cardiac α_1-adrenoceptor responsiveness and expression. *Eur J Pharmacol* 1991;208:231–238.
24. Noguchi A, Whitsett JA, Dickman L. Ontogeny of myocardial α_1-adrenergic receptor in the rat. *Dev Pharmacol Ther* 1981;3:179–188.
25. Kojima M, Ishima T, Taniguchi N, Kimura K, Sada H, Sperlakis N. Developmental changes in β-adrenoceptors, muscarinic cholinoceptors and Ca^{2+} channels in rat ventricular muscles. *Br J Pharmacol* 1990;99:334–339.
26. Katano Y, Akera T, Temma K, Kennedy RH. Enhanced ouabain sensitivity of the heart and myocardial sodium pump in aged rats. *Eur J Pharmacol* 1984;105:95–103.
27. Gu XH, Ou RC, Casley DJ, Daly MJ, Nayler WG. Effects of age on endothelin-1 binding sites in rat cardiac ventricular membranes. *J Cardiovasc Pharmacol* 1992;19:764–769.
28. Endoh M. Signal transduction of myocardial α_1-adrenoceptors: regulation of ion channels, intracellular calcium, and force of contraction: a review. *J Appl Cardiol* 1991;6:379–399.
29. Fedida D, Braun AP, Giles WR. α_1-Adrenoceptors in myocardium: functional aspects and transmembrane signaling mechanisms. *Physiol Rev* 1993;73:469–487.
30. Triassic A, Pucéat M, Vassort G, Vogel SM. Cardiac α_1-adrenoceptors: an overview. *Pharmacol Rev* 1993;45:147–175.
31. Fujita S., Endoh M. Effects of endothelin-1 on $[Ca^{2+}]_i$-shortening trajectory and Ca^{2+} sensitivity in rabbit single ventricular cardiomyocytes loaded with indo-1/AM: comparison with the effects of phenylephrine and angiotensin II. *J Cardiac Failure* 1996;2:545–557.
32. Damron DS, Wagoner DRV, Moravec CS, Bond M. Arachidonic acid and endothelin potentiate Ca^{2+} transients in rat cardiac myocytes via inhibition of distinct K^+ channels. *J Biol Biochem* 1993;268:27335–27344.
33. Lakatta EG, Gerstenblith G, Angell CS, Shock NW, Weisfeldt ML. Prolonged contraction duration in aged myocardium. *J Clin Invest* 1975;55:61–68.
34. Taffet GE, Tate CA. CaATPase content is lower in cardiac sarcoplasmic reticulum isolated from old rats. *Am J Physiol* 1993;264:H1609–H1614.

PART V

Effect of Increased Workload

The Developing Heart,
edited by Bohuslav Ošťádal et al.
Lippincott-Raven Publishers,
Philadelphia © 1997.

23

Excitation–Contraction Coupling in Cardiac Dysmorphogenesis

Tony L. Creazzo, Jarrett L. Burch, and Marco A. P. Brotto

Department of Cellular Biology and Anatomy and Heart Development Group, Medical College of Georgia, CA 4004, Augusta, GA 30912-2640

The embryonic heart must supply circulatory support for the developing embryo even while undergoing morphogenesis itself. Although there has been some progress toward understanding the mechanisms that influence structural development of the heart, very little is known with regard to the influence these mechanisms may have on the development of function at the level of a single myocyte. Over the past 12 years it has become clear that one of the more important contributors to structural heart development is the cardiac neural crest (neural crest extending from mid-otic placode to caudal region of somite 3) (1–5). Bilateral ablation of the cardiac neural crest in chick embryos, prior to migration, leads to aortic arch anomalies that generally include failure of the arch arteries to develop to their normal size as well as inappropriate patterning of persistent arch arteries early in development (6,7). Later in the development of the neural crest–ablated embryos, there is a failure of septation of the cardiac outflow tract that produces a severe defect known as persistent truncus arteriosus (PTA) (1). These observations in the chick have led to the classification of a series of severe human congenital heart defects as neural crest related (2–5). In 1992, the Pediatric Cardiac Care Quality Assurance Consortium, with 60 participating U.S. centers, reported that three of the four congenital heart defects associated with the highest mortality (25–38%) are persistent truncus arteriosus, double outlet right ventricle, and interrupted aortic arch. All these structural anomalies of the cardiac outflow tract are included in the neural crest spectrum of defects. The study of neural crest–related heart defects has recently been facilitated by the addition of three new mouse genetic models in which neural crest development is disrupted (2,4) (see "Discussion" later). In all the animal models of neural crest–related heart defects, prenatal mortality is too high to be attributed to structural defects of the heart alone, suggesting that there is altered development of the myocardium.

Myocardial function in neural crest–related heart defects has been best characterized in the embryonic chick heart following complete bilateral ablation of the premigratory cardiac neural crest, which leads to PTA. Following this ablation, it was found that hemodynamic abnormalities occur well before the period when normal septation occurs and involve decreased contractility of the myocardium (8). These embryos compensate for decreased contractility by ventricular dilation, enabling them to maintain an adequate cardiac output for survival (9). It is thought that these functional compensations in very early cardiac development may play an etiologic role in the subsequent development of structural heart defects. At older ages, when septation would normally be complete, these embryos have reduced ejection fraction, suggesting that the myocardium shows poor contractility (10,11). Poor cardiac function is further indicated by reduced embryo weight and edema (12).

One likely explanation for the gross signs of cardiac dysfunction observed in the intact heart could be impairment of myocardial contractility caused by a defect in one or more of the mechanisms involved in excitation–contraction coupling (EC coupling). Contraction of the myocardium is initiated by depolarization of the membrane, followed by net entry of calcium through voltage-gated Ca^{2+} channels. In the adult heart, this calcium causes a further release of calcium from the sarcoplasmic reticulum (SR) via a mechanism termed Ca^{2+}-induced Ca^{2+} release (CICR). The subsequent rise in intracellular Ca^{2+} activates cyclic interactions between the contractile proteins myosin and actin, which give rise to force production and shortening of the muscle cell. Relaxation of the cell is caused primarily by a decrease in the intracellular level of Ca^{2+} caused by active uptake of Ca^{2+} back into the SR. The processes linking depolarization of the membrane and the ensuing rise in intracellular Ca^{2+} is termed EC coupling (reviewed in ref. 13). Indeed, hearts destined to develop PTA have reduced L-type Ca^{2+} current ($i_{Ca,L}$) as early as embryonic day 3 (14), which continues to later ages (15,16). The reduction in $i_{Ca,L}$ is associated with a reduction in the number of functional L-type Ca^{2+} channels (16). These reports indicate that EC coupling may be impaired. To further investigate this possibility, we measured Ca^{2+} transients in field-stimulated isolated myocytes loaded with the Ca^{2+} fluorescent indicator, fura-2. The following results indicate that impaired myocardial function in hearts with PTA may be due to a reduction in SR function as well as to a reduction in $i_{Ca,L}$.

METHODS

Animal Surgery

Fertilized Arbor Acre chicken eggs (Seaboard Hatchery, Athens, GA) were incubated in forced-draft incubators maintained at 90% humidity and 38°C. The eggs for sham-operated and experimental animals were windowed at Hamburger-Hamilton stages 8–10 (approximately 30 hours of development). The embryos were stained with neutral red and the cardiac neural crest cells (neural crest cells extending from the mid-otic placode to the caudal region of somite 3) were ablated bilaterally with a pulsed nitrogen/dye laser (model VSL-337/DLM-110, Laser Science, Inc.), as previously described in detail by Kirby and colleagues (17). This lesion produces PTA in more than 90% of embryos that survive to day 15 as the cardiac neural crest normally provides ectomesenchymal cells essential for septation of the cardiac outflow tract (18). The microsurgery was performed by a surgery Core Unit, under the supervision of Dr. Margaret L. Kirby, using procedures that are standardized to produce PTA. Only those diagnosed with PTA were used. The hearts from sham-operated embryos were considered "normal" if no outflow tract anomalies were detected at the time of macroscopic inspection. PTA was never observed in sham-operated embryos.

Myocyte Preparation

Sham-operated and experimental embryos at embryonic age day 15 were sacrificed by decapitation. The hearts were rapidly removed and trimmed of the atria and great vessels; then the ventricles were cleaned of connective tissue. The myocyte dissociation procedure was done as previously reported and is described in detail elsewhere (15,16). After the dissociation, approximately 5×10^5 cells were plated in DeHaan's 21212 medium (19) onto either 35-mm plastic culture dishes for patch clamp experiments or plastic petri dishes containing a glass cover slip (25-mm diameter and 0.16-mm thickness) for Ca^{2+} transient measurements. The cultures were used within 12–24 hours following the dissociation. All experiments were carried out at room temperature.

Fura-2 Loading and Fluorescence Measurements

After washing the cells with Ringer solution they were loaded with fura-2/AM, as previously described elsewhere in detail (20). A SPEX microspectrofluorometer with dual monochrometers was used to collect the fura-2 calcium transients (340/380 nm ratios). The transients were then calibrated in terms of $[Ca^{2+}]_i$ with the ratiometric procedure described by Grynkiewicz et al. (21).

We previously determined that under our experimental conditions cytoplasmic fura-2 concentrations ranging from 16 to 60 μM did not affect the size and the shape of the Ca transients (20). In the present study we have estimated a fura-2 cytoplasmic concentration of approximately 20 μM using the methods described by Moore et al. (22).

Patch Clamp Procedure

The voltage clamp protocols and solutions used in this report were the same as those described previously (15,16). Briefly the extracellular solution was comprised of (in mM): 1.8 $CaCl_2$, 20 CsCl, 120 tetraethylammonium chloride, 1.8 $MgCl_2$, 10 HEPES, 3 μM tetrodotoxin (approx. 500 times K_I for the chick cardiac sodium channel [23]); 5 dextrose, adjusted to pH 7.4 with CsOH. The perforated patch configuration was achieved using nystatin essentially as described by Horn and Marty (24) and routinely used in this laboratory (20,25). The perforated patch solution in the pipette was comprised of (in mM): 55 KCl, 70 K_2SO_4, 7 $MgCl_2$, 10 HEPES, and 5 dextrose (pH 7.3, KOH). In some experiments Cs_2SO_4 was used instead of K_2SO_4 with no noticeable difference in the Ca current.

RESULTS

The current–voltage (*I–V*) relationships shown in Fig. 23–1 demonstrated reduced L-type Ca^{2+} current ($i_{Ca,L}$) in ventricular myocytes from hearts with persistent truncus arteriosus (PTA) at day 15 of incubation when compared with aged-matched sham-operated controls. The reduction was about 50% at the peak of the *I–V* curves, which occurred at +10 mV. These results at this later age of development confirm previous reports from this laboratory that indicated a reduction of $i_{Ca,L}$ at day 11 in chick hearts with PTA (15,16). The reduction in $i_{Ca,L}$ implies that there should be a corresponding reduction in the peak of the transient increase in intracellular Ca^{2+} that occurs with stimulation of action potentials. To verify this prediction, Ca^{2+} transients elicited by field stimulation were studied in fura-2-loaded myocytes. Despite numerous attempts, Ca^{2+} transients were never observed above baseline noise in myocytes from hearts with PTA, indicating that, if present, the transients peaked at less than 100 nM. Figure 23–2A shows a typical response to field stimulation in a myocyte from a heart with PTA. Ca^{2+} transients were always observed in myocytes from sham-operated embryos (Fig. 23–2B). The average peak of these transients was 465 ± 22 nM (± standard error, $n = 15$). The diastolic Ca^{2+} level, on the other hand, was not significantly different (Sham: 177 ± 15 nM vs. PTA: 135 ± 10 nM; $p > 0.05$, Student's t-test).

The decreased Ca current shown in Fig. 23–1 could account for the reduced Ca^{2+} transients because there would have been less extracellular Ca^{2+} entering the myocyte and, consequently, less Ca^{2+} to trigger CICR. If this were the only defect in PTA myocytes, it should be possible to restore the Ca transient by increasing L-type current comparable to the level found in normal hearts. Figure 23–3 shows that the Ca current can be elevated to a level equal to or greater than that observed in myocytes from normal hearts using 100 μM isoproterenol (ISO). The average peak of the Ca^{2+} transients in myocytes from sham-operated embryos in the presence of 100 μM ISO increased nearly twofold in the presence of ISO (825 ± 43 nM, $n = 15$; Fig. 23–4). However, exposure to ISO did not restore the Ca^{2+} transient in myocytes from hearts with PTA (Fig. 23–4). With PTA the average peak

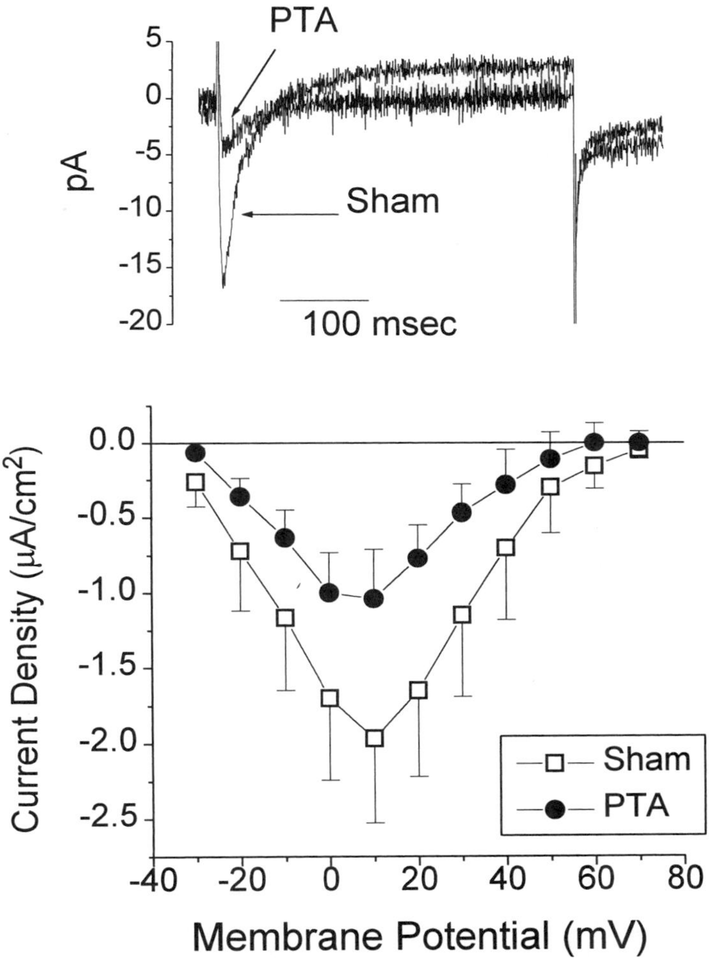

FIG. 23–1. L-type Ca current in ventricular myocytes from normal hearts from sham-operated embryos (Sham) and hearts with PTA. Examples of Ca current records are shown in the absence of isoproterenol (ISO). The currents were elicited by a 500-msec prepulse to −40 mV from a holding potential followed by a 400-msec test pulse to +10 mV (15,16). Mean current–voltage relationships showing peak Ca current are illustrated. Peak Ca current is measured as the difference between the peak inward current and the current at the end of the 400-msec voltage step. $N = 10 - 15$ myocytes per point. Bars indicate standard error.

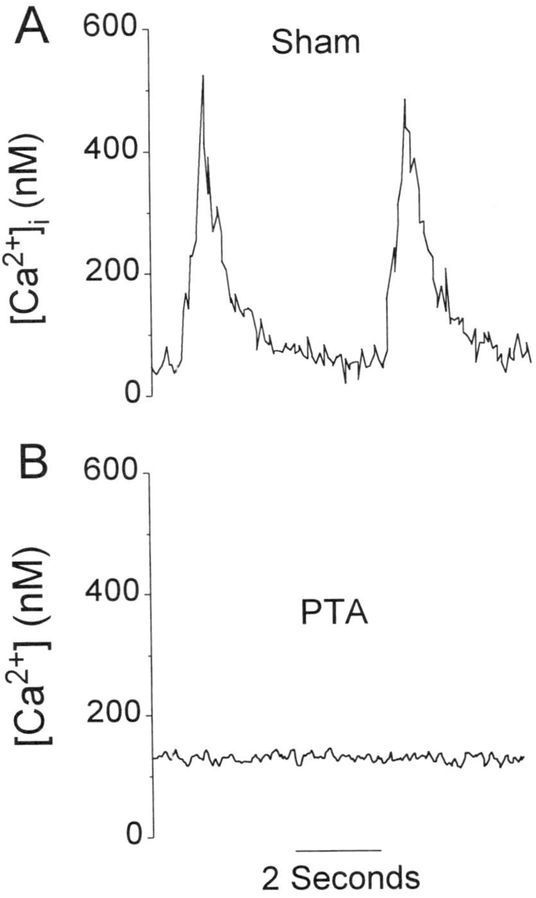

FIG. 23–2. Ca^{2+} transients in ventricular myocytes from a normal heart from a sham-operated embryo and a heart with PTA in the absence of ISO at embryonic day 15. (**A**) A myocyte from a sham-operated embryo (Sham). (**B**) A myocyte from a heart with PTA. The transients were elicited by field stimulation at 0.2 Hz. Note that transients were not observable in the PTA myocytes above background noise when field stimulated.

was only 300 ± 40 nM ($n = 12$), which was 35% less than the average for sham-operated embryos in the absence of ISO ($p < 0.05$, Student's t-test). Thus, although ISO could restore the level of Ca current in hearts with PTA, the Ca^{2+} transient was significantly less than in the sham-operated group in the absence of ISO. These results suggest that, in addition to reduced $i_{Ca,L}$, other mechanisms involved in EC coupling may also be impaired. Other possibilities include alterations in SR CICR, SR Ca^{2+} uptake and/or Na–Ca exchange.

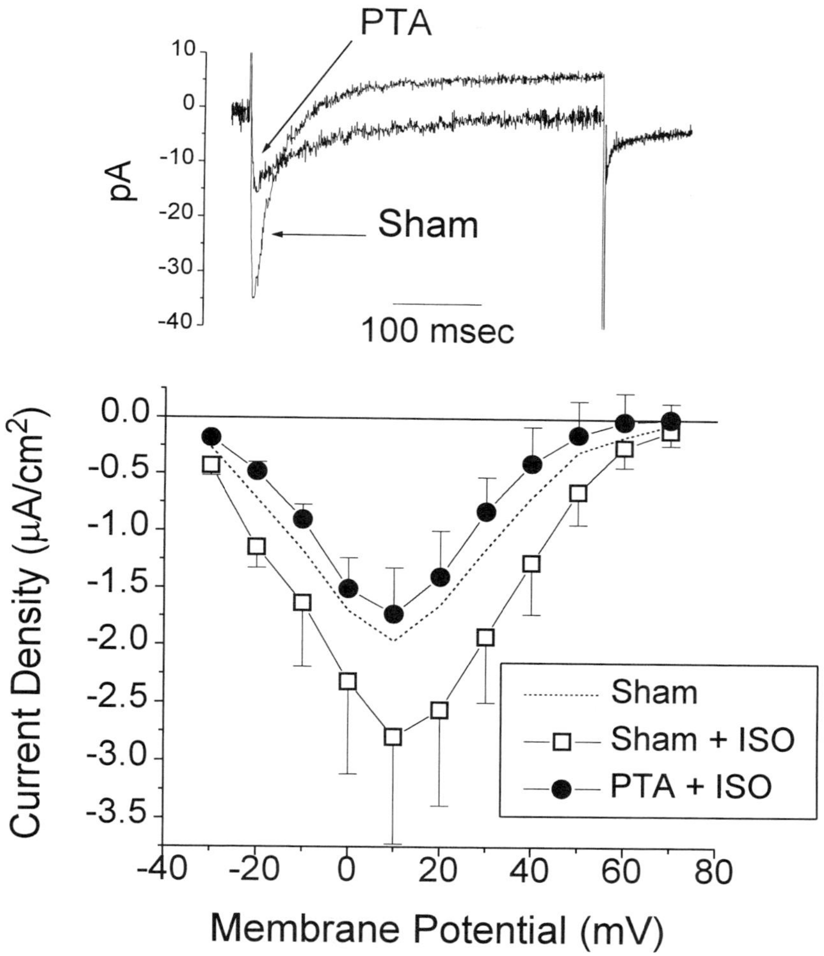

FIG. 23–3. L-type Ca current in ventricular myocytes in the presence of 100 μM ISO. Examples of Ca current records are from the same myocytes used as examples in Fig. 23–1 and with the same voltage clamp protocol. Mean current–voltage relationships showing peak Ca current are illustrated in the presence of ISO. For comparison, the data in Fig. 23–1 for Sham in the absence of ISO are represented as a dotted line. In this example the decay of the current in the PTA myocyte appears slower than the Sham. However, this is not a consistent finding. $N = 5 - 7$ myocytes per point. Bars indicate standard error.

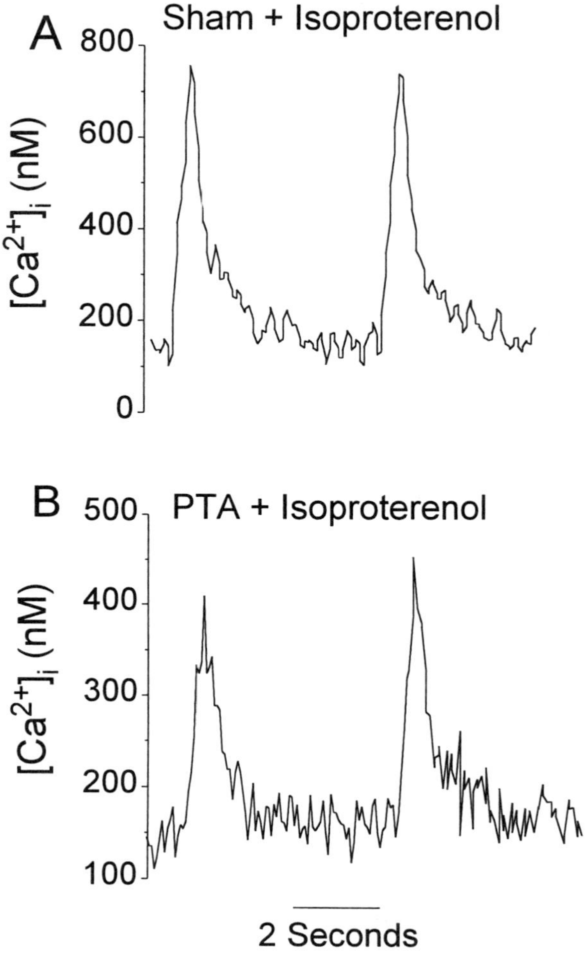

FIG. 23–4. Ca^{2+} transients in same ventricular myocytes used as examples in Fig. 23–2 but in the presence of 100 μM ISO. (**A**) Myocyte from the sham-operated embryo (Sham). (**B**) A myocyte from the heart with PTA. Note that transients are now observable in the PTA myocyte. However, the transients are smaller than those from Sham in the absence of ISO (see text). The transients were elicited by field stimulation at 0.2 Hz.

DISCUSSION

A number of experimental observations of embryonic hearts with PTA, a severe cardiac neural crest–related heart defect, indicate poor myocardial function that is suggestive of impaired EC coupling (see the introductory discussion). Previous reports from this laboratory as well as the data given in the present study indicate a reduction of $i_{Ca,L}$ in embryonic hearts with PTA (15,16). Consistent with these findings, the present study shows that Ca^{2+} transients are reduced in hearts with PTA. However, stimulation of L-type Ca current with ISO to levels that approximate the level of $i_{Ca,L}$ found in normal hearts from the sham-operated controls did not restore the Ca^{2+} transient in hearts with PTA. Thus, in addition to reduced L-type current, there appears to be an impairment of SR function. This may be due to reduced Ca^{2+} uptake by the SR Ca^{2+}–ATPase and/or to reduced CIRC via ryanodine receptor–Ca^{2+} release channels. Another possibility could be a reduction in Ca^{2+} entry via reverse Na–Ca exchange, which may occur during the peak of the membrane depolarization (26).

SR function is well developed in the chick heart by embryonic day 11. Immunofluorescence labeling indicates the presence of SR Ca^{2+}–ATPase in the developing chick myocardium at stages 9–10 ($\approx$36 hours of incubation), when the primitive heart tube begins contracting (27). Ca^{2+} sequestration by SR has been detected at low levels at day 2.5 and the level increases in a near linear fashion through to hatching (28). Ryanodine receptor binding studies indicate the presence of Ca^{2+} release channels by day 4 of incubation (29). We have found that 100 μM ryanodine inhibits Ca^{2+} transients by 30% at day 11 (20) and that the inhibition increases to about 60% by day 15 (Creazzo, unpublished). Phosphorylation of the SR protein phospholamban has also been detected as early as day 4 in the chick embryo (30). ISO would be expected to stimulate Ca^{2+} uptake and loading of the SR via phosphorylation of phospholamban, thereby increasing the amount of Ca^{2+} available for release (31–33). Despite the possibility that loading of the SR may be enhanced in addition to elevation of Ca current, ISO was not able to restore the Ca transients to normal levels, further suggesting impairment of SR function. Impaired SR function in chick hearts with PTA has been further demonstrated in two recent preliminary reports. One report indicated that caffeine-releasable Ca^{2+} was decreased in myocytes (34); the second demonstrated a nearly identical impairment of Ca^{2+} transients in fura-2-loaded intact trabeculae in the ventricles of day 15 embryos with PTA (35).

The foregoing discussion and the introductory section clearly indicates that the mechanisms of EC coupling are affected with adverse consequences for the developing chick embryo. But are these findings in chicks relevant in terms of the human fetus with structural heart anomalies? Like the human fetus, chick embryos are protected from left to right shunting *in ovo* by high pulmonary vascular resistance and *in ovo* circulatory pathways that are quite similar to those in human fetuses. However, chick embryos with PTA are edematous and have low body weight as well as a large heart with respect to body weight (12). *In ovo* survivability to late embryonic ages is poor and presumably due to heart failure. The embryos never hatch. These observations in the chick embryo parallel the phenomenon of "fetal wastage" often observed during prenatal life in humans with outflow tract defects (36,37). And as with our chick model, recent evidence indicates that children with congenital heart defects have a primary myocardial dysfunction that is not corrected by surgical repair of the structural defects (38–40). Moreover, despite being hemodynamically protected from the effects of structural anomalies, a number of clinical studies indicate significant cardiac symptoms in human fetuses in utero, with significantly elevated *in utero* and neonatal mortality (41–43).

More recently in a preliminary study, we have found similar impairment of EC coupling in a mouse model of neural crest–related heart defects. Mice with mutations at the *splotch* locus (*Pax3* gene) exhibit a phenotype consistent with disruption of the neural crest (44). About half of the embryos homozygous for the *splotch*^{2H} mutation (sp^{2H}/sp^{2H}) develop PTA. All the sp^{2H}/sp^{2H} embryos with PTA die by 14.5 days post coitum (dpc). On day 13.5 dpc, ventricular myocytes from sp^{2H}/sp^{2H} embryos show about a 2.5-fold reduction in the peak magnitude of the Ca^{2+} current (unpublished data). Thus, disruption of the cardiac neural crest, either genetic or surgical, results in abnormal development of EC coupling, which leads to poor cardiac function and subsequent embryo death.

Although it is becoming increasingly clear that structural defects of the heart alter the normal developmental program for cellular mechanisms in the myocardium in a deleterious way, the factors that initiate these alterations remain unknown. The possibilities include a direct effect on the myocardium via a factor secreted, or induced to be secreted, by the neural crest and/or an indirect effect caused by neural crest–related alterations in hemodynamic parameters in the aortic arch arteries and in the cardiac outflow tract.

SUMMARY

It is now well established that the cardiac neural crest makes major contributions to normal cardiovascular development. This is supported by extensive work in an embryonic chick model of defective heart development that has led to the classification of a series of human congenital heart anomalies as neural crest related. Bilateral ablation of the cardiac neural crest in the chick embryo (neural crest extending from mid-otic placode to the caudal region of somite 3) prior to migration leads to aortic arch anomalies and, later in development, to failure of septation of the cardiac outflow tract into aortic and pulmonary arteries. This is referred to as persistent truncus arteriosus (PTA). Survivability of embryos with PTA is poor, suggesting impaired myocardial function. Most embryos die well before hatching, and the few that do survive to near term are never able to hatch. Recent studies of the chick heart model indicate a reduction in L-type Ca current ($i_{Ca,L}$) and not only support the hypothesis that there is impaired ventricular function, but also indicate that the depressed function is due at least in part to defects in excitation–contraction (EC) coupling. In this study, intracellular Ca^{2+} was measured in fura-2-loaded myocytes. It was found that the peak of the Ca^{2+} transient was depressed in hearts with PTA, at day 15 of incubation, and not observable above background noise. Treatment with isoproterenol (ISO) restored $i_{Ca,L}$ to the level found in normal hearts (≈ -1.7 μA/cm^2 at +10 mV without ISO) but could only partially restore the Ca^{2+} transient (300 $\pm$ 40 nM in PTA with ISO versus 465 $\pm$ 22 nM in normal hearts with no ISO; $\pm$ standard error). The possible relevance of these findings to human congenital heart defects is discussed.

ACKNOWLEDGMENTS

I wish to thank Dr. Robert Godt for helpful discussions of the data and reading the manuscript. Additional thanks go to the members of the Heart Development

Group and the Medical College of Georgia; in particular, we thank Dr. Kirby, Ms Harriet Stadt, and Ms Donna Kumiski for the help and support of the Microsurgery Core Unit in producing the neural crest–related heart defects. This work was supported by National Heart, Lung, and Blood Institute Grant HL-36059 and a Grant-in-Aid from the American Heart Association, Georgia Affiliate.

REFERENCES

1. Kirby ML, Gale TF, Stewart DE. Neural crest cells contribute to normal aorticopulmonary septation. *Science* 1983;220:1059–1061.
2. Kirby ML, Creazzo TL. Cardiovascular development: neural crest and new perspectives. *Cardiol Rev* 1995;3:226–235.
3. Kirby ML, Waldo KL. Role of neural crest in congenital heart disease. *Circulation* 1990;82:332–340.
4. Kirby ML, Waldo KL. Neural crest and cardiovascular patterning. *Circ Res* 1995;77:211–215.
5. Payne RM, Johnson MC, Grant JW, Strauss AW. Toward a molecular understanding of congenital heart disease. *Circulation* 1995;91:494–504.
6. Bockman DE, Redmond ME, Waldo KL, Davis H, Kirby ML. Effect on neural crest ablation on development of the heart and arch arteries in the chick. *Am J Anat* 1987;180:332–341.
7. Nishibatake M, Kirby ML, Van Mierop LHS. Pathogenesis of persistent truncus arteriosus and dextroposed aorta in chick embryo after neural crest ablation. *Circulation* 1987;75:255–264.
8. Leatherbury L, Gauldin HE, Waldo K, Kirby ML. Microcinephotography of the developing heart in neural crest–ablated chick embryos. *Circulation* 1990;81;1047–1057.
9. Tomita H, Connuck DM, Leatherbury L, Kirby ML. Relation of early hemodynamic changes to final cardiac phenotype and survival after neural crest ablation in chick embryos. *Circulation* 1991;84:1289–1295.
10. Lutin WA, Aliff CL, Creazzo TL, Connuck DM. Possible mechanism for increased mortality in embryos with persistent truncus arteriosus. *Pediatr Res* 1995;37:29A. Abstract.
11. Godt RE, Chu JC, Merry H, Lutin WA. Depressed ventricular in an experimental heart defect in the embryonic chick is not associated with an elevated microtubule content. In: Ostadal B, Nagano M, Takeda N, Dhalla NS, eds. *The developing heart.* New York: Raven Press, 1997;373–383.
12. Creazzo TL, Burch J, Redmond S, Kumiski D. Myocardial enlargement in defective heart development. *Anat Rec* 1994;239:170–176.
13. Bers DM. *Excitation–contraction coupling and cardiac contractile force.* Boston: Kluwer Academic Publishers, 1991.
14. Creazzo TL, Brotto MAP, Burch J. Reduced Ca^{2+} transients and Ca^{2+} currents during early and late cardiac dysmorphogenesis. *FASEB J* 1995;9:A557. Abstract.
15. Creazzo TL. Reduced L-type calcium current in the embryonic chick heart with persistent truncus arteriosus. *Circ Res* 1990;66:1491–1498.
16. Aiba S, Creazzo TL. Calcium currents in hearts with persistent truncus arteriosus. *Am J Physiol Heart Circ Physiol* 1992;262:H1182–H1190.
17. Kirby ML, Kumiski DH, Myers T, Cerjan C, Mishima N. Backtransplantation of chick cardiac neural crest cells cultured in LIF rescues heart development. *Dev Dyn* 1993;198:296–311.
18. Kirby ML, Gale TF, Stewart DE. Neural crest cells contribute to normal aorticopulmonary septation. *Science* 1983;220:1059–1061.
19. Nathan RD, DeHaan RL. Voltage clamp analysis of embryonic heart cell aggregates. *J Gen Physiol* 1979;73:175–198.
20. Brotto MAP, Creazzo TL. Calcium transients in embryonic chick heart: contributions from calcium channels and the sarcoplasmic reticulum. *Am J Physiol Heart Circ Physiol* 1995.
21. Grynkiewicz G, Poenie M, Tsien RY. A new generation of calcium indicators with greatly improved fluorescence properties. *J Biol Chem* 1985;260:3440–3450.
22. Moore EDW, Becker PL, Fogarty KE, Williams DA, Fay FS. Ca^{2+} imaging in single living cells: theoretical and practical issues. *Cell Calcium* 1990;11:157–179.
23. Marcus NC, Fozzard HA. Tetrodotoxin sensitivity in the developing and adult chick heart. *J Mol Cell Cardiol* 1981;13:335–340.
24. Horn R, Marty A. Muscarinic activation of ionic currents measured by a new whole cell recording method. *J Gen Physiol* 1988;92:145–159.

25. Brotto MAP, Fogaça RTH, Creazzo TL, Godt RE, Nosek TM. The effect of 2,3-butanedione 2-monoxime (BDM) on ventricular trabeculae from the avian heart. *J Muscle Res Cell Motil* 1995;16:1–10.
26. Levi AJ, Spitzer KW, Kohmoto O, Bridge JHB. Depolarization-induced Ca entry via Na–Ca exchange triggers SR release in guinea pig cardiac myocytes. *Am J Physiol Heart Circ Physiol* 1994;266:H1422–H1433.
27. Jorgensen AO, Bashir R. Temporal appearance and distribution of Ca^{2+} + Mg^{2+} ATPase of the sarcoplasmic reticulum in developing chick myocardium as determined by immunofluorescence labeling. *Dev Biol* 1984;106:156–165.
28. Vetter R, Will H. Sarcolemmal Na–Ca exchange and sarcoplasmic reticulum calcium uptake in developing chick heart. *J Mol Cell Cardiol* 1993;18:1267–1275.
29. Dutro SM, Airey JA, Beck CF, Sutko JL, Trumble WR. Ryanodine receptor expression in embryonic avian cardiac muscle. *Dev Biol* 1993;155:431–441.
30. Will H, Küttner I, Vetter R, Will-Shahab L, Kemsies C. Early presence of phospholamban in developing chick heart. *FEBS Lett* 1983;155:326–330.
31. Sasaki T, Inui M, Kimura Y, Kuzuya T, Tada M. Molecular mechanism of regulation of Ca^{2+} pump ATPase by phospholamban in cardiac sarcoplasmic reticulum: effects of synthetic phospholamban peptides on Ca^{2+} pump ATPase. *J Biol Chem* 1992;267:1674–1679.
32. Kirchberger MA, Toda M, Katz AM. Adenosine 3′ : 5′-monophosphate-dependent protein kinase-catalyzed phosphorylation reaction and its relationship to calcium transport in cardiac sarcoplasmic reticulum. *J Biol Chem* 1974;249:6166–6771.
33. James P, Inui M, Tada M, Chiesi M, Carafoli E. Nature and site of phospholamban regulation of the Ca^{2+} pump of sarcoplasmic reticulum. *Nature* 1989;342:90–92.
34. Creazzo TL, Brotto MAP. Excitation–contraction coupling in cardiac dysmorphogenesis. *J Mol Cell Cardiol* 1995;27:A81. Abstract.
35. Nosek TM, Fogaça RTH, Allee PL, Brotto MAP, Godt RE. Cardiac neural crest ablation (CNCA) decreases calcium uptake and release by the cardiac sarcoplasmic reticulum. *J Mol Cell Cardiol* 1995;27:A82. Abstract.
36. Machado MV, Crawford DC, Anderson RH, Allan L. Atrioventricular septal defect in prenatal life. *Br Heart J* 1988;59:352–355.
37. Allan LD. Echocardiographic detection of congenital heart disease in the fetus: present and future. *Br Heart J* 1995;74:103–106.
38. Helbing WA, Regergen SA, Maliepaard C, Hansen B, Ottenkamp J, Reiber JHC. Quantification of right ventricular function with magnetic resonance imaging in children with normal hearts and with congenital heart disease. *Am Heart J* 1995;130:828–837.
39. Redington AN, Olderhaw PJ, Shinebourne EA, Rigby ML. A new technique for the assessment of pulmonary regurgitation and its application to the assessment of right ventricular function before and after repair of tetrology of Fallot. *Br Heart J* 1988;60:57–65.
40. Redington AN, Rigby ML, Olderhaw PJ, Gibson DG, Shinebourne EA. Right ventricular function 10 years after the Mustard operation for transposition of the great arteries, analysis of size, shape and wall motion. *Br Heart J* 1989;62:455–461.
41. Vergani P, Mariani S, Ghidini A, Schiavina R, Cavallone M, Locatelli A, Strobelt N, Cerruti P. Screening for congenital heart disease with the four-chamber view of the fetal heart. *Am J Obstet Gynecol* 1992;167:1000–1003.
42. Samanek M, Goetzova J, Benesova D. Distribution of congenital heart malformations in autopsied child population. *Int J Cardiol* 1985;8:235–250.
43. Gough JD, Keeling JW, Castle B, Lliff PJ. The obstetric management of non-immune hydrips. *Br J Obstet Gynaecol* 1986;130:828–837.
44. Franz T, Kothary R. Characterization of the neural crest defect in Splotch (Sp (1H)) mutant mice using a lacZ transgene. *Dev Brain Res* 1993;72:99–105.

The Developing Heart,
edited by Bohuslav Ošťádal et al.
Lippincott-Raven Publishers,
Philadelphia © 1997.

24

Neonatal Cardiac Myocytes: Experimental Systems for Study of Cardiac Hypertrophy

Howard E. Morgan and Cathy J. Beinlich

Sigfried and Janet Weis Center for Research, Geisinger Clinic, 100 N. Academy Avenue, Danville, PA 17822-2601

Neonatal cardiac muscle cells are frequently used experimental systems in which to study cardiac growth during the first few days of life. The most commonly used experimental system is cultured neonatal rat cardiac muscle cells from 1–3-day-old rat pups. Three phases of growth occur in the neonatal rat heart: (a) a hyperplastic phase during the first 4–5 days of life that is characterized by a doubling of heart weight, (b) a transitional phase during which both hyperplasia and hypertrophy occur, and (c) a hypertrophic phase during which the heart grows by increasing myocyte volume (1). During the hyperplastic phase (1–5 days), the number of left and right ventricular myocytes increases 57% and 25%, respectively, while the increase in myocyte volume is similar in the left ventricle (LV) and right ventricle (RV) (2). Binucleated myocytes increase from 2.7% to 48% during the first 11 days of life. Thus, in vivo, the left ventricle of rat heart increases in size more rapidly than the right ventricle primarily by faster cellular proliferation during the first 3 days of life, when hearts are harvested for cell culture experiments.

Recently, methods were developed to culture cardiac muscle cells from the newborn pig heart (3). In contrast to the neonatal rat, the 4.3-fold increase in weight of the pig LV during the first 14 days of life is associated with a 3.4-fold increase in myocyte volume and a 1.3-fold increase in number of cells (Table 24–1; 4). Thus, approximately 80–90% of the growth of the LV is accounted for by cellular hypertrophy. The weight of the RV increases 1.75-fold, and the volume of RV myocytes increases 1.62-fold. The number of RV myocytes does not change significantly, indicating that nearly all growth of the RV during this period is by hypertrophy. Approximately 10% of the myocytes are binucleated at birth, and the percentage increases to 53% and 67% for the RV and LV, respectively, by 14 days of age. In contrast to the neonatal rat heart, the newborn pig heart grows by cellular hypertrophy rather than by hyperplasia during the period that the tissue is used for cell culture experiments.

TABLE 24–1. *Effect of piglet age on ventricular weight, myocyte volume, and myocyte number*[a]

Parameter	12 hr (5)	4.5 days (5–6)	14 days (5–7)
Body weight, kg	1.07 ± 0.08	1.49 ± 0.12	3.79 ± 0.28
Ventricle weight, g			
RVFW	2.03 ± 0.24	2.13 ± 0.22	3.56 ± 0.41*
LVFW	2.22 ± 0.10	4.05 ± 0.33*	9.62 ± 1.01*
Protein/DNA			
RVFW	39.2 ± 2.8	45.0 ± 1.6	45.2 ± 3.1
LVFW	30.4 ± 3.3	48.1 ± 1.0*	61.8 ± 3.4*
Myocyte volume, μm^3			
RVFW	1511 ± 57	1814 ± 143	2454 ± 259*
LVFW	1075 ± 59	1858 ± 40*	3688 ± 215*
Myocytes/ventricle $X10^{-8}$			
RVFW	10.1 ± 0.6	N.D.	12.4 ± 2.4
LVFW	16.9 ± 1.4	N.D.	21.7 ± 1.0*

[a]Hearts were removed from weight-matched littermate piglets at 12 hr, 4.5 days or 14 days after birth. The left and right ventricular free walls were collected and processed as previously described (4). Myocytes were isolated of the LVFW and RVFW of piglets of the same age, and size parameters were determined as previously described. Results represent the mean ± SEM for the number of piglets in parentheses.

*$P < 0.02$ as compared to the same ventricle from piglets less than 24 hr old, using Student's t-test.

The purpose of this article is to evaluate systems of neonatal cardiac myocytes for studies of increased myocardial cell size with particular attention to tissues and cells from rats and pigs. The indices of hypertrophy that are used are increased muscle cell volume and protein/DNA ratios. Studies of myocardial cell growth are to be distinguished from studies of signal transduction in response to cellular deformation or agonist/receptor binding without documented cellular hypertrophy. The latter experiments should not be construed to represent studies of the mechanisms of cardiac cellular hypertrophy.

CARDIAC ORIGINS AND DEVELOPMENT

Formation of the heart during embryogenesis of vertebrates involves commitment of mesodermal precursor cells to the cardiac lineage. Early events in formation of the chick heart include commitment of cells from the anterior lateral plate mesoderm to the cardiogenic lineage at approximately stages 3–4 (5,6). Morphologically, there is no sign that these cells will become heart cells, but when the cells are removed from embryos and grown in culture, differentiated cardiac myocytes appear 2 days later (7). When it is first recognizable morphologically, the heart precursor is a paired structure formed of premyocardial cells, pre-endocardial cells, and associated extracellular material (8,9). Fusion of the right and left cardiac precursors gives rise to the primitive heart tube, a structure with two concentric cellular layers, an inner endocardium, and an outer myocardium, separated by extracellular matrix. The heart tube loops, forms the outflow tract and atrial and ventricular cavities, and septates to produce the mature four-chambered heart. In the zebrafish, individual blastomeres can be filled with fluorescent dextran and their migratory path can be traced (10,11). By late blastula, different blastomeres have their progeny restricted to a single chamber, indicating that different chambers arise from different progenitors. Polarity is evident as early as the precardiac mesoderm in that more posterior tissue will form atria and more anterior tissue will form ventricles (8). Thus, the neonatal heart is made up of chambers of different cellular origin and phenotype. For example, an atrium-specific myosin heavy-chain isoform is expressed only in the posterior progenitors that lead to formation of atria (12). Another myosin heavy-chain isoform is expressed in all differentiated myocytes at early stages of heart formation. The possibility exists that cells of different lineage will respond in different ways to factors that may modify cardiac muscle cell growth.

In the neonatal rat heart, the usual procedure is to culture cells from the RV and LV together because of the small size of the organ and the difficulty in separating the free walls of the RV and LV. At 1 day of age in the rat, the RV and LV are approximately equal in size (2). In the newborn pig heart, weighing about 8 g, the free walls of RV and LV are also of approximately equal size and are easily dissected and provide sufficient tissue for culture of RV and LV myocytes.

Each ventricle is made up of muscle and nonmuscle cells, including fibroblasts, vascular cells, conduction tissue, and endocardium. During preparation of cardiac muscle cells, this cell type is enriched and constitutes 70–90% of the cells on the plate (3,13). As a result, heterogeneity is a problem in the interpretation of results as representing the properties of LV muscle cells. This problem is particularly acute in cultures of neonatal rat heart cells, where at least half the cells are derived from the RV or are nonmuscle cells.

EXPERIMENTAL MODELS FOR STUDY OF NEONATAL CARDIAC GROWTH

Criteria for Use of Cellular/Tissue Preparations

Common criteria for the suitability of tissue or cellular preparations for studies of growth are as follows (14). Cells of the preparation must be intact and capable of being supplied with saturating quantities of oxygen and oxidative substrate. When saturating quantities of these substances are available, tissue/cellular contents of ATP and creatine phosphate either are stable for several hours or may increase in quantity in cultured cells if creatine (5 mM) is included in the media. Rates of protein synthesis should be able to be made equal to rates of proteolysis and be similar to rates that occur in vivo. Isolated neonatal pig hearts perfused as

Langendorff preparations meet the criteria of cellular integrity, substrate delivery, and stable energy levels (15). Although rates of protein synthesis are stable during perfusion, in vivo rates of protein synthesis in hearts of newborn pigs are not available for comparison.

Cultured neonatal cardiomyocytes from pigs are made up of both rod-shaped (70–90%) and rounded cells, indicating that some cells may have lost their membrane integrity. Delivery of oxygen and substrates is easy and energy levels can be maintained if the cells from pigs or rats are cultured in the presence of creatine, taurine, carnitine, pyruvate, and insulin (3,16). Rates of protein synthesis in cultured cells reflect their calcium tolerance, the presence or absence of contractions, and addition of agonists. In cultured rat cardiomyocytes that beat spontaneously, arrest of contraction with 50 mM KCl decreases the rate of protein synthesis (17). Rates of protein synthesis have not been measured in isolated perfused neonatal rat hearts or in vivo for comparison with rates that are measured in cell culture. Thus, the extent to which the protein synthesis rate in cultured rat cardiomyocytes simulates the *in vivo* situation in neonatal rats is unknown. In cultured neonatal pig cardiomyocytes, freshly prepared cells usually do not beat regularly but may contract infrequently (3). Rates of protein synthesis in cultured cells can be compared to rates in the isolated perfused pig heart, but synthesis rates in the newborn pig are not available for comparison.

Another factor that may influence the suitability of tissue/cellular systems for studies of cardiomyocyte growth is the mechanical activity of the cells. The isolated perfused neonatal pig heart beats spontaneously, but a systematic study has not been undertaken to determine whether beating affects the rate of protein synthesis. In isolated perfused hearts of adult rats that also beat spontaneously, arrest of cardiac contraction has no effect on rates of protein synthesis even if arrest is combined with drainage of the left ventricle (18). In this preparation, rates of protein synthesis are increased by raising the perfusion pressure from 60 to 120 mmHg in beating, arrested, and arrested-drained preparations. These effects appear to depend upon stretch of the ventricular wall. Similar studies have not been undertaken in the perfused neonatal pig heart.

In cultured cells, mechanical activity and cell stretching increase rates of protein synthesis in rat cardiomyocytes (for reviews see refs. 13 and 19). Agonists such as norepinephrine also enhance contraction of rat cardiomyocytes, raising the question of whether the agonist effect is via induction of contraction or directly upon the pathway of protein synthesis. In rat cardiomyocytes this question was answered by demonstrating that norepinephrine accelerates protein synthesis in cultured cells in which contraction is arrested with 50 mM KCl (17). The basic question is whether the tissue/cellular preparation is still suitable for a meaningful evaluation of potential effects of a particular experimental variable after its imposition. (For example, does contraction of cells result in energy depletion that obscures the stimulatory effect of contraction on protein synthesis?)

Knowledge of the specific radioactivities of precursor pools of amino acids that serve protein synthesis and nucleotide pools that are incorporated into RNA is required for studies of cell growth if incorporation of radioactive precursors is to be interpreted reliably. In the perfused pig heart, the specific radioactivity of phenylalanine bound to transfer RNA is 92.5% of the specific activity of phenylalanine in the perfusate (20). These findings are similar to those in the perfused adult rat heart where complete equilibration of the specific radioactivities of tRNA-bound and perfusate phenylalanine is observed (21). In cultured cells, equilibration of tRNA-bound and medium phenylalanine is only about 60% complete (17; Beinlich, unpublished observations). Incomplete equilibration must be taken into account in comparing rates of protein synthesis in perfused newborn pig hearts and cultured neonatal pig cardiomyocytes. The possibility that an experimental variable affects the calculated rate of protein synthesis by changing the equilibration of tRNA-bound and medium phenylalanine in cultured cells must be considered. Characterization of precursor nucleotide pools for RNA synthesis has been achieved in cultured rat myocytes (17) but has not been studied in pig cardiomyocytes.

Finally, an important criterion for rigorous studies of cell growth is availability of cDNA probes and antibodies for identification of gene products. Since rats are one of the most commonly studied species, many more reagents for identification of RNAs and proteins are available for rats than pigs. These reagents are used to follow contents of messenger RNAs, to specifically measure the synthesis of ribosomal RNA by hybridization with ribosomal DNA and to follow the appearance of newly made proteins, such as transcription factors, and their phosphorylation or other posttranslational modification.

Criteria for Assessing Cellular Hypertrophy

The gold standard for assessment of hypertrophy is measurement of myocyte volume. In rat and pig hearts, cardiomyocytes are dissociated enzymatically, they are fixed with buffer that contains glutaraldehyde, and their size is determined with a Coulter counter or morphometrically (4). When DNA content per heart portion is constant, as is the case in the first 4.5 days of a piglet's life, protein/DNA ratios also reflect cellular hypertrophy. As seen in Table 24–1, myocyte volume increases by a factor of 1.2 and 1.72 in RVFW and LVFW, respectively, from 12 hours to 4.5 days of life. In these heart portions, protein/DNA increases by a factor of 1.15 and 1.58. From 4.5 to 14 days in the newborn pig, approximately 60% of cardiac myocytes become binucleated, and DNA content per heart portion increases proportionally. In this situation, protein/DNA ratios are unreliable indices of cellular hypertrophy. For example, myocyte volume increases 1.35 and 1.98 times in the RVFW and LVFW, respectively, between 4.5 and 14 days of age. In these heart portions, protein/DNA is unchanged in the RVFW and increases only 1.28 times in the LVFW.

In cultured cells, measurement of cell volume is the most reliable index of hypertrophy, but protein/DNA ratios are a suitable surrogate, especially if the DNA content per culture dish is unchanged over the duration of the experiment. Morphometric measurements of cellular area are often unreliable indices of cell volume because of thinning and spreading of cultured cells.

EXPERIMENTAL MODELS

Isolated Perfused Neonatal Pig Heart

The isolated perfused heart is a useful experimental system in which to assess the mechanisms of rapid growth of the pig heart during the first 2 weeks of life (15). In this physiologic example of growth, the slow-growing RV is an intra-organ control for the rapidly growing LV to account for differences in animal size and nutritional status. During the first 2 weeks of life, the weight of the left ventricular free wall (LVFW) approximately doubles in 4.5 days and increases 4.3 times in 14 days (Table 24–1; 4). Rapid growth of LVFW is accompanied by a 3.6-fold increase in total protein and 3.2-fold greater RNA content. The RVFW weight increases 1.75-fold during the first 14 days of life, and total protein and RNA change to a similar extent. As the cells binucleate, DNA increases 1.63-fold in the RVFW and 2.24-fold in the LVFW during the first 14 days of life.

Growth of the newborn pig heart can be manipulated in vivo with oral administration of angiotensin-converting enzyme (ACE) inhibitors such as enalapril maleate (22). The ACE inhibitor restrains growth of the LVFW by partially preventing hypertrophy of the muscle cells, but enalapril has no effect on RVFW myocyte growth (4). Whether the lack of effect of an ACE inhibitor on the RV is due to a phenotypic difference between RV and LV myocytes that reflects different cellular origins or to a difference imposed by the mechanical loading of these cells in vivo remains to be determined.

Hearts are removed from control and enalapril-treated animals at various days of age and are perfused in vitro as Langendorff preparations for measurement of rates of protein synthesis and ribosome formation (22,23). As noted earlier, the specific radioactivity of tRNA-bound phenylalanine relative to perfusate phenylalanine is known, so that meaningful synthetic rates can be calculated using radioactive precursors. The perfused heart is hemodynamically stable for 1–2 hours and allows for effects of hormonal agents to be assessed. Sufficient tissue is available in both the RVFW and LVFW for measurements of rates of protein synthesis and for preparation of ribosomal subunits to assess rates of ribosome formation.

Neither adrenergic agonists, angiotensin II, bradykinin, glucagon, nor a phosphodiesterase inhibitor (IBMX) that increases cellular cyclic AMP has an effect on rates of protein synthesis or ribosome formation when added to the perfusate of control piglet hearts (24). Some of these agents (adrenergic agonists, angiotensin II, and IBMX) accelerate heart rate in these same preparations, demonstrating that they are active on other physiologic events. These observations led to the suggestion that protein synthesis and ribosome formation are maximally stimulated in control hearts and, as a result, are insensitive to further stimulation.

In hearts from enalapril-treated pigs in which LV growth is restrained, ribosome formation in the LVFW is 33% lower than in control hearts, but this rate is unchanged in the RVFW (25). Addition of norepinephrine to the perfusate accelerates ribosome formation in the LVFW of the enalapril-treated piglet but has no effect on ribosome formation in the RVFW of the same heart. Addition of angiotensin II has no effect on ribosome formation. Rates of protein synthesis are not increased in the first hour after norepinephrine addition because the effect on ribosome formation must persist for several hours to increase ribosome content before rates of protein synthesis can change. In this context, the effect of norepinephrine is on the capacity for synthesis via ribosome formation rather than on the efficiency with which existing protein synthetic components are used.

In contrast to cultured cells that will be discussed in the next section, isolated hearts are perfused with Krebs-Henseleit bicarbonate buffer that contains 5 mM glucose and 5 mM lactate as substrate at a perfusion pressure of 60 mmHg (20). Insulin is not added to the perfusate of control hearts. Under similar conditions in the isolated perfused adult rat heart, a partial block in peptide chain initiation develops after about 1 hour of perfusion that is corrected by addition of insulin (14). In the perfused neonatal pig heart, a partial block in peptide chain initiation may be present throughout perfusion because approximately 16–20% of RNA is in ribosomal subunits in untreated piglets in vivo and during perfusion as compared to approximately 9% of RNA in subunits in vivo in piglets that have been treated with insulin (20). Addition of insulin to the perfusate has no significant effect on rates of protein synthesis or ribosomal subunit content in the LVFW during the first hour of perfusion, but the hormone raises the rate of synthesis approximately 40% in the RVFW and decreases ribosomal subunit content (20). We must explore whether the differential responsiveness of the RVFW and LVFW during in vivo treatment with the ACE-inhibitor enalapril and exposure to norepinephrine and insulin during in vitro perfusion represent phenotypic differences that are accounted for by different cellular origins.

The isolated perfused neonatal pig heart is a useful preparation in which to monitor changes in rates of protein synthesis and ribosome formation during the rapid hypertrophic growth of the LV and modest hypertrophy of the RV. Sufficient tissue is available to measure both rates in the LVFW and RVFW. The cells are intact, energy levels are maintained, and the heart beats spontaneously. Short-term effects of potential growth-promoting agents can be explored by their addition to the perfusate. If differential effects occur in the RV compared to those in the LV, as is the case with norepinephrine and insulin, these effects are easily detected.

Cultured Neonatal Pig Cardiomyocytes

Cardiac muscle cells are isolated from the LVFW and RVFW of the piglet heart following perfusion as a Langendorff preparation with nominally Ca^{2+}-free buffer that contains 2,3-butanedione monoxime (BDM) to inhibit contraction and collagenase A and hyaluronidase to digest extracellular components (3). The LVFW and RVFW are harvested from the digested heart, minced, and incubated for 15 min at 37°C in protease-free buffer containing deoxyribonuclease II. The Ca^{2+} concentration is gradually restored to 1 mM as the BDM is gradually removed. The cell suspensions are filtered and repeatedly sedimented to remove nonviable myocytes and nonmuscle cells. The cardiomyocytes are suspended in serum-free Dulbecco minimal essential medium supplemented with 0.2% bovine serum albumin, creatine (5 mM), taurine (5 mM), carnitine (2 mM), sodium pyruvate (2 mM), insulin (10^{-7} M), penicillin (100 IU/ml), and streptomycin (100 μg/ml). Myocytes are plated on laminin-coated 100-mm culture dishes for 15–30 min at a density of 1.5×10^6 rod-shaped cells per dish. Sufficient cells are obtained from a single heart for more than 25 dishes of cells from both the RVFW and LVFW. Nonadherent cells are washed from the plate, and fresh media are added. In some experiments this medium contains 40 mM KCl. Cells are maintained for up to 3 days with daily changes of media. The cultures generally contain 60–80% rod-shaped cells after 3 hours in culture, and cross-striations are visible on the generally quiescent cells that are observed without 40 mM KCl addition. After 1 day in culture, the cells remain elongated, but the ends become rounded. In the presence of 40 mM KCl, the cells spread during the first day of incubation (Beinlich, unpublished observations).

The growth-promoting effects of endothelin-1 (1×10^{-7} M) and norepinephrine (1×10^{-5} M) and propranolol (2×10^{-6} M) are assessed by addition to the media (3). Rates of protein synthesis are measured by addition of [^{3}H] phenylalanine (1 μCi/ml) to culture media that contains 0.4 mM phenylalanine. The specific radioactivity of t-RNA-bound phenylalanine is approximately 60% of the specific radioactivity of phenylalanine in the media in both RV and LV myocytes (Beinlich, unpublished observations). Contents of ATP and creatine phosphate are relatively constant at values similar to those found in the intact heart (3).

Incorporation of [^{3}H] phenylalanine into protein increases linearly during the first 24 hours of culture in cells incubated in media with or without 40 mM KCl. When the rate of protein synthesis is compared to rates that are observed in perfused hearts from piglets of the same age, the rates during the first day of culture in myocytes from the RVFW and LVFW are approximately 60% of the rate observed during the first hour of perfusion of the isolated heart (Beinlich, unpublished observations). During days 2 and 3 of culture of LV myocytes in the absence of 40 mM KCl, the rates of protein synthesis falls by 29% and 37%, respectively. When 40 mM KCl is present, rates of protein synthesis are unchanged during days 2 and 3 of incubation (Beinlich, unpublished observations).

Inclusion of endothelin-1 in media containing 40 mM KCl increases the rates of protein synthesis in LV myocytes by 50% and 78% during days 2 and 3, respectively (Beinlich, unpublished observations). Without addition of 40 mM KCl, percentage changes in relation to control cells are similar, but absolute rates are less because of the decline in control values. Inclusion of norepinephrine/propranolol has a smaller effect on rates of protein synthesis (approximately 15%) in LV myocytes that are cultured for 3 days in media containing 40 mM KCl. Endothelin-1 and norepinephrine induce cell spreading and contraction of the cells during incubation in the absence of 40 mM KCl (3). Endothelin-1 enhances cell spreading in LV myocytes that are cultured in media with 40 mM KCl. The effects of beating and cell stretch have not been studied.

Cultured neonatal pig cardiomyocytes are a useful experimental system in which to explore longer-term effects of such growth-promoting agents as endothelin-1 and norepinephrine. The cultured myocyte system is much less heterogeneous than the intact heart, and sufficient cells are obtained from the LVFW and RVFW for separate measurements of rates of protein synthesis. Rates during the first 24 hours of culture are approximately 60% of rates observed in the RVFW and LVFW of isolated perfused piglet hearts despite the fact that the cultured cells are quiescent.

Cultured Neonatal Rat Cardiomyocytes

Since their introduction in the early 1980s cultured neonatal rat heart cardiomyocytes have been used extensively for studies of cardiac cellular growth and signal transduction (26–29). Generally 30–40 newborn rat pups, preferably 1–2 days of age, are used to prepare sufficient cells for 30 or more 60-mm dishes of cells (17). The right and left ventricles are minced together in Ca^{2+}-Mg^{2+} free Hanks' salt solution buffered with 30 mM HEPES and incubated with a mixture of partially purified trypsin, chymotrypsin, and elastase. The cells are dissociated and mixed with minimum essential medium EAGLE (MEM) containing 10% newborn calf serum and 0.1 mM 5-bromo-2′-deoxyuridine (BrdU). The cells are filtered and plated as described earlier (17). The cells may be plated sparsely (1.5×10^6 cells per 60-mm dish) so that there is little contact between cells or more densely (4×10^6 cells per 60-mm dish) so that most cells are in contact and beat synchronously. As noted earlier, at 1 day of age the RV and LV are approximately equal in size, suggesting that approximately equal numbers of RV and LV myocytes are present in the culture. After an overnight incubation, the attached cells are rinsed and maintained in serum-free medium (17). The standard MEM is supplemented with MEM amino acids, vitamins, penicillin-streptomycin, glutamine, $NaSeO_4$, transferrin, BrdU, and ascorbic acid. The supplemented MEM contains fatty substrates and leucine in concentrations that stimulate peptide chain initiation in isolated perfused hearts of adult rats (14). As a result, accelerated rates of protein synthesis follow formation of new ribosomes and the resulting increase in capacity for synthesis (17).

The muscle cells do not divide in culture, although the rat heart grows by cellular proliferation in the first 4–5 days of life. Under culture conditions, the mixed cardiomyocyte population grows by cellular hypertrophy, which is usually assessed by measurement of protein/DNA ratios. The specific radioactivities of tRNA-bound phenylalanine and UTP have been measured so that rates of protein and RNA synthesis can be calculated (17). These rates cannot be compared with rates in the intact heart either in vitro or in the newborn rat pup because these measurements have not been made.

Hypertrophy of cultured neonatal rat cardiomyocytes is induced by mechanical, neural, endocrine, paracrine, and autocrine mechanisms (19). These factors include contractile activity, cell stretch, α- and β-adrenergic agonists, thyroid hormone, endothelin-1, angiotensin II, and agents that activate protein kinase C, such as phorbol esters. Accelerated ribosome formation depends upon faster transcription of ribosomal DNA that is controlled by activity of a RNA polymerase I transcription factor, upstream binding factor (UBF) (13).

Cultured neonatal rat cardiomyocytes are a useful experimental system in which to study the mechanisms of cardiac hypertrophy. The cells are intact, are easily supplied with nutrients and oxygen, and maintain their ATP and creatine phosphate contents over several days of culture (16). The specific radioactivity of precursor pools for protein and RNA synthesis is characterized so that radioactive precursors can be used for measurements of rates of synthesis. Antibodies and cDNA probes are available to characterize a wide range of gene products. The major disadvantage of the system is that it contains a heterogeneous mixture of right and left ventricular myocytes together with some nonmuscle cells. No data are available to indicate whether RV and LV myocytes respond in the same way to growth-promoting agents. The system is not a model for growth of the newborn rat heart during the first 4–5 days of life because the heart *in vivo* grows by cellular proliferation not hypertrophy, as occurs in the culture system. A mixture of right and left ventricular myocytes from 1–2-day-old rat pups probably is not a model for hypertrophic growth of the left ventricle that begins at about 1 week of life. At this time, LV myocytes hypertrophy much more than RV myocytes that constitute 50% of the cultured cells. The phenotype of cells from 7–14-day-old rats is certainly quite different from that of cultured cells. The cardiomyocytes from older hearts do not proliferate but do undergo nuclear division to become binucleated. Cells from adult animals express different phenotypes from cells from newborn animals (30), so that neither cultured neonatal rat nor pig cardiomyocytes may demonstrate the same responses to growth-promoting stimuli as adult cardiomyocytes.

CONCLUSIONS

Cultured neonatal rat cardiomyocytes are the most frequently used model because of the convenience of obtaining and culturing the cells. Hypertrophy is induced in a cell preparation that would normally divide. The preparation is grossly heterogeneous because it consists of right and left ventricular muscle cells and nonmuscle cells. The extent to which heterogeneity affects responses to mechanical factors and hormones is unknown. The magnitude of effects on hypertrophy of left ventricular myocytes is unknown because of the heterogeneity.

The isolated perfused neonatal pig heart retains normal morphologic relationships of an organ whose left ventricle is growing by hypertrophy. Differential rates of growth of the right and left ventricle are observed in vivo, and these rates respond differentially to treatment with ACE-inhibitors. In control hearts, protein synthesis and ribosome formation in the RV or LV do not respond to usual growth stimuli during perfusion, but in hearts from enalapril-treated animals, rates of ribosome formation increase in LV, but not in RV, in response to an α-adrenergic agonist. Effects of mechanical stimuli have not been explored, and the stability of the preparation is limited to 2 hours.

The newborn pig heart is sufficiently large to allow for separation and culture of cardiomyocytes from LVFW and RVFW. Although the cells maintain or increase their ATP and creatine phosphate contents during culture, rates of protein synthesis fall over 3 days of culture. The rate of protein synthesis is stable if cells are exposed to 40 mM KCl to arrest the minimal contractions. Cell spreading is increased by arrest with KCl, adrenergic agonists, and endothelin. Cultured pig cardiomyocytes offer the opportunity to study cellular hypertrophy of RVFW and LVFW cardiomyocytes from an organ that grows in vivo by hypertrophy rather than by cellular proliferation.

SUMMARY

Experimental systems from rats and pigs are used to study rapid growth of the heart in the neonatal period. These systems have both advantages and disadvantages. Overall, the focus of studies must be on the mechanisms of cardiomyocyte growth. Hypertrophy of cells will occur only if total protein is made more rapidly than it is degraded. The purpose must be to define molecular mechanisms that either increase the efficiency or capacity of total protein synthesis or decrease the rate of degradation. Studies of the expression of surrogate markers for hypertrophy, such as oncogene products and myosin light and heavy chains, may obscure the determination of molecular mechanisms of hypertrophy if the mechanisms of surrogate gene expression are extrapolated to represent mechanisms of growth of the heart.

REFERENCES

1. Clubb FJ Jr, Bishop SP. Formation of binucleated myocardial cells in the neonatal rat. *Lab Invest* 1984;50:571–577.
2. Anversa P, Olivetti G, Loud AV. Morphometric study of early postnatal development in the left and right ventricular myocardium of the rat. 1. Hypertrophy, hyperplasia and binucleation of myocytes. *Circ Res* 1980;46:495–502.
3. Beinlich CJ, Morgan HE. Development of a cell culture system for neonatal pig cardiomyocyte growth studies. In: Yazaki Y, ed. *Cardiac development and gene regulation.* Tokyo: Excerpta Medica; 1995:65–75.
4. Beinlich CJ, Rissinger CJ, Morgan HE. Mechanisms of rapid growth in the neonatal pig heart. *J Mol Cell Cardiol* 1995;27:273–281.

5. Hamburger V, Hamilton HL. A series of normal stages in the development of the chick embryo. *J Morphol* 1951;88:49–67.
6. Garcia-Martinez V, Schoenwolf GC. Primitive-streak origin of the cardiovascular system in avian embryos. *Dev Biol* 1993;159:706–719.
7. Gonzalez-Sanchez A, Bader D. In vitro analysis of cardiac progenitor cell differentiation. *Dev Biol* 1990;139:197–209.
8. DeHaan RL. Morphogenesis of the vertebrate heart. In: DeHaan RL, Ursprung H, eds. *Organogenesis.* New York: Holt, Rinehart and Winston; 1964:377–419.
9. Rosenquist GC. A radioautographic study of labeled grafts in the chick blastoderm: development from primitive-streak stages to stage 12. *Carnegie Inst Wash Contrib Embryol* 1966;38:71–110.
10. Stainer DYR, Lee RK, Fishman MC. Cardiovascular development in the zebrafish. I: Myocardial fate map and heart tube formation. *Development* 1993;119:31–40.
11. Stainier DYR, Fishman MC. The zebrafish as a model system to study cardiovascular development. *Trends Cardiovasc Med* 1994;4:207–212.
12. Yutzey KE, Rhee JT, Bader D. Expression of the atrial-specific myosin heavy chain AMHC1 and the establishment of anteroposterior polarity in the developing chicken heart. *Development* 1994;120:871–883.
13. Hannan RD, Rothblum LI. Regulation of ribosomal DNA transcription during neonatal cardiomyocyte hypertrophy. *Cardiovasc Res* 1995;30:501–510.
14. Morgan HE, Chua BHL, Russo L. Protein synthesis and degradation. In: Fozzard HA, Haber E, Jennings RB, Katz A, Morgan HE, eds. *The heart and cardiovascular system.* New York: Raven Press; 1992:1505–1524.
15. Beinlich CJ, Morgan HE. Growth of the neonatal pig heart. In: Dhalla NS, Pierce GN, Panagia V, Beamish RD, eds. *Heart hypertrophy and failure.* Boston: Kluwer Academic Publishers; 1995: 171–182.
16. Allo SN, Carl LL, Morgan HE. Acceleration of growth of cultured cardiomyocytes and translocation of protein kinase C. *Am J Physiol* 1992;263:C319–C325.
17. McDermott PJ, Morgan HE. Contraction modulates the capacity for protein synthesis during growth of neonatal heart cells in culture. *Circ Res* 1989;64:542–553.
18. Kira Y, Kochel PJ, Gordon EE, Morgan HE. Aortic perfusion pressure as a determinant of cardiac protein synthesis. *Am J Physiol* 1984;246:C247–C258.
19. Morgan HE, Baker KM. Cardiac hypertrophy: mechanical, neural and endocrine dependence. *Circulation* 1991;83:13–25.
20. Peterson CJ, Whitman V, Watson PA, Schuler HG, Morgan HE. Mechanisms of differential growth of heart ventricles in newborn pigs. *Circ Res* 1989;64:360–369.
21. McKee EE, Cheung JY, Rannels DE, Morgan HE. Measurement of the rate of protein synthesis and compartmentation of heart phenylalanine. *J Biol Chem* 1978;253:1030–1040.
22. Beinlich CJ, White GJ, Baker KM, Morgan HE. Angiotensin II and left ventricular growth in newborn pig hearts. *J Mol Cell Cardiol* 1991;23:1031–1038.
23. Camacho JA, Peterson CJ, White GJ, Morgan HE. Accelerated ribosome formation and growth in neonatal pig hearts. *Am J Physiol* 1990;258:C86–C91.
24. Beinlich CJ, Baker KM, White GJ, Morgan HE. Control of growth in neonatal pig heart. *Am J Physiol* 1991;261(suppl 1):3–7.
25. Beinlich CJ, Baker KM, Morgan HE. α-Adrenergic receptor agonists stimulate ribosome formation in hearts from enalapril-treated piglets. *J Mol Cell Cardiol* 1993;25:395–406.
26. Clark WA, Zak R. Assessment of fractional rates of protein synthesis in cardiac muscle cultures after equilibrium labeling. *J Biol Chem* 1981;256:4863–4870.
27. Frelin C. The regulation of protein turnover in newborn rat heart cell cultures. *J Biol Chem* 1980;255:11149–11155.
28. Simpson P, Savion S. Differentiation of rat myocytes in single cell cultures with and without proliferating nonmyocardial cells. *Circ Res* 1982;50:101–116.
29. Simpson P, McGrath A, Savion S. Myocyte hypertrophy in neonatal rat heart cultures and its regulation by serum and by catecholamines. *Circ Res* 1982;51:787–801.
30. Chien KR. Molecular analysis of cardiac developmental phenotypes: problems, progress and prospects. In: Yazaki Y, ed. *Cardiac development and gene regulation.* Tokyo: Excerpta Medica; 1995:1–28.

The Developing Heart,
edited by Bohuslav Ošťádal et al.
Lippincott-Raven Publishers,
Philadelphia © 1997.

25

Cardiac Hypertrophy in Newborn Rats with Genetic or Experimental Hypertension

Jaroslav Kuneš, Zdenka Dobešová, and Josef Zicha

Institute of Physiology, Academy of Sciences of the Czech Republic, Vídeňská 1083, CZ-142 20 Prague 4, Czech Republic

It has been suggested that there are two components in the etiology of essential hypertension: an initiating process and an amplifying one (1). The initiating process should start the mechanisms leading to the blood pressure rise, and the amplifying process should progressively magnify the blood pressure difference throughout the life. If this is true, the initiating abnormality could be difficult to detect because it would have only a small effect on blood pressure and other systems in the beginning of the disease. The development of hypertension should be therefore studied with respect to the maturation of the organism. There is considerable evidence for important ontogenetic changes of structure and function of the cardiovascular and renal systems (for details see ref. 2). Thus, the prevention of the development of hypertension and its cardiovascular complications would require the detailed analysis of all factors that can influence the organism during early developmental periods.

Embryonic and fetal life is a characteristic period for the growth of the vertebrate heart. Strong hyperplasia is typical for fetal life and persists shortly after birth (to the fourth day of postnatal life). In this period the heart grows more rapidly than the rest of the animal, so that the heart weight/body weight ratio maximizes at 4–5 days of age and then declines (3). During this phase of rapid growth, left ventricle (LV) grows faster than right ventricle (RV); thus, LV weight exceeds RV weight in the first week of postnatal life in both rat (4) and human (5) hearts. It is evident that the response of the heart to increased metabolic demands or to an increased workload depends on the age of the animal when the stress is imposed. Increased myocardial workload due to higher blood pressure, chronic hypoxia, or carbon monoxide exposure during fetal or early neonatal life leads to cardiac enlargement. It is generally accepted that hyperplasia of myocardial cells does not occur in mature hearts, the enlargement of which is due to cell hypertrophy. Several mechanisms triggering cardiac enlargement in the neonatal period can be involved (6–8). In the present review we shall focus on the role of blood pressure as a primary event in this process.

BLOOD PRESSURE IN NEWBORN RATS

In normotensive strains mean arterial blood pressure of newborn rats is about 14 mmHg, and it increases to 85 mmHg within the next 3 weeks (9).

The development of hypertension has been studied extensively in spontaneously hypertensive rats (SHR), which are hemodynamically similar in many aspects to humans with essential hypertension (10). This genetic model offers a big advantage because the genetic basis for hypertension development became more established in SHR than did that for essential hypertension in humans. The number of studies on neonatal manifestations of hypertension in various experimental models is increasing (for a review see ref. 11).

The first values of systolic blood pressure in the early postnatal life of hypertensive rats were received by Jones and Dowd in 2-day-old rats of New Zealand hypertensive strain (12). The tail-cuff pressure in ether-anesthetized rats was 41.6 ± 1.6 mmHg, and it was significantly higher than in appropriate control animals (36.4 ± 1.5 mmHg, $p < 0.05$). Recently, servo-null micropipette transducer system helped to measure blood pressure in newborn rats. By this technique, several investigative groups have recorded discrepant results in newborn SHR in comparison with Wistar-Kyoto (WKY) controls. Lais et al. (13) found no differences in blood pressure between SHR and WKY newborns (SHR: 36 ± 2 mmHg, WKY: 37 ± 3 mmHg). The animals were restrained on a heated table and blood pressure was measured in the femoral artery under local intracutaneous anesthesia with 1% procaine. On the other hand, Bruno et al. (14) recorded 26.0 ± 0.7 mmHg in Inactin-anesthetized SHR and 22.0 ± 0.4 mmHg in WKY rats ($p < 0.001$). All pressure readings were done in the femoral artery and were started within 30–40 min after the injection of the anesthetic. The similar results were obtained by Gray (15,16) in sodium pentobarbitol-anesthetized pups. In this case, the carotid artery was used for blood pressure determination and the blood pressure values were 30.8 ± 0.9 mmHg for SHR and 24.2 ± 1.0 mmHg for WKY pups ($p < 0.05$). Finally, Clubb et al. (17) have also used micropressure servo-null system for blood pressure measurement in restrained newborn rats. Animals were locally anesthetized with 1% lidocaine injected subcutaneously into the femoral area and blood pressure was recorded in the femoral artery. Mean arterial blood pressure of SHR pups was 24.6 ± 0.7 mmHg, and this was significantly higher from that of WKY ones (18.4 ± 1.9 mmHg). The reasons for the preceding results are unclear but may be related to the use of different substrains of SHR and to some differences in the methodology.

The developmental increase of arterial blood pressure is dependent on two fundamental hemodynamic variables, cardiac output and total peripheral resistance, which are changing progressively during the postnatal period. At birth, there are major changes in the circulation, when the lungs are becoming functional and placental circulation ceases. Thus, there is reduced peripheral resistance to the right side of the heart, whereas the left side has increased peripheral resistance. It is not known whether the changes in peripheral resistance or cardiac output play a significant role in the increase of blood pressure in SHR newborns. There is some evidence that heart rate is always higher in newborn SHR compared to WKY controls (14,16), but because of a high variability in the individual values within each group the difference between SHR And WKY did not reach statistical significance.

The increased blood pressure in SHR newborns may be simply due to a more advanced stage of maturation. This is supported by the observation that sympathetic influence on heart rate in newborn SHR was enhanced (18). Moreover, higher blood pressure might also be the result of a more advanced stage of mononuclear cardiomyocyte development in newborn SHR (17). There is still a question of whether the accelerated hyperplastic growth of cardiomyocytes in SHR fetus could influence blood pressure level or increased pressure in fetal SHR could accelerated myocyte growth.

CARDIAC HYPERPLASIA AND/OR HYPERTROPHY IN NEWBORN RATS

Cardiac muscle growth can be regulated by two sets of factors: those that during normal growth maintain the proper allometric ratio of heart to body size, and those that are responsible for matching the heart size to the functional load during adaptation to altered hemodynamic requirements (19). Because cardiac myogenesis takes place prior to any apparent physiologic influence from the undeveloped circulatory system, it may be speculated that all steps in heart development are controlled by a time-dependent developmental program. Certainly, it is difficult to determine the distinction between endogenous developmental program and the influence of circulation on cardiac myogenesis. However, hemodynamic factors seem to influence the progression of morphogenesis, and the importance of hemodynamic factors in the regulation of cardiac growth following birth is clearly established. This can be well documented by increased left ventricular growth after the postnatal increase in peripheral resistance.

The dissociation between elevated blood pressure and cardiac hypertrophy that has been demonstrated in animals and humans suggests the existence of stimuli other than blood pressure that are responsible for the development of cardiac hypertrophy (20–23). Several investigators have suggested that sympathetic inervation of cardiac muscle is also involved in the control of myocyte proliferation and differentiation (24–26). Alternatively, it has been shown that such inervation is not always necessary for the normal development of heart (27). But there is some evidence that despite the lack of functional neurotransmission, adrenergic receptors are already present in the neonate (28). When examining the early role of nervous influence on the heart, two different effects must be considered: the actual nervous transmission and the humoral influences. Experiments using tissue cultures have suggested that, at least in vitro, nervous tissue can influence contractile protein production in both cardiac and skeletal muscle (29,30) and that both biochemical and physiologic characteristics of myocytes can be modified by nervous influences (23). Although the nervous system is one of the factors that control cell proliferation, the ultimate mechanism responsible for the decline in the mitotic activity of cardiac myocytes is unknown. Several hypotheses have been proposed, but none of them is entirely satisfactory (31).

It can be suggested that cardiac hypertrophy involves a sequence of events, including initiating signals, coupling mechanisms, and regulation of gene expression (Fig. 25–1). The adaptive hypertrophy and altered contractility are physiologic consequences of these events. Although several stimuli have been shown to induce cardiac hypertrophy, the exact mechanisms mediating the hypertrophic process are still unclear.

There is some evidence that the mechanism for the increased heart weight in SHR newborns is an accelerated rate of hyperplasia in utero. Clubb et al. (17) have

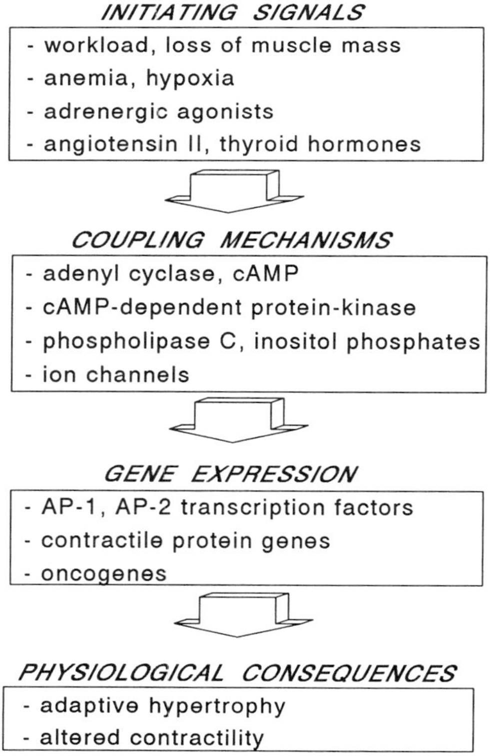

FIG. 25–1. Possible mechanisms associated with the process of cardiac hypertrophy.

demonstrated that, despite the lack of difference in cell size between SHR and WKY at birth, there was a larger number of SHR cardiomyocytes at birth. The estimated myocardial cell number in newborn SHR was $15.4 \pm 1.1 \times 10^6$ compared to $10.8 \pm 0.9 \times 10^6$ in WKY. This difference was even reversed at the third postnatal day and disappeared by the fifteenth postnatal day. This is in good agreement with our previous results (32), suggesting that relative DNA content in newborn hearts was significantly higher in SHR than in WKY pups. Because the relative protein content was only slightly higher in SHR, one can speculate that hearts of SHR newborns contain more cells that are smaller or that have more binucleated cells. Clubb et al. (17) demonstrated that at birth all cardiomyocytes were mononucleated in both SHR and WKY hearts. Moreover, we have demonstrated (33) that the diameter across the cell, measured at the level of the nucleus in nondividing cells, was significantly smaller in cardiomyocytes from SHR (6.45 ± 0.08 vs 6.95 ± 0.09 μm, $p < 0.01$). This supports the idea that SHR hearts contain more cells at birth.

Several investigative groups studied SHR hearts at early developmental stages and all concluded that cardiac hypertrophy occurs very early in the hypertensive process (for review see ref. 11). Table 25–1 summarizes the data on the relative heart weight in newborn spontaneously hypertensive rats. As can be seen, relative heart weight was always significantly higher in SHR newborns when compared either with WKY control pups or Brown Norway (BN) ones. On the contrary, Pang et al. (34) demonstrated that comparison of Kyoto stroke-prone SHR (SHRSP) with their normotensive WKY controls did not reveal any difference in relative heart weight between hypertensive and normotensive babies (SHRSP: 5.6 ± 0.1 mg/g, WKY: 5.6 ± 0.1 mg/g). This was due not to the difference between SHRSP and other SHR substrains but to the difference between particular control substrains. This suggested that the genetic background might play a very significant role in the determination of cardiac enlargement. This idea is supported by other results of Pang et al. (34). Cardiac enlargement in newborns was also seen in some other ge-

TABLE 25–1. *Relative heart weight (mg/g) in newborn SHR and normotensive controls*

Author	SHR		Ref.
		WKY	
Cutilletta et al. (1978)	4.27 ± 0.08	3.69 ± 0.08	50
Hamet et al. (1982)	5.52 ± 0.08	4.60 ± 0.09	32
Gray (1984)	3.82 ± 0.18	3.24 ± 0.09	16
Kuneš et al. (1984)	5.50 ± 0.06	4.54 ± 0.06	33
Clubb et al. (1987)	4.6 ± 0.1	3.7 ± 0.1	17
		BN	
Dobešová et al. (1995)	5.13 ± 0.10	4.20 ± 0.10	38

SHR, spontaneously hypertensive; WKY, Wistar-Kyoto normotensive controls; BN, Brown Norway normotensive strain.
Data are means ± SEM.

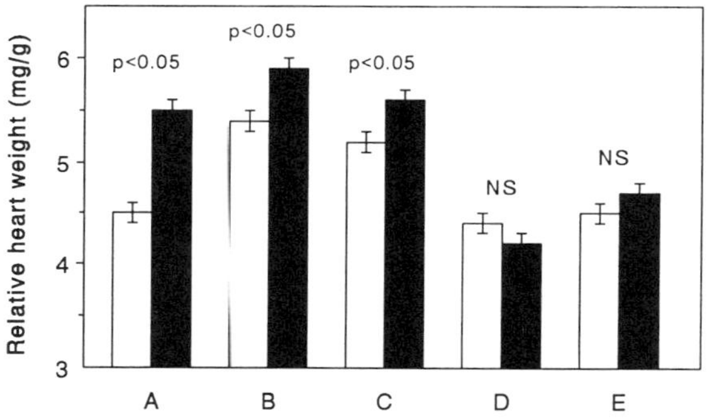

FIG. 25–2. Relative heart weight in newborn rats of different strains with genetic or experimental hypertension (*full columns*) and their respective normotensive controls (*open columns*). (**A**) WKY vs SHR. (**B**) New Zealand hypertensive strain. (**C**) Lyon hypertensive strain. (**D**) Milan hypertensive strain. (**E**) DCCA–salt-treated rats. (For more details see ref. 34.)

netic models with spontaneous hypertension (Fig. 25–2) (e.g., in New Zealand genetically hypertensive rats and Lyon hypertensive rats). On the other hand, this was not true for the Milan hypertensive strain, which is known to have renal abnormalities. In addition, we have included the offspring of genetically normotensive Wistar rats in which severe DOCA-salt hypertension was induced. There was no difference in relative heart weight between offspring of normotensive mothers and mothers with DOCA-salt hypertension (Fig. 25–2). It has been proven that even in adult rats a significant left ventricular hypertrophy already occurred after 1 week of DOCA-salt treatment prior to blood pressure elevation, suggesting that blood pressure, a determinant of left ventricle wall tension, is not a primary trigger for the initiation of left ventricular hypertrophy, at least in this experimental model (35). Recently, we have found (36) that the relative heart weight was even significantly lower in newborns of Prague hypertensive rats in comparison with the appropriate normotensive controls (4.49 $\pm$ 0.05 vs 4.71 $\pm$ 0.05 mg/g, $p < 0.05$). Similarly, we have demonstrated (37) in Dahl rats that the relative heart weight was always higher in newborns of Dahl salt-resistant dams when compared to those of Dahl salt-sensitive (DS) dams irrespective of the fact that DS dams had higher blood pressure. On the other hand, heart weight of newborns correlated significantly with maternal blood pressure only in that part of recombinant inbred strains (SHR $\times$ BN) that were derived from SHR mother (38). Taking all these results together, it is again evident that other factors besides blood pressure play a significant role in the determination of cardiac weight in newborn hypertensive rats.

CONCLUSION

Cardiac hypertrophy associated with hypertension does not appear to be a simple functional response of the myocardium to the mechanical stress after overload.

Several studies have shown the dissociation between the degree of cardiac hypertrophy and blood pressure level in both human and animal models of hypertension (20–24).

The existence of critical developmental periods stimulates the research in very early developmental periods to document hypertensive changes at the earliest significant level and their relationship to cardiac enlargement. Blood pressure may always be higher in SHR babies, even in utero, and thus could influence heart weight. But several developmental studies have also reported the early increase of adrenal medullary function (39), vasopressin (40), and renin-angiotensin system (41–43) in the fetal and neonatal periods. These factors are important for blood pressure regulation in spontaneous hypertension of the rat as well as in essential hypertension of humans. Moreover, a transfer of potential hypertensive humoral factor via breast milk was also demonstrated (44).

To assess the molecular mechanisms of cardiac hypertrophy, the expression of cellular oncogenes and the early change in the translational activity of specific cardiac mRNA were studied (45). It was demonstrated that there are some early responsive genes in cardiac hypertrophy and that mechanical loading directly stimulates gene expression, probably via protein kinase C activation.

Neonatal cardiac enlargement may be distinctly different from secondary myocardial hypertrophy. It is evident that the higher DNA/protein ratio in most studies of newborn hypertensive rats does not persist throughout the development of hypertension and cardiac hypertrophy (i.e., cell hyperplasia shifts to cell hypertrophy). This is also probably true for other organs of the cardiovascular system because we have demonstrated renal hyperplasia in SHR newborns as well (33). This was documented not only by higher DNA/protein ratio but also by higher incorporation of ^{3}H-thymidine into DNA in vivo (46). Moreover, arterial hypertrophic changes were documented in neonatal SHR (for a review see ref. 11). Thus, it is very difficult to answer the question of whether blood pressure per se is the major factor in determining cardiac size during early developmental periods. It is evident also that other factors may play a significant role and that all depends on genetic background.

In general, the study of early developmental periods is very important for better understanding of primary events or secondary response to the disease (47). Recently, it has been shown in humans that the intrauterine growth and development as well a the "maternal environment" could be responsible for and/or could predict blood pressure level in adulthood (48,49).

SUMMARY

The prevention of hypertension and its cardiovascular complications requires the detailed analysis of factors that can influence the organism during early developmental periods. Several studies have shown higher blood pressure and cardiac enlargement in newborns of genetically hypertensive rats in comparison with controls. This was, however, not revealed in rats with experimental hypertension. Thus, genetic predisposition rather than blood pressure of mothers per se could play a significant role. Moreover, the dissociation of elevated blood pressure and neonatal cardiac enlargement that has been demonstrated in some genetic studies on segregating populations suggests that both abnormalities are not coded by identical genes. More results are needed for better understanding of primary or secondary events in hypertension.

ACKNOWLEDGMENTS

We are indebted to our colleagues whose many scientific contribution made this report possible. The work was partially supported by research grants No. 71109 and 711104 from Academy of Sciences of the Czech Republic.

REFERENCES

1. Folkow B. Cardiovascular structural adaptation: its role in the initiation and maintenance of primary hypertension. *Clin Sci* 1978;55:3s–22s.
2. Zicha J, Kuneš J, Jelínek J. Experimental hypertension in young and adult animals. *Hypertension* 1986;8:1096–1104.
3. Clubb FJ Jr., Bishop SP. Formation of binucleated myocardial cells in the neonatal rat: an index for growth hypertrophy. *Lab Invest* 1984;50:571–577.
4. Penney DG, Baylerian MS, Thill JE, Yedavally S, Fanning CM. Cardiac response of the fetal rat to carbon monoxide exposure. *Am J Physiol* 1983;244:H289–H297.
5. Recavarren S, Arias-Stella J. Growth and development of the ventricular myocardium from birth to adult life. *Br Heart J* 1964;26:187–192.
6. Trávníčková E, Heller J. Plasma and blood volume of infant rats during the first postnatal month. *Physiol Bohemoslov* 1963;12:541–547.
7. Oparil S, Bishop S, Clubb FJ Jr. Myocardial cell hypertrophy or hyperplasia. *Hypertension* 1984;6(suppl III):III-38–III-43.
8. Morgan HE, Baker KM. Cardiac hypertrophy: mechanical, neural, and endocrine dependence. *Circulation* 1991;83:13–25.
9. Litchfield JB. Blood pressure in infant rats. *Physiol Zool* 1958;31:1–6.
10. Trippodo NC, Frohlich ED. Similarities of genetic (spontaneous) hypertension: man and rat. *Circ Res* 1981;48:309–319.
11. Gray SD. Spontaneous hypertension in the neonatal rat: a review. *Clin Exp Hypertens A* 1984; 6:755–781.
12. Jones DR, Dowd DA. Development of elevated blood pressure in young genetically hypertensive rats. *Life Sci* 1970;9:247–250.
13. Lais LT, Rios LL, Boutelle S, DiBona GF, Brody MJ. Arterial pressure development in neonatal and young spontaneously hypertensive rats. *Blood Vessels* 1977;14:277–284.
14. Bruno L, Azar S, Weller D. Absence of a pre-hypertensive stage in post-natal Kyoto hypertensive rats. *Jpn Heart J* 1979;20(suppl I):90–92.
15. Gray SD. Early postnatal differences between WKY and SHR in anatomical and physiological parameters. *Fed Proc* 1982;41:1589.
16. Gray SD. Pressure profiles in neonatal spontaneously hypertensive rats. *Biol Neonate* 1984;45: 25–32.
17. Clubb FJ, Bell PD, Kriseman JD, Bishop SP. Myocardial cell growth and blood pressure development in neonatal spontaneously hypertensive rats. *Lab Invest* 1987;56:189–197.
18. Tucker DC, Johnson AK. Development of autonomic control of heart rate in genetically hypertensive and normotensive rats. *Am J Physiol* 1984;246:R570–R577.

19. Bugaisky L, Zak R. Biological mechanisms of hypertrophy. In: Fozzard HA, Haber E, Jennings RB, Katz AM, Morgan HE, eds. *The heart and cardiovascular system.* New York: Raven Press; 1986:1491–1506.
20. Sen S, Tarazi RC, Khairallah PA, Bumpus FM. Cardiac hypertrophy in spontaneously hypertensive rats. *Circ Res* 1976;10:775–781.
21. Tanase H, Yamori Y, Hansen CT, Lovenberg W. Heart size in inbred strains of rats. Part 1: Genetic determination of the development of cardiovascular enlargement in rats. *Hypertension* 1982;4:864–872.
22. Kuneš J, Křen V, Klír P, Zicha J, Pravenec M. Genetic determination of heart and kidney weights studied using a set of recombinant inbred strains: the relationship to blood pressure. *J Hypertens* 1990;8:1091–1095.
23. Harrap SB, Mitchell GA, Norman TL. Is cardiovascular hypertrophy in young SHR the result of a recessive gene? In: Sassard J, ed. *Genetic hypertension.* Colloque INSERM/John Libbey Eurotext; 1992:341–343.
24. Bareis DL, Slotkin TA. Responses of the heart ornithine decarboxylase and adrenal catecholamines to methadone and sympathetic stimulans in developing and adult rats. *J Pharmacol Exp Ther* 1978;205:164–174.
25. Claycomb WC. Biochemical aspects of cardiac muscle differentiation: possible role of deoxyribonucleic acid synthesis and cell differentiation by adrenergic innervation and cyclic adenosine 3′ : 5′-monophosphate. *J Biol Chem* 1976;251:6082–6089.
26. Morgan HE, Baker KM. Cardiac hypertrophy: mechanical, neural and endocrine dependence. *Circulation* 1991;83:13–24.
27. Bareis DL, Morgan RE, Lau C, Slotkin TA. Maturation of sympathetic neurotransmission in the rat heart. VI. The effects of guanethidine-induced sympathectomy in neonatal development of synaptic vesicles, synaptic terminal function and heart growth. *Dev Neurosci* 1981;4:15–24.
28. Deskin R, Mills E, Whitmore WL, Seidler FJ, Slotkin TA. Maturation of sympathetic neurotransmission in the rat heart. VI. The effect of neonatal central catecholaminergic lesions. *J Pharmacol Exp Ther* 1980:215:342–347.
29. Ecob MS, Butler-Browne GS, Whalen RG. The adult fast isoenzyme of myosin is present in tissue culture system. *Differentiation* 1983;25:84–87.
30. Toyota N, Shimada Y. Isoform variants of troponin in skeletal and cardiac muscle cells cultured with and without nerves. *Cell* 1983;33:297–304.
31. Bishop SP. Ultrastructure of the myocardium in physiologic and pathophysiologic hypertrophy in experimental animals. *Perspect Cardiovasc Res* 1983;7:127–147.
32. Hamet P, Kune˛s J, Fletcher K, Cantin M, Genest J. Hypertrophy and hyperplasia of heart and kidney in newborn hypertensive rats. In: Rascher W, Clough D, Ganten D, eds. *Hypertensive mechanism: the spontaneously hypertensive rat as a model to study human hypertension.* Stuttgart: Schattauer Verlag; 1982:161–164.
33. Kuneš J, Pang SC, Cantin M, Genest J, Hamet P. Cardiac and renal hyperplasia in newborn spontaneously hypertensive rats. *Clin Sci* 1987;72:271–275.
34. Pang SC, Long C, Poirier M, Tremblay J, Kune˛s J, Vincent M, Sassard J, Duzzi L, Bianchi G, Ledingham J, Phelan EL, Simpson FO, Ikeda K, Yamori Y, Hamet P. Cardiac and renal hyperplasia in newborn genetically hypertensive rats. *J Hypertens* 1986;4(suppl 3):S119–S122.
35. Yokota N, Bruneau BG, Fernandez BE, Kuroski de Bold ML, Piazza LA, Eid H, de Bold AJ. Dissociation of cardiac hypertrophy, myosin heavy chain isoform expression, and natriuretic peptide production in DOCA-salt rats. *Am J Hypertens* 1995;8:301–310.
36. Dobešová Z, Zicha J, Heller J, Kuneš J. The lack of cardiac hypertrophy in newborn Prague hypertensive rats. *Physiol Res* 1991;40:373–376.
37. Dobešová Z, Zicha J, Kuneš J. The influence of prenatal exposure to the different salt diets on body and organ weights in newborn Dahl rats. *J Dev Physiol* 1993;19:17–21.
38. Dobešová Z, Zicha J, Kuneš J. Newborn organ weight and spontaneous hypertension: recombinant inbred strain study. *Clin Exp Hypertens* (submitted).
39. Grobecker H, Saavedra JM, Weise VK. Biosynthesis enzyme activities and catecholamines in adrenal glands of genetic and experimental hypertensive rats. *Circ Res* 1982;50:742–746.
40. Crofton JT, Share L, Shade RE, Allen C, Tarnowski D. Vasopressin in the rat with spontaneous hypertension. *Am J Physiol* 1978;235:H361–H366.
41. Sen S, Smeby RR, Bumpus FM. Renin in rats with spontaneous hypertension. *Circ Res* 1972;31: 876–880.

42. Sinaiko A, Mirkin BL. Ontogenesis of the renin-angiotensin system in spontaneously hypertensive and normal Wistar rats. *Circ Res* 1974;34:693–696.
43. Mullins MM, Kleinman LI, Russell PT, Srivastava LS. Plasma aldosterone concentrations in neonatal spontaneously hypertensive rats. *Life Sci* 1982;31:2751–2755.
44. McMurtry JP, Wright GL, Wexler BC. Spontaneous hypertension in cross-suckled rats. *Science* 1981;211:1173–1175.
45. Komuro I, Kurabayashi M, Shibazaki Y, Katoh Y, Hoh E, Kaida T, Ieki K, Takaku T, Yazaki Y. Molecular mechanism of cardiac hypertrophy. *Jpn Circ J* 1990;54:526–534.
46. Walter SV, Hamet P. Enhanced DNA synthesis in heart and kidney of the newborn spontaneously hypertensive rats. *Hypertension* 1986;8:520–525.
47. Hamet P, Tremblay J, Pang SC, Walter SV, Wen YI. Primary versus secondary events in hypertension. *Can J Physiol Pharmacol* 1984;63:380–386.
48. Barker DJP, Bull AR, Osmond C, Simmonds SJ. Fetal and placental size and risk of hypertension in adult life. *Br Med J* 1990;301:259–262.
49. Barker DJP, Osmond C, Golding J, Kuh D, Wadsworth MEJ. Growth in utero, blood pressure in childhood and adult life, and mortality from cardiovascular disease. *Br Med J* 1989;296:564–567.
50. Cutilletta AF, Benjamin M, Culpepper WS, Oparil S. Myocardial hypertrophy and ventricular performance in the absence of hypertension in spontaneously hypertensive rats. *J Mol Cell Cardiol* 1978;10:689–703.

The Developing Heart,
edited by Bohuslav Ošťádal et al.
Lippincott-Raven Publishers,
Philadelphia © 1997.

26

Adaptive Changes of the Rat Myocardium Exposed to Pressure Overload During First Postnatal Week

Jan Černohorský, Václav Pelouch, František Kolář,
Marie Milerová, and Bohuslav Ošťádal

*Institute of Physiology, Academy of Sciences of the Czech Republic,
Vídeňská 1083, 142 20 Prague 4, Czech Republic*

During postnatal development, the cardiac myocyte rapidly loses its ability to proliferate and subsequent growth of the heart is based on the enlargement of preexisting myocytes. When subjected to a chronic increase in pressure load, the myocardium adapts by increasing its mass (1). Rakušan and Korecký (2) have reported that the contribution of cell hyperplasia and cell hypertrophy to the total increase in cardiac mass after constriction of the abdominal aorta in 5-day-old animals is approximately the same. In contrast, Campbell et al. (3) have observed almost no increase in myocyte number in the left ventricle in the same experimental model.

It has been demonstrated, however, that the period of the most intensive hyperplastic growth, typical for fetal life, terminates in rats by the fifth day of postnatal life (4). This phase of rapid growth is accompanied by a dramatic development of contractile function and its regulation at the level of calcium transport (5) as well as by significant protein remodeling of atrial and ventricular myocardium (6–9). It was therefore of interest to compare the effect of increased workload imposed during and after the period of hyperplastic growth. For this purpose a gradual pressure overload was induced in either 2-day-old or 6-day-old animals by constriction of the abdominal aorta. Particular attention was paid to the adaptive changes in the weight, contractile function, and protein profiling of this overloaded immature heart.

METHODOLOGICAL REMARKS

Gradual pressure overload was induced in either 2-day-old (A2) or 6-day-old (A6) male Wistar rats by constricting the abdominal aorta under ether anesthesia;

the aorta was constricted by a silk suture around a steel template (diameter 0.25 mm in A2 and 0.45 mm in A6 group) (10). Control rats (C) underwent sham operation. Assessment of cardiac function and biochemical analyses were carried out in all groups at the age of 60 days. In A2 animals the protein profiling was examined also at the age of 1 month.

The rats were weighed and then anesthetized with thiopental. Systemic arterial pressure was measured in the left coronary artery and the functional performance of the left ventricle (LV) was assessed in open-chest animals using acute ligation of the ascending aorta as a loading test (11,12). The difference in the left ventricular systolic pressure (LVSP) or maximum rate of pressure development [(+*dP/dt*)index max] after and before ligation was considered as the functional reserve.

Then the hearts were removed and dissected into the right ventricle (RV), LV, and septum. Samples of both the control and the experimental RV and LV were treated consecutively with different buffers (9,13). The procedure yielded three basic fractions: (a) sarcoplasmic proteins (various enzymes of aerobic and anaerobic metabolic pathways), (b) contractile proteins (complex of proteins transducing the chemical energy of ATP into mechanical work), (c) structural collagenous proteins (extracellular matrix and cytoskeleton—the fraction includes collagens, elastins, proteoglycans, and glycoproteins). This latter fraction can be divided into two subfractions: (a) soluble collagenous proteins, constituted mainly by collagen I and III, and (b) insoluble collagenous proteins that include collagen aggregates, elastins, and other proteins of the extracellular matrix. While concentration of noncollagenous proteins was the sum of sarcoplasmic and contractile proteins, collagenous proteins represent the sum of both soluble and insoluble subfractions.

Separate groups of both control and experimental animals ($n = 5$ for each group) were used for the extraction of myosin (14); β-mercaptoethanol and azide were added into an extraction solution. Ca–ATPase activity of myosin was determined by measuring enzymatically released phosphate after 5 min incubation at 30°C.

Qualitative changes of myosin and collagenous proteins were estimated by SDS electrophoresis performed on polyacrylamide gel (5–15% gradient). Whereas myosin was stained with Coomassie Blue R-450, silver staining was used for the detection of collagenous proteins.

RESULTS

Weight Parameters

Pressure overload induced in either 2-day-old or 6-day-old male rats did not significantly affect body weight of these animals (Table 26–1). On the other hand, cardiac enlargement was found in both aortic constricted groups. In the A2 animals the LV weight increased by 49% in 30-day-old and by 63% in 60-day-old rats, and the RV weight increased by 24% and 13%, respectively. In the A6 group, the con-

TABLE 26–1. *Body weight (BW), heart weight (HW), and the weight of the left (LV) and right (RV) ventricles of experimental (A2,A6) and control (C) 30-day-old and 60-day-old rats.*[a]

Age (days)	C/A	BW (g)	HW (mg)	LV (mg)	RV (mg)	RV/LV
30	A2	93.4	529.9*	300.0*	109.1*	0.39
	(n = 12)	±3.3	±42.9	±29.1	±6.2	±0.03
	C	99.6	364.6	200.7	87.9	0.44
	(n = 7)	±3.0	±5.3	±2.8	±2.4	±0.02
60	A2	236.2	986.5*#	634.6*#	169.4*#	0.28*
	(n = 20)	±7.7	±51.1	±37.6	±8.0	±0.01
	A6	241.2	804.0*	503.8*	147.5	0.30*
	(n = 25)	±4.5	±29.3	±21.2	±4.0	±0.01
	C	245.2	664.9	389.4	149.8	0.38
	(n = 22)	±5.3	±19.7	±11.5	±5.2	±0.01

[a]Values are means ± SEM. Significant differences ($p < .05$): *A2 (A6) vs. C; #A2 vs. A6.

striction induced enlargement of the LV only (by 29% at 60 days of age) (Table 26–1).

Hemodynamics

At 60 days of age, the systemic arterial pressure increased by 28% in A6 and by 67% in A2 groups. Both resting and maximum LVSP, attained after acute ligation of the aorta, were significantly increased in aortic constricted rats; this increase was more pronounced in the A2 group. For both LVSP and *dP/dt,* the functional reserve was slightly but significantly increased in animals with constriction, while no difference was observed between groups A2 and A6 (Table 26–2). Whereas in the A6 group the values of maximum LVSP after loading positively correlated with

TABLE 26–2. *Systemic blood pressure and LV hemodynamics in experimental (A2,A6) and control (C) 60-day-old rats*

Group	C (n = 20)	A6 (n = 18)	A2 (n = 13)
SAP (mmHg)	169.4 ± 3.5	217.0 ± 5.8*	283.3 ± 8.4*#
LVSP (mmHg)	269.5 ± 4.5	321.3 ± 5.8*	344.2 ± 6.8*#
LVSP reserve (mmHg)	181.7 ± 5.6	211.8 ± 6.8*	219.5 ± 12.3*
dP/dt reserve (mmHg/s)	4091 ± 232	5244 ± 286*	5068 ± 520*

SAP, systemic arterial pressure (systolic); LVSP, maximum LV systolic pressure after acute ligation of the aorta; LVSP reserve, difference between LVSP after and before acute ligation of the aorta; *dP/dt* reserve, difference between (+*dP/dt*)index max after and before acute ligation of the aorta.

Values are means ± SEM.

Significant differences ($p < .05$): *A2 (A6) vs. C; #A2 vs. A6.

the degree of LV enlargement, a negative correlation was observed in the A2 group (data not shown).

Quantitative Changes of Proteins

Whereas the LV of 30-day-old rats exhibited no significant changes in the concentration of noncollagenous (sarcoplasmic and contractile) proteins, decreased concentrations, as compared with controls, were observed in both banded groups (A2 and A6) at 60 days of age (Fig. 26–1 upper part). Aortic banding had no effect

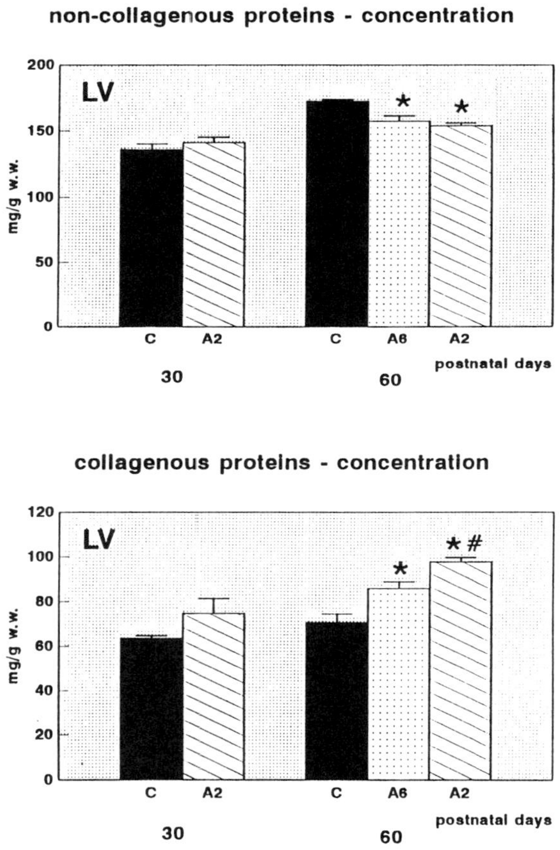

FIG. 26–1. Protein profiling of the left ventricle (LV). Concentration of noncollagenous (*upper part*) and collagenous proteins (*lower part*) in the LV of experimental (A2,A6) and control (C) rats at 30 and 60 days of age. Values (expressed as milligrams of proteins/wet weight of the LV) are means ± SEM. Student's t-test was used for statistical evaluation. Significant differences ($p < 0.05$): *A2 (A6) vs. C; # A2 vs. A6. (Data from ref. 10.)

on the concentration of noncollagenous proteins in the RV. The concentration of collagenous proteins in the LV was enhanced in both experimental groups on day 60, but this change was more pronounced in the A2 group than in the A6 animals (Fig. 26–1 lower part).

The Ca–ATPase activity of myosin isolated from the LV of 30-day-old experimental animals was significantly higher than in controls. On the other hand, decline in the Ca–ATPase activity was observed in 60-day-old rats with aortic constriction (both A2 and A6 groups). Similar changes were found in the RV of banded animals (Fig. 26–2).

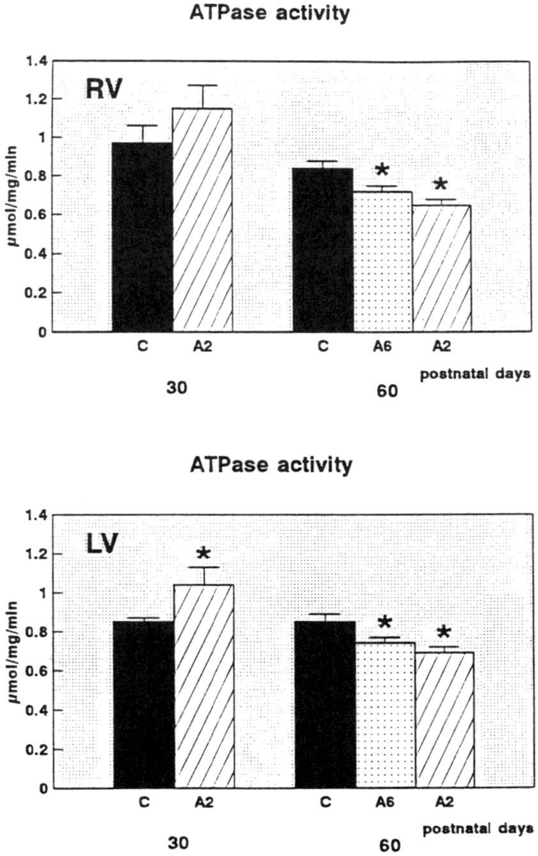

FIG. 26–2. Ca–ATPase activity of myosin extracted from the right (RV, *upper part*) and left (LV, *lower part*) ventricles of 30-day-old and 60-day-old experimental (A2,A6) and control (C) rats. Values (expressed as μmolP mg^{-1} of protein min^{-1}) are means $\pm$ SEM. Student's t-test was used for statistical evaluation. Significant differences ($p < 0.05$): *A2 (A6) vs. C; # A2 vs. A6.

Qualitative Changes of Proteins

Electrophoresis of myosin samples (Fig. 26–3) revealed that aortic constriction caused remodeling of myosin heavy chains (αHC and βHC) in the LV. At the age of 30 days both α- and βHCs were detected in the control group; on the other hand, only αHC was observed in A2 animals. Unlike the A6 group, a higher proportion of βHC was found in A2 animals at 60 days of age.

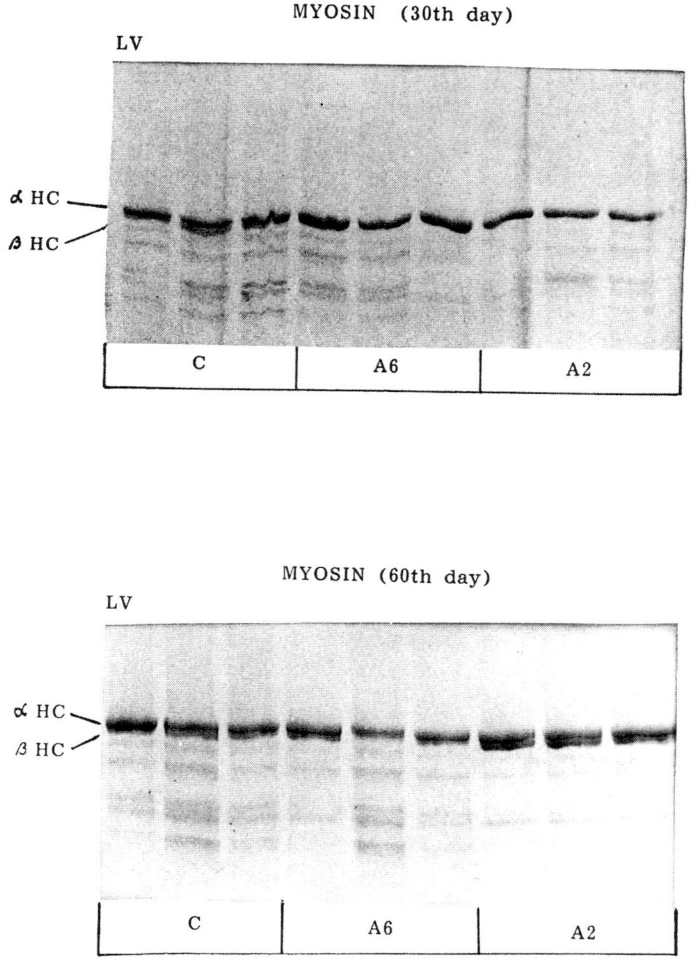

FIG. 26–3. SDS polyacrylamide gel electrophoresis of myosin extracted from the left ventricle (LV) of 30-day-old (*upper part*) and 60-day-old (*lower part*) experimental (A2,A6) and control (C) rats. HC, myosin heavy chains.

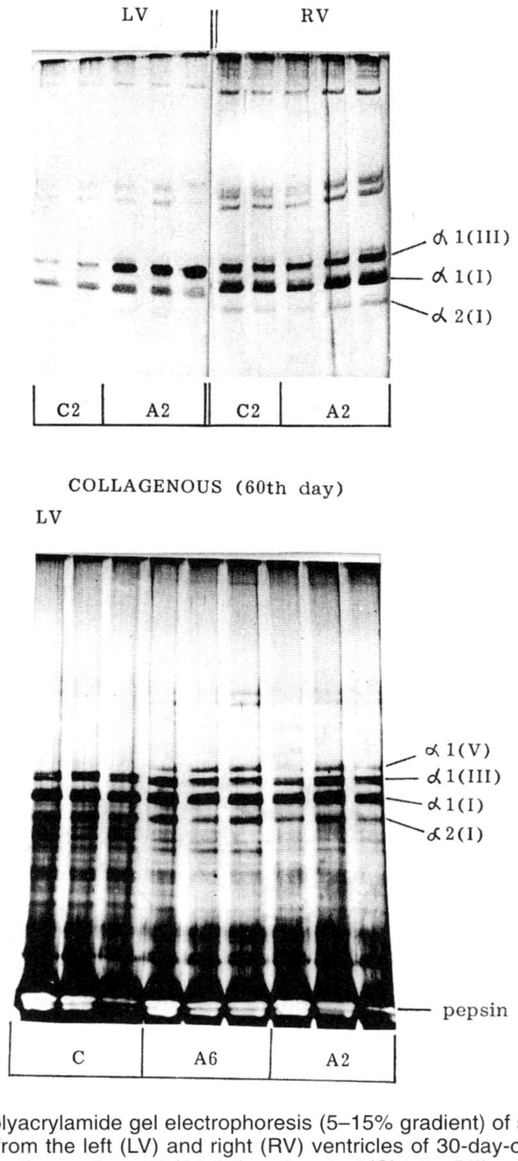

FIG. 26–4. SDS polyacrylamide gel electrophoresis (5–15% gradient) of soluble collagenous proteins extracted from the left (LV) and right (RV) ventricles of 30-day-old (*upper part*) and 60-day-old (*lower part*) experimental (A6,A2) and control (C) rats. Different α-chains of collagen types were characterized by using collagen standards (Sigma). (Data from ref. 10.)

An electrophoretic pattern of soluble collagenous proteins is shown in Fig. 26–4. Ventricular collagen is composed of a mixture of types I, III, and V. The proportion of these different collagen types was affected by pressure overload. At the age of 30 days, a higher amount of collagen III and a lower amount of collagen I was observed in the LV of the A2 group, whereas no such changes were found in the RV of these animals (Fig. 26–4 upper part). At 60 days of age, an increased proportion of collagen V was found in the LV of both experimental groups (Fig. 26–4 lower part); however, no significant difference was detected between A2 and A6 rats. Proportions of collagen types I, III, and V in the RV remained unaffected. Furthermore, increased proportion of collagenous α2(I) chain was observed in the LV of both control and experimental animals during postnatal development (from day 30 to day 60).

DISCUSSION

It is well known that cardiac enlargement in rats exposed to pressure overload from the first postnatal week is significantly greater than that in those banded in adulthood (2). In the present study, we compared the effects of abdominal aortic constriction induced in either 2-day-old or 6-day-old neonatal rats. In A6 animals the enlargement of LV only was observed at the age of 30 and 60 days. This result is in good agreement with the observation of Rakušan and Korecký (2), who reported increased LV weight in 30-day-old animals banded on postnatal day 5. On the other hand, A2 animals exhibited more pronounced enlargement of the LV as compared with that of A6 rats, and their RV weight increased as well. It is likely that the hyperplastic growth of cardiac myocytes was more stimulated by aortic constriction performed on day 2 than it was by that on day 6, and this may have contributed to greater cardiac growth in the former group. However, it should be taken into account that the aorta of the A2 group was constricted to a smaller diameter than it was in the A6 group. Therefore, not only a different onset of pressure loading, but also a different degree of load can be partly responsible for the distinct response in these two experimental groups. This view is supported by the observation of higher systemic blood pressure in the A2 group as compared with that in A6 rats. Furthermore, the RV enlargement in the A2 group may be the result of the developing LV dysfunction in some of the animals, though the mean parameters of LV performance did not differ from those of the A6 group. However, the RV weight increased only in those animals that exhibited most severe LV enlargement and signs of dysfunction. It should be mentioned that in a recent study on rats banded on day 2 and examined on day 90, the pronounced RV enlargement was clearly associated with indices of cardiac failure (15).

Pressure overload induced in the neonatal hearts significantly influenced the protein composition of the myocardium. Our data show that changes in cardiac myosin HCs after aortic constriction varied in different periods of postnatal development and correlated with myosin Ca–ATPase activity, in agreement with previous observations (9,16,17). Whereas in 30-day-old A2 rats only αHC was detected together with an elevated Ca–ATPase activity, a decrease of Ca–ATPase activity was observed in 60-day-old aorta-constricted animals. This change was more pronounced in A2 rats because of a higher proportion of βHC than that in the A6 group.

At the age of 60 days, the LV enlargement was associated with a significantly increased concentration of collagenous proteins in both A2 and A6 banded groups. The higher concentration of these extracellular proteins in the A2 group corresponded with the greater cardiomegaly of these animals than was found in the A6 group. However, these changes occurred at the expense of noncollagenous sarcoplasmic proteins that play a crucial role in the production of ATP (9,18). Detailed analysis revealed that although the concentrations of newly synthesized extracellular matrix proteins (soluble collagenous fraction) in the LV was elevated already in 30-day-old aorta-constricted animals, higher concentrations of both soluble and insoluble collagenous proteins were found in experimental 60-day-old rats only (10,19). This finding suggests that the extent of extracellular posttranslational modifications of the secreted collagen molecules is greater in the LV of experimental rats than in that of controls (20). These modifications consist of intermolecular and intramolecular covalent cross-linking that leads to the formation of collagen aggregates during postnatal development (21). Unlike the collagenous proteins, the myocardial concentration of collagen, determined as hydroxyproline, was unchanged after aortic constriction in both experimental groups, suggesting that its formation was proportional to cardiac enlargement (12,19). Moreover, aortic constriction affected the proportion of distinct collagen types in the LV (higher collagen III in 30-day-old and higher collagen V in both A2 and A6 60-day-old rats). Our results are in a good agreement with our previous findings (22) that the ratio of collagen types I and III increases during postnatal development. We have particularly observed elevated synthesis of the collagenous α2(I) chain in the LV of both control and experimental 60-day-old rats as compared with 30-day-old animals. This means that higher synthesis of collagen I heterotrimer participated in remodeling of the developing myocardium.

SUMMARY

It may be concluded that a gradual pressure overload induced by abdominal aortic constriction in neonatal rats results in cardiac enlargement, increase in systemic arterial pressure, and myocardial protein remodeling. Cardiac alterations were significantly more expressed in the LV. The intensity of adaptive changes depends on the onset and degree of pressure overload as much as on the age when the examination is performed.

ACKNOWLEDGMENT

This work was supported by Grant No. 2039-3 of the Ministry of Health of the Czech Republic.

REFERENCES

1. Bilsen M, Chien KR. Growth and hypertrophy of the heart: towards an understanding of cardiac specific and inducible gene expression. *Card Res* 1993;27:1140–1149.
2. Rakušan K, Korecký B. Regression of cardiomegaly induced in newborn rats. *Can J Cardiol* 1985;1:217–222.
3. Campbell SE, Rakušan K, Gerdes AM. Change in cardiac myocyte size distribution in aortic-constricted neonatal rats. *Basic Res Cardiol* 1989;84:247–258.
4. Clubb FJ Jr, Bishop SP. Formation of binucleated myocardial cells in the neonatal rat: an index for growth hypertrophy. *Lab Invest* 1984;50:571–577.
5. Ošt'ádalová I, Kolář F, Ošt'ádal B, Rohlíček V, Rohlíček J, Procházka J. Early postnatal development of contractile performance and responsiveness to Ca^{2+}, verapamil and ryanodine in the isolated rat heart. *J Mol Cell Cardiol* 1993;25:733–740.
6. Borg TM, Burgess ML. Holding it all together: organization and function of the extracellular matrix in the heart. *Heart Failure* 1992/1993;8:230–238.
7. Brodsky VY, Pelouch V, Arefyeva AM, Milerová M, Ošt'ádal B. Lack of proportionality between gene dosage and total muscle protein content in the rat heart. *Int J Dev Biol* 1992;36:339–342.
8. Weber KT, Brilla CG, Janicki JS. Myocardial fibrosis: functional significance and regulatory factors. *Cardiovasc Res* 1993;27:341–348.
9. Pelouch V. Molecular aspects of regulation of cardiac contraction. *Physiol Res* 1995;44:53–60.
10. Černohorský J, Pelouch V, Milerová M, Ošt'ádal B. Protein profiling of the myocardium exposed to pressure overload from birth. *Physiol Res* 1995;44:139–142.
11. Čihák R, Kolář F, Pelouch V, Procházka J, Ošt'ádal B, Widimský J. Functional changes in the right and left ventricle during development of cardiac hypertrophy and after its regression. *Cardiovasc Res* 1992;26:845–850.
12. Kolář F, Papoušek F, Pelouch V, Procházka J, Ošt'ádal B. Left ventricular performance in cardiomegaly due to pressure overload induced in neonatal rats. *Physiol Res* 1993;42:9P.
13. Pelouch V, Milerová M, Ošt'ádal B, Šamánek M, Hučín B. Protein profiling of human atrial and ventricular musculature: the effect of normoxaemia and hypoxemia in congenital heart diseases. *Physiol Res* 1993;42:235–242.
14. Declayre C, Swynghedauw B. A comparative study of heart myosin ATPase and light subunits from different species. *Pflugers Arch* 1975;255:39–47.
15. Zheng L, Wibo M, Kolář F, Godfraind T. Calcium channels and cation transport ATPase in cardiac hypertrophy induced by aortic constriction in newborn rats. *Mol Cell Biochem* 1996;163/164:23–29.
16. Tsuchimochi H, Takaku F, Yoshida K, Kawana M, Yazaki Y. Expression of myosin isozymes during the developmental stage and their redistribution induced by pressure overload. *Jpn Circ J* 1985;50:1044–1052.
17. Hannan RD, Rothblum LI. Regulation of ribosomal DNA transcription during neonatal cardiomyocyte hypertrophy. *Cardiovasc Res* 1995;30:501–510.
18. Bass A, Šamánek M, Ošt'ádal B, Hučín B, Stejskalová M, Pelouch V. Differences between atrial and ventricular energy supplying enzymes in children. *J Appl Cardiol* 1988;3:397–405.
19. Černohorský J. Pelouch V, Ošt'ádal B, Milerová M. Protein changes in the rat heart exposed to pressure overload from birth. *J Mol Cell Cardiol* 1995;27:A85.
20. Doering CW, Jalil JE, Janicki JS, Pick R, Aghili S, Abrahams C, Weber KT. Collagen network remodelling and diastolic stiffness of the rat left ventricle with pressure overload hypertrophy. *Cardiovasc Res* 1988;22:686–695.
21. Chapman D, Weber KT, Eghbali M. Regulation of fibrillar collagen types I and III and basement membrane type IV collagen gene expression in pressure overloaded rat myocardium. *Circ Res* 67:787–794.
22. Pelouch V, Milerová M, Ošt'ádal B, Procházka J. Ontogenetic development of the protein composition of the right and left ventricular myocardium. In: Ježek V, Morpurgo M, Tramarin R, eds. *Right ventricular hypertrophy and function in chronic lung disease.* London: Springer Verlag, 1992:39–54.

The Developing Heart,
edited by Bohuslav Ošťádal et al.
Lippincott-Raven Publishers,
Philadelphia © 1997.

27

Protein Remodeling of Malformed Human and Mouse Heart

*Václav Pelouch, †T. Pexieder, ‡Marie Milerová,
*Bohuslav Ošťádal, ‡Milan Šamánek

**Institute of Physiology, Academy of Sciences of the Czech Republic, Prague,
†Institute of Histology and Embryology, University of Lausanne, Lausanne,
Switzerland, and ‡Centre of Pediatric Cardiology and Cardiovascular Surgery,
University Hospital Motol, Prague, Czech Republic*

Complex biological structures such as the developing cardiovascular system are characterized by the integration of multiple levels of organization ranging from organ through tissue and cell composition to the molecular level. Congenital heart disease is caused by abnormalities in the first 6–8 weeks of fetal life, a period when the fetal cardiovascular system is being formed; the incidence of heart malformations is approximately eight out of 1,000 (1). The embryogenetic theories about their origin are, however, purely speculative. One reason for this is the absence of an adequate animal model for experimental analysis of pathogenesis of congenital heart disease. Whereas a lot of data are available concerning the morphology of cardiac congenital malformations (2–6), much less is known about the possible protein remodeling (7) that may accompany the structural changes. Furthermore, many congenital heart defects have hypertrophic myocardium as a consequence; it has been repeatedly described that increased pressure and volume load substantially modified the quantitative and qualitative properties of contractile and collagenous proteins (8–15). In this survey, we would like to summarize some of our data dealing with the protein composition of the structurally changed myocardium: (a) in human hypoxemic and normoxemic congenital heart disease (16,17) and (b) in experimental cardiac malformations induced by retinoic acid in mice (6,18).

SUBJECT OF STUDY

The study was performed on samples obtained during surgery of children with congenital heart disease and by analyzing retinoic acid–induced malformation of mouse myocardium. During surgery the samples were taken from right atria and right ventricles of both normoxemic (ventricular septal defect and atrial septal defect) and hypoxemic patients (tetralogy of Fallot) age 6 months to 16 years. The atrial tissue was excised before commencement of cardiopulmonary bypass; the ventricular samples were taken 2–80 min after the heartbeat had been arrested; no in vitro aging of collagenous and noncollagenous proteins was observed during this time (16,17). To analyze the retinoic acid–induced malformation of mouse myocardium the samples were taken from cardiac tissue of embryos on the fifteenth embryonic day (e.d.), fetuses on e.d. 19, and newborns. Intraperitoneal injection of 20 mg/kg all-*trans* RA dissolved in 200 μl vehicle solution (composed of 7.6 ml absolute C_2H_5OH, 0.4 ml of 2 M NaOH, and 92 ml of soybean oil, pH 10.79) was given to the pregnant mice on the e.d. 8. Three experimental groups were analyzed: untreated (UNTREAT) controls without any intervention, controls treated with 200 μl of vehicle (VEHICLE), and RA-treated group composed of three subgroups: (a) morphologically normal (NON-M) fetuses, (b) fetuses with transposition of great arteries (TGA), or (c) double outlet of the right ventricle (DORV). No attempt was made to separate the atria from the ventricles as well as the right and left half of the mouse heart. This decision was made on the basis of preliminary biochemical analysis of individual cardiac chambers that did not show any significant differences of the cardiac protein profiles at the stages studied (6,18).

CHARACTERIZATION OF PROTEIN FRACTIONS FROM CARDIAC MUSCLE

Pieces of the cardiac tissue were rapidly transferred into precooled test tubes and frozen to −80°C. The tissue samples were later thawed, and their volume was made up to 20-fold with buffer (50 mmol/L sodium potassium phosphate, pH = 7.4, containing 10 mmol/L EDTA and 1% Triton X-100). They were then subjected to shaking (2 hours at 4°C) and then centrifuged at 7000 *g*; the supernatant was used for the determination of sarcoplasmic proteins. In subsequent steps the pellet was resuspended and fractions of contractile and collagenous proteins were obtained in a stepwise manner by extracting (24 hours 4°C under mild shaking) contractile proteins into a supernatant with TRIS–HCl buffer containing 1.1 mol/L NaCl (pH = 7.5). The pellet was extracted with 10-fold volume of 0.5 mol/L acetic acid containing 1 mg of pepsin /ml, pH = 1.45. The extracts were centrifuged after 24 hours at 4°C; the supernatants contained the fraction of soluble collagenous proteins. The pellet was further suspended in 1.1 mol/L NaOH and heated two times for 10 min at 105°C. This fraction contained pepsin-insoluble collagenous proteins (10,20). Protein and hydroxyproline concentration was determined in individual fractions; total protein was the sum of total noncollagenous (sum of sarcoplasmic and contractile proteins) and collagenous proteins (sum of pepsin-soluble and pepsin-insoluble fractions). The results are expressed in milligrams per gram of wet weight.

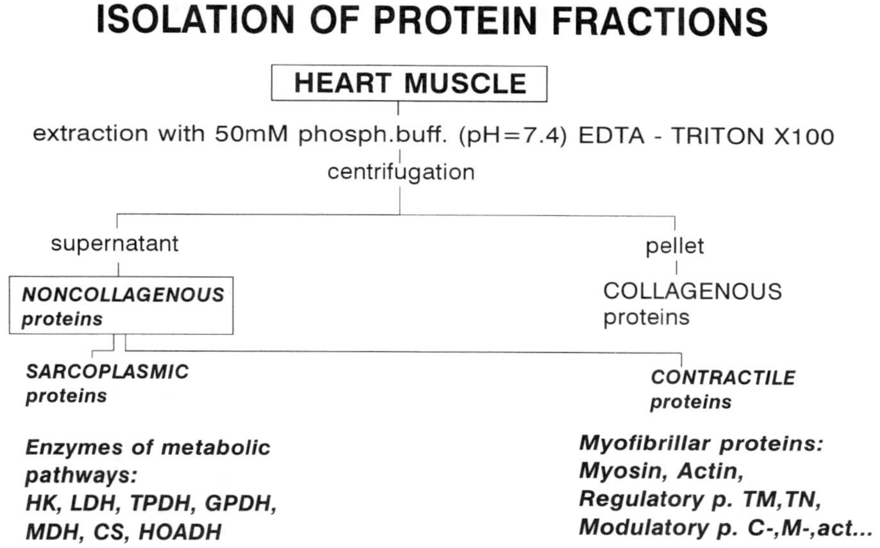

FIG. 27–1. Scheme of isolation of a protein fraction from the heart muscle: preparation of noncollagenous proteins. Sarcoplasmic protein fraction contained different metabolic pathways: HK, hexokinase; LDH, lactatedehydrogenase; TPDH, triosephosphate dehydrogenase; GPDH, glycerolphosphate dehydrogenase; MDH, malate dehydrogenase; CS, citrate synthase; HOADH, 3-hydroxyacyl-CoA dehydrogenase; contractile protein fraction contained the main contractile proteins (myosin and actin), regulatory proteins (TM, tropomyosin; TN, troponin) and different modulatory proteins (e.g., C-, M-proteins) (for details see refs. 19, 21).

Two categories of proteins occupied the noncollagenous compartment (Fig. 27–1): metabolic proteins (recovered in the fraction of sarcoplasmic proteins) and myofibrillar proteins (recovered in the fraction of contractile proteins). We have previously shown (19) that the fraction of sarcoplasmic proteins is composed of various enzymes of metabolic pathways: glycolytic enzymes (e.g., hexokinase, lactate dehydrogenase, triosephosphate dehydrogenase, glycerol-3-phosphate dehydrogenase), Krebs cycle enzymes (citrate synthase, malate dehydrogenase), and free fatty acid degradation enzymes (3-hydroxyacyl-CoA dehydrogenase). The fraction of contractile proteins contains (as judged from SDS-electrophoresis; see refs. 20–22) actin, regulatory proteins (the troponin–tropomyosin complex), and different modulatory proteins.

The extracellular matrix compartment (populated by pluripotent, highly undifferentiated cells—cardiac fibroblasts, blood and lymphatic vessels, and proteins—and by different collagenous fibrilar and nonfibrilar proteins) is a dynamic entity, and alterations in this structure result in the development of heart dysfunction and affect cardiac contractility. The cardiac collagenous proteins were recovered in the fraction of soluble and insoluble collagenous proteins (Fig. 27–2). Whereas the

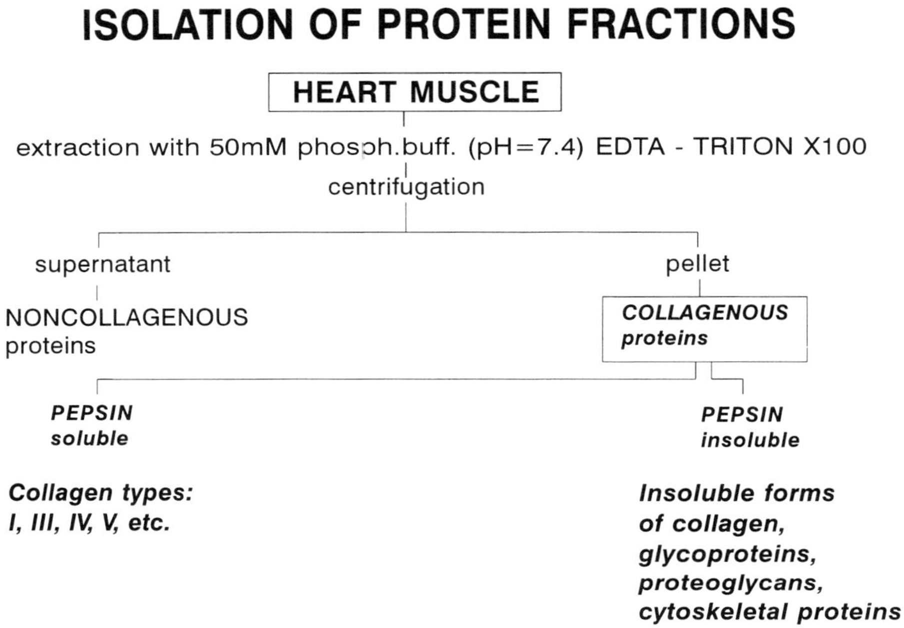

FIG. 27–2. Scheme of isolation of a protein fraction from the heart muscle: preparation of pepsin-soluble (newly synthesized extracellular matrix proteins) and insoluble collagenous proteins (collagen aggregates, glycoproteins, and other cardiac interstitial proteins).

fraction of pepsin-soluble collagenous proteins contained different types of collagen (where collagen types I and III are major, and types IV, V, VI are minor cardiac collagen forms [10,22], the pepsin-insoluble fraction contains predominantly highly cross-linked collagenous aggregates and different glycoproteins (10,20,21).

VENTRICULAR AND ATRIAL PROTEIN PROFILING IN CHILDREN WITH CONGENITAL HEART DISEASE

All human congenital heart defects have, however, hypertrophic myocardium as a consequence. In hypoxemic defects this is occasioned by the increased pressure load; in normoxemic disease the volume load is the prime factor (15,23). Cardiac mammalian muscle is a heterogeneous tissue composed of distinct muscle cell populations. The existence of significant differences between ventricular and atrial fibers has been described: the large ventricular myocytes are organized into layers, whereas atrial cells are more slender (24–26). The atrioventricular differences were also observed at the levels of contractile proteins (27–29) and of collagenous proteins (28,30). Furthermore, it was shown that ventricular musculature of human myocardium has a higher capacity of all enzymes that catalyze the aerobic and anaerobic splitting of various substrates. On the other hand, the utilization of glucose is much higher in the atrial muscle (19).

Quantitative Protein Profiles

The concentration of total atrial protein in normoxemic patients exceeded the ventricular value (Fig. 27–3); in the hypoxemic group this atrioventricular difference disappeared. There was no statistical atrioventricular difference in the concentration of noncollagenous proteins in the normoxemic group. The concentration of noncollagenous proteins in hypoxemic atrial samples was, however, significantly lower. The higher concentration of total atrial proteins in normoxemic patients is due to a higher concentration of collagenous proteins. In hypoxemic congenital heart disease the concentration of total atrial collagenous proteins is slightly higher than ventricular values. However, the mean value of atrial collagenous protein is significantly lower than the atrial value of the normoxemic group (Fig. 27–3).

Qualitative Protein Profiles

Qualitative atrioventricular differences in both collagenous and noncollagenous proteins were observed already in normoxemic patients. The higher proportion of total hydroxyproline (as a marker of collagen) in atrial musculature was due to a higher concentration of hydroxyproline derived from pepsin-insoluble collagenous material (Fig. 27–4). Hypoxemia elevated only the concentration of hydroxyproline in atrial soluble collagenous proteins; the concentration of hydroxyproline in insoluble collagenous proteins of hypoxemic atrial muscle was significantly lower (Fig. 27–4). Our previous papers (16,17) have revealed that atrioventricular differences are due not only to a higher quantity of total collagen, but also to a qualitatively distinct collagen structure. Both atrial and ventricular samples are composed of a mixture of collagens I, III, and V, but a contamination of collagen fraction with protein fragments (29–35 kDa) was found only in the ventricular samples from both hypoxemic and normoxemic myocardium (16). Elevated concentration of pepsin-insoluble collagenous material in atria may have originated from a higher amount of basic growth factors detected as a rule in the atrial part of myocardium (30). The changes of concentration of hydroxyproline in the fraction of soluble collagenous proteins in the atria of hypoxemic patients attests to fasted collagen synthesis; higher posttranslation modification of atrial collagen cannot be ruled out (31).

The electrophoretic pattern of myofibrillar proteins derived from the atrial and ventricular part of human myocardium is different. Both ventricular and atrial samples of contractile proteins contained heavy chains of myosin, actin, and tropomyosin. On the other hand, the electrophoretic pattern of the myosin light

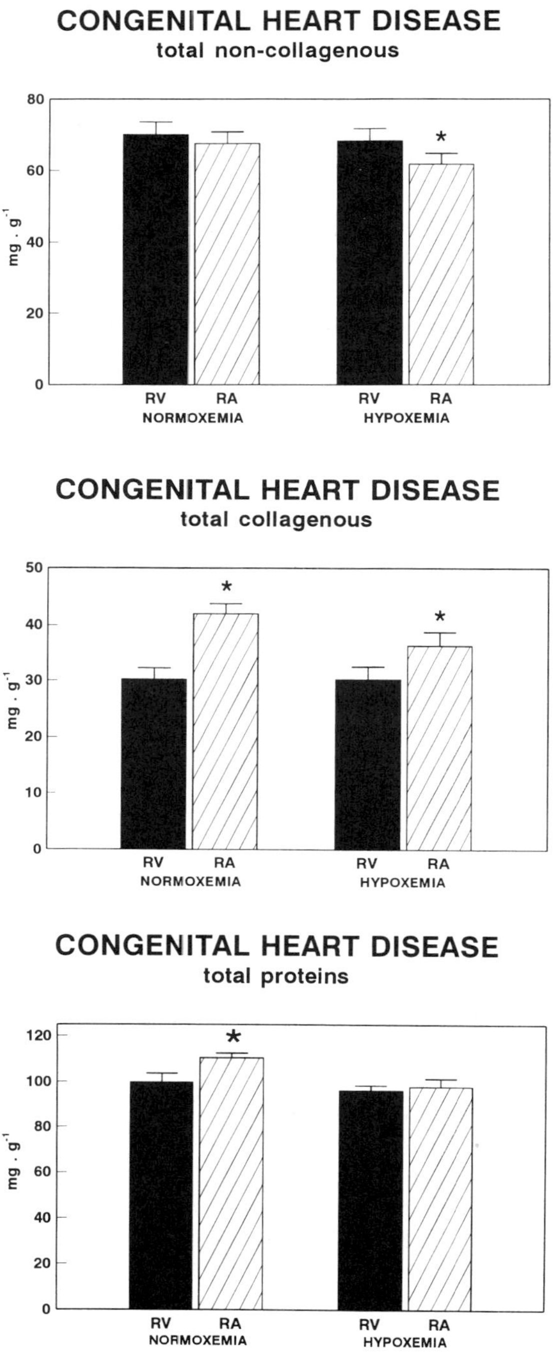

FIG. 27–3. Protein profile in congenital heart disease. Concentration of total protein, total noncollagenous, and total collagenous proteins in the human right ventricle (RV) and right atrium (RA) of normoxemic and hypoxemic patients. Values are means ± SEM (expressed as milligram per gram wet weight). Significance * $p < 0.05$ or less vs RA.

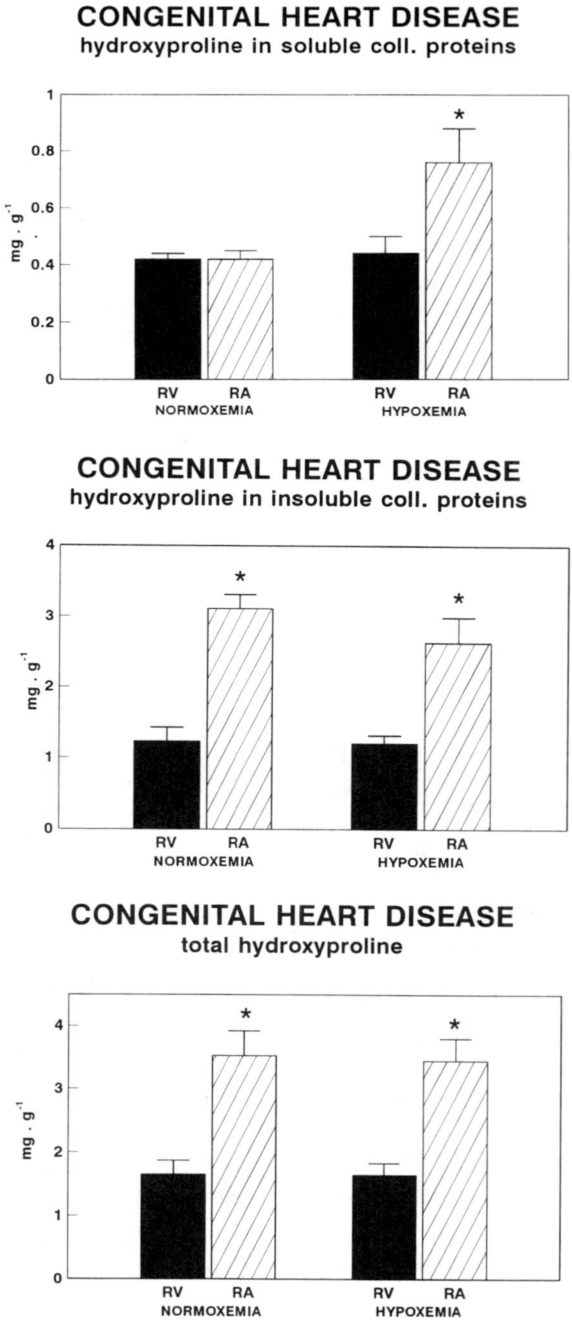

FIG. 27–4. Protein profile in congenital heart disease. Concentration of total hydroxyproline (a marker of total collagen), hydroxyproline in soluble collagenous proteins (a marker of newly synthesized collagen), and hydroxyproline in insoluble collagenous proteins (highly cross-linked collagen) in the human right ventricle (RV) and right atrium (RA) of normoxemic and hypoxemic patients. Values are means ± SEM (expressed as milligrams per gram wet weight). Significance * $p < 0.05$ or less vs RA.

chains was not identical; ventricular samples were contaminated with atrial light chains, but the amount of contamination in normoxemic and hypoxemic patients was not different (Fig. 27–5). It was demonstrated that the reappearance of atrial types in ventricles and vice versa is typical for diseased myocardium (32,33). Whereas the function and structure of different myofibrillar protein isoforms have been the subject of numerous reviews (10,27,34), the function and biochemical properties of extracellular matrix proteins of cardiac muscle (a mixture of different collagen types, elastin, glycoproteins, glycosaminoglycans, and growth factors that form an extensive network of myocardial connective tissue) are less understood (7,10,13,14,35,36).

In summary:

1. The proportion of individual protein fractions in congenital heart disease is significantly different in right ventricular and atrial musculature of human myocardium. The concentration of contractile proteins is significantly higher in ventricles, whereas collagenous proteins are more abundant in atria. On the other hand, the concentration of metabolic proteins was not different (17).

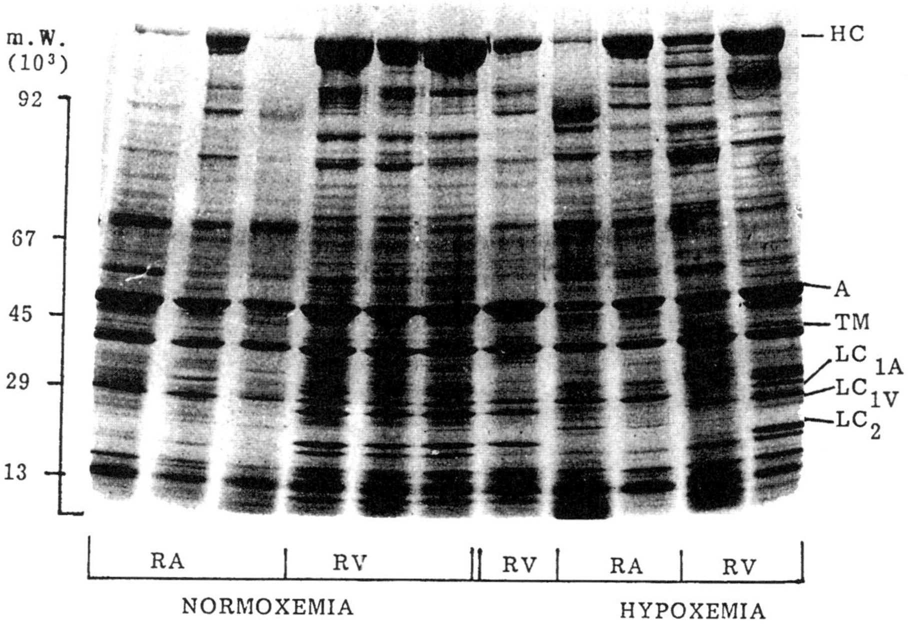

FIG. 27–5. SDS-polyacrylamide gel electrophoresis of contractile proteins of human cardiac muscle. Molecular weight standards and contractile proteins extracted from human right atrium (RA) and right ventricle (RV) were run. The positions of main contractile proteins are identified: HC, myosin heavy chains; A, actin; TM, tropomyosin; LC_1, LC_2 of atrial (A) and ventricular (V) origin. (Data from ref. 16.)

2. There were significant atrioventricular differences in enzymes connected with aerobic metabolism: higher activity of citrate synthase, malate dehydrogenase, and hydroxyacyl-CoA dehydrogenase was found in ventricular myocardium. Hypoxemia lowered the capacity of oxidative enzymes in both parts. The changes were more pronounced in atrial tissue (19,37).
3. The concentration of total atrial protein in normoxemic patients exceeded the ventricular value. In the hypoxemic group this atrioventricular difference disappeared. The contractile fractions derived from both normoxemic and hypoxemic patients were contaminated with myosin light chain of atrial origin. Newly synthesized collagenous proteins, predominantly collagen I and III, derived from all ventricular samples, were contaminated by 29–35-kDA protein fragments. The electrophoretic pattern did not allow us to determine whether these fragments originate from degradation of collagen molecules [35] or from the intermediate filament network of the myocyte cytoskeleton material [16].)
4. Chronic hypoxia did not elevate the concentration of total collagen, but atria contained a higher proportion of collagenous soluble forms. It seems, therefore, that lower oxygen saturation affects the synthesis of collagen preferentially in atrial tissue (16,17).

THE PROTEIN PROFILING OF MALFORMED MOUSE HEART

There are different experimental possibilities of how to affect normal cardiovascular development; one of them is application of all-*trans* retinoic acid (RA). RA belongs to the membrane-permeant substances that bind to ligand-specific receptors in the nucleus and that directly bring about alterations in target gene transcription. A variety of retinoid receptors—such as RA receptors, retinoid X receptors, and potential receptors with nonidentified ligands—have been described. RA receptors regulate many developmental control genes, including homeobox genes and growth factor genes (for a review see ref. 38). All these receptors, however, bind to the RA response elements.

Recently, we have shown (6,18) that RA applied to pregnant mice on the eighth e.d. induced cardiovascular malformations in fetuses. Most frequent lesions were transposition of great vessels (TGA) and double outlet of the right ventricle (DORV). One of the initial pathogenetic changes is looping anomalies. Apparently RA does not allow the heart tube to form normal D-loops; therefore, A-loops are created. Later, some of the A-loops become D-loops; others transform into L-loops (6). Whereas morphologic data are available, data on the protein composition of cardiac muscle in RA-induced malformations are virtually absent (18).

Quantitative Protein Profiles

There are significant differences in cardiac proteins in the groups of untreated and vehicle-treated embryos (Fig. 27–6). A higher amount of total proteins was in

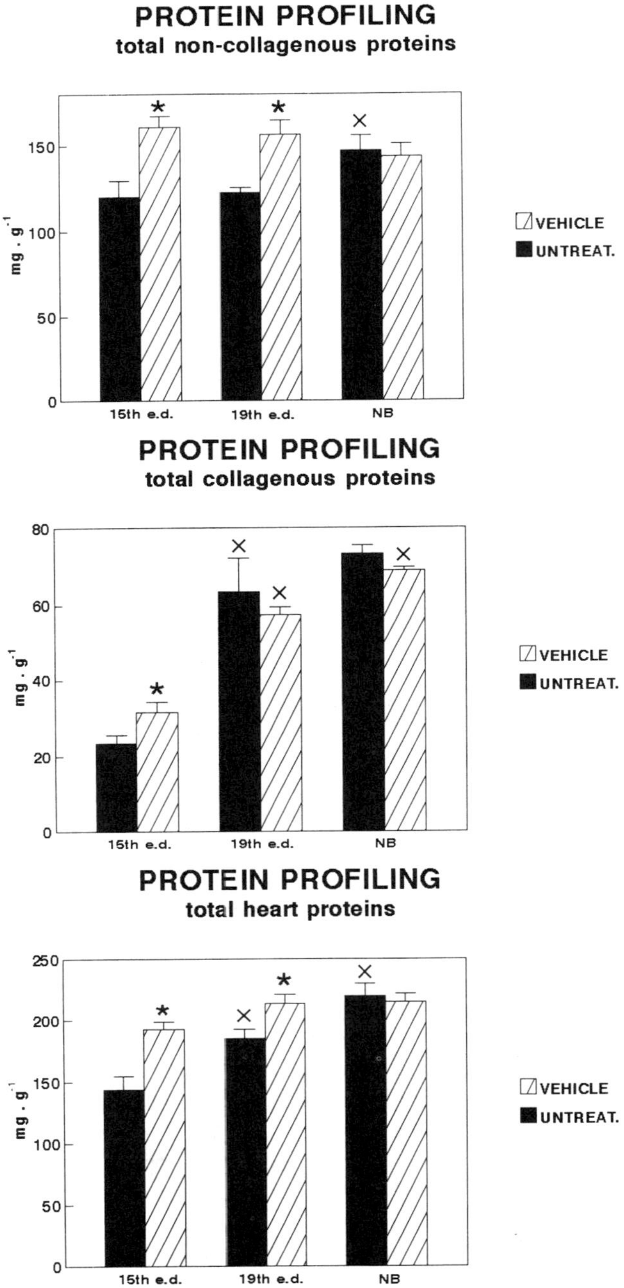

FIG. 27–6. Protein profile in retinoic acid–induced malformation of cardiac muscle. The effect of the vehicle on the concentration of total proteins, total noncollagenous, and total collagenous mouse heart protein. Values are means ± SEM (expressed as milligrams per gram wet weight) in vehicle-treated (vehicle, white bars) and controls (untreated, without any intervention, untreat., black bars). Significance: * $p < 0.05$ or less vs untreat, untreated (black column); * $p < 0.05$ or less vs fifteenth embryonic day (e.d.) in the particular group.

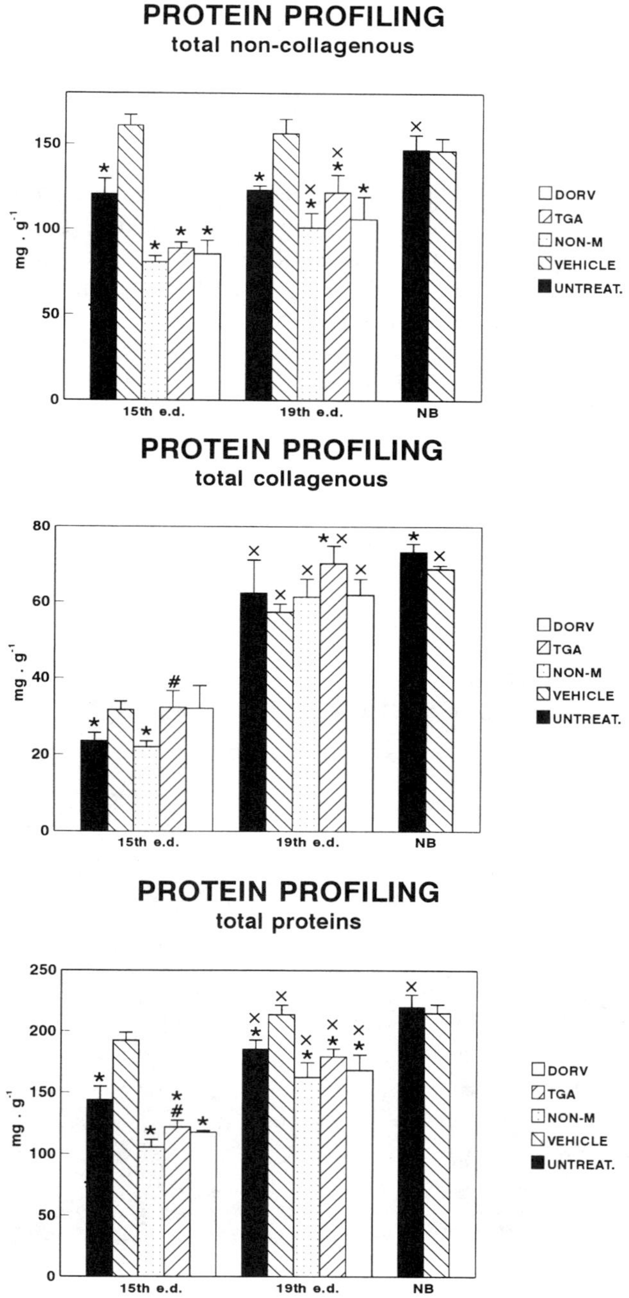

FIG. 27–7. Protein profile in retinoic acid (RA)–induced malformation of cardiac muscle. The concentration of total proteins, total noncollagenous proteins, and total collagenous proteins in heart muscle on embryonic day (e.d.) 15, on e.d. 19, and in newborn mice (NB). Controls (untreated, without any intervention, untreat), vehicle-treated (vehicle), RA-treated but morphologically normal (Non-M), RA-treated with transposition of great arteries (TGA) and RA-treated with double outlet of the right ventricle (DORV). Significance: * $p < 0.05$ or less vs untreated; * $p < 0.05$ or less vs. e.d. 15. In given group: # $p < 0.05$ or less vs Non-M.

the vehicle-treated group. This difference disappeared in newborn animals. From the analysis of noncollagenous and collagenous proteins it followed that the differences between both groups were due to a higher amount of noncollagenous proteins. No quantitative difference was detected in the fraction of collagenous proteins (Fig. 27–6). We have no explanation for the effect of the vehicle alone. However, the changes of pH in the vicinity of myofibrils, induced by vehicle application, might affect the level of high-energy phosphate and then, secondarily, the protein synthesis (9,39). Higher water content on e.d. 15 in vehicle-treated offspring could also be taken into consideration (6). A significantly higher concentration of total protein was found in both untreated and vehicle-treated groups as compared with RA-treated groups, because of elevated concentration of both noncollagenous and collagenous proteins (Fig. 27–7). During the late fetal development of cardiac muscle a stepwise elevation of collagenous proteins was detected in all experimental groups (Fig. 27–7). Whereas no differences of total noncollagenous proteins were observed between RA-treated, morphologically normal em-

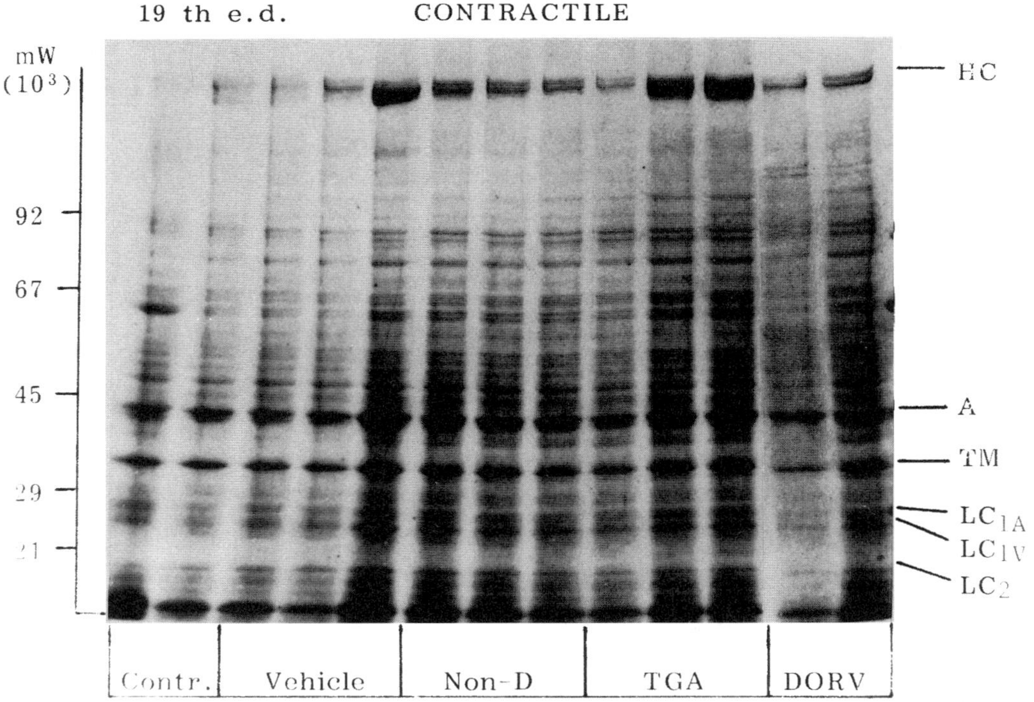

FIG. 27–8. SDS-polyacryamide gel electrophoresis of cardiac contractile proteins: effect of retinoic acid (RA). Samples were derived from cardiac muscle (e.d. 19) of control, vehicle-treated, and RA-treated groups (both TGA and DORV) and RA-treated group without morphologic damage (Non-D). The positions of the main contractile proteins are identified: HC, myosin heavy chains; A, actin; TM, tropomyosin, LC_1, LC_2-myosin light chains of atrial (A) and ventricular (V) origin.

bryos (Non-D) and RA-treated, morphologically damaged fetuses (TGA and DORV), a higher concentration of cardiac collagenous proteins was observed on e.d. 15 in both DORV and TGA groups. On the other hand, the amount of cardiac collagenous proteins in the RA-treated groups on e.d. 19 was the same (Fig. 27–6).

Qualitative Protein Profiles

The electrophoretic pattern of contractile proteins on e.d. 15 is relatively primitive, with predomination of α and β heavy chains of myosin, actin and light chains of myosin (data not shown). During the further embryonic development (Fig. 27–8) the pattern becomes more complex. On e.d. 19 not only the bands of the main contractile proteins, but also regulatory and modulatory proteins were visible. This maturation of myofibrils persists until delivery (40). The extracellular proteins—collagens, glycoproteins, and sulfated or undersulfated glycosaminoglycans—are secreted in the atrioventricular canal region of the heart (36,41–43). Whereas the electrophoretic pattern of cardiac collagen on e.d. 15 is composed of one band only (a homotrimer of collagen type I [data not given]), on e.d. 19 the heterotrimers of collagen I (bands: α_1 [I]and α_2 [II]), and of collagen III (α_1 [III]) were detected (Fig. 27–9). A higher proportion of collagen III, as compared with untreated controls, was in the TGA and DORV groups.

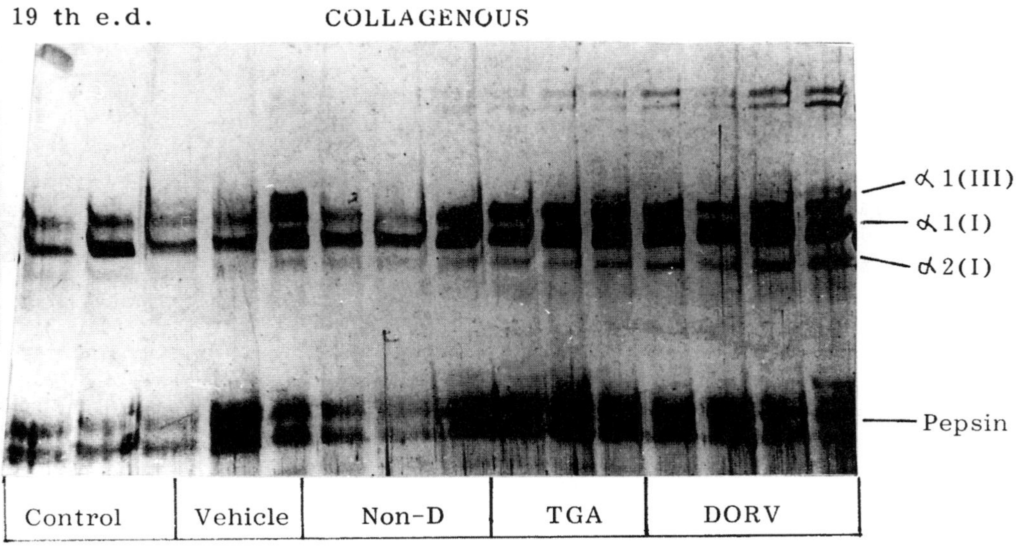

FIG. 27–9. SDS-polyacrylamide gel electrophoresis of the pepsin-soluble fraction of collagen: effect of retinoic acid (RA). Reference grade collagen type I (α_1[I] and α_2) and collagen III (α_1[III]) standards and collagen extracted from cardiac muscle (e.d. 19). Groups included untreated (control), vehicle-treated, and RA-treated mothers both without morphologic damage (Non-D) and with damage structure (TGA and DORV). The position of pepsin is identified.

SUMMARY

1. Application of an oily vehicle results in an increase of total protein of the fetal hearts; this increase is mainly due to a higher concentration of noncollagenous proteins (18).
2. Retinoic acid significantly decreases the amount of total protein in both morphologically normal and malformed hearts. This change is significantly lower on e.d. 19, particularly in the TGA group. The fraction of noncollagenous proteins (metabolic and contractile proteins) is more affected by retinoic acid than by collagenous proteins on both e.d. 15 and e.d. 19.
3. The concentration of contractile proteins is significantly higher in the malformed hearts than it is with RA-treated nondamaged myocardium (6,18).
4. Whereas the electrophoretic picture of the contractile fraction derived from a 15th e.d. myocardium contains only main myofibrillar components, many regulatory and modulatory protein bands besides myosin and actin are present on e.d. 19. The maturation is observed also in the collagenous fraction, which contained the *homotrimer* of collagen I on e.d. 15 and the *heterotrimer* of collagen I and homotrimer of collagen III on e.d. 19.
5. Surgeons who are reconstructing cardiac anatomy should be aware that they are dealing with biochemically abnormal tissue. This might explain some of the failures or late problems in children who had surgery for congenital heart disease.

REFERENCES

1. Pexieder T. Conotruncus and its septation at the advent of the molecular biology era. In: Clark EB, Markwald RR, Takao A, eds. *Developmental mechanisms of heart disease.* New York: Futura Publishing; 1995:227–247.
2. Icardo JM, Manasek FJ. Cardiogenesis: development mechanism and embryology. In: Fozzard HA, Haber E, Jennings RB, Katz AM, Morgan HE, eds. *The heart and cardiovascular system.* New York: Raven Press; 1992:1563–1586.
3. Markwald RR. Overview: formation and early morphogenesis of the primary heart tube. In: Clark EB, Markwald RR, Takao A, eds. *Developmental mechanisms of heart disease.* Mount Kisco, NY: Futura Publishing; 1995:149–156.
4. Gittenberger-deGroot AC, Bartelings MM, Poelmann RE. Normal and abnormal morphogenesis of the outflow tract. In: Clark EB, Markwald RR, Takao A, eds. *Developmental mechanisms of heart disease.* Mount Kisco, NY: Futura Publishing; 1995:249–254.
5. Chien KR. Overview: molecular analysis of cardiac developmental phenotypes: Problems, progress and prospects. In: Clark EB, Markwald RR, Takao A, eds. *Developmental mechanisms of heart disease.* Mount Kisco, NY: Futura Publishing; 1995:3–27.
6. Pexieder T, Blank O, Pelouch V, Ošťádalová I, Milerová M, Ošťádal B. Late fetal development of retinoic acid–induced transposition of great arteries: morphology, physiology, and biochemistry. In: Clark EB, Markwald RR, Takao A, eds. *Developmental mechanisms of heart disease.* Mount Kisco, NY: Future Publishing; 1995:297–308.
7. Borg TK, Nakagawa M, Carver W, Terracio L. Overview: Extracellular matrix, receptors and heart development. In: Clark EB, Markwald RR, Takao A, eds. *Developmental mechanisms of heart disease.* Mount Kisco, NY: Futura Publishing; 1995:175–184.
8. Pelouch V, Ošťádal B, Procházka, J, Urbanová D, Widimský J. Effect of high altitude hypoxia on the protein composition of the right ventricular myocardium. *Prog Respir Res* 1985;20:41–48.
9. Pelouch V, Kolář F, Khuchua ZA, Elizarova GV, Milerová M, Ošťádal B, Saks VA. Cardiac phosphocreatine deficiency induced by GPA during postnatal development in rat. *Mol Cell Biochem* 1996 (in press).

10. Pelouch V, Dixon IC, Golfman L, Beamish RE, Dhalla NS. Role of extracellular matrix proteins in heart function. *Mol Cell Biochem* 1994;129:101–120.
11. Hoffman U, Siegert E. Atrial and ventricular myosins from human hearts. I: Isoenzyme distribution during development and in adults. *Basic Res Cardiol* 1987;82:348–358.
12. Hoffman U, Axmann C, Palm N. Atrial and ventricular myosins from human hearts. II: Isoenzyme distribution after myocardial infarction. *Basic Res Cardiol* 1987;82:359–369.
13. Weber K. Cardiac interstitium: Extracellular space of the myocardium. In: Fozzard HA, Haber E, Jennings RB, Katz AM, Morgan HE, eds. *The heart and cardiovascular system.* New York: Raven Press; 1992:1465–1480.
14. Borg TK, Burgess ML. Holding it all together: organization and function of the extracellular matrix in the heart. *Heart Failure* 1992;8:230–238.
15. Morgan HF, Baker KM. Cardiac hypertrophy: mechanical, neural, and endocrine dependence. *Circulation* 1991;83:13–25.
16. Pelouch V, Milerová M, Ošt'ádal B, Hučín B, Šamánek M. Differences between atrial and ventricular protein profiling in children with congenital heart disease. *Mol Cell Biochem* 1995;147:43–49.
17. Pelouch V, Milerová M, Ošt'ádal B, Šamánek M, Hučín B. Protein profiling of human atrial and ventricular musculature: the effect of normoxemia and hypoxemia in congenital heart diseases. *Physiol Res* 1993;42:235–242.
18. Pelouch V, Pexieder T, Milerová M, Ošt'ádal B. Protein remodeling of the normal and malformed fetal heart. *J Mol Cell Cardiol* 1995;27:A274.
19. Bass A, Šamánek M, Ošt'ádal B, Hučín B, Stejskalová M, Pelouch V. Differences between atrial and ventricular energy supplying enzymes in children. *J Appl Cardiol* 1988;3:397–405.
20. Pelouch V, Jirmář R. Biochemical characterization of cardiac collagen and its role in ventricular remodelling following infarction. *Physiol Res* 1993;42:283–292.
21. Pelouch V. Molecular aspects of regulation of cardiac contraction. *Physiol Res* 1995;44:53–60.
22. Černohorský J, Pelouch V, Milerová M, Ošt'ádal B. Protein profiling of the myocardium exposed to pressure overload from the birth. *Physiol Res* 1995;44:139–142.
23. Burn J. Overview: Heart malformation: the human model. In: Clark EB, Markwald RR, Takao A, eds. *Developmental mechanisms of heart disease.* Mount Kisco, NY: Futura Publishing; 1995:489–504.
24. Sommer JR, Jennings RB. Ultrastructure of cardiac muscle. In: Fozzard HA, Haber E, Jennings RB, Katz AM, Morgan HE, eds. *The heart and cardiovascular system.* New York: Raven Press; 1992:3–50.
25. Gorza L, Sartore S, Schiaffino S. Myosin types and fiber types in cardiac muscle. II: Atrial myocardium. *J Cell Biol* 1982;95:838–845.
26. Sartore S, Gorza L, Bormioli SP, Dalla-Libera L, Sciaffino S. Myosin types and fiber types in cardiac muscle. I: Ventricular myocardium. *J Cell Biol* 1981;88:226–233.
27. Swynghedauw B. Developmental and functional adaptation of contractile proteins in cardiac and skeletal muscles. *Physiol Rev* 1986;66:710–771.
28. Imataka K, Naito S, Seko Y, Fujii J. Hydroxyproline in all part of rabbit heart in the hypertension and in its reversal. *J Mol Cell Cardiol* 1989;21(suppl V):133–139.
29. Yazaki Y, Tsuchimochi H, Kurabayashi M, Komuro I. Molecular adaptation to pressure overload, in human and rat hearts. *J Mol Cell Cardiol* 1989;21:91–101.
30. Kardami E, Fandrich RR. Basic fibroblast growth factor in atria and ventricles of the vertebrate heart. *J Cell Biol* 1989;109:1865–1874.
31. Kivirikko KI. Collagens and their abnormalities in wide spectrum of diseases. *Ann Med* 1993;2:113–126.
32. Trahair T, Yeoh T, Cartmill T, Keogh A, Spratt P, Chang V, dos Remedios CG, Gunning P. Myosin light chain gene expression associated with disease states of the human heart. *J Mol Cell Cardiol* 1993;26:577–585.
33. Hirzel HO, Tuchschmid CR, Schneider J, Krayenbuehl HP, Schaub MC. Relationship between myosin isoenzyme composition, hemodynamics and myocardial structure in various forms of human cardiac hypertrophy. *Circ Res* 1985;57:729–740.
34. Malhotra A, Siri FA, Aronson R. Cardiac contractile proteins in hypertrophied and failing guinea pig heart. *Cardiovasc Res* 1992;26:153–162.
35. Laurent GJ. Dynamic state of collagen: pathways of collagen degradation in vivo and their possible role in regulation of collagen mass. *Am J Physiol* 1987;252:C1–C9.
36. Fisher SA, Periasamy M. Collagen synthesis inhibitors disrupt embryonic cardiocyte myofibrillogenesis and alter the expression of cardiac specific genes in vitro. *J Mol Cell Cardiol* 1994;26:721–731.
37. Šamánek M, Bass A, Ošt'ádal B, Hučín B, Stejskalová M. Effect of hypoxaemia on enzymes supplying myocardial energy in children with congenital heart disease. *Int J Cardiol* 1989;25:265–270.

38. Means AL, Gudas LJ. The roles of retinoic acid in vertebrate development. *Annu Rev Biochem* 1995;64:201–233.
39. Sugden PH, Fuller SJ. Correlation between cardiac protein synthesis rates, intracellular pH and the concentrations of creatine metabolites. *Biochem J* 1991;273:339–346.
40. Lim SS, Woodroofe MN, Lemanski LF. An analysis of contractile proteins in developing chick heart by SDS polyacrylamide gel electrophoresis and electron microscopy. *J Embryol Exp Morphol* 1983;77:1–14.
41. Manasek FJ, Lacktis J, Aiton J, Lieberman M. Synthesis and distribution of glycopeptides and glycosaminoglycans in cultures of embryonic heart cells. In: Pexieder T, ed. *Perspectives in cardiovascular research.* New York: Raven Press; 1981:181–195.
42. Leivo I, Vaheri A, Timpl R, Wartiovaara J. Appearance and distribution of collagens and laminin in the early mouse embryo. *Dev Biol* 1980;76:100–114.
43. Linask KK, Lash JW. Precardiac cell migration: fibronectin localization at mesoderm–endoderm interface during movement. *Dev Biol* 1986;114:87–101.

The Developing Heart,
edited by Bohuslav Ošťádal et al.
Lippincott-Raven Publishers,
Philadelphia © 1997.

28

Depressed Ventricular Contractility in an Experimental Heart Defect in the Embryonic Chick Is Not Associated with an Elevated Microtubule Content

Robert E. Godt, Jane C. Chu, *E. Howard Merry, and *William A. Lutin

*Departments of Physiology & Endocrinology and *Pediatrics and Heart Development Group, Medical College of Georgia, Augusta GA 30912*

Ablation of cells from the cardiac neural crest in the early chick embryo (Hamilton-Hamburger stages 8–10) produces structural heart defects later in development (around embryonic day 9 [1]). Chief among these is persistent truncus arteriosus (PTA), in which division of the common outflow tract into aorta and pulmonary artery does not occur. Ablation of the neural crest also causes early changes in myocardial contractility as monitored either with microcinephotography (at stages 14–25 [2]) or with echocardiography (at embryonic days 11–19 [3,4]). These studies showed that hearts from neural crest–ablated chicks had reduced left ventricular ejection fraction (i.e., the fraction of diastolic volume ejected with systole). End diastolic volume was normal but end systolic volume was increased, that is, less blood volume was expelled with each beat.

Using pressure-overloaded right ventricle of cat, Tsutsui et al. (5,6) found reduced isotonic shortening of myocytes was associated with a doubling of microtubule content, and suggested that excessive microtubules caused the reduced shortening. Inasmuch as microtubules have been shown to run parallel to, as well as to encircle, the myofibrils in mammalian heart cells (7), it is plausible that excessive quantities of microtubules may place a mechanical load on the sarcomeres.

As is well established, tubulin is the major protein of the microtubules and exists in a wide variety of cells as heterodimers of α- and β-tubulin in dynamic equilibrium with microtubules. To examine whether increased microtubule content could explain the decreased ventricular contractility in chick hearts showing PTA, we compared the content of β-tubulin in left ventricles of hearts whose left ventricular volume ejection fraction had been determined previously with *in ovo* echocardiography. If excessive microtubules dramatically influence ventricular performance, we expected that ejection fraction should show a strong negative correlation with tubulin content and that PTA hearts should contain significantly more β-tubulin. Ventricular contraction could also be influenced by differences in the amount of contractile proteins. This possibility was tested by estimating the content of myosin and actin in each ventricular sample as well.

METHODS

Production of Experimental Heart Defect

Fertilized Arbor Acre chicken eggs (Seaboard Hatchery, Athens, GA) for sham-operated and experimental animals were windowed at Hamburger-Hamilton stages 8–10 (approximately 24 hours of development). The embryos were stained with Neutral Red and the cardiac neural crest cells were ablated bilaterally with a pulsed nitrogen/dye laser as previously described (8). This lesion produces PTA in more than 90% of embryos that survive to day 11 as the cardiac neural crest normally provides ectomesenchymal cells essential for septation of the cardiac outflow tract (9). The microsurgery was performed by a Microsurgery Core Unit under the supervision of Dr. Margaret L. Kirby, using procedures that are standardized to produce PTA. For sham-operated control embryos, the vitelline membrane was ruptured and the embryos stained with Neutral Red but the laser ablation was not done. All eggs were sealed with cellophane tape and reincubated until used.

Echocardiography

Ventricular function was assessed using standard echocardiographic techniques, as we have previously adapted to chick embryonic myocardium (4). The air space in previously windowed embryos was partially filled with ultrasound gel warmed to 37°C. Noninvasive imaging of these embryos was performed using a 7.5-MHz dual-frequency ultrasound transducer and a Hewlett-Packard (Palo Alto, CA) SONOS 2000 ultrasound machine. All hemodynamic measurements were made with the egg in a sand bath, to maintain an embryo temperature from 36.5 to 37.0°C during the period of monitoring. Two-dimensional imaging and color flow Doppler allowed identification of the left and right ventricles, ascending aorta, main pulmonary artery, and descending aorta. Two-dimensional images of the right and left ventricles were traced to determine the inner boundaries of the ventricles. From these the long- and short-axis dimensions of the ventricle, area, and volume were calculated for five cardiac cycles in systole and diastole. Systole and diastole were defined as the image frames in which the ventricular size is at its minimum and maximum values, respectively. Ventricular volume was estimated using Simpson's rule, applied to a four-chamber view of the ventricles, by the method of Schmidt et al. (10). From ventricular volume estimations the ventricular volume ejection fraction was derived by standard methods. These methods are well validated in small fetal hearts in animal models (10).

Biochemical Analysis

Once echocardiographic measurements had been made, the left ventricle of the heart was dissected and weighed, before processing for biochemical analysis. The embryo was also weighed and immersed in fixative for anatomic evaluation of the outflow and great vessels to verify PTA.

To determine the content of the major contractile proteins a small strip (diameter ~300 μm, length ~1000 μm) was dissected from the left ventricle in chick Ringer solution. This strip was placed overnight in an ATP-containing solution with EGTA and no added calcium, which also contained 0.5% Triton X-100 detergent to remove all membranes and diffusible proteins, leaving the myofibrils and a few other cytoskeletal proteins remaining. Elimination of extraneous proteins from the sample ensured that the protein bands corresponding to myosin and actin were prominent, which facilitated quantification by densitometry. The next day the strip was transferred to SDS sample buffer in a microcentrifuge tube and heated in boiling water for 3 min. After determination of total protein content using a Pierce (Rockford, IL) BCA assay kit, samples containing 300 μg total protein were loaded into wells of a polyacrylamide electrophoresis apparatus (Bio-Rad, Richmond, CA). Gels with 7.5% acrylamide concentration were run for approximately 3.5 hours, after which proteins were stained with Coomassie Blue. To estimate the content of the contractile apparatus, the myosin and actin bands were digitized with a scanning densitometer and normalized to total protein content in the sample for statistical comparisons.

The remainder of the ventricle was used for determination of total β-tubulin. It was placed directly into SDS sample buffer in a microcentrifuge tube and heated, without intervening treatment with Titron detergent. After determination of total protein content, samples containing 300 μg total protein were loaded into wells of a polyacrylamide electrophoresis apparatus. Gels with 7.5% acrylamide concentration were run for approximately 3.5 hours, after which proteins were transferred to nylon membranes in a Hoefer (San Francisco, CA) blotting unit. The content of total β-tubulin was determined using Western analysis with commercially available antibodies (Amersham, Arlington Heights, IL) and a Bio-Rad chemiluminescence assay kit. The content of β-tubulin was normalized to total protein concentration in the sample for statistical comparisons. To enable comparison of absolute β-tubulin concentrations from gel to gel with Western analysis and chemiluminescent detection, one lane on each gel contained a known concentration of β-tubulin (Molecular Probes, Eugene, OR). From serial dilution of samples, we found the protein concentration ranges in which Coomassie Blue and Western blot analysis with chemiluminescence detection were linear and all experimental samples were loaded in these ranges on the gels.

Statistics

Statistical comparisons were performed using SigmaStat software (Jandel Scientific, San Rafael, CA) using $p < 0.05$ as criterion.

RESULTS

1. *Contractility is not reduced because of a reduction in amount of contractile proteins.* The content of myosin and actin in our ventricular samples as a function of embryonic age is shown in Figs. 28–1 and 28–2. Note that, as expected in growing hearts, there is a tendency for myosin and actin content to increase with embryonic age. The myofibrillar content, as reflected by myosin and actin

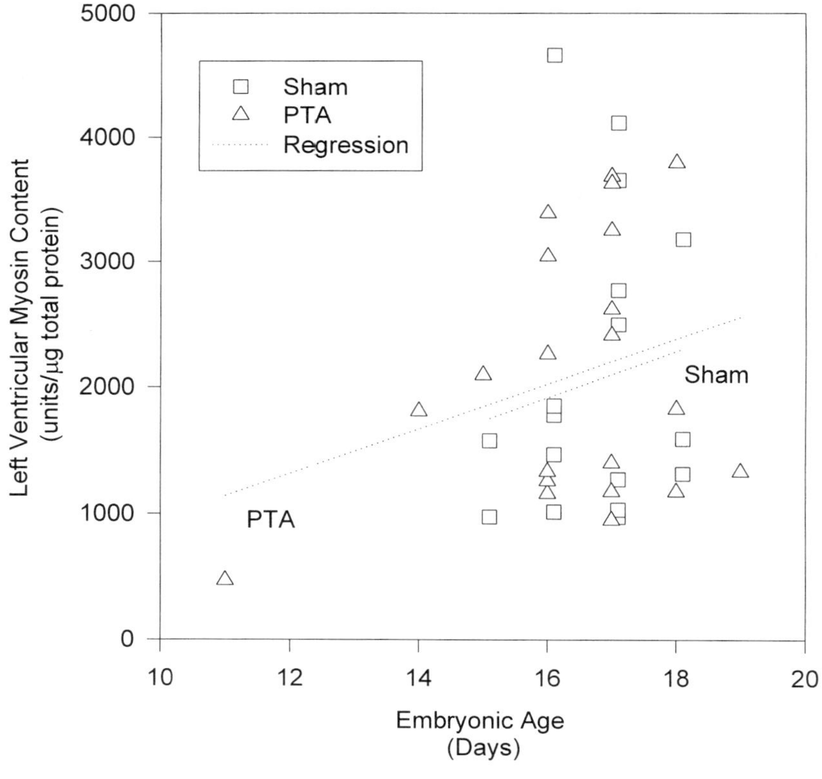

FIG. 28–1. Myosin content of chick left ventricles (normalized to total protein in the sample; see text for details) as a function of embryonic age. Content is expressed as arbitrary density units per microgram total protein loaded on the gel. The data for sham-operated control and PTA hearts have been offset slightly for clarity. The dotted regression lines were calculated by SigmaPlot plotting software (Jandel Scientific, San Rafael, CA) for each data set.

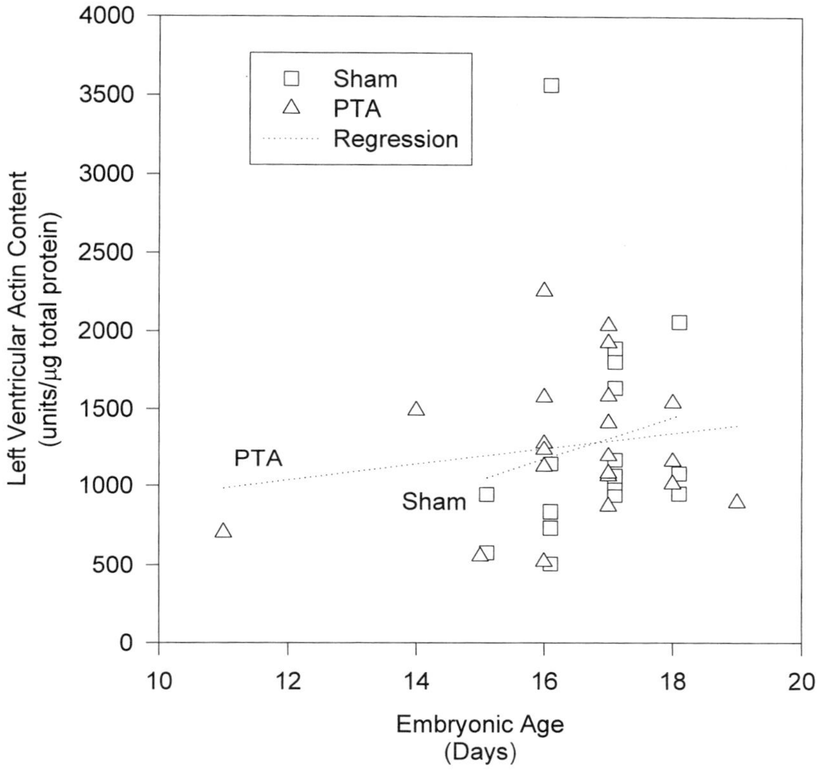

FIG. 28–2. Actin content of chick left ventricles as a function of embryonic age. Content, data offset, and regression lines as in Fig. 28–1.

concentration, is not statistically different in sham-operated and PTA ventricles, however. Previous electron-micrographic studies on a different group of chick hearts showed that the organization and orientation of the sarcomeres was also similar in sham-operated and PTA ventricles (M. L. Kirby, D. E. Bockman, R. T. H. Fogaça, and R. E. Godt, unpublished observations; data not shown).

2. *Unlike the pressure-overloaded cat ventricle, total tubulin levels are not significantly different in sham and PTA hearts.* If microtubules can influence ventricular performance, we expected that PTA ventricles should contain significantly more β-tubulin than sham-operated controls. Figure 28–3 shows the relation between total β-tubulin content and embryonic age in our ventricular samples. There was a general tendency for the amount of total β-tubulin to decline relative to total protein content as the embryos aged. Comparison of the regressions, however, indicated no statistical difference between the values from sham-operated and PTA ventricles.

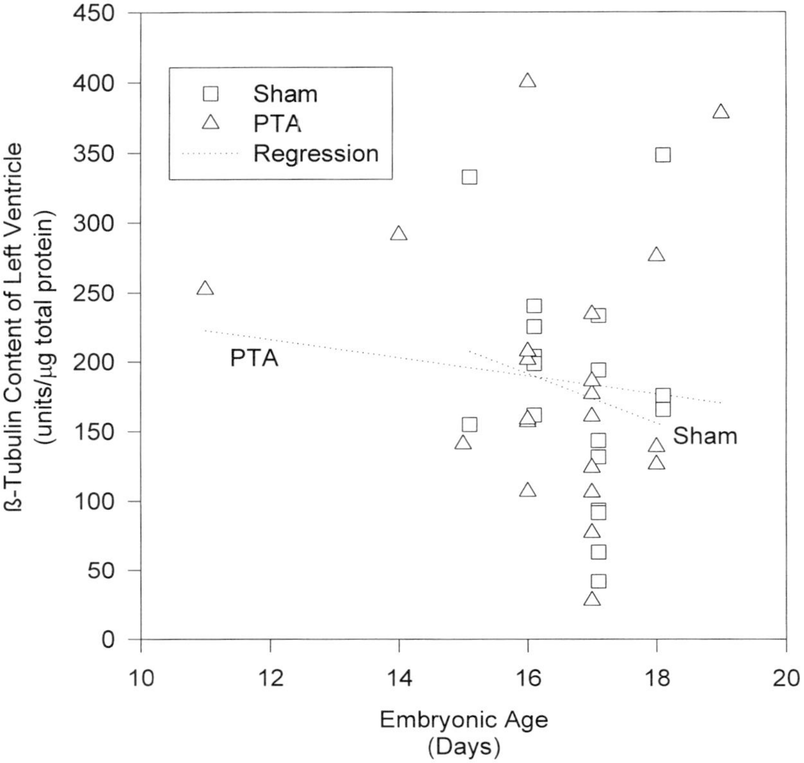

FIG. 28–3. Relation between β-tubulin content of chick left ventricles (normalized to total protein loaded on the gel; see text for details) as a function of embryonic age. Content, data offset, and regression lines as in Figs. 28–1 and 28–2.

3. *There is no statistical correlation between decreased ejection fraction and increased tubulin content.* If microtubules play a significant role in ventricular contractility in vivo, we expected that ejection fraction should show a strong negative correlation with β-tubulin content in both sham-operated and PTA hearts. A graphical representation of this prediction is given in Fig. 28–4. The actual data, shown in Fig. 28–5, are quite different. There is no statistical correlation between reduced ejection fraction and increased β-tubulin content (Pearson Product Moment Correlation, $p < 0.05$). Moreover, it is clear that sham-operated and PTA populations do not fall along the same trend line. This suggests that other mechanisms play a more substantial role in the depression of contractility in PTA hearts.

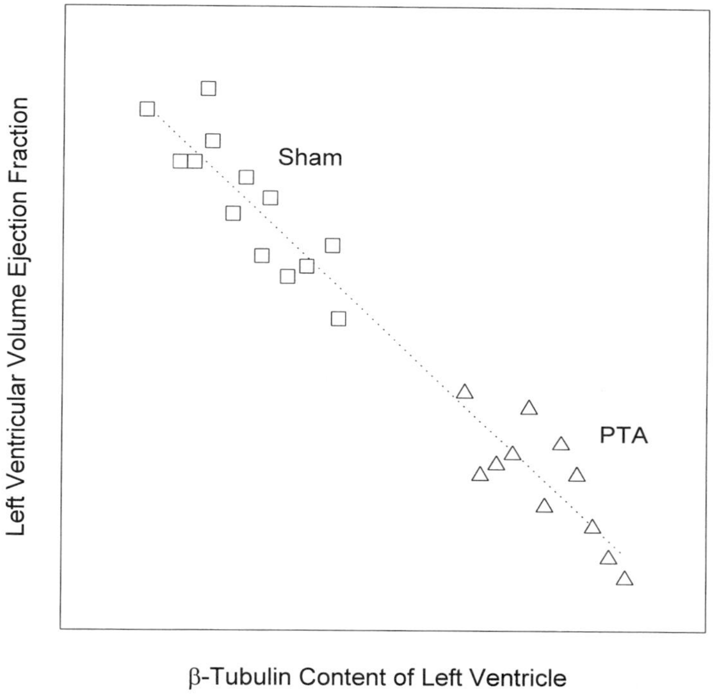

FIG. 28–4. Hypothetical relation between left ventricular volume ejection fraction and β-tubulin content of chick left ventricles if microtubules play a significant role in ventricular contractility in vivo. (Please note that these are not actual data.)

DISCUSSION

In the present work, we are attempting to understand the mechanisms that underlie the reduced in vivo contractility observed in the experimental heart defect (persistent truncus arteriosus) produced in embryonic chicks by surgical ablation of the cardiac neural crest. As has been shown in previous work, this defect is associated with a reduced ejection fraction at both early and late stages of embryonic development (2–4,11), wherein diastolic volume was normal but end systolic volume was increased. Recent work by Tsutsui et al. (5,6) suggested a role for the cytoskeleton in the contractile dysfunction associated with myocardium hypertrophied in response to pressure overload. Using cat heart, they demonstrated that banding of the pulmonary artery led to increased expression of microtubules in myocytes isolated from the right ventricle, whereas microtubule content was unchanged in myocytes from the left ventricle. They found that total tubulin concentration in the right ven-

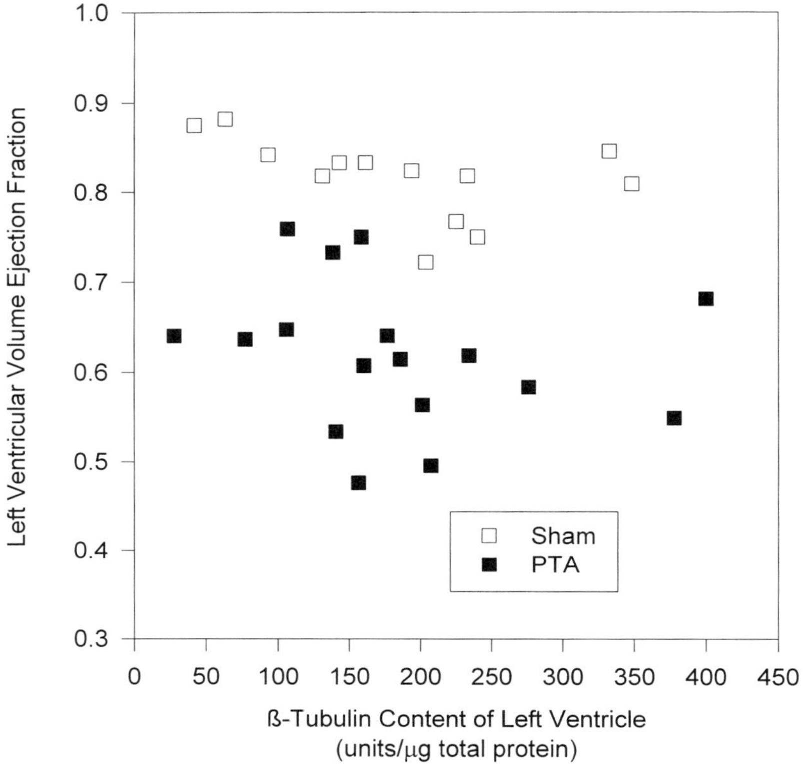

FIG. 28–5. Actual relation between left ventricular volume ejection fraction estimated from echocardiography and β-tubulin content measured in samples of the same chick left ventricles. Content expressed as in Fig. 28–3.

tricle doubled within 2 weeks, although the fraction of total tubulin polymerized into microtubules (approximately one-third) was similar in right and left ventricles. Changes in microtubule content were not observed when hypertrophy was induced by atrial septotomy resulting in volume overload, indicating that pressure overload is the required trigger. When isolated myocytes were stimulated electrically, the maximum extent and velocity of shortening as well as the maximum rate of relaxation were markedly less in right ventricular myocytes with elevated microtubular content. By analogy, reduced ejection fraction as a result of an increase in end systolic volume represents a decrease in the maximum extent of shortening of the ventricular myocytes. Thus, it was plausible to test whether microtubular content was elevated in our defective chick hearts.

As can be seen in Fig. 28–5, although the average ejection fraction in PTA hearts is well below the average for sham-operated controls, some of the PTA hearts had ejection fractions in the normal range. Thus, to adequately test the excessive microtubule hypothesis, it was essential to measure the tubulin content in each ventricle after its function had been determined in vivo. For the same reason, it was also important to measure myosin and actin in each characterized ventricle.

We found that myosin and actin content was not significantly different in sham-operated and PTA ventricles. This appears to rule out the possibility that reduced ejection fraction was a consequence of reduced content of contractile proteins. Although we did not observe the myofibrillar structure in these preparations, previous work from our group indicates that sarcomeres appear normal in PTA hearts (Kirby, Bockman, Fogaça, and Godt, unpublished observations).

If excessive microtubules played a major role in the depression of ejection fraction in our defective chick hearts, we expected the tubulin content to be significantly elevated in these hearts. Moreover, it was reasonable to expect that ejection fraction should be correlated in some fashion with the content of tubulin. Such correlation might occur in both normal and defective hearts if microtubules pose a load on myofibrillar shortening. A naïve prediction of such a correlation is shown in Fig. 28–4. Figure 28–5, however, shows that there was no obvious correlation between ejection fraction and β-tubulin content in either sham-operated or PTA ventricles. This does not support a role for excessive microtubules in the depression of in vivo ventricular contractility in embryonic chicks with PTA.

This conclusion should be tempered by the following caveat. In a variety of tissues, microtubules exist as dynamic structures, assembling and disassembling in equilibrium with the pool of free α-β-tubulin dimers. This turnover process proceeds at widely differing speeds in various cell types. Microtubules can be stabilized by a variety of microtubule-associated proteins (MAPs). Tubulin can be posttranslationally modified by phosphorylation, acetylation, or removal of the terminal tyrosine of α-tubulin (Tyr-tubulin), which results in Glu-tubulin. More stable microtubules (i.e., those that turn over slowly) contain α-tubulin subunits that are acetylated and detyrosinated (12). In a recent abstract, Sato et al. (13) reported finding little or no Glu-tubulin in ventricular myocytes from normal cat ventricle, suggesting that most of the microtubules were quite labile. In myocytes from hypertrophied right ventricle, however. Glu-tubulin increased markedly, indicating that more stable microtubules are formed under these conditions. They hypothesized that this increase in the content of stable microtubules leads to contractile dysfunction. If the fraction of total tubulin polymerized in stable microtubules is substantially higher in PTA hearts, this might impose a higher mechanical load on the contractile machinery. At present, however, we cannot answer this question because we measured only total β-tubulin and not the content of stable microtubules in our preparations.

Even if microtubules play no role in myocardial contractility in chicks with PTA, there are other mechanisms that are likely to decrease ejection fraction in these hearts. It is known that excitation–contraction (EC) coupling is impaired in PTA hearts. L-type Ca^{2+} current (14), Ca^{2+}-induced Ca^{2+} release from the sarcoplasmic reticulum (15), and, consequently, the intracellular Ca^{2+} transient (16,17) are reduced in the ventricular myocardium of PTA hearts. This results in decreased twitch force in ventricular strips prepared from PTA hearts (18). In addition, when ventricular strips are exposed to Triton detergent to remove the membranes (i.e., they are "skinned"), they can be contracted in experimental solutions with known concentrations of Ca^{2+}, bypassing the normal steps of the EC coupling process. We found that the maximal Ca^{2+}-activated force (F_{max}) of skinned strips from PTA hearts at embryonic day 7 was about half of that from equivalent skinned strips from sham-operated control hearts (18). This indicates a defect at the level of the contractile machinery as well. Recently, however, we found that F_{max} of skinned strips from PTA hearts at embryonic days 11 and 15 was not significantly different from that of control hearts (Godt, Fogaça, and T. M. Nosek, unpublished observations), indicating that contractile defects may not be playing a role during the period of embryonic development covered by the present study. The molecular mechanisms that underlie these impairments in EC coupling and contraction are still unclear but are the focus of our current investigations.

SUMMARY

Ablation of cardiac neural crest at about stage 9 produces a structural heart defect (persistent truncus arteriosus, PTA) in embryonic chicks. PTA is associated with decreased myocardial contractility, as indicated by decreased left ventricular ejection fraction determined using microcinephotography (at stages 14–25 in the early embryo) or echocardiography (in the later embryo at embryonic days 11–19). In pressure-overloaded right ventricle of cat, it has been reported that reduced isotonic shortening of myocytes was associated with a doubling of microtubule content, which suggested that excessive microtubules might cause the reduced shortening. To examine whether increased microtubule content could explain the decreased ventricular contractility in chick hearts showing PTA, we compared the content of β-tubulin in left ventricles from hearts whose left ventricular volume ejection fraction had been determined previously with *in ovo* echocardiography. We also estimated the amount of myosin and actin in these ventricles to ascertain any differences in myofibrillar content. In studies at embryonic days 11–19, we found no statistically significant differences in left ventricular content of myosin, actin, or β-tubulin between control hearts and those showing PTA, even though the PTA hearts had a significantly decreased ejection fraction. In either normal or abnormal hearts, there was no statistical correlation between β-tubulin content and left ventricular ejection fraction, and the two populations did not fall along the same regression line. These observations do not support a major role for elevated microtubules in the depression of ventricular contractility in this heart defect. Depressed contractility in PTA hearts over the embryonic period studied is more likely to be due predominantly to inhibition of excitation–contraction coupling by mechanisms that remain to be elucidated.

ACKNOWLEDGMENTS

The authors are members of the Heart Development Group at the Medical College of Georgia. We would like to thank the other members of the Heart Development Group for their support, in particular Dr. T. L. Creazzo for help with this manuscript, and Dr. M. L. Kirby, Ms. Harriett Stadt, and Ms. Donna Kumiski for the assistance of the Microsurgery Core Unit in producing our experimental preparations. This work is supported by USPHS grant HL36059.

REFERENCES

1. Kirby ML, Waldo KL. Role of neural crest in congenital heart disease. *Circulation* 1990; 82:332–340.
2. Leatherbury L, Connuck DM, Gauldin HE, Kirby ML. Microcinephotography of the developing heart in neural crest-ablated chick embryos. *Circulation* 1990;1:1047–1057.
3. Lutin WA, Aliff CL, Creazzo TL, Connuck DM. Possible mechanism for increased mortality in embryos with persistent truncus arteriosus. *J Invest Med* 1995;43:27A. Abstract.
4. Lutin WA, Aliff CL, Creazzo TL, Connuck DM. Possible mechanism for increased mortality in embryos with persistent truncus arteriosus. *Pediatr Res* 1995;37:29A. Abstract.
5. Tsutsui H, Ishihara K, Cooper G. Cytoskeletal role in the contractile dysfunction of hypertrophied myocardium. *Science* 1993;260:682–687.
6. Tsutsui H, Tagawara H, Kent RL, McCollam PL, Ishihara K, Nagatsu M, Cooper G. Role of microtubules in contractile dysfunction of hypertrophied cardiocytes. *Circulation* 1994;90:533–555.
7. Goldstein MA, Entman ML. Microtubules in mammalian heart muscle. *J Cell Biol* 1979;80: 183–195.
8. Kirby ML, Kumiski DH, Myers T, Cerjan C, Mishima N. Backtransplantation of chick cardiac neural crest cells cultured in LIF rescues heart development. *Dev Dyn* 1993;198:296–311.
9. Kirby ML, Gale TF, Stewart DE. Neural crest cells contribute to normal aorticopulmonary septation. *Science* 1983;220:1059–1061.
10. Schmidt KG, Silverman NH, VanHare GF, Hawkins JA, Cloez JL, Rudolph AM. Two-dimensional echocardiographic determination of ventricular volumes in the fetal heart: validation studies in fetal lambs. *Circulation* 1990;81:325–333.
11. Tomita H, Connuck DM, Leatherbury L, Kirby ML. Relationship of early hemodynamic changes to survival and cardiac phenotype after neural crest ablation in chick embryos. *Circulation* 1991;84:1289–1295.
12. Kreis T, Vale R. *Guidebook to the cytoskeleton and motor proteins.* Oxford: Oxford University Press, 1993.
13. Sato H, Tagawa H, Koide M, Cooper G. Enhanced microtubule stability as a mechanism for excess microtubule density in pressure overload cardiac hypertrophy. *Circulation* 1994;90:I264. Abstract.
14. Aiba S, Creazzo TL. Calcium currents in hearts with persistent truncus arteriosus. *Am J Physiol Heart Circ Physiol* 1992;262:H1182–H1190.
15. Nosek TM, Fogaça RTH, Allee PL, Godt RE. Depressed myocardial function secondary to cardiac neural crest ablation (CNCA) in the embryonic chick is associated with a decrease in function of the sarcoplasmic reticulum. *FASEB J* 1994;8:A612. Abstract.
16. Nosek TM, Fogaça RTH, Allee PL, Brotto MAP, Godt RE. Cardiac neural crest ablation (CNCA) decreases calcium uptake and release by the cardiac sarcoplasmic reticulum. *J Mol Cell Cardiol* 27:A821995. Abstract.
17. Creazzo TL, Burch J, Brotto MAP. Excitation–contraction coupling in cardiac dysmorphogenesis. In: Ostadal B, Nagano M, Takeda N, Dhalla NS, eds. *The developing heart.* New York: Lippincott-Raven Press, 1997.
18. Fogaça RTH, Warren KS, Lin JJ-C, Nosek TM, Godt RE. Contractile alterations during myocardial development in the chick subsequent to ablation of the cardiac neural crest. *J Cell Biochem* 1993;17D(suppl):211. Abstract.

PART VI

Effect of Hypoxia and Ischemia

The Developing Heart,
edited by Bohuslav Ošťádal et al.
Lippincott-Raven Publishers,
Philadelphia © 1997.

29

Effects of Hypoxia on Adenylyl Cyclase Activity in Developing Human Heart

Milan Šamánek and Bohumil Hučín, *Věra Klenerová, and *Sixtus Hynie

*Kardiocentrum FN Motol, Prague; *1st Medical School, Charles University, Prague, Czech Republic*

Exposure to hypoxia may stimulate favorable cardiopulmonary adaptation and impose a stress the magnitude of which depends upon the intensity and duration of hypoxia stimulus (for review see ref. 1).

In this paper we focus on the effect of hypoxia on adenylyl cyclase, an enzyme that catalyzes the formation of an important second messenger cAMP from ATP. We were able to find differences in the basal and stimulated activity of adenylyl cyclase in human myocardium exposed during its postnatal development to normal or decreased oxygen supply.

SUBJECTS OF STUDY

In total, 28 myocardial samples were used for the assessment of adenylyl cyclase activity. The myocardial tissue was harvested during corrective surgery of congenital heart defects from 21 patients (12 boys and 9 girls). In 11 patients with tetralogy of Fallot and double outlet right ventricle of the tetralogy type the heart developed under hypoxemic conditions. Oxygen saturation of the arterial blood never reached 80%. In 10 patients the arterial oxygen saturation of the myocardium remained normal during its whole postnatal development. These patients suffered from congenital heart malformations with a left-to-right shunt—defects of atrial, atrioventricular, or ventricular septum. The age of patients at myocardial tissue sampling ranged from 2 to 15 years. The mean age in the hypoxemic cohort was 5.5 years. A sample from the normoxemic myocardium was obtained at the mean age of 6.9 years.

METHODS

The myocardial tissue samples were immediately frozen in liquid nitrogen and processed. The time interval between the sampling and analysis did not exceed 3 months. Adenylyl cyclase activity was assayed in a crude homogenate by using 32p-α-ATP as the substrate (2). The product was separated using aluminium column chromatography. The enzyme activity was measured under basal conditions and after several grades of stimulation by forskolin (Calbiochem, U.S.A.). The results are expressed in pmol/mg protein. A double-blind approach was used in evaluating individual results. All data are presented as mean and SEM values. The significance of differences of mean values of the basal activity between normoxemic atria and hypoxemic atria and ventricles was evaluated using the t-test. Two-way analysis of variance (ANOVA) was performed to evaluate differences in dose–response curves between myocardium exposed to normal or low oxygen tension during its development.

RESULTS

Basal Activity of Adenylyl Cyclase

Cyclic AMP production caused by the nonstimulated activity of adenylyl cyclase in *hypoxemic atria* was 116.3 (SEM $\pm$ 13.0) pmol/mg protein. It was significantly higher than the cAMP value of 63.2 (SEM $\pm$ 6.0) pmol/mg protein measured in *normoxemic atria* ($p < 0.05$). Basal activity of adenylyl cyclase in right ventricular samples was higher than in the hypoxemic atria. Cyclic AMP mean value was 163.5 (SEM $\pm$ 14.0) pmol/mg protein. The value in hypoxemic ventricles was significantly higher than in the atria of normoxemic patients ($p < 0.001$), and also higher than in the hypoxemic atria ($p < 0.05$).

Activity of Adenylyl Cyclase After Stimulation

The stimulation by forskolin elicited a highly statistically significant increase of adenylyl cyclase activity in *all atrial and ventricular samples* expressed by an increased concentration of cAMP produced (Fig. 29–1). Activity response to the stimulation was significantly higher in hypoxemic ventricles and atria than in atria that were not subjected to hypoxia during development. The difference in dose–response curves between normoxemic and hypoxemic atrial and ventricular tissue was highly significant ($p < 0.001$).

DISCUSSION

Our results have shown that human myocardial cells respond to a decreased oxygen supply during postnatal development by increasing the activity of adenylyl

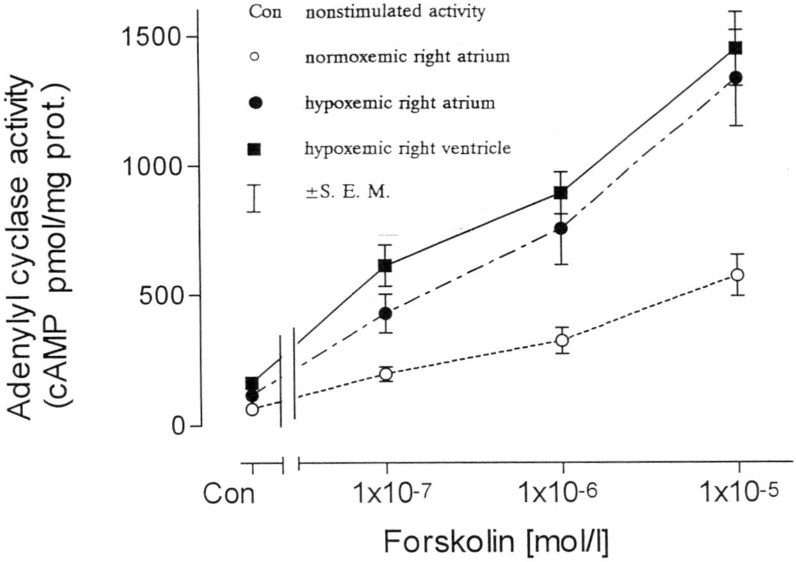

FIG. 29–1. Adenylyl cyclase activity before and after stimulation by forskolin in normoxemic and hypoxemic human myocardium.

cyclase. The increase of the catalytic activity of this enzyme results in an enhanced breakdown of ATP and consequently in an increased production of cAMP, with its important effect on myocardial function (3,4).

Myocardial ischemia has been the most widely used model of myocardial hypoxia. There are several experimental studies on effects of myocardial ischemia and reperfusion on β-adrenergic receptors and signal transduction. Reported changes are often contradictory and dependent on the method and species used (5). On the other hand, direct inhibition of adenylyl cyclase but not adrenergic β-blockade itself was shown recently to protect ischemic hearts from infarction in open-chest pigs (6).

Changes of the β-adrenergic receptor density and sensitivity and postreceptor mechanisms were found in heart failure. They are responsible for an insufficiency in the response of myocardium to catecholamines (3). In end-stage heart failure, not only β-adrenoceptors, but also G-proteins involved in the cAMP-dependent signal transduction using cAMP are altered (7,8). Oddis and Finkel (9) have shown that cAMP regulates the expression of nitric oxide synthase in myocytes of rat hearts. They believe that the enhancement of the nitric oxide production may contribute to the deleterious effects of cAMP elevation in patients with congestive heart failure.

Our previous study demonstrated that the developing human heart exposed to hypoxemia can adapt to a decreased oxygen supply on the cellular level by changing its energetic metabolism (10). A low activity of citrate synthase, NAD dehydrogenase, and triosophosphate dehydrogenase in hypoxemic as compared to normoxemic atria in children with congenital heart diseases can be interpreted as a decreased capacity of aerobic metabolism and a decrease in aerobic carbohydrate breakdown caused by hypoxia. Moreover, a low level of lactate dehydrogenase indicated a disturbed lactate metabolism in the hypoxemic myocardium. A change in the adenylyl cyclase activity in human myocardium exposed to hypoxemia during its development demonstrated in this study has not been reported yet.

We are not able, however, to answer two important questions. First, at what stage of myocardial development can hypoxia change the activity of adenylyl cyclase; second, how long a period of hypoxemia is needed to elicit these changes. We know from our previous experimental study that marked changes in the energetic metabolism enzymes were present in rats after only 24 exposures to 4-hour-long high-altitude hypoxia (11).

The difference in the response to hypoxia between the right ventricle and right atrium was not surprising. We were able to prove its existence in our previous studies. Activity of the energy metabolism enzymes in ventricles differed from that in atria of children with both normoxemic and hypoxemic congenital heart diseases. The right ventricle was able to utilize all the main nutrients, whereas the right atrium utilized primarily glucose. These atrioventricular differences were independent of the type of congenital heart disease and oxygen saturation of the arterial blood (12). Right atria and ventricles differed also in their protein fractions and in their response of collagen synthesis to hypoxia. The effect of hypoxemia in patients with a cyanotic heart disease on the synthesis of collagen was more pronounced in the atrial than in the ventricular tissue (13).

SUMMARY

Adenylyl cyclase activity was measured in 28 samples of myocardial tissue harvested during open heart surgery from 21 children with congenital heart disease aged 2–15 years.

The adenylyl cyclase activity in hypoxemic atria was 116.3 (SEM ± 13.0) pmol/mg protein. It was significantly ($p < 0.05$) higher than in normoxemic atria (63.2 ± 6.0 pmol/mg protein). The value of 163.5 (SEM ± 14.0) measured in hypoxemic right ventricles was even significantly higher than in the atria of normoxemic patients ($p < 0.001$) and in the hypoxemic atria ($p < 0.05$). Increase of the adenylyl cyclase activity after stimulation by forskolin was significantly more pronounced in ventricles and atria subjected to hypoxia during development than in normoxemic atria ($p < 0.001$).

In conclusion, human myocardial cells respond to hypoxemic exposure during development by increasing activity of the adenylyl cyclase.

ACKNOWLEDGMENT

This project was supported by the grant from the Ministry of Health IGA No. 2040-3.

REFERENCES

1. Oštádal B, Kolář F, Pelouch V, Procházka J, Widimský J. Intermittent high altitude and the cardiopulmonary system. In: Nagano M, Takeda N, Dhala NS, eds. *The adapted heart.* New York: Raven Press; 1994:173–182.
2. Čepelík J, Hynie S. Inhibitory effects of clonidine and dopamine on adenylate cyclase of rabbit ciliary processes. *Curr Eye Res* 1990;9:111–120.
3. Brodde OE. β1- and β2-adrenoreceptors in the human heart: properties, function, and alterations in chronic heart failure. *Pharmacol Rev* 1991;43:203–242.
4. Heusch G, Ross JR, eds. Adrenergic mechanisms in myocardial ischemia. *Basic Res Cardiol* 1990;85(suppl 1):1–371.
5. van den Ende R, Batink HD, Michel MC, van Zwieten PA. Influence of ischemia and reperfusion on cardiac signal transduction. G protein content, adenylyl cyclase activity, cyclic AMP content, and forskolin and dibutyryl cyclic AMP-induced inotropy in the rat Langerdorf heart. *Fundam Clin Pharmacol* 1994;8:408–416.
6. Vogt A, Ando H, Weihrauch D, Arras M, Elsasser A, Podzuweit T, Schaper W. An inhibitor of adenylate cyclase but not beta-blockade protects ischemic pig hearts. *J Mol Cell Cardiol* 1995;27:Tu 144.
7. Ungerer M, Böhm M, Elce JS, Erdmann E, Lohse MJ. Altered expression of β-adrenergic receptor kinase and β_1-adrenergic receptors in the failing human heart. *Circulation* 1993;87:454–463.
8. Neumann J, Schmitz W, Scholz H, von Meyerinck L, Döring V, Kalmár P. Increase in myocardial G1-proteins in heart failure. *Lancet* 1988;2:936–937.
9. Oddis CV, Finkell MS. cAMP regulates nitric synthase expression in cardiac myocytes. *Circulation* (suppl 1)1995;92:1–6.
10. Šamánek M, Bass A, Oštádal B, Hučín B, Stejskalová M. Effect of hypoxemia on enzymes supplying myocardial energy in children with congenital heart disease. *Int J Cardiol* 1989;25:265–270.
11. Bass A, Oštádal B, Procházka J, Pelouch V, Šamánek M, Stejskalová M. Intermittent high altitude–induced changes in energy metabolism in the rat myocardium and their reversibility. *Physiol Bohemoslov* 1989;38:155–161.
12. Bass A, Šamánek M, Oštádal B, Hučín B, Stejskalová M, Pelouch V. Differences between atrial and ventricular energy supplying enzymes in children. *J Appl Cardiol* 1988;3:397–405.
13. Pelouch V, Milerová M, Oštádal B, Hučín B. Differences between atrial and ventricular protein profiling in children with congenital heart disease. *Mol Cell Biochem* 1995;147:43–49.

The Developing Heart,
edited by Bohuslav Ošťádal et al.
Lippincott-Raven Publishers,
Philadelphia © 1997.

30

Effect of Respiratory Inhibition and Ischemia on Nucleotide Metabolism in Newborn Swine Cardiac Myocytes

Charlene M. Hohl

The Ohio State University, Department of Medical Biochemistry
Columbus, OH 43210

There are numerous studies describing the effects of ischemia and hypoxia on cardiac metabolism and function in adult species, yet corresponding information is lacking for the neonate. Furthermore, many of the existing reports are conflicting, probably because of species differences and varying maturity levels of the neonatal models. Mitochondrial enzymes, especially those involved in fatty acid oxidation, may be less active in the neonate (1,2), thus limiting the number of pathways for energy production. By contrast, neonatal isoforms of phosphofructokinase (3) and lactate dehydrogenase (4) allow for greater rates of anaerobic glycolysis. Indeed, it has been suggested that increased tolerance of the neonatal heart to hypoxia may be accounted for by increased glycolytic capacity (5). On the other hand, younger hearts are generally more susceptible to ischemic damage (6, and references therein). This has been partially attributed to an immature contractile apparatus, resulting in decreased systolic and diastolic functional reserve compared to adult myocardium (7). However, it is not yet clear to what extent altered metabolism contributes to postischemic contractile dysfunction in the neonate.

In vitro hypoxia and ischemia are often simulated in isolated perfused hearts where experimental conditions such as substrate deprivation and coronary flow can be highly controlled. However, it is difficult to eliminate differences in neurohumoral influences, contractile activity, and perfusion variability that are also affected by hypoxia and ischemia, and that consequently contribute to the metabolic status of the myocardium. In an effort to overcome these problems and to define properties intrinsic to the muscle cells, in the present study, energy metabolism was examined in myocytes isolated from the ventricles of newborn piglet hearts. The piglet was chosen because cardiac mechanical function and metabolism of this larger, slow-heart-rate mammal closely parallel those of humans. Furthermore, in contrast to neonatal rabbits and rats, the piglet is relatively mature at birth and may therefore be a more suitable model for the human infant.

The purpose of the present work was to investigate pathways for ATP synthesis and degradation in newborn piglet ventricular cardiomyocytes. Furthermore, the effects of respiratory inhibition and ischemia on nucleotide metabolism and glycolytic activity were examined. Because of existing controversies regarding the ability of the neonate to utilize certain substrates, particularly fatty acids, substrate preferences were also evaluated in piglet myocytes.

MATERIALS AND METHODS

Isolation of Myocytes

Newborn mixed-breed piglets less than 24 hours old were used for all experiments. The piglets were obtained from Dawson Farms, Delaware, Ohio. Piglets were anesthetized with 100 mg/kg sodium pentobarbital, the heart removed, and the aorta cannulated. The heart was perfused with Medium 199 (GIBCO) until cleared of blood and then placed on a Langendorff apparatus and perfused without recirculation for 10 min at 37°C with Krebs-Henseleit buffer (gased with 95% O_2/5% CO_2; pH 7.3) containing the following in mM): 110 NaCl, 4.8 KCl, 1.2 $MgSO_4$, 1.2 KH_2PO_4, 1 $CaCl_2$, 26 $NaHCO_3$, 11 glucose, 5 pyruvate, 10 taurine, 10 creatine, 0.68 glutamine, 0.001 insulin, a complete amino acid mixture (BME and MEM, GIBCO) and penicillin–streptomycin. The perfusate was changed to a recirculating Ca-free Krebs-Henseleit containing collagenase (1 mg/ml, type II, Worthington Biochemicals) and BSA (1 mg/ml, Fraction V, Miles). After 15 min, $CaCl_2$ was added in small increments over a 10-min period to achieve a final concentration of 1 mM. After an additional 5 min of perfusion, the softened tissue was removed from the apparatus, the ventricles minced, and the dispersed cells filtered through cheesecloth. The cells were washed twice and resuspended in medium (pH 7.3) containing the following (in mM): 110 NaCl, 4.8 KCl, 1.2 $MgSO_4$, 1.2 KH_2PO_4, 1 $CaCl_2$, 5 $NaHCO_3$, 25 HEPES, 11 glucose, 5 pyruvate, 20 taurine, 10 creatine, 0.68 glutamine, 0.001 insulin, amino acids, vitamins, and penicillin–streptomycin. All incubations were carried out in this medium unless stated otherwise.

Isolation of Cardiac Mitochondria

Mitochondria were prepared using the procedure of Vercesi et al (8). Piglet heart ventricles were minced in cold medium (4°C) containing 250 mM sucrose, 1 mM EGTA and 15 mM HEPES (pH 7.3). The tissue suspension was then treated with nagarse (1 mg/g wet weight heart tissue) for 18 min. Following removal of the protease, the tissue was homogenized and centrifuged at 600 $\times$ *g* for 12 min and the resulting supernatant was centrifuged at 10,000 × *g* for 18 min. The pellet was resuspended in 250 mM sucrose buffered with 15 mM HEPES (pH 7.2) and again centrifuged at 10,000 × *g* for 12 min. This final step was repeated and the resulting mitochondria were stored in HEPES-buffered sucrose medium at 4°C.

Analysis

Protein was determined by the method of Lowry et al (9). Cellular creatine, phosphocreatine, and lactate contents were estimated according to Bergmeyer (10).

Nucleotides and nucleosides were extracted by sedimenting mitochondria and intact myocytes through 0.5 ml bromododecane into perchloric acid as described previously (11). Acid extracts were neutralized with freon–trioctylamine (1.1:3.9 v:v) and separated on a Whatman Partisil SAX HPLC column using a pH and phosphate elution gradient (11).

Oxygen Consumption

Oxygen consumption was measured at 37°C with a Clark electrode (Yellow Springs Instrument). Mitochondria were suspended in medium containing 100 mM KCl, 15 mM HEPES, 1.2 mM KH_2PO_4, and 1.0 mM $MgCl_2$ (pH 7.0) and the indicated substrates. Myocytes were suspended in Ca^{2+}-free medium containing 110 mM NaCl, 4.8 mM KCl, 1.2 mM $MgSO_4$, 1.2 mM KH_2PO_4, 25 mM HEPES, 0.6 glutamine, amino acids, and the indicated substrates. Bovine serum albumin (1%) was included when β-hydroxybutyrate, palmitate, or palmitoylcarnitine were present in the medium. Respiration rates in the absence of added substrates averaged 18 ng atom O_2 min^{-1} mg^{-1} myocyte protein and were unaffected by the presence of bovine serum albumin. Rotenone (16 μM) was present in incubations containing succinate.

Induction of Ischemia

Myocytes suspended in HEPES-buffered Krebs-Henseleit medium that did not contain glucose or pyruvate were sedimented in conical microfuge tubes and extracellular medium was removed to achieve a concentrated slurry of cells at 25 mg protein/ml. 5-Ethyl-5-isoamylbarbituric acid (amytal, 3 mM), a reversible NADH dehydrogenase blocker, was added to prevent reaeration effects during sampling (12) and the cell pellet was incubated without agitation for up to 60 min at 37°C. After samples were taken for metabolite analysis, the remaining cells were washed twice to remove amytal, resuspended at 2 mg/ml in medium containing glucose and pyruvate, and incubated for a further 25 min in an orbital shaking water bath (37°C) under air.

Statistics

Values reported are means ± SE for *n* different myocyte preparations. Data were evaluated using Students' *t*-test, and differences and were considered significant at $P < 0.05$.

RESULTS

Preparations of freshly isolated piglet myocytes were 86 ± 2% viable as estimated by cellular exclusion of trypan blue. These cells contained an average of 33 nmol/mg protein ATP and 37 nmol/mg total adenine nucleotides (Table 30–1). In addition to components listed in Table 30–1, 0.4 nmol/mg adenosine, 0.6 nmol/mg inosine, and trace amounts of GMP were recovered from acid extracted myocytes.

The total adenine nucleotide content of mitochondria isolated from newborn piglet hearts averaged 15.1 ± 0.9 nmol/mg mitochondrial protein ($n = 9$) and total pyridine nucleotide levels [NAD(H) + NADP(H)]approximated 16 nmol/mg protein. These values are comparable to published results for adult swine mitochondria (13).

Substrate Dependence of Oxygen Consumption by Piglet Mitochondria

Oxygen consumption was determined in myocytes isolated from newborn piglets presented with a variety of substrates (Table 30–2). The results demonstrate that substrates entering the citric acid cycle are readily utilized by piglet myocytes. Fatty acids are also oxidized by these neonatal cells, but at rates that are significantly lower than oxidation of succinate or other potential precursors of the citric acid cycle. Oxygen consumption in the presence of palmitate was not further stimulated by including 1 mM carnitine in the incubation medium, indicating that carnitine levels were not deficient. Respiration rates measured in isolated piglet mitochondria support the findings in myocytes (Table 30–3). State 3 respiratory rates were maximal in the presence of succinate, while slightly lower rates were obtained in mitochondria oxidizing pyruvate or glutamate. In subsequent studies using intact myocytes, cells were routinely incubated with pyruvate, since it is highly

TABLE 30–1. *Metabolite profile of isolated piglet myocytes*[a]

ATP	ADP	AMP	ΣAN	IMP	GTP	NAD(H)	PCr	Total Cr
32.5	4.09	0.53	37.1	0.38	1.74	6.97	44.7	85.3
1.9	0.16	0.07	1.9	0.08	0.07	0.33	3.6	4.6

[a]Values are mean ± SEM in nmol/mg myocyte protein for eight preparations. ΣAN = AMP + ADP + ATP.

TABLE 30–2. *Effect of substrate on oxygen consumption in isolated myocytes*[a]

Substrates	*n*	+ digitonin (32 μg/mg)	+ ADP (1.1 mM)
5 mM pyruvate, 5 mM malate	5	67.6 ± 18.9	168.2 ± 34.1
5 mM glutamate, 5 mM malate	3	93.9 ± 24.1	162.3 ± 48.5
5 mM succinate	11	115.6 ± 13.2	177.8 ± 20.8
5 mM β-hydroxybutyrate	7	57.6 ± 5.7	103.0 ± 11.0
30 μM palmitoly-carnitine	6	52.1 ± 7.2	88.0 ± 17.7
100 μM palmitate	4	48.8 ± 10.1	58.3 ± 14.0

[a]Values are mean ± SEM (ngatom O_2 $min^{-1}mg^{-1}$ myocyte protein) for *n* preparations.

permeable (in contrast to succinate) and was oxidized efficiently by piglet ventricular cells.

Effect of Respiratory Inhibition on Piglet Myocytes

Piglet cardiac myocytes suspended in medium containing glucose and pyruvate, and incubated at 37°C under air produced approximately 14 nmol lactate per milligram of protein per minute. In the presence of 16 μM rotenone, an inhibitor of NADH dehydrogenase, lactate production increased to 25 nmol lactate per milligram of protein per minute (Fig. 30–1).

Rotenone-treated myocytes maintained ATP stores at 95% of control levels for up to 30 min by stimulating anaerobic glycolysis (Fig. 30–2). However, phosphocreatine content fell by 50% during this period (Fig. 30–2), without a change in total creatine content. Both ATP and phosphocreatine increased slightly in respiring piglet myocytes incubated at 37°C. As expected, NAD/NADH ratios were significantly decreased in rotenone-treated myocytes (control NAD/NADH = 2.36 6 0.39; rotenone-treated cells NAD/NADH = 0.78 6 0.04; $p < 0.05$). Compartmentation studies indicated that mitochondrial pyridine nucleotides, but not those of the cytosol, were highly reduced in myocytes maintaining ATP stores through anaero-

TABLE 30–3. *Respiratory rates of piglet mitochondria*[a]

Substrates	*n*	State 3
5 mM pyruvate, 5 mM malate	4	387.7 ± 11.8
5 mM glutamate, 5 mM malate	4	263.3 ± 29.0
5 mM succinate	5	578.1 ± 31.35
5 mM β-hydroxybutyrate	5	79.0 ± 18.6

[a]Values are mean ± SEM (ngatom O_2 $min^{-1}mg^{-1}$ mitochondrial protein) for *n* preparations.

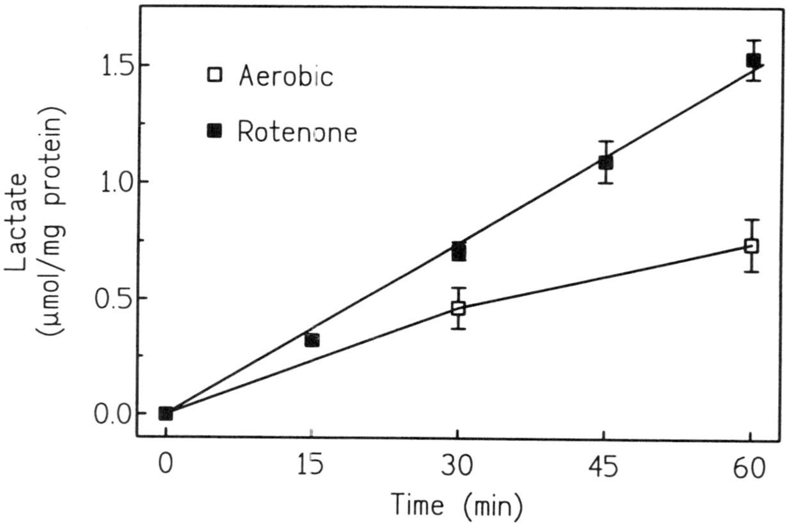

FIG. 30–1. Lactate production by isolated piglet myocytes. Lactate production was determined in suspensions of myocytes incubated in the presence of glucose with (*closed squares*) or without (*open squares*) the respiratory inhibitor, rotenone (16 μM). Points are mean ± SEM for five myocyte preparations.

bic glycolysis (data not shown). Other nucleotide and nucleoside levels were not altered by respiratory inhibition in glycolyzing myocytes.

Glycolytic Activity of Piglet Myocytes

As demonstrated earlier, glycolysis is stimulated in myocytes that are treated with inhibitors of electron transport. Glycolytic activity can be further accelerated in nonrespiring myocytes by increasing ATP turnover. The effects of titrating piglet myocytes with carbonyl cyanide m-chlorophenylhydrazone (CCCP), a protonophore that promotes the dephosphorylation of ATP by stimulating mitochondrial ATPase activity, on ATP and lactate content of rotenone-treated myocytes is shown in Fig. 30–3A. In the presence of glucose, rotenone and 10^{-7} M CCCP, cellular ATP content declined by 70%, resulting in a corresponding elevation of lactate production to 48 nmol mg^{-1} min^{-1}. In this case ATP hydrolysis exceeded glycolytic ATP production, whereas higher concentrations of CCCP were less effective at reducing cellular ATP; consequently, lactate accumulation was also reduced (Fig. 30–3A). The ratio of ATP to ADP closely paralleled changes in ATP content and was inversely related to lactate production (Fig. 30–3B, $r = -.97$). Since glycolytic activity has been shown to be dependent on ATP/ADP (14), extrapolation of the plot of lactate production rate as a function of ATP/ADP gives a theoretical

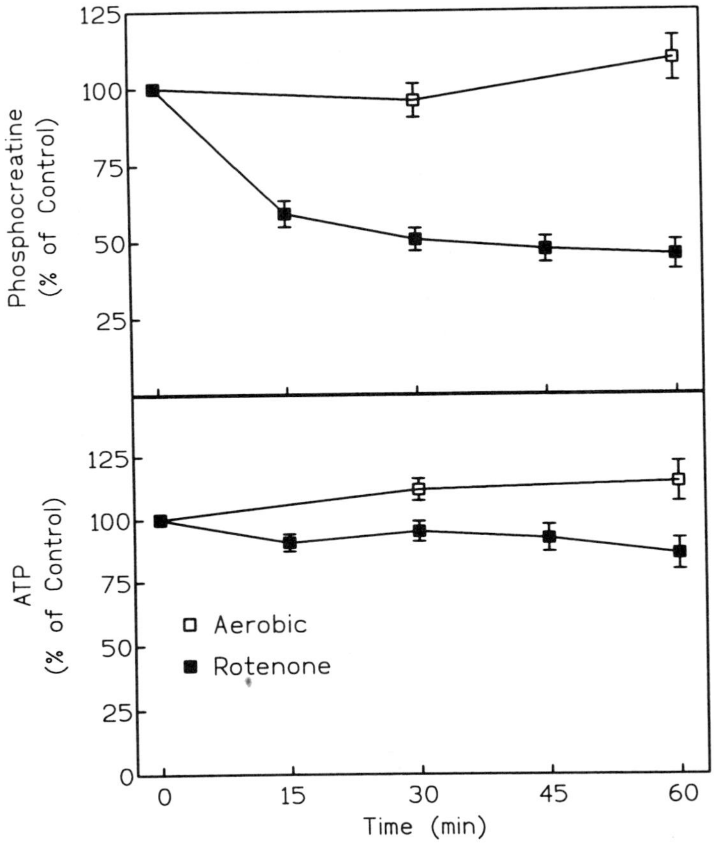

FIG. 30–2. Retention of ATP and phosphocreatine contents in piglet myocytes after treatment with rotenone. All conditions are as stated for Fig. 30–1.

maximum for glycolytic capacity in piglet cardiac myocytes of 58 nmol mg^{-1} min^{-1}.

Effect of Stimulated Ischemia on Myocytes

To simulate ischemia, myocytes were incubated in a concentrated slurry (25 mg cell protein/ml) at 37°C in the presence of 3 mM amytal, a reversible inhibitor of NADH dehydrogenase, and without any added substrates. Under these conditions 6.4 nmol lactate mg^{-1} min^{-1} was produced, most likely from glycogen metabolism. However, as depicted in Fig. 30–4, glycolytic ATP production was not sufficient to maintain ATP stores under these conditions. ATP content of myocytes de-

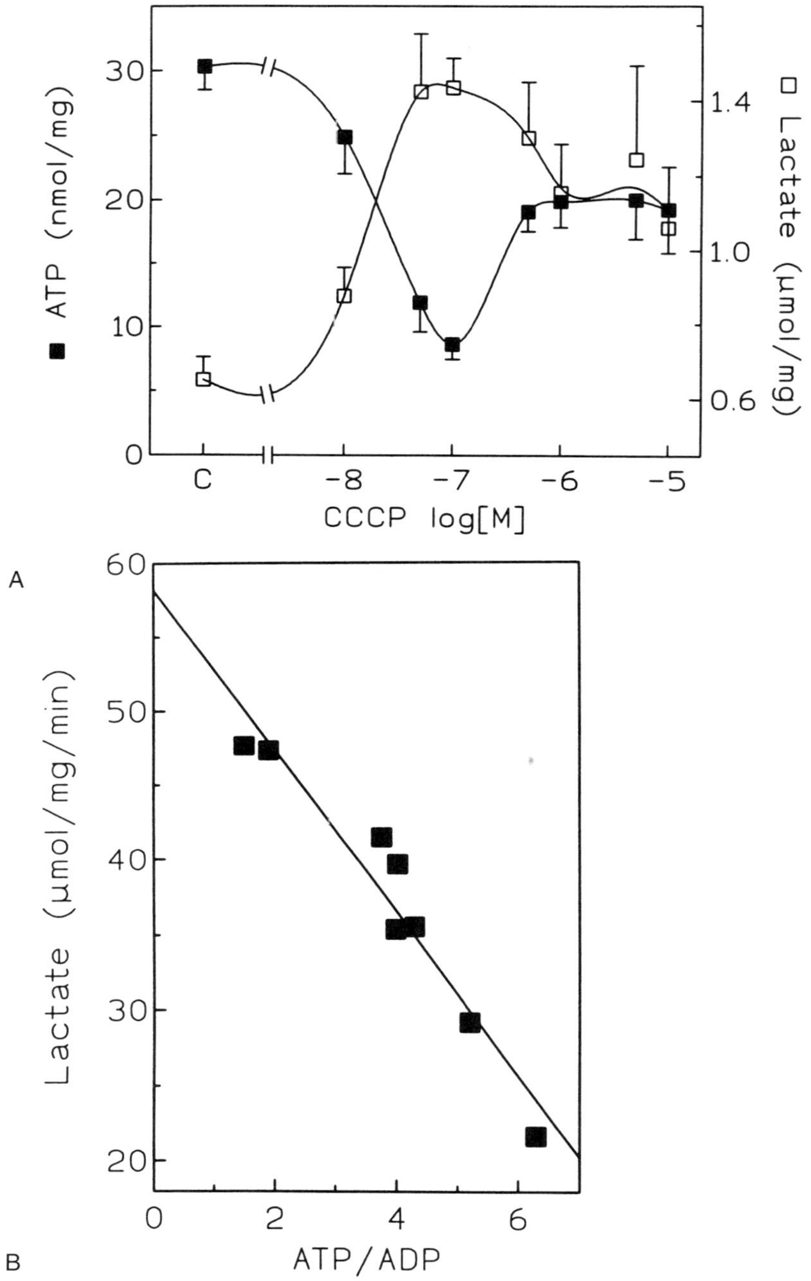

FIG. 30–3. Effect of CCCP on ATP content and lactate production in respiratory inhibited piglet myocytes. Lactate formation (*open squares*) and ATP content (*closed squares*) were analyzed in myocytes incubated for 30 min at 37°C with 11 mM glucose and 16 µM rotenone in the presence of varying concentrations of the ionophore, CCCP. Values are mean ± SEM for six preparations.

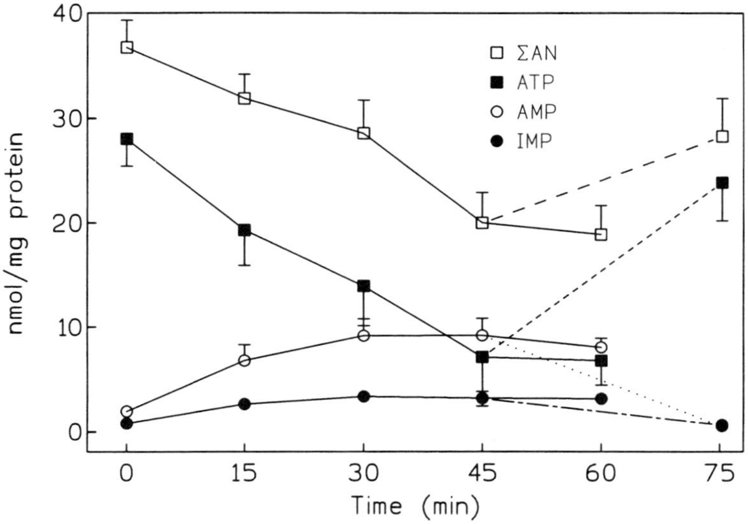

FIG. 30–4. Effect of ischemia and reperfusion on nucleotide content of piglet myocytes. Myocytes were suspended in substrate-free medium, sedimented to a dense pellet (~25 mg/ml), and incubated without shaking for up to 60 min at 37°C. After 45 min myocytes were washed twice, resuspended in medium supplemented with glucose and pyruvate at 2 mg protein/ml, and incubated for a further 30 min (values at 75 min). Points are mean ± SEM for six preparations.

clined to 2.8 ± 0.8 nmol ATP/mg after 60 min incubation in a substrate-free dense slurry. Phosphocreatine was rapidly depleted (data not shown) and AMP levels increased, whereas ADP remained relatively constant. Piglet myocytes formed approximately 3 nmol/mg IMP after 60 min ischemia compared to less than 1 nmol IMP/mg in control aerobic cells. Intracellular adenosine and inosine rose to 4 and 6 nmol/mg, respectively. An approximately equal amount of inosine was recovered in the extracellular medium, suggesting that considerable efflux of inosine (and/or adenosine) occurred.

"Reperfusion" of ischemic myocytes by removal of amytal and resuspension in medium supplemented with glucose and pyruvate at 2 mg/ml resulted in restoration of the ATP pool to the extent possible by the existing nucleotide pools (Fig. 30–4).

DISCUSSION

The isolation procedure for piglet myocytes yielded cells having adenine nucleotide content similar to published values for intact neonatal piglet cardiac tissue (15,16). When cellular ATP values in Table 30–1 are corrected upward to account for the 14% of cells that are nonviable, we estimate that freshly isolated viable myocytes contain approximately 40 nmol/mg ATP. Furthermore, nucleotide profiles obtained from neonatal piglet myocytes are similar to those of adult swine myocardial tissue (17).

Substrate Utilization by Piglet Cardiac Mitochondria

The data in Tables 30–2 and 30–3 demonstrate that citric acid cycle intermediates are readily oxidized by newborn piglet mitochondria at rates that are comparable to those established for adult (18–20) and neonatal (15,21,22) hearts. Although palmitoyl-carnitine was utilized to some degree by all piglet myocyte preparations tested, the rates of fatty acid oxidation varied considerably. Similarly, palmitate was poorly oxidized by piglet cardiac myocytes. These findings are in agreement with other groups studying age-related differences in fatty acid metabolism (2,23). Carnitine-dependent oxidation of palmitoyl-CoA was reduced in newborn piglet heart (21), yet developmental changes in carnitine palmitoyltransferase I activity were not observed in this species (24). Decreased long-chain fatty acid oxidation in 1-day-old rabbit hearts has been linked to age-related changes in acetyl-CoA carboxylase catalyzed production of malonyl-CoA, a potent inhibitor of carnitine palmitoyltransferase I (25). Moreover, insulin potentiates malonyl-CoA inhibition (25,26) and lactate (27) suppresses palmitate utilization. The effect of these compounds was not assessed in this study; however, carnitine deficiency does not appear to have a role, since addition of carnitine to the myocyte suspending medium did not improve oxygen consumption rates in the presence of palmitate.

Glycolytic Capacity in Newborn Piglet Myocytes

Rouslin (28) has demonstrated an ATP-sparing effect in ischemic hearts of species having heart rates of less than or equal to 200 beats/min. Larger adult mammals such as pig, dog, and human have a full complement of a mitochondrial ATPase inhibitor protein that slows the hydrolysis of ATP during nonenergizing conditions, whereas the mitochondria of rodents and other fast heart rate animals exhibit very little in situ ATPase inhibition (28). The smaller species compensate for the increased ATPase activity by stimulating glycolytic flux (29). We have previously described differences in glycolytic activity in nonrespiring adult canine and rat myocytes (7 [canine] vs 16 [rat]) nmol lactate mg^{-1} min^{-1} in the presence of glucose, pyruvate, and rotenone [12,19]). Rotenone-treated myocytes isolated from newborn piglet hearts produced lactate at a slightly higher rate of 25 nmol mg^{-1} min^{-1} in the presence of glucose, whereas rotenone-treated adult swine cardiac myocytes produced only 9.5 + 1.3 nmol lactate mg^{-1} min^{-1} (C. Hohl, unpublished data). Greater basal energy expenditure, as indicated by higher basal glycolytic rates in nonrespiring cells compared to adult swine myocytes, is in line with evidence that resting heat production is inversely related to body-to-surface volume ratio (30). Furthermore, estimates of maximum glycolytic capacity of piglet myocytes (58 nmol lactate mg^{-1} min^{-1}) were intermediate between those established for adult canine (35 nmol lactate mg^{-1} min^{-1}) and rat heart cells (95 nmol lactate mg^{-1} min^{-1}, [19]). These findings are in agreement with reports of significantly higher lactate levels in normothermic ischemic neonatal piglet hearts compared to adult swine hearts (16,31).

EFFECT OF ISCHEMIA ON PIGLET MYOCYTE NUCLEOTIDES

Under conditions of simulated ischemia where substrate availability was limited and metabolic products were allowed to accumulate, cellular ATP content was significantly reduced. As expected, the primary degradation product was AMP; however, further breakdown to adenosine and inosine was also apparent. A striking finding was the deamination of AMP to inosine monophosphate (IMP). Although AMP deaminase is quite active in rodent hearts (32,33), little conversion of AMP to IMP is observed in myocardium of adult large mammals. Furthermore, we have evidence that AMP deaminase is enhanced by adenosine (32) and activators of protein kinase C (33), suggesting that this alternate pathway for AMP degradation may be important in the neonate, especially during certain disease states.

SUMMARY

The present studies establish that ATP generating pathways in newborn piglet myocytes are highly developed at birth. Mitochondria oxidize citric acid cycle intermediates at rates comparable to adults of this species. By contrast, utilization of fatty acids by piglet hearts is quite variable immediately after birth, but reports from other laboratories indicate that impairments in fatty acid oxidation are attributable to an increase in inhibitory factors rather than to a deficiency of the enzymes required for these reactions. Although nucleotide profiles of well-energized piglet myocytes are similar to adults of this species, we have evidence that AMP deaminase is more active in the neonate (34), suggesting that routes for ATP degradation are different. In conclusion, ventricular myocytes isolated from newborn piglet hearts are ideal for studying nucleotide metabolism in a relatively mature neonatal species. In this regard, piglet hearts are an excellent model for comparison to the human infant.

ACKNOWLEDGMENTS

These studies were supported by Grant-in-Aid CO9313I from the Ohio Affiliate of the American Heart Association and by National Institutes of Health Grants HL36240 and HL52793. I thank Beth Livingston for technical assistance.

REFERENCES

1. Warshaw JB, Terry ML. Cellular energy metabolism during fetal development. II. Fatty acid oxidation by the developing heart. *J Cell Biol* 1970;44:354–360.
2. Lopaschuk GD, Spafford MA. Energy substrate utilization by isolated working hearts from newborn rabbits. *Am J Physiol* 1990;258:H1274–H1280.
3. Jones CT, Rolph TP. Metabolism during fetal life: a functional assessment of metabolic development. *Physiol Rev* 1985;65:357–423.
4. Dawson DM, Goodfriend TL, Kaplan ND. Lactic dehydrogenases: functions of the two types. *Science* 1964;143:929–933.
5. Jarmakani JM, Nagatomo T, Nakazawa M, Langer GA. Effect of hypoxia on myocardial high-energy phosphates in the neonatal mammalian heart. *Am J Physiol* 1978;235:H475–H481.
6. Riva E, Hearse DJ. *The developing myocardium.* Mount Kisco, NY: Futura Publishing, 1991.
7. Friedman WF. The intrinsic physiologic properties of the developing heart. *Prog Cardiovasc Dis* 1972;15:87–110.
8. Vercesi A, Reynafarje B, Lehninger AL. Stoichiometry of H^+ ejection and Ca^{2+} uptake coupled to electron transport in rat heart mitochondria. *J Biol Chem* 1978;253:6379–6385.
9. Lowry OH, Rosebrough NJ, Farr AL, Randall RJ. Protein measurement with the folin phenol reagent. *J Biol Chem* 1951;183:265–272.
10. Bergmeyer HU. *Methods of enzymatic analysis.* New York: Academic Press, 1977.
11. Geisbuhler T, Altschuld RA, Trewyn RW, Ansel AZ, Lamka K, Brierley GP. Adenine nucleotide metabolism and compartmentalization in isolated adult rat heart cells. *Circ Res* 1984;54:536–546.
12. Hohl C, Ansel A, Altschuld R, Brierley GP. Contracture of isolated rat heart cells on anaerobic to aerobic transition. *Am J Physiol* 1982;242:H1022–H1030.
13. Jung DW, Apel LM, Brierley GP. Transmembrane gradients of free Na^+ in isolated heart mitochondria estimated using a fluorescent probe. *Am J Physiol* 1992;262:C1047–C1055.
14. Racker E. *Mechanisms in bioenergietics.* New York: Academic Press; 1965:193–208.
15. Werner JC, Whitman V, Fripp RR, Schuler HG, Morgan HE. Carbohydrate metabolism in isolated, working newborn pig heart. *Am J Physiol* 1981;241:E364–E371.
16. Wittnich C, Peniston C, Ianuzzo D, Abel JG, Salerno TA. Relative vulnerability of neonatal and adult hearts to ischemic injury. *Circulation* 1987;76(suppl V):156–160.
17. Neumar RW, Brown CG, Van Ligten P, Hoekstra J, Altschuld RA, Baker P. Estimation of myocardial ischemic injury during ventricular fibrillation with total circulatory arrest using high-energy phosphates and lactate as metabolic markers. *Ann Emerg Med* 1991;20:222–229.
18. Jurkowitz M, Scott KM, Altschuld RA, Merola AJ, Brierley GP. Ion transport by heart mitochondria: retention and loss of energy coupling in aged heart mitochondria. *Arch Biochem Biophys* 1974;165:98–113.
19. Hohl CM, Altschuld RA. Response of isolated adult canine cardiac myocytes to prolonged hypoxia and reoxygenation. *Am J Physiol* 1991;260:C383–C391.
20. Rouslin W, Millard RW. Mitochondrial inner membrane enzyme defects in porcine myocardial ischemia. *Am J Physiol* 1981;240:H308–H313.
21. Honeyfield DC, Froseth JA. Evaluation of energy sources with and without carnitine in newborn pig heart and liver. *J Nutr* 1991;121:1117–1122.
22. Werner JC, Whitman V, Musselman J, Schuler HG. Perinatal changes in mitochondrial respiration of the rabbit heart. *Biol Neonate* 1982;42:208–216.
23. Ascuitto TJ, Ross-Ascuitto NT, Chen V, Downing SE. Ventricular function and fatty acid metabolism in neonatal pig heart. *Am J Physiol* 1989;256:H9–H15.
24. Wolfe RG, Maxwell CV, Nelson EC. Effect of age and dietary fat level on fatty acid oxidation in the neonatal pig. *J Nutr* 1978;108:1621–1634.
25. Lopaschuk GD, Witters LA, Itoi T, Barr R, Barr A. Acetyl-CoA carboxylase involvement in the rapid maturation of fatty acid oxidation in the newborn rabbit heart. *J Biol Chem* 1994;269:25871–25878.
26. Hudson EK, Liu MH, Buja LM, McMillin JB. Insulin-associated changes in carnitine palmitoyltransferase in cultured neonatal rat cardiac myocytes. *J Mol Cell Cardiol* 1995;27:599–613.
27. Werner JC, Sicard RE, Schuler HG. Palmitate oxidation by isolated working fetal and newborn pig hearts. *Am J Physiol* 1989;256:E315–E321.
28. Rouslin W. The mitochondrial adenosine 5′-triphosphatase in slow and fast heart rate hearts. *Am J Physiol* 1987;252:H622–H627.

29. Rouslin W, Broge CW. Mechanisms of ATP conservation during ischemia in slow and fast heart rate hearts. *Am J Physiol Cell Physiol* 1993;264:C209–C216.
30. Ponce-Hornos JE, Parker JM, Langer GA. Heat production in isolated heart myocytes: differences among species. *Am J Physiol* 1990;258:H880–H886.
31. Coles JG, Watanabe T, Wilson GJ, Benson LN, Kent GM, Mickle DA, Romaschin AD, Villamater J, Ujc H, Williams WG, Trusler GA. Age-related differences in the response to myocardial ischemic stress. *J Thorac Cardiovasc Surg* 1987;94:526–534.
32. Hu B, Altschuld RA, Hohl CM. Adenosine stimulation of AMP deaminase activity in adult rat cardiac myocytes. *Am J Physiol Cell Physiol* 1993;264:C48–C53.
33. Hu B, Altschuld RA, Hohl CM. Phorbol esters and cyclic AMP activate AMP deaminase in adult rat cardiac myocytes. *Arch Biochem Biophys* 1991;291:100–106.
34. Hohl CM, Livingston B. Hormonal stimulation of neonatal pig cardiac AMP deaminase. *J Mol Cell Cardiol* 1994;26:clxxv.

The Developing Heart,
edited by Bohuslav Ošťádal et al.
Lippincott-Raven Publishers,
Philadelphia © 1997.

31

Myocardial Ischemic Tolerance: Differences Between Immature and Adult Rats

Narcisa Tribulová, L'udmila Okruhlicová,
Barbara Ziegelhöffer Mihalovičová, Ján Slezák

*Institute for Heart Research, Slovak Academy of Sciences,
Bratislava, Slovak Republic*

Development and maturation are characterized by considerable changes in metabolism, structure, and function of the heart. Many of the developmental changes have been already quite well documented (1–7). However, a more detailed description of peculiarities in the metabolism of the neonatal heart that characterize the differences in its ischemia tolerance (8,9) in comparison to mature myocardium was still missing.

Much controversy exists about whether the neonatal myocardium is more (10–12), less (13–16), or similarly (17,18) susceptible to ischemic damage when compared with its adult counterpart. Experimental studies dealing with this problem have focused largely on functional (14,18) or metabolic (11,19) recovery of the heart after global ischemia. Studies dealing with morphologic alterations are, however, more scarce, and studies dealing with fine structural alterations in the immature myocardium are almost completely lacking.

The aim of the present study was to determine, by investigation on the ultrastructural level, whether global ischemia (20 min) is inducing similar alterations in rat hearts that are in different phases of postnatal development up to maturation. The ultrastructural study was accompanied by cytochemical examination of two marker enzymes: that of 5-nucleotidase (EC. 3.1.3.5), a marker of the sarcolemmal membrane, and that of glucose-6-phosphatase (EC. 3.1.3.9), a marker of the sarcoplasmic reticulum.

MATERIAL AND METHODS

All studies were performed in accordance with the *Guide for the Care and Use of Laboratory Animals* published by the U.S. National Institutes of Health (NIH - Publication No. 85-23, revised 1985).

Experiments were performed on 35 male Wistar rats. Experimental groups consisted of animals 1, 4, 8, 22, and 90 days old. Animals 1–4 days old were classified as newborn; those 8 days old, as neonatal; those 22 days old, after weaning as weanlings or juvenile rats; and those 90 days old as adult rats. Animals were killed by cervical dislocation. Hearts of control rats were rapidly excised and prepared for electron-microscopic investigation by immersing into ice cold fixation solution consisting of 2.5% glutaraldehyde buffered with 0.1 M sodium cacodylate to pH 7.4.

Electron Microscopic Investigation

The left ventricle was dissected and cut into small pieces from subepi-, mid-, and subendocardial regions and fixed for 3 hours in the same fixation solution as controls. After fixation in glutaraldehyde, tissue was washed in 0.1 M cacodylate buffer, pH 7.4, supplemented with 0.22 M sucrose, postfixed in 1% OsO_4, dehydrated in alcohol, and embedded in Epon 812.

Cytochemical Investigation

The tissue of left ventricle was fixed for 10 min in freshly prepared, ice cold, 4% solution of formaldehyde buffered with 0.1 M sodium cacodylate, pH 7.4. After subsequent washing in ice cold 0.1 M cacodylate buffer, containing 0.22 M sucrose, the left ventricle was frozen in liquid nitrogen. Frozen sections (50 μm thick) were used for estimation of 5-nucleotidase (5′NC) and of glucose-6-phosphatase (G-6-Pase) by means of the procedures adapted from Borgers et al. (20). The incubation applied was 45 min for 5′NC and 60 min for G-6-Pase at 37°C. After incubation the sections were washed in 0.1 M sodium cacodylate buffer supplemented with 0.22 M sucrose pH 7.4. Next, they were postfixed in 1% OsO_4, then dehydrated, and routinely embedded in Epon 812. Reactions performed in the absence of glucose-6-phosphate (substrate for G-6 Pase) and/or addition of 10 mM sodium fluoride (to inhibit 5′NC activity) were used as controls.

The hearts of the ischemic group were subjected to 20 min of global ischemia at 37°C. After this period tissue samples were processed for cytochemistry or conventional electron microscopy as in the control groups.

Semithick sections (1 μm thick) from the left ventricle, stained with toluidine blue, were used for light-microscopic examination. Representative tissue blocks from each group were thin-sectioned and stained with uranyl acetate and lead citrate. For enzyme cytochemistry unstained thin sections were used. All specimens were analyzed in transmission electron microscope Tesla 500.

Semiquantitative scoring of the enzyme activities was based on gradation of the amount of electrondense precipitate created in specific reactions coupled to the enzyme reaction. Semiquantitative evaluation of ischemic ultrastructural changes was performed as well.

All reagents were of the highest purity grade and were purchased from Sigma, St. Louis, or Serva, Heidelberg, FRG.

RESULTS

Control Groups

Myocytes from hearts of newborn 1-day-old rats (Fig. 31–1) were characterized by a great volume of sarcoplasm and by a high number of glycogen granules and ribosomes. Some nuclei contained dense chromatine material. Intensive formation of new myofilaments, numerous small mitochondria with simple cristae, and development of the longitudinal sarcoplasmic reticulum were also observed. Simple but differentiated intercellular junctions of intercalated discs were present in the first postnatal day. The activity of membrane-bound 5′NC was localized predomi-

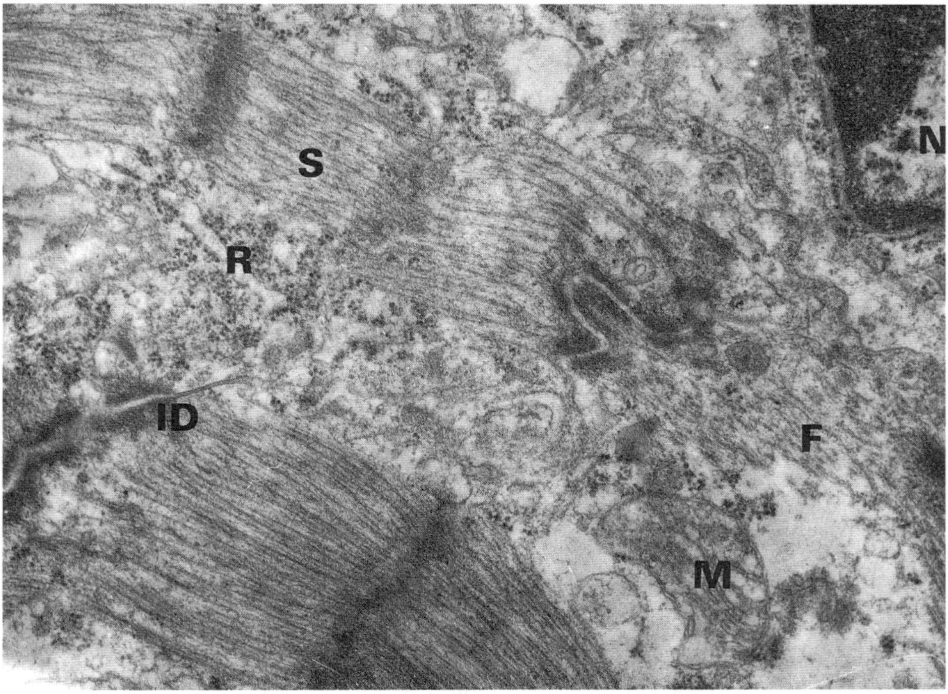

FIG. 31–1 Electron microscopic picture of 1-day-old cardiomyocytes shows a high amount of polyribosomes (R), nondifferentiated sarcomeres (S), neoformation of myofilaments (F), simple mitochondria (M), intercalated disc (ID), and nucleus (N) with dense chromatin material on the periphery. 30,000×.

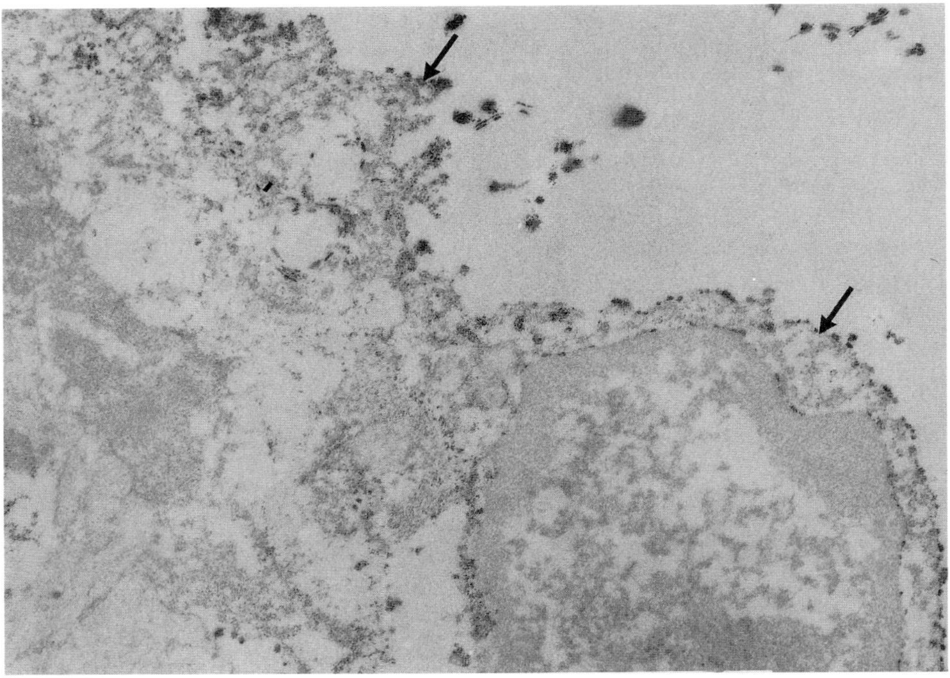

FIG. 31–2. 5′NC activity in 1-day-old heart. Reaction product is present predominantly on membrane of capillary endothelium (*arrows*). Unstained section. 27,000×.

nantly in the capillary endothelium (Fig. 31–2) and appeared only sporadically on the sarcolemma of some myocytes. In animals immediately after the birth, the sarcoplasmic reticulum was purely developed and exhibited low activity of G-6-Pase.

In myocytes from 4-day-old rats (Fig. 31–3) persisting myofibrillogenesis and development of the sarcoplasmic reticulum could be observed. This period was also characterized by further differentiation of the sarcolemmal membrane into transversal T-tubular system. High amounts of ribosomes indicated intensive proteosynthesis. The quantity of mitochondria was also increasing. Electrondense material in the nuclei frequently resembled high mitotic activity. In this stage of development cytochemical labeling revealed more positive sites for G-6-Pase and 5′NC (Fig. 31–4) than were seen in 1-day-old rats.

In the eighth postnatal day (Fig. 31–5) myocytes were markedly better differentiated than in newborn hearts. A relatively high number of mitochondria, longitudinal orientation of the myofibrils, and abundant structures of the sarcoplasmic reticulum as well as presence of T-tubules started to resemble the cytoarchitecture of juvenile hearts. Electrondense precipitate originating from reactions for G-6-

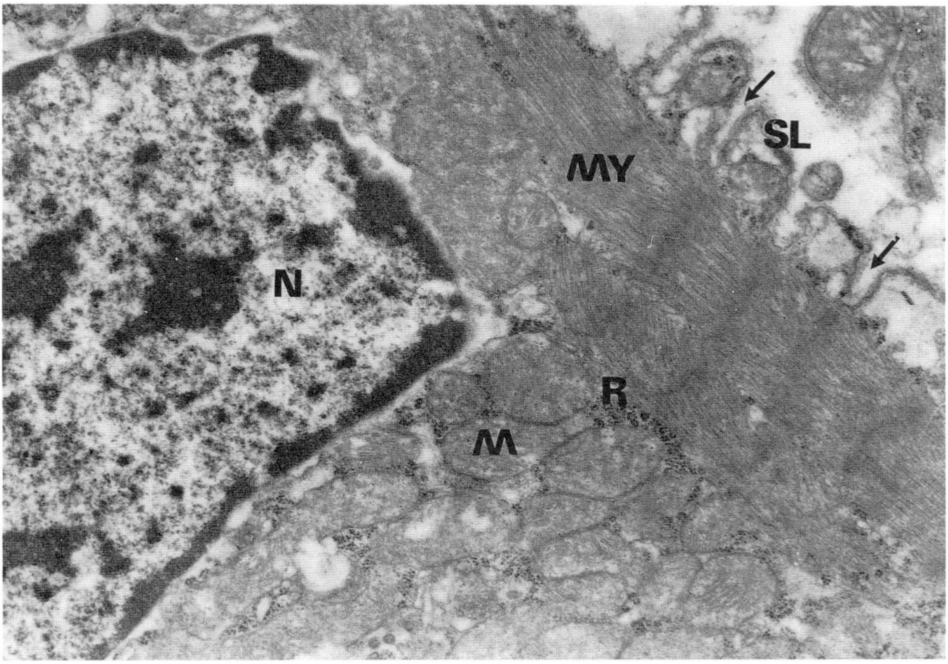

FIG. 31–3. Ultrastructure of 4-day-old myocytes of the heart. Invagination of the sarcolemma (SL) to T-tubules (*arrows*). Longitudinal orientation of myofibrils (MY). Mitotically active nucleus (N), perinuclear localization of mitochondria (M), ribosomes (R). 23,000×.

Pase and 5′NC occurred more frequently. 5′NC could be permanently detected in the capillaries and relatively frequently in the sarcolemma.

On the twenty-second postnatal day, cardiomyocytes were already fully differentiated (Fig. 31–6), just as in adult animals. Much electrondense precipitate originating from the cytochemical reaction for demonstration of 5′NC was present both in endothelial cells of the capillary network and in the sarcolemma of each myocyte (Fig. 31–7). Glucose-6-phosphatase activity was cytochemically demonstrated not only in the longitudinal sarcoplasmic reticulum but also in the junctional sarcoplasmic reticulum (Fig. 31–8).

Ischemic Groups

Twenty minutes of global ischemia exerted no particular influence on fine structure (Fig. 31–9) and cytochemical picture of the hearts of 1-day-old animals. Only mitochondria exhibited a slightly electronlucent matrix.

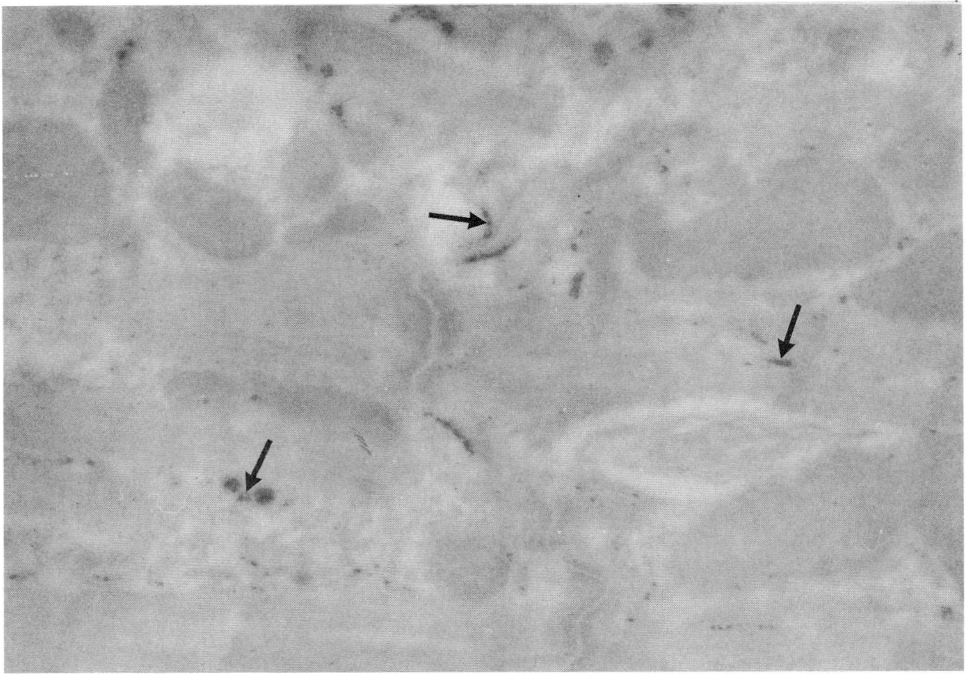

FIG. 31–4. G-6-pase activity in myocytes of 4-day-old heart. Reaction product is localized in developing sarcoplasmic reticulum (*arrows*). Unstained section. 27,000×.

On the fourth day, however, ischemia of the same duration induced already moderate alterations in fine structure in the majority of myocytes (Fig. 31–10). Cardiomyocytes were slightly edematous and contained both normal and altered mitochondria. Some mitochondria exhibited disintegrated cristae. Besides normal sarcomeres that have been predominating, hypercontraction bands could also be seen. But no effect of ischemia on cytochemically demonstrated activities of 5′NC and G-6-Pase could be detected.

Ischemia-induced changes were more pronounced in hearts of 8-day-old rats. In addition to the altered mitochondria and hypercontracted myofibrils (Fig. 31–11) in these hearts, a slight reduction in precipitate originating from the cytochemical estimation of G-6-Pase activity could be found. Nevertheless, the reaction for 5′NC seemed not be much influenced by ischemia.

In 22-day-old rats 20-min ischemia induces both moderate (Fig. 31–12) and marked (Fig. 31–13) damage in the myocytes. Inhomogeneity in the ischemia-caused damage was the most characteristic feature of hearts in this group. Gener-

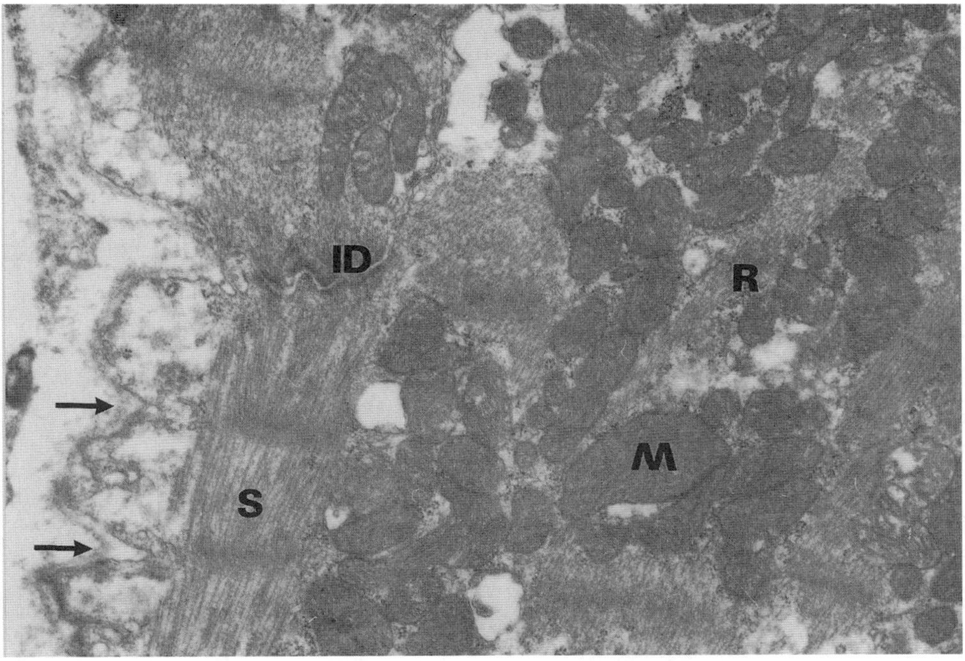

FIG. 31–5. Partially differentiated myocardium of 8-day-old rat exhibits an increased amount of mitochondria (M). Ribosomes (R) are less frequently observed in comparison to those in a newborn heart. Purely differentiated sarcomeres (S) are present. Sarcolemma (SL), T-tubules (*arrows*), intercalated disc (ID). 22,000×.

ally, intracellular edema was more pronounced and less precipitate originating from cytochemical estimation of 5′NC (Fig. 31–14) and G-6-Pase (Fig. 31–15) activities could be observed.

From the point of view of ultrastructural and cytochemical alterations, 20-min ischemia at 37°C induced no further changes in adult hearts, that would be considerably different from those seen in hearts of juvenile animals. Tables 31–1 and 31–2 summarize semiquantitative evaluation of ischemia-induced changes in ultrastructure and cytochemically estimated activities of 5′NC and G-6-Pase.

DISCUSSION

Immature myocardium is a matter of persistent interest from both experimental and clinical points of view. Since the mortality rate in neonates exceeds that in adults, clinicians are keenly interested in proper protection of neonatal hearts

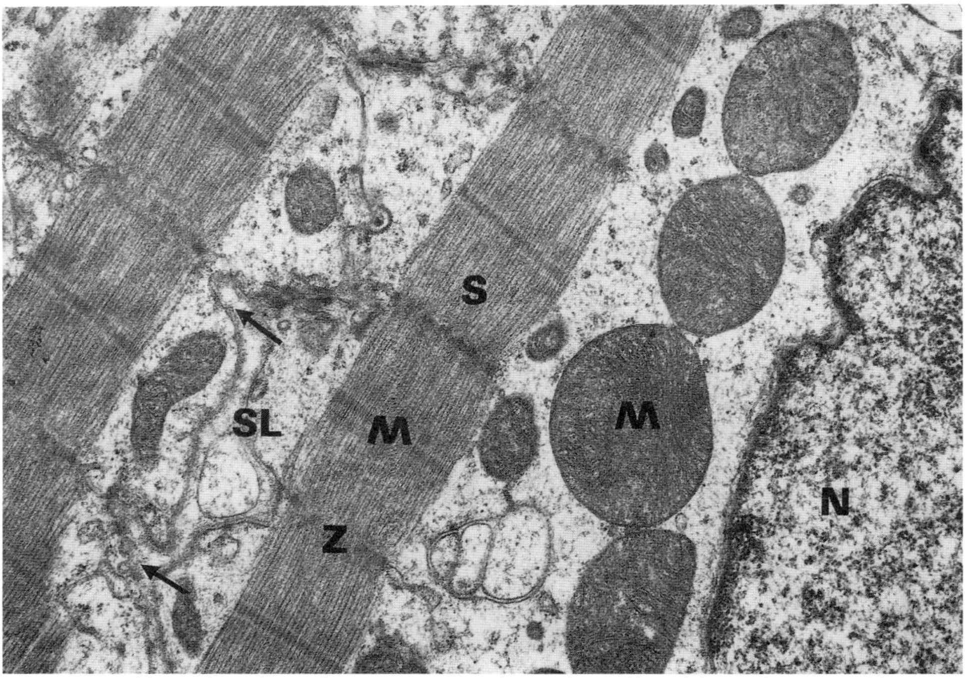

FIG. 31–6. Fully differentiated cardiomyocytes from 22-day-old heart. Nucleus (N) with dispersed chromatin. Well-differentiated sarcomeres (S) containing Z band, M band. Electron-dense mitochondria (M). Sarcolemma (SL), T-tubules (*arrows*). 24,000×.

against ischemia during open heart surgery (21). However, the protection of neonatal hearts may require different precautions from the protection of adult hearts. This follows from the experience that the impetuous development of structure and metabolism of subcellular systems that characterizes the hearts in early stages of their postnatal development may be closely associated with peculiarities in their response to various physiologic and/or pathophysiologic stimuli, including ischemia.

The essential task of the present study was to investigate the effect of ischemia on the ultrastructural and cytochemical characteristics of the heart in various phases of its development. As concerns the dynamics of postnatal development of cardiac ultrastructure and the study of 5′NC and G-6-pase activities, our results could be summarized as follows (see Tables 31–1 and 31–2):

High resistance to ischemia was observed in the time interval up to the fourth postnatal day, which is characterized with the fastest rate of heart growth (22–24), increased workload imposed on the left ventricle and cardiac metabolism that is

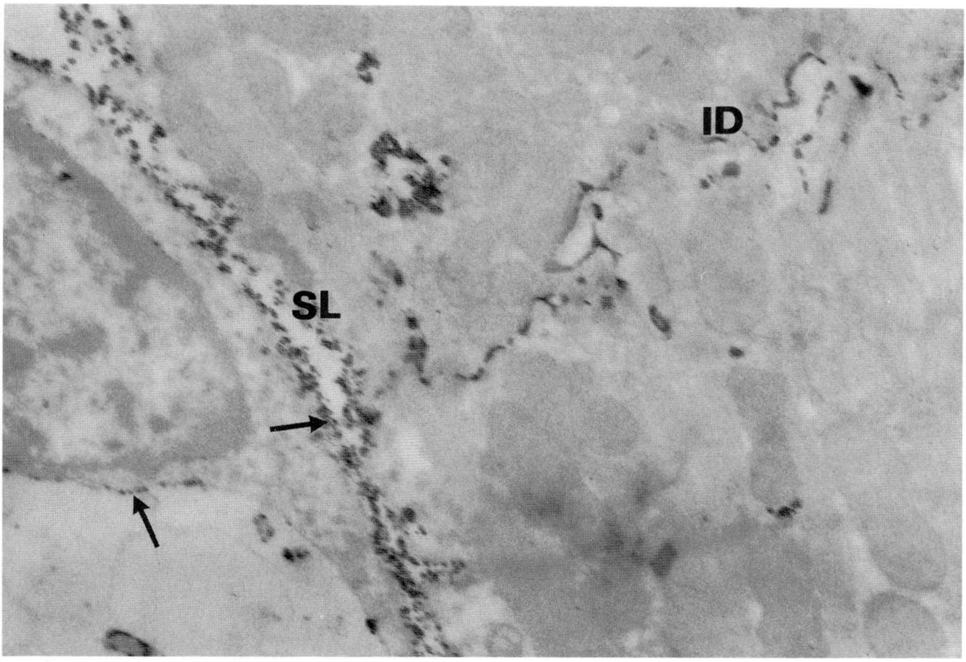

FIG. 31–7. Activity of 5′NC in 22-day-old heart. Heavy electrondense precipitate is localized on sarcolemma (SL), intercalated disc (ID), and capillary endothelium (*arrows*). Unstained section. 25,000×.

TABLE 31–1. *Semiquantitative evaluation of ischemia-related ultrastructural changes in various stages of the postnatal development*

	Mitochondria			Myofilaments		
Postnatal days	Matrix light	Cristae broken	Nucleus, swelling	Contr. bands	Contr. or rel.	Edema, intracellular
1	+	–	–	–	contr.	–
4	+	+	(+)	(+)	contr.	+
8	+++ or ++	++	+	++	contr.	+
22	++ or +++	++ or +++	+	–	rel.	++
90	++ or +++	++ or +++	+	–	rel.	++

Gradation of changes: –, absent; +, slight; ++, moderate; +++, marked; contr., contraction of sarcomere; rel, relaxation of sarcomere.

TABLE 31–2. *Semiquantitative evaluation of the cytochemical reactions in control and ischemic rat hearts of different age*

	1d		4d		8d		22d		90d	
	C	I	C	I	C	I	C	I	C	I
G-6-P										
SR	+	+	++	++	++	+	+++	+	+++	+
5′NC										
SL	–	–	+	+	++	++	+++	++	+++	++
CCM	+	+	++	++	++	++	+++	++	+++	++

Gradation of the amount of reaction precipitate: –, no; +, small amount; ++, moderate amount; +++, great amount. SR, sarcoplasmic reticulum; SL, sarcolemma; CCM, capillary cell membrane; C, control heart; I, ischemic heart.

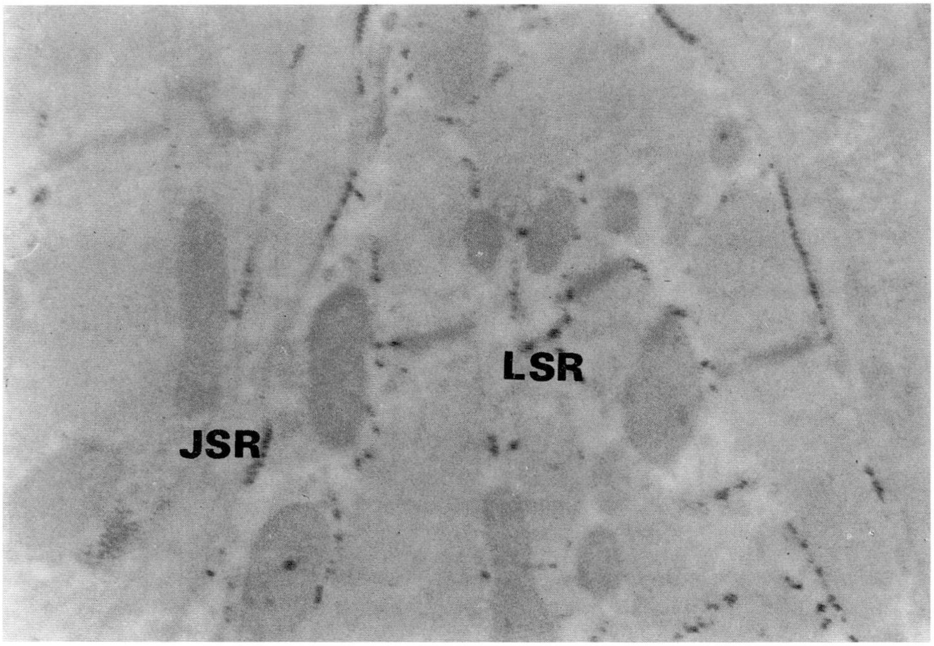

FIG. 31–8. Activity of G-6-pase is localized in longitudinal (LSR) and junctional structures (JSR) of well-developed sarcoplasmic reticulum in cardiomyocytes of a juvenile heart. Unstained section. 28,000×.

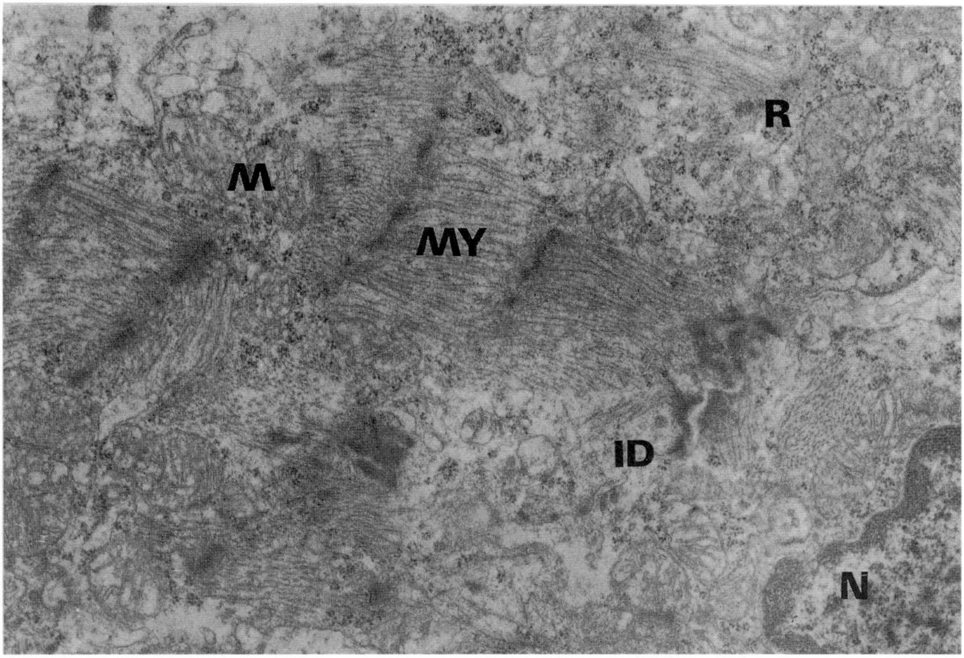

FIG. 31–9. No apparent fine structural changes in myocytes of 1-day-old hearts treated by 20 min of global ischemia. Slight clearing of the mitochondrial matrix (M), intercalated disc (ID), polyribosomes (R), nucleus (N), myofibrils (MY). 24,000×.

gradually shifted from an anaerobic to an aerobic one. At 22 days of age and later, minor age-dependent differences were seen in ischemic tolerance of the rat heart.

Twenty min of global ischemia did not induce any apparent ultrastructural damage in newborn hearts, nor were any changes in distribution of activities both 5′NC and G-6-Pase found. This period of postnatal life is characterized by a high amount of glycogen and a greater capacity for glycolysis (13), which might be beneficial during ischemia, because glycolysis is a predominant source of myocardial ATP production in newborn hearts (25,26). Glycogen stores, the principal source of energy during ischemia, can be beneficial for preservation of the viability not only of contractile cardiomyocytes (19) but also specialized conducting cells (27,28). The latter ultrastructurally and metabolically resemble immature contractile myocytes. Moreover, the newborn heart is less vulnerable to accumulation of glycolytic product, lactate (13), and particularly acidosis since it possesses a greater intrinsic pH_i, buffering capacity (5,29). As the heart matures, sensitivity to acidosis increases.

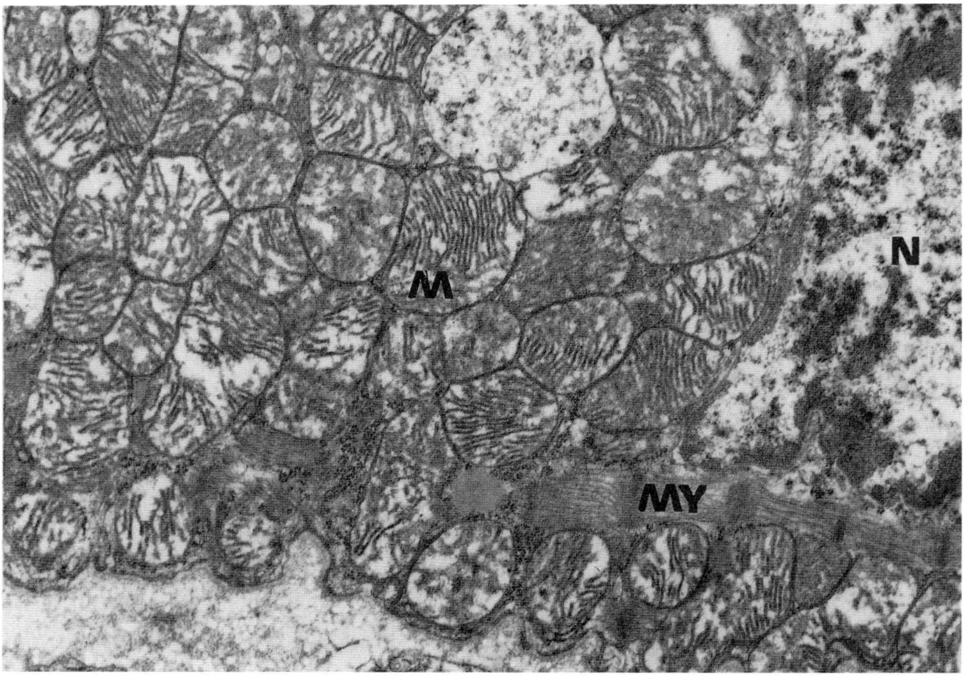

FIG. 31–10. Four-day-old ischemic heart exhibits moderate ultrastructural changes. Slightly edematous mitochondria (M), occasionally with broken cristae, cleared nucleoplasm (N), contracted myofibrils (MY). 18,000×.

Hyperplastic growth of rat cardiomyocytes starts to decrease between days 4 and 5 of postnatal life, which is connected with a shift from hyperplastic to hypertrophic growth (7,24). In accordance with intensive myofibrilogenesis and maturation of sarcoplasmic reticulum structures, an enhancement of cytochemical detection of G-6-Pase activity was observed. An increase of sarcoplasmic reticulum Ca–ATPase activity was also reported (18). Development of the sarcolemmal transverse tubular system is apparent in this period. This might be associated with functional maturation of sarcolemmal systems, accompanied also by changes in transsarcolemmal Ca fluxes (25) that predominate in newborn hearts (5). The heart in this stage of development responds to ischemia by moderate injury of the majority of the myocytes. However, a few cardiac cells with hypercontraction were also present. The cytochemically determined activities of both 5′NC and G-6-Pase were almost unchanged. Electron microscopic observation correlates with our previous histochemical studies (30) and supports the finding of better resistance of the heart to ischemia during the first postnatal week.

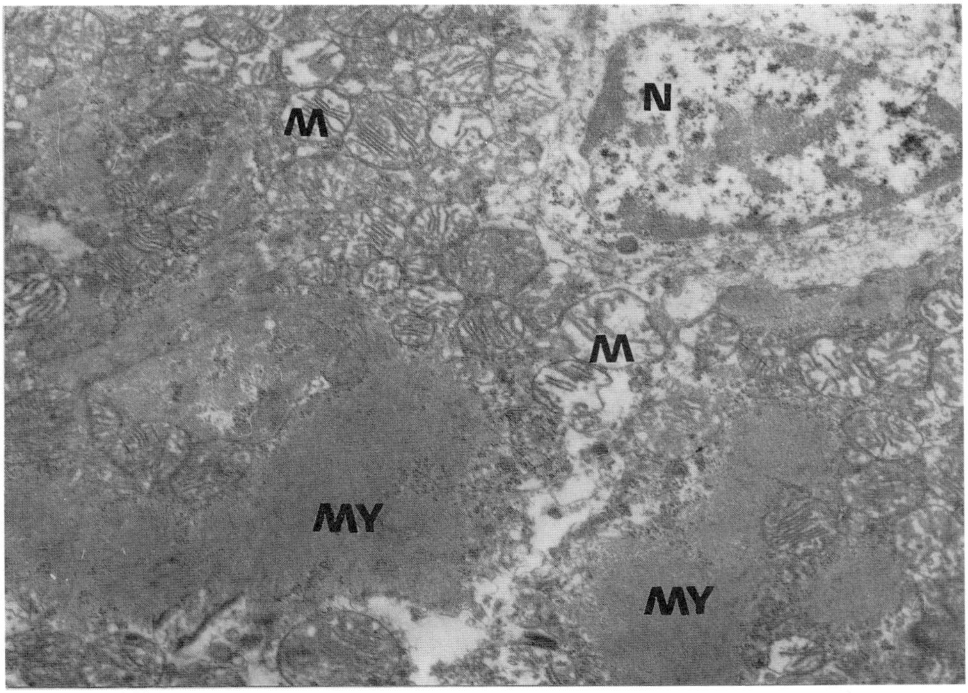

FIG. 31–11. More pronounced structural changes in cardiomyocytes from ischemia-treated 8-day-old rat. Homogenization of myofibrils (MY). Mitochondria (M) in different stages of deterioration. 16,000×.

Parallel with the decrease of the glycolytic rate, a dramatic increase in the ability to oxidize fatty acids occurs (26), starting from the second postnatal week. In this stage cardiomyocytes are morphologically and cytochemically more differentiated. In neonatal heart (8 days old) ischemia induced more evident ultrastructural changes in the myocytes than in newborn (1–4-day-old) hearts. They were characterized predominantly by mitochondrial alterations and by hypercontractions of myofibrils. The presence of contractures might indicate greater sensitivity of contractile proteins to acidosis (5) as well as to disturbances in Ca homeostasis. The latter may be induced by insufficiently mature Ca-transporting enzyme systems. Hypercontraction and ischemic contracture occur when the actin–myosin uncoupling is impaired and also result from an injury of mitochondria caused by abnormal Ca influx (31). The time when contractures occur is shorter in neonatal than in adult hearts (16,18,19,31). However, neonatal hearts have a more rapid return of function because of a greater capacity to recover (18,32,33).

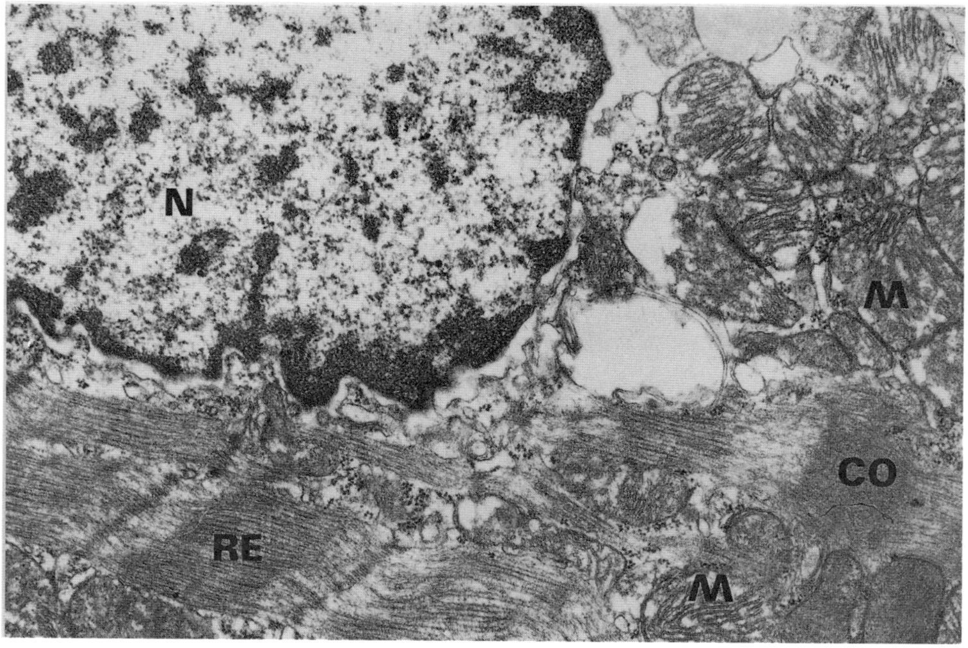

FIG. 31–12. Moderate ischemic injury in cardiomyocytes of the 22-day-old rat. Clearing of the mitochondrial matrix (M), margination of nuclear chromatine (N), relaxed (RE), and contracted (CO) myofibrils. 18,000×.

Although defense mechanisms resulting from increased glycogen stores and a higher rate of glycolysis in newborn hearts disappear in the neonatal period, the production of anaerobic energy through substrate level phosphorylation of amino acids (14,15) might partially account for ischemic tolerance associated with this age.

The tolerance of immature hearts to ischemia can also contribute to less breakdown of the adenine nucleotides as a result of lower 5-nucleotidase activity determined cytochemically. Low activity was also found in tissue homogenates of control hearts (11,34). The age-dependent increase in enzyme activity during cardiac development was observed histochemically in our previous study (30), which indicates increased turnover of adenine nucleotides.

The full morphologic differentiation of cardiac muscle cells was observed in the hearts of juvenile 22-day-old rats. Cardiomyocytes were well equipped with longitudinal and junctional sarcoplasmic reticulum. T-tubular and contractile systems were also well developed. Generally, the ultrastructural features of the myocytes

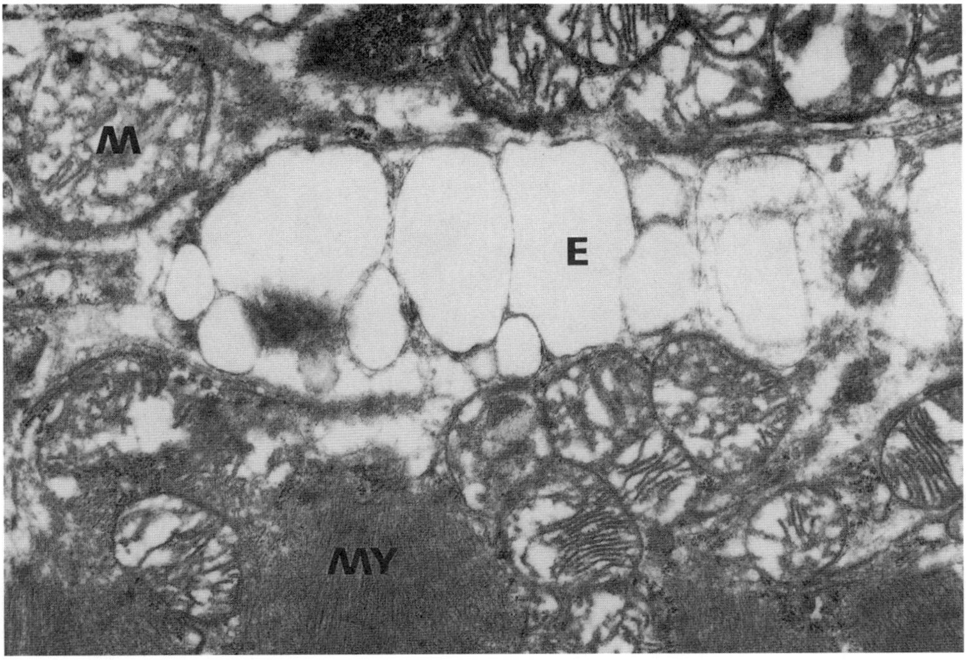

FIG. 31–13. Marked ischemia-induced ultrastructural changes in myocytes from the heart of 22-day-old rat. Hypercontraction of myofibrils (MY), injured mitochondria (M), and extracellular edema (E). 18,000×.

were similar to adult hearts. This was accompanied by the same distribution of activities of both investigated enzymes as in the hearts of adult animals. The response of the myocardium to ischemia in this period of postnatal life was different to that of newborn hearts and resembled the ischemia-induced structural and enzyme–cytochemical changes of the adult hearts. Slightly decreased 5′NC activity indicates decreased but persisting nucleotide degradation. Decreased G-6-Pase activity as well as decrease of sarcoplasmic Ca–ATPase activity (35) may contribute to disturbances in Ca homeostasis.

We can conclude that the greatest resistance to ischemia occurs in the rat heart immediately after birth, when the main source of energy is glycogen. Lowered resistance was observed in the second postnatal week. At that time developmental changes progressed and the metabolism shifted from glycolytic to fatty acid oxidation. Later, when cardiomyocytes are fully differentiated and functionally and metabolically mature, the tolerance to ischemia is decreased.

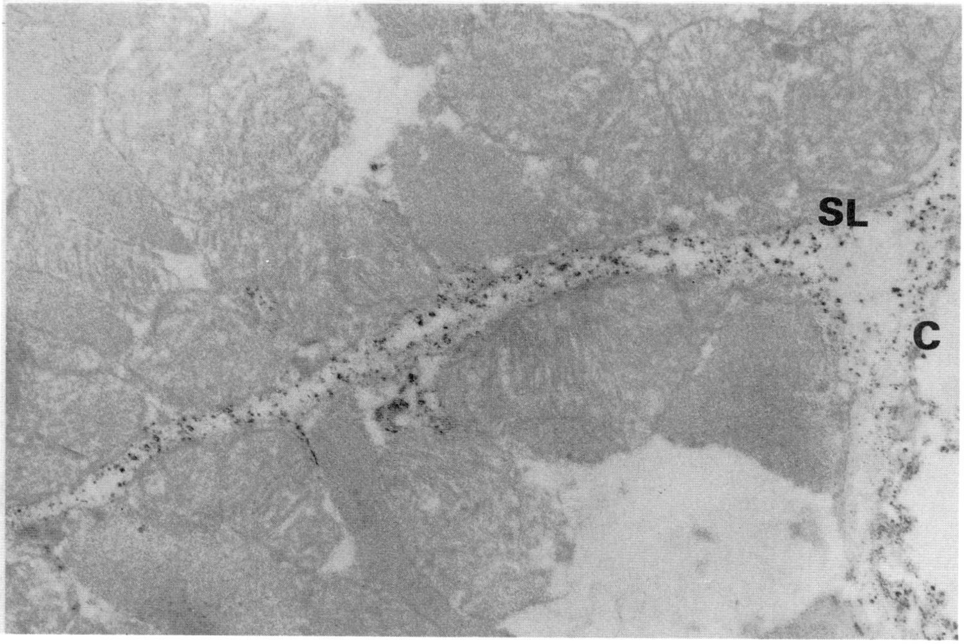

FIG. 31–14. Decreased but persistent activity of 5′NC on the sarcolemma of myocytes (SL) and cell membrane of capillaries (C) in the ischemic 22-day-old heart. Unstained section. 23,000×.

SUMMARY

The ischemic tolerance of immature versus adult rat myocardium with reference to ultrastructural and enzyme cytochemical developmental changes was studied. The age-related response of the heart to 20 min of normothermic global ischemia was evaluated using newborn (1 and 4 days old), neonate (8 days old), weanlings (22 days old), and adult (90 days old) rats. In the newborn, purely differentiated cardiomyocytes with nonregular distribution and low activities of 5′-nucleotidase and glucose-6-phosphatase the mildest ischemia induced fine structural alterations and cytochemical changes. Alterations were characterized predominantly by damage of mitochondria, presence of hypercontractions, intracellular edema, and decrease of glucose-6-phosphatase activity. Ischemic injury in the full morphologically and cytochemically differentiated heart of weanlings was manifested by moderate and more pronounced structural alterations of the myocytes. However, contractures did not occur. Activity of 5′-nucleotidase was decreased and glucose-6-phosphatase was decreased even more. A similar picture was observed in the adult heart. Our results indicate that tolerance of the myocardium to ischemia de-

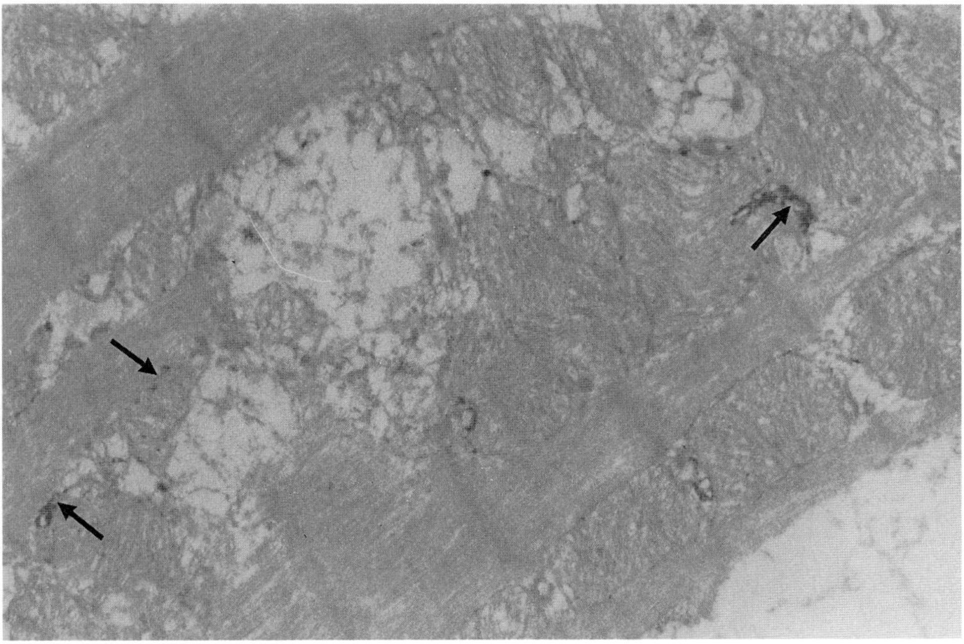

FIG. 31–15. Apparent decreasing of the enzyme-positive sites for G-6-Pase activity (*arrows*) after ischemic injury in 22-day-old heart. Unstained section. 23,000×.

creases shortly after birth, when the newborn heart is most resistant to ischemia. Later, ischemia-induced changes progressed with age. We suggest that differences in tolerance to ischemia might be associated with and reflect the actual metabolic and maturity state of the heart.

ACKNOWLEDGMENT

This study was supported by Slovak Grant Agency for Science, grants No. 21/1001/95, 2/1258/95.

REFERENCES

1. Achtenberg PW. Development of myocardial energy metabolism. *Myocardial Energ Metab* 1988;43:9–16.
2. Breuer E, Barta E, Pappova E, Zlatoš L. Developmental changes of myocardial metabolism. I. Peculiarities of cardiac carbohydrate metabolism in the early postnatal period in dogs. *Biol Neonate* 1967;11:367–377.
3. Breuer E, Barta E, Zlatoš L, Pappova E. Developmental changes of myocardial metabolism. II. Myocardial metabolism of fatty acids in the early postnatal period of dogs. *Biol Neonate* 1968; 12:54–64.

4. Bugaisky L, Zak R. Cellular growth of cardiac muscle after birth. *Texas Rep Biol Med* 1979;39: 123–138.
5. Nakanishi T, Seguchi M, Takao A. Development of the myocardial contractile system. *Experientia* 1988;44:935–944.
6. Oštádalová I, Kolář F, Oštádal B, Rohliček V, Rohliček J, Procházka J. Early postnatal development of contractile performance and responsiveness to Ca^{2+}, verapamil and ryanodine in the isolated rat heart. *J Mol Cell Cardiol* 1993;25:733–740.
7. Rakusan K, Jelinek J, Korecky B, Soukupová M, Poupa O. Postnatal development of muscle fibres and capillaries in the rat heart. *Physiol Bohemoslov* 1965;14:32–37.
8. Avkiran M, Hearse DJ. Protection of the myocardium during global ischemia: is crystalloid cardioplegia effective in the immature myocardium. *J Thorac Cardiovasc Surg* 1989;97:220–228.
9. Magovern JA, Pae WE Jr, Miller CA, Waldhausen JA. The immature and mature myocardium: responses to multidose crystalloid cardioplegia. *J Thorac Cardiovasc Surg* 1988;95:618–624.
10. Chiu RCJ, Bindon W. Why are newborn hearts vulnerable to global ischemia. *Circulation* 1987; 76:146–149.
11. Grosso MA, Banarjee A, Cyr JAS, Rogers KB, Brown JM, Clarke DR, Campbell DN, Harken AH. Cardiac 5′-nucleotidase activity increases with age and inversely relates to recovery from ischemia. *J Thorac Cardiovasc Surg* 1992;103:206–209.
12. Parrish MD, Payne A, Fixler DE. Global myocardial ischemia in the newborn, juvenile and adult isolated isovolumic rabbit heart: age related differences in systolic function, diastolic stiffness, coronary resistance, myocardial oxygen consumption and intracellular pH. *Circ Res* 1987;61:609–615.
13. Itoi T, Huang L, Lopaschuk GR. Glucose use in neonatal rabbit hearts reperfused after global ischemia. *Am J Physiol* 1993;265:427–433.
14. Julia PL, Kofsky ER, Buckberg GD, Young HH, Bugyi HI. Studies myocardial protection in the immature heart. *J Thorac Cardiovasc Surg* 1990;100:879–887.
15. Julia PL, Kofsky ER, Buckberg GD, Young HH, Bugyi HI. Studies myocardial protection in the immature heart. III. Models of ischemic and hypoxic/ischemic injury in the immature puppy heart. *J Thorac Cardiovasc Surg* 1991;101:14–22.
16. Cooley DA, Reul GJ, Wukasch DC. Ischemic contracture of the heart: "stone heart." *Am J Cardiol* 1972;29:575–577.
17. Hoffmeister HM, Seipel L. Tolerance of myocardium of aged animals to repeated oxygen deficiency. *Basic Res Cardiol* 1992;87:161–172.
18. Quantz M, Tchervenkov H, Chiu RCJ. Unique response of immature heart to ischemia. *J Thorac Cardiovasc Surg* 1992;103:927–935.
19. Goodwin GW, Taegtmeyer H. Metabolic recovery of isolated working rat heart after brief global ischemia. *Am J Physiol* 1994;267:H462–H470.
20. Borgers M, Schaper J, Schaper W. Localization of specific phosphatase activities in canine coronary blood vessels and heart muscle. *J Histol Cytochem* 1971;19:526–539.
21. Bull C, Cooper J, Stark J. Cardioplegic protection of the child's heart. *J Thorac Cardiovasc Surg* 1984;88:948–952.
22. Slevak J, Zlatoš L, Randhawa A, Singal PK. Age-dependent differences in cardiac growth response to workload. In: Nagano M, Takeda N, Dhalla NS, eds. *The cardiomyopathic heart.* New York: Raven Press; 1994:345–360.
23. David H, Marx I. Quantitative und qualitative Veränderungen der Herzmuskulatur des linken ventrikels männlicher Ratten während der Entwicklung und Reifung in den ersten 6 Lebensmonaten. *Z Mikrosk-Anat Forsch* 1987;91:709–736.
24. Oštádal B, Wachtlova M, Bili J, Rakusan K, Poupa O. Weight of the heart in the rat before and after birth. *Physiol Bohemoslov* 1967;16:111–115.
25. Hanson GL, Schilling WP, Michael LH. Sodium–potassium pump and sodium–calcium exchange in adult and neonatal canine cardiac sarcolemma. *Am J Physiol* 1993;264:320–326.
26. Lopaschuk GD, Spafford MA. Differences in myocardial ischemic tolerance between 1- and 7-day-old rabbits. *Can J Physiol Pharmacol* 1992;70:1315–1323.
27. Slezak J, Tribulova N, Ravingerova T, Singal PK. Myocardial heterogeneity and regional variations in response to injury. *Lab Invest* 1992;67:322–330.
28. Tribulova N, Slezak J, Ravingerova T, Styk J, Gabauer I. Vulnerability of specialized conductive tissue to ischemia and reperfusion related injury. *Bratislava Med J (Bratisl Lek Listy)* 1990;92:1–4.
29. Carr LJ, Vanderwerf QM, Anderson SE, Kost GL. Age-related response of rabbit heart to normothermic ischemia: a ^{31}P-MRS study. *Am J Physiol* 1992;262:391–398.

30. Tribulova N, Ziegelhöffer B, Slezak J. Histochemical characterization of the developing rat myocardium in physiologic and ischemic conditions. In: Haunso S, Kjeldsen K, eds. *Proceedings of XV European Section Meeting of the International Society for Heart Research.* Monduzzi Editore; 1994:711–715.
31. Hearse DJ, Garlic PB, Humphrey SM. Ischemic contracture of the myocardium, mechanisms and prevention. *Am J Physiol* 1977;39:986–993.
32. Witnich C, Torrance SM. Does the severity of acute hypoxia influence neonatal myocardial metabolism and sensitivity to ischemia? *J Mol Cell Cardiol* 1994;26:675–682.
33. Magovern JA, Pae WE, Miller CA, Waldhausen JA. The mature and immature heart: response to normothermic ischemia. *J Surg Res* 1989;46:366–369.
34. Abd-Elfattah AS, Murphy ChE, Salter DR, Louis AB, Goldstein JP, Wechsler AS. Development role of myocardial 5′-nucleotidase and AMP-deaminase isoenzymes in the increased tolerance of immature hearts to ischemic injury. *Circulation* 1986;74:492.
35. Dhalla NS, Ziegelhöffer A, Harrow JAC. Regulatory role of membrane system in heart function. *Can J Physiol Pharmacol* 1977;55:1211–1234.

The Developing Heart,
edited by Bohuslav Ošťádal et al.
Lippincott-Raven Publishers,
Philadelphia © 1997.

32

Age-Related Differences in the Cardiac Response to Ischemia and Free Radical Production on Reperfusion

Richard Southworth, Michael J. Shattock, and Frank J. Kelly

Cardiovascular Research, The Rayne Institute, St. Thomas' Hospital, Lambeth Palace Road, London, SE1 7EH, United Kingdom

BACKGROUND

There is now a vast literature concerning adult heart disease and its treatment. The improved understanding of cardiac function and biochemistry has facilitated the evolution of new cardiac surgical techniques, which have in turn decreased morbidity and mortality associated with adult heart surgery. Because of the refinement of surgical techniques, increasingly complex procedures are now being applied to surgery in the very young.

Protective techniques such as cardioplegia, a pivotal component of adult heart surgery, have been designed and implemented based on knowledge of the biochemistry, physiology, and pharmacology of the mature heart. During the first few years of life, however, these parameters are known to change markedly (1,2). It is now clear that certain cardioplegic regimes, known to be beneficial in the mature myocardium, are less beneficial or even detrimental when used in the immature myocardium (3–5). Improved understanding of the biology of the immature heart is therefore essential prior to identification of means of improving its protection during surgery.

It has been suggested that reperfusion of the globally ischemic heart following bypass may not be entirely benign (6–8). Restoration of blood flow to the arrested ischemic heart may also impose a degree of "reperfusion injury," distinct from the injury caused by the preceding ischemia. Increased free radical production has been observed immediately on reperfusion in a number of studies using a variety of experimental models (9–11). Several investigators have also demonstrated alleviation of the effects of reperfusion injury through the use of exogenous antioxidants, coupled with decreased detection of free radical species in the coronary effluent (12,13). Reperfusion injury is therefore thought to be mediated at least in part by the generation of reactive oxygen species, including free radicals, formed from the rapid influx of oxygen during reperfusion. The degree of structural and functional damage caused by reactive oxygen species formation on reperfusion is modified by both endogenous and exogenous antioxidants (14,15).

In this short review we examine the developmental differences in cardiac response to ischemia/reperfusion injury with respect to the heart's capacity to produce, and defend itself against, reactive oxygen species.

ISCHEMIA PRIMES THE HEART FOR RADICAL PRODUCTION ON REPERFUSION

While the processes underlying ischemic injury are numerous, interrelated, and complex, in its simplest form, the three major components of ischemia are (a) lack of oxygen; (b) lack of substrate delivery, and (c) accumulation of metabolites. Hypoxia causes metabolic disruption, leading to increased glycogen breakdown, calcium imbalance, and ATP degradation (16–18). Reduction of coronary flow also limits the washout of waste products such as lactate, resulting in acidemia (19). Because of these effects, extended periods of ischemia result in loss of cellular membrane integrity and tissue necrosis (20). Individually and collectively, these components create conditions that promote free radical production on reperfusion.

During ischemia, cellular antioxidants are depleted while the precursors of radical generating pathways accumulate. Several investigators have proposed a link between the degree of ischemic injury and the extent of free radical production on reperfusion (21,22). In the following sections we review several processes known to occur during ischemia that may play an important role in governing free radical production on reperfusion.

Conversion of Xanthine Dehydrogenase to Xanthine Oxidase

Xanthine dehydrogenase, an enzyme bound to the capillary endothelium, is responsible for the conversion of xanthine and hypoxanthine into uric acid, using NAD^+ as an electron acceptor. During ischemia, xanthine dehydrogenase is converted to xanthine oxidase by either oxidation of thiol groups or partial proteolysis by calcium-activated protease's (23,24). Xanthine oxidase converts xanthine and hypoxanthine into uric acid, but in using oxygen as an oxygen acceptor, it generates the superoxide anion ($O_2^{\cdot -}$) and hydrogen peroxide (H_2O_2). During ischemia, oxygen is not available for this process to occur. Upon reperfusion, the influx of oxygen leads to an increase in xanthine oxidase activity. At this point hypoxanthine is metabolized to urate by xanthine oxidase, and $O_2^{\cdot -}$ and H_2O_2 are produced as a consequence. This process is represented in Fig. 32–1.

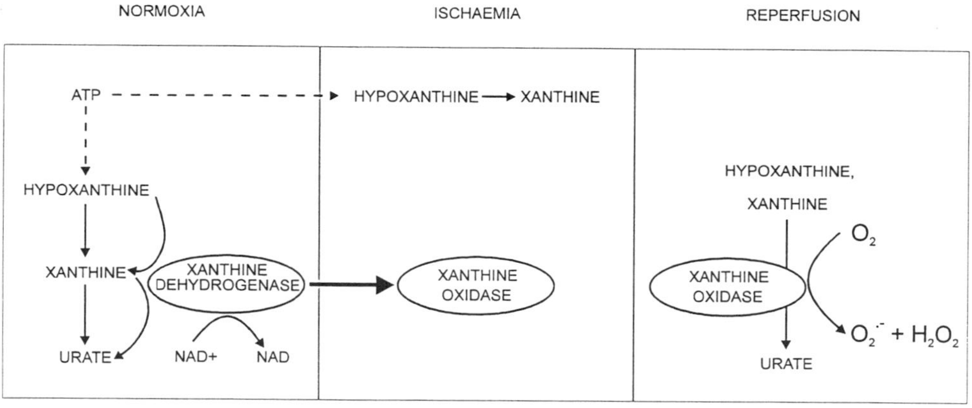

FIG. 32–1. The priming of the xanthine oxidase mechanism for reactive oxygen species production during ischemia and reperfusion. Xanthine dehydrogenase is converted to xanthine oxidase during ischemia by calcium-activated proteases. Reperfusion provides the oxygen necessary for xanthine oxidase to produce the superoxide anion ($O_2^{\cdot -}$) and hydrogen peroxide (H_2O_2).

The importance of xanthine oxidase as a source of radical production during reperfusion has been investigated by several groups (25,26), including our own. In our study, isolated Langendorff perfused adult guinea pig hearts were reperfused with bicarbonate buffer containing 10 μM succinylated ferricytochrome *c* (cyt *c*) following 20-min global ischemia. Leakage of $O_2^{\cdot -}$ into the vascular lumen was detected by its SOD-inhibitable reductive effect on cyt *c* in the coronary perfusate. This response was quantified as a decreased optical absorbance of the perfusate at 550 nm. The countereffect of cytochrome *c* oxidation by H_2O_2 was removed by perfusing with buffer-containing catalase, as described in Fig. 32–2. Using this system, reperfusion of hearts with allopurinol, a competitive xanthine oxidase inhibitor, resulted in significant inhibition of $O_2^{\cdot -}$ production on reperfusion, indicating that xanthine oxidase was the major source of $O_2^{\cdot -}$ in the reperfused adult guinea pig heart (Fig. 32–3).

The clinical importance of myocardial xanthine oxidase is, however, controversial, as several investigators have found little evidence of xanthine oxidase activity in the human myocardium (27,28). Xanthine oxidase activity may well be high in the endothelium. The direct relevance of this particular free radical generating system during reperfusion is therefore unclear. However, as an indication of the priming of ischemic tissue for free radical production, the conversion of xanthine dehydrogenase to xanthine oxidase during ischemia may be representative of the general upregulation of other, possibly more clinically relevant, free radical generating systems during ischemia, such as neutrophil activation, or the increased mitochondrial leakage of $O_2^{\cdot -}$.

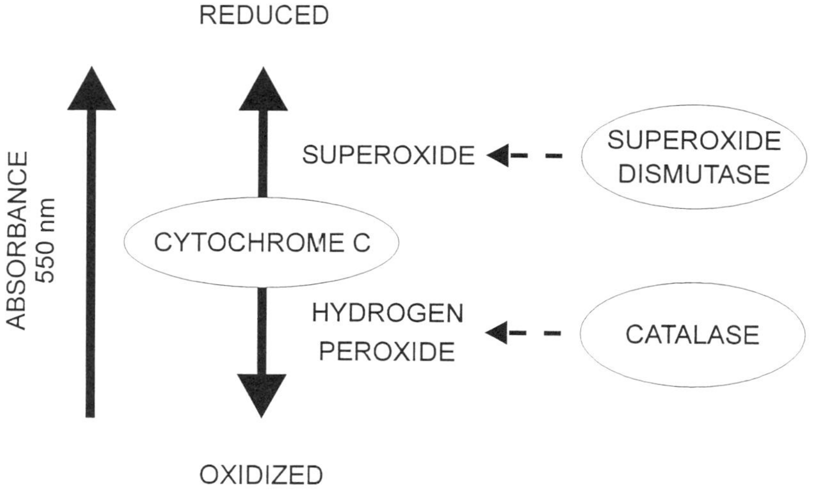

FIG. 32–2. The cytochrome *c* assay for superoxide production. Superoxide is capable of reducing cytochrome *c,* resulting in its increased optical absorbance at 550 nm. Conversely, hydrogen peroxide is capable of oxidizing cytochrome *c,* resulting in decreased absorbance. If both reactive oxygen species are present in equal quantities, then no net change in cytochrome *c* absorbance will result. Therefore, to obtain an accurate estimation of superoxide production, the conflicting effect of hydrogen peroxide–mediated oxidation is removed by addition of catalase. The component of the remaining signal that is inhibitable by superoxide dismutase can then be attributed to superoxide action.

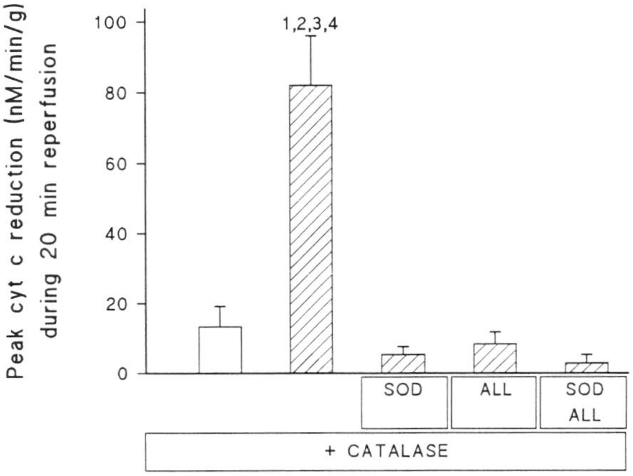

FIG. 32–3. Characterization of the cytochrome *c* detection system in the isolated mature guinea pig heart. Hearts ($n = 6$/group) were made globally ischemic (hatched bars) for 20 min and then reperfused with cytochrome *c* and either catalase alone; catalase and superoxide dismutase (SOD); catalase and allopurinol (ALL); or catalase, superoxide dismutase, and allopurinol. An additional time-matched aerobic control group was included (*open bar*). 1, signif. diff from control; 2, signif. diff. from CAT + SOD; 3, signif. diff. from CAT + ALL; 4, signif. diff from CAT + SOD + ALL ($p < 0.05$).

Leukocyte Action

The cytotoxic action of leukocytes is mediated by the release of proteases, hypochlorous acid, and large quantities of $O_2^{\cdot -}$ (29). When triggered, they undergo a "respiratory burst" consisting of an accelerated uptake of oxygen and increased glucose consumption. Oxygen is reduced to $O_2^{\cdot -}$ by the pentose phosphate pathway in the cytosol (30). This process may play a role in free radical production during reperfusion injury (31). Leukocyte infiltration into the ischemic myocardium has been recorded in a number of cases and appears to occur in an ischemic-duration-dependent accumulative manner (32). Hearts irreversibly injured with a short ischemic period exhibited little or no leukocyte accumulation, whereas with extended periods of ischemia, leukocyte influx and activation occurred during both late ischemia and reperfusion (33). Leukocyte activation occurs via a number of mechanisms. These include complement activation, contact with leukotrienes and subcellular membrane fragments, increased expression of endothelial leukocyte activation molecules (ELAM-1) on endothelial cells (32), and release of products of xanthine oxidase metabolism (34). All these events are thought to occur during both ischemia and reperfusion. Thus, although most leukocyte infiltration and injury occur on reperfusion, the necessary activating and chemoattractant cofactors are governed to some degree by the extent of the preceding ischemic injury.

Electron Transport Chain Leakage

Mitochondrial electron transport chain leakage has been proposed as a possible mechanism for the observed increase in free radical production on reperfusion. Leakage of electrons from electron transport chains has been recorded during both aerobic and ischemic/reperfused conditions (35). These free electrons are able to bind to molecular oxygen without further reduction to water, thus forming $O_2^{\cdot -}$. During ischemic injury and the ensuing loss of organelle integrity and uncoupling of electron transport chains (36), electron transport chain leakage and hence $O_2^{\cdot -}$ production may increase. High mitochondrial concentrations of SOD, however, may be sufficient to compensate for any detrimental effects of this $O_2^{\cdot -}$ production (37). With the relatively low levels of $O_2^{\cdot -}$ production detected from this mechanism and the high local antioxidant defense, electron transport chain leakage is considered a relatively minor source of radical production during reperfusion.

Summary

The mechanisms for the production of free radicals on perfusion so far described are all triggered or primed by the ischemic insult. It is therefore possible that each system has a threshold of ischemic injury, before which the pathway is not activated. Beyond this critical ischemic period, the induction and activity of the radical generating system will require a finite time before maximal activity is

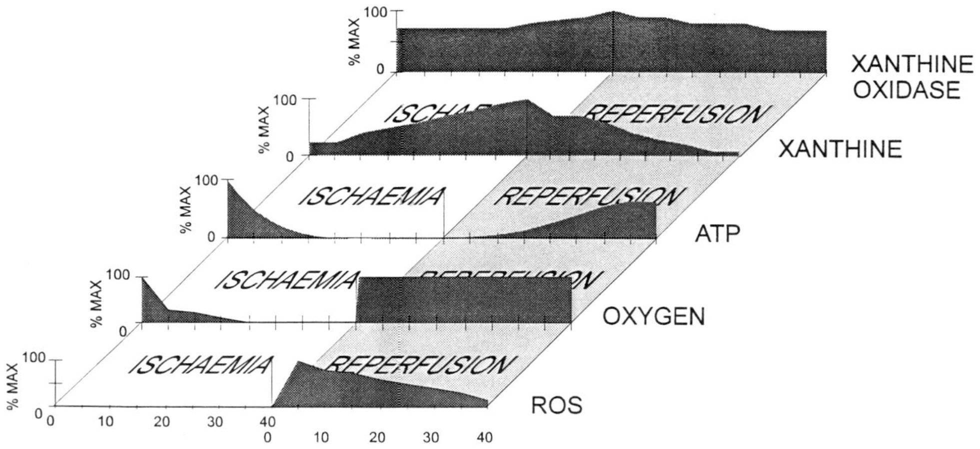

FIG. 32–4. Schematic of the possible interrelation between components responsible for superoxide production via xanthine oxidase. During ischemia, xanthine oxidase concentration increases as a result of conversion from xanthine dehydrogenase. Xanthine concentration also increases because of increased ATP catabolism. Reactive oxygen species (ROS) production proceeds at a very low, if not negligible, rate. All these processes occur in an ischemic duration-dependent manner. On reperfusion, xanthine oxidase activity remains high, xanthine levels are elevated, and the influx of oxygen activates the burst of production of ROS. The magnitude of ROS production may depend upon how far each of the priming mechanisms had progressed during the preceding ischemia, which in turn is governed by ischemic duration and relative resistance to ischemic injury.

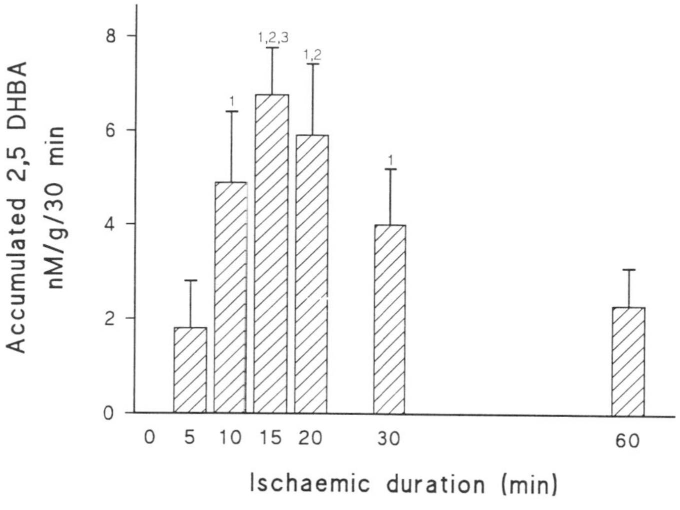

FIG. 32–5. The relationship between ischemic duration and the accumulated amount of hydroxyl radical product (2,5-dihydroxybenzoic acid [DHBA]). Isolated perfused rat hearts were exposed to a range of ischemic durations and reperfused for 30 min with 1 mM salicylic acid. 1, signif. diff. from aerobic control (0 min); 2, signif. diff. from 5 min ischemic group; 3, signif. diff. from 60-min ischemic group. (Redrawn, with permission, from Takemura et al., 1992 [22].)

achieved. For example, the time required for the conversion of xanthine dehydrogenase to xanthine oxidase or the accumulation of hypoxanthine (Fig. 32–4). It is therefore likely that the extent of radical production, on reperfusion, is related to the relationship between the number of threshold events that have been exceeded. These events in turn are related to the duration of the preceding ischemic insult. Such a relationship has been shown by Takemura et al. (22) in the isolated rat heart (Fig. 32–5). Following reperfusion, radical production was proportional to the preceding ischemic duration up to a peak value achieved after 20 min of ischemia. With ischemic durations exceeding 20 min, radical production slowly decreased. This was most likely due to a combined loss of cell viability, enzyme activity, and decreased oxygen availability resulting from the no-reflow phenomenon. A bell-shaped relationship between ischemic period duration and radical production on reperfusion is evident. This parallels a similar relationship between ischemic period duration and the incidence of reperfusion-induced arrhythmias (Fig. 32–6) (1,38). This temporal association supports the concept that free radicals are involved in the pathogenesis of arrhythmias on reperfusion.

The duration of the ischemic period is unlikely to be the sole determinant of the extent of radical production on reperfusion. The resistance of the heart to ischemic injury may also modify this response. Understanding the developmental differences in cardiac response to ischemic injury should therefore facilitate an appreciation of the importance of these priming effects on mature and immature hearts and how they influence radical production on reperfusion following comparable ischemic insults.

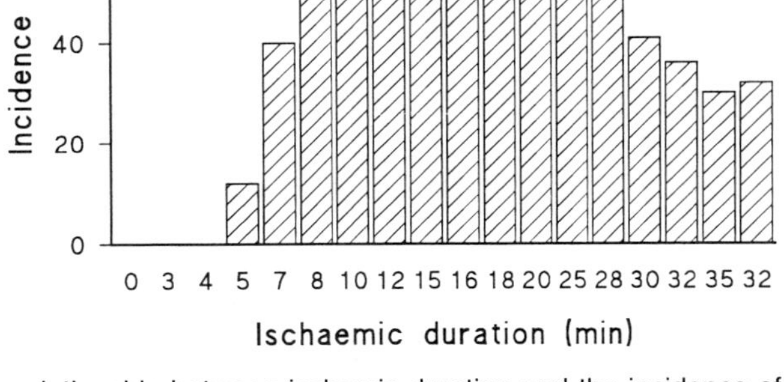

FIG. 32–6. The relationship between ischemic duration and the incidence of reperfusion-induced ventricular fibrillation (V.F.). These data were compiled from a large number of different studies, and show a bell-shaped relationship between ischemic duration and the incidence of V.F. (Reproduced with permission from ref. 1.)

CHANGE IN ISCHEMIC TOLERANCE DURING CARDIAC DEVELOPMENT

Several investigators have shown the immature heart to be inherently more resistant to the effects of ischemia than the mature heart (1,2). This increased resistance may be due in part to its more efficient energy metabolism under conditions of suboptimal blood flow, which may exist as an adaptation to the relatively hypoxic in utero environment.

The major energy sources used by the heart change during development. Whereas the mature heart is able to utilize lipids, carbohydrates, and amino acids, long-chain fatty acids seem to be the favored source (39). Long-chain fatty acids are not, however, a significant energy source in the developing heart. The two major fetal energy sources are lactate and glucose, and it is these that are responsible, in part, for the increased resistance of the immature heart to ischemia (40). The ability of the immature heart to utilize lactate enables it to maintain anaerobic metabolism and continue to create ATP. One significant consequence of this is that it also delays the onset of acidosis during ischemia (41). In addition, ATP synthesis by glycolysis in the immature heart can continue longer in conditions of reduced blood supply because it has a greater tissue glycogen content (42).

The ATP catabolic pathways also change during development (43,44). During normoxia, the adult heart releases 80% of total purine release as urate and 7% as inosine, whereas the immature heart releases 64% hypoxanthine and 15% inosine. These data are indicative of a lower activity of xanthine oxidoreductase in the developing heart, which has now been confirmed enzymatically (45). Hypoxanthine and inosine, produced by the immature heart, can be recycled into the ATP pool, whereas xanthine and urate are not recyclable. As a consequence, ATP depletion occurs much more rapidly in the mature heart. In addition, AMP accumulates in the immature heart during ischemia, which allows a rapid replenishment of ATP on reperfusion, whereas de novo synthesis of ATP is required in the mature heart. Combined, these observations suggest that the immature heart is better adapted to ATP synthesis than to its breakdown—a situation that may be advantageous in conditions of low substrate availability. In conclusion, the immature heart suffers less ischemic injury than the mature heart after the same ischemic insult.

DEVELOPMENTAL DIFFERENCES IN ISCHEMIC TOLERANCE MAY GOVERN FREE RADICAL PRODUCTION ON REPERFUSION

Thus far, we have described three major factors that may influence developmental differences in the response of the heart to ischemia/reperfusion injury: first, that free radicals are produced on reperfusion, and that these species may play an important role in governing the recovery of cardiac function on reperfusion; second, that the degree of preceding ischemic insult may play a governing role in the activation of free radical generating systems on reperfusion; and third, that the immature heart endures less ischemic injury than the mature heart during a comparable ischemic insult. It is therefore possible that when exposed to an ischemic insult, the immature heart suffers less injury than the mature heart and, as a consequence, produces fewer free radicals on reperfusion. Hence, the immature heart's inherent resistance to ischemic injury may also endow it with increased resistance to free radical–mediated reperfusion injury. Recently we have investigated this proposal experimentally. Using the cyt *c* assay for $O_2^{\cdot -}$ production described in the section entitled "Conversion of Xanthine Dehydrogenase to Xanthine Oxidase," the capacity of mature (7-week-old) and immature (3 days premature delivered by caesarean section) isolated guinea pig hearts to produce $O_2^{\cdot -}$ on reperfusion following a range of ischemic periods was determined.

The data obtained are shown in Fig. 32–7. Both mature and immature hearts exhibited a bell-shaped relationship between ischemic period duration and peak free radical production on reperfusion. This relationship exhibited a similar time course to the ischemic period–related profile of hydroxyl radical production described by Takemura et al. (Fig. 32–5) (22). The mechanisms that may contribute to this relationship are the same as those discussed earlier, in the discussion of ischemia and its effect in priming the heart for radical production on reperfusion. Briefly, we

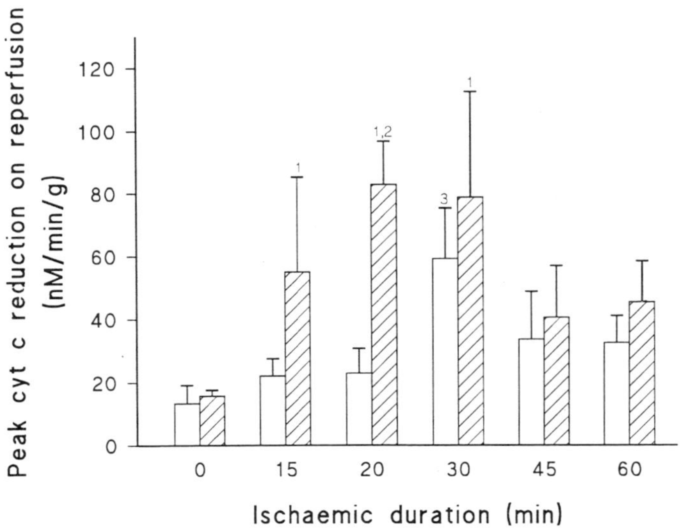

FIG. 32–7. Relationship between ischemic duration, cardiac maturity, and superoxide production on reperfusion. Mature (7-week-old, hatched bars) and immature (3 days premature, by caesarean section, open bars) isolated perfused guinea pig hearts were made globally ischemic for a range of durations (n = 6/group) and reperfused with the cytochrome *c* detection system for 20 min. Cytochrome *c* reduction was proportionate to superoxide leakage into the coronary vasculature. 1, signif. diff. from mature aerobic control (0 min); 2, signif. diff. from immature 20-min ischemic group; 3, signif. diff. from immature aerobic control ($p < 0.05$).

found that peak capacity for $O_2^{\cdot -}$ production was observed following 20 min of ischemia in the mature heart and 30 min in the immature heart. Mature hearts consistently produced more $O_2^{\cdot -}$ than immature hearts over the range of ischemic durations examined. The biggest difference was observed after 20 min ischemia, when mature hearts produced four times more $O_2^{\cdot -}$ than immature hearts. $O_2^{\cdot -}$ production, on reperfusion, following 45 and 60 min of ischemia was not significantly different from that measured in aerobically perfused control hearts in both age groups.

In our preliminary work characterizing the cyt *c* assay in this experimental model (Figs. 32–2 and 32–3), we showed that the major source of $O_2^{\cdot -}$ detected in this preparation was xanthine oxidase, known to be present in high concentrations in the guinea pig endothelium (46). Thus, the developmental differences in capacity for free radical production on reperfusion can be explained in terms of priming the xanthine oxidase system during ischemia. The greater maximal rate of radical production in mature heart tissue may be due to its greater xanthine oxidase activity, as reported previously (45,47). It is also possible that increased xanthine oxidase activity in the mature heart may be due to increased hypoxanthine availability because of greater catabolism of ATP during ischemia. It is therefore possible that relationships such as those shown in Fig. 32–4 are shifted to the right in the immature heart, suggesting that a longer ischemic period is required to up-regulate free radical production mechanisms. This may explain not only why mature hearts produce more $O_2^{\cdot -}$ by this mechanism, but also why peak radical production on reperfusion occurs after a shorter ischemic insult in the mature heart.

It is not presently clear if similar developmental changes occur in other free radical generating mechanisms that may be important in the pathogenesis of ischemia/reperfusion injury. As already mentioned, xanthine oxidase may play a role in leukocyte chemotaxis and activation; this may indirectly modulate developmental differences in response to ischemia and reperfusion. Although neutrophil depletion has proven protective in the immature heart during ischemia and reperfusion (48), the relationship between neutrophil capacity for causing injury and cardiac maturity has yet to be investigated.

RADICAL PRODUCTION IS NOT THE ONLY DETERMINANT OF POSTISCHEMIC FUNCTIONAL RECOVERY

Although we have demonstrated strong developmental differences in free radical productive capacity, the exact relationship between free radical production on reperfusion and recovery of contractile function remains unclear. The extent and rate of recovery of contractile function depend on the extent of ischemic injury and the degree of reperfusion injury (free radical–mediated myocardial stunning), respectively. We have found that recovery of contractile function is closely related to ischemic duration rather than to the bell-shaped profile of radical production (Fig. 32–8). This suggests that ischemic injury is a more important factor in influencing recovery of cardiac function than free radical production. Similarly, the inherent

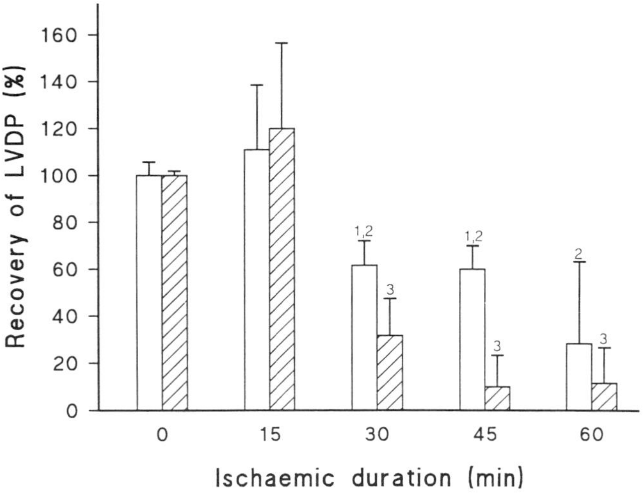

FIG. 32–8. Relationship between ischemic duration, cardiac maturity, and recovery of left ventricular developed pressure (LVDP). Hearts were treated as described in Fig. 32–7, except that they were reperfused with buffer only. Hatched bars = mature hearts; open bars = immature hearts. 1, signif. diff. from immature aerobic control (0 min); 2, signif. diff. from immature 15 min ischemic; 3, signif. diff. from mature aerobic control (0 min).

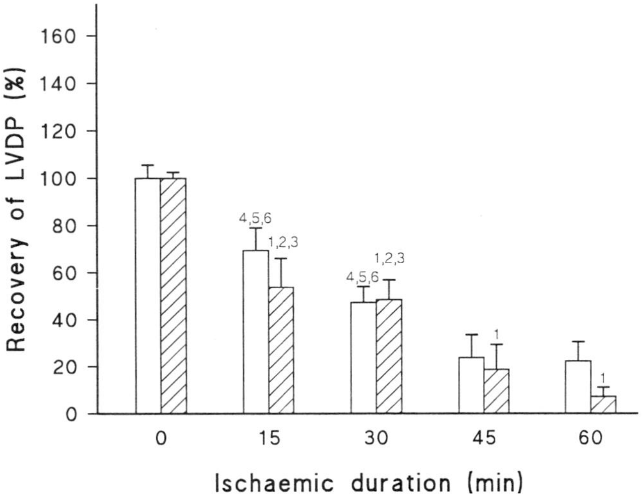

FIG. 32–9. Relationship between ischemic duration, cardiac maturity, and recovery of left ventricular developed pressure (LVDP) when reperfused with free radical scavengers. Hearts were treated as described in Fig. 32–7. Hatched bars = mature hearts; open bars = immature hearts. 1, signif. diff. from mature aerobic control (0 min); 2, signif. diff. from mature 45 min ischemic; 3, signif. diff. from mature 60 min aerobic; 4, signif. diff. from immature aerobic control (0 min); 5, signif. diff. from immature 45-min ischemic; 6, signif. diff. from 60-min immature ischemic ($p < 0.05$).

resistance of the immature heart to ischemic injury enables it to recover contractile function better than mature hearts after the same ischemic duration. The relative roles of ischemic injury and free radical–mediated reperfusion injury in governing recovery of function are difficult to resolve within 20 min of the onset of reperfusion, as both stunning and irreversible ischemic injury are likely to play a role. However, comparison of recovery of function between hearts reperfused with buffer only (Fig. 32–8) and those reperfused with free radical scavengers (cyt *c* and catalase, Fig. 32–9) shows that the developmental difference in tolerance to ischemia/reperfusion injury can be removed by free radical scavengers. This implies that the increased production of free radicals in the mature heart may contribute to its poor recovery of function during early reperfusion. However, free radical production per se is not the sole determinant of the extent of free radical–mediated reperfusion injury. Free radicals will only have a biological effect if their production rate exceeds the local antioxidant defense network.

Antioxidant Defenses

Although it is clear that there are developmental differences in the mechanisms underlying free radical generation in the heart, the ability of the heart to defend itself against oxidative stress also changes with maturation. A number of antioxidant enzymes are not at their full complement until relatively late in the development of

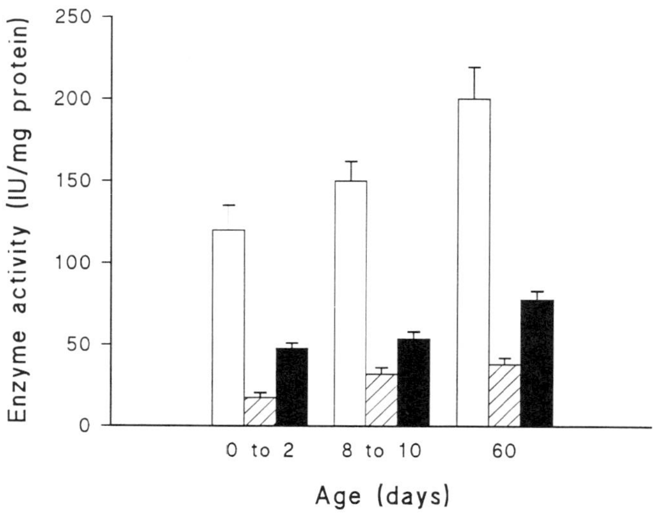

FIG. 32–10. Relationship between cardiac maturity and antioxidant enzyme activity in the pig heart. Open bars, glutathione peroxidase; hatched bars, glutathione reductase; solid bars, superoxide dismutase. (Redrawn with permission from ref. 52.)

the heart. For example, glutathione, catalase and glutathione peroxide all increase with age in the rat (49). Likewise, superoxide dismutase, glutathione peroxidase, and glutathione reductase activities all increase in the pig heart as it develops (Fig. 32–10) (50). Other studies have shown that although antioxidants are lost during ischemia in both adults and newborns (51), the preischemic activities of superoxide dismutase and catalase are significantly lower in newborns (52). Increased free radical production by the mature, in comparison with the immature, myocardium may be combatted to some extent by the mature heart's increased complement of antioxidant defenses. However, if antioxidant defenses in the immature myocardium are incapable of defending the heart against even the smaller burst of free radical production on reperfusion, then it may be at more risk from free radical–mediated injury than the mature heart.

SUMMARY

The possible relationships among ischemic injury, reperfusion injury, and cardiac development are as complex and potentially controversial as the proposed mechanisms for either ischemic injury or reperfusion injury alone. In this review we have explored, from the perspective of oxidative stress, the potential mechanisms for the developmental differences in responses to ischemia/reperfusion injury reported by a number of investigators. Free radical production is only one pathogenic mechanism of tissue injury during such an episode, and it is likely that other factors not discussed here, such as calcium overload, will also play a role. We suggest that the immature heart's increased resistance to ischemic injury provides it with a further advantage over the mature heart, namely a reduced capacity to produce free radicals on reperfusion. However, the biochemical immaturity from which it gains this advantage may also be responsible for its decreased (antioxidant) capacity to defend itself against lower levels of oxidative stress. Tissue survival following an ischemia/reperfusion episode in the immature heart is therefore finely balanced, and antioxidant therapy may prove to be useful in increasing the protection of the immature heart during surgery.

ACKNOWLEDGMENTS

These studies were supported in part by the Leopold Muller Foundation and the British Heart Foundation. RS is a BHF postgraduate student.

REFERENCES

1. Riva E, Hearse DJ. *The developing myocardium.* New York: Futura Publishing, 1991.
2. Murashita T, Borgers M, Hearse DJ. Developmental changes in tolerance to ischaemia in the rabbit heart: disparity between interpretations of structural, enzymatic and functional indices of injury. *J Mol Cell Cardiol* 1992;24:1143–1154.

3. Avkiran M, Hearse DJ. The vulnerability of the immature myocardium to ischaemia and its responsiveness to cardioplegic protection. In: Crupi G, Anderson RH, Parenzan L, eds. *Perspectives in pediatric cardiology.* Mount Kisco, NY: Futura Publishing; 1990:219–222.
4. Watanabe H, Yokosawa T, Eguchi S, Imai S. Functional and metabolic protection of the neonatal myocardium from ischaemia: insufficient protection by cardioplegia. *J Thorac Cardiovasc Surg* 1989;97:50–58.
5. Avkiran M, Hearse DJ. Protection of the myocardium during global ischaemia: is crystalloid cardioplegia effective in the immature myocardium? *J Thorac Cardiovasc Surg* 1989;97:220–228.
6. Downey JM. Free radicals and their involvement during long-term myocardial ischaemia and reperfusion. *Ann Rev Physiol* 1990;52:487–504.
7. Becker LC, Ambrosio G. Myocardial consequences of reperfusion. *Prog Cardiovasc Dis* 1987;30: 23–44.
8. Hearse DJ. Ischaemia, reperfusion, and the determinants of tissue injury. *Cardiovasc Drugs Ther* 1990;4:767–776.
9. Hearse DJ, Tosaki T. Free radicals and reperfusion-induced arrhythmias: protection by spin trap agent PBN in the rat heart. *Circ Res* 1987;60:375–383.
10. Powell SR, Hall D. Use of salicylate as a probe for .OH formation in isolated ischaemic rat hearts. *Free Rad Biol Med* 1990;9:133–141.
11. Henry TD, Archer SL, Nelson D, Weir EK, From AHL. Enhanced chemiluminescence as a measure of oxygen-derived free radical generation during ischaemia and reperfusion. *Circ Res* 1990;67:1453–1461.
12. Bolli R, Jeroudi MO, Patel BS, Aruoma OI, Halliwell B, Lai EK, McCay PB. Marked reduction of free radical generation and contractile dysfunction by antioxidant therapy begun at the time of reperfusion: evidence that myocardial "stunning" is a manifestation of reperfusion injury. *Circ Res* 1989;65:607–622.
13. Blasig IE, Shuter S, Garlick P, Slater T. Relative time-profiles for free radical trapping, coronary flow, enzyme leakage, arrhythmias, and function during myocardial reperfusion. *Free Rad Biol Med* 1994;16:35–41.
14. Pucheu SP, Coudray C, Tresallet N, Favier A, de Leiris J. Effect of dietary antioxidant trace element supply on cardiac tolerance to ischaemia-reperfusion in the rat. *J Mol Cell Cardiol* 1995; 27:2303–2314.
15. Galinanes M, Ferrari R, Qui Y, Cargoni A, Ezrin A, Hearse DJ. PEG-SOD and myocardial antioxidant status during ischaemia and reperfusion: dose–response studies in the isolated blood perfused rabbit heart. *J Mol Cell Cardiol* 1992;24:1021–1030.
16. Opie LH. Myocardial ischaemia: metabolic pathways and implications of increased glycolysis. *Cardiovasc Drugs Ther* 1990;4:777–790.
17. Hearse DJ. Oxygen deprivation and early myocardial contractile failure: a reassessment of the possible role of adenosine triphosphate. *Am J Cardiol* 1979;44:1115–1120.
18. Kihara Y, Grossman W, Morgan JP. Direct measurement of changes in intracellular calcium transients during hypoxia, ischaemia and reperfusion of the intact mammalian heart. *Circ Res* 1989;65:1029–1044.
19. Cobbe SM, Poole-Wilson PA. The time of onset and severity of acidosis in myocardial ischaemia. *J Mol Cell Cardiol* 1980;12:745–760.
20. Williamson JR, Schaffer SW, Ford C, Safer B. The cellular basis of ischaemia and infarction: contribution of tissue acidosis to ischaemic injury in the perfused rat heart. *Circulation* 1976;53:I-3–I-13.
21. Henry TD, Archer SL, Nelson D, Weir EK, From AHL. Postischaemic oxygen radical production varies with duration of ischaemia. *Am J Physiol* 1993;264:H1478–H1484.
22. Takemura G, Onodera T, Ashraf M. Quantification of hydroxyl radical and its lack of relevance to myocardial injury during early reperfusion after graded ischaemia in rat hearts. *Circ Res* 1992;71: 96–105.
23. Parks DA, Williams TR, Beckman JS. Conversion of xanthine dehydrogenase to oxidase in ischaemic rat intestine: a reevaluation. *Am J Physiol* 1988;254:G768–G774.
24. Engerson TD, McKelvey TG, Rhyne DB, Boggio EB, Snyder SJ, Jones HP. Conversion of xanthine dehydrogenase to oxidase in ischaemic rat tissues. *J Clin Invest* 1987;79:1564–1570.
25. Kvietys PR, Inauen W, Bacon BR, Grisham MB. Xanthine oxidase-induced injury to endothelium: role of intracellular iron and hydroxyl radical. *Am J Physiol* 1989;257:H1640–H1646.
26. Abd-Elfattah AS, Jessen ME, Lekven J, Doherty NE, Brunsting LA, Wechsler AS. Myocardial reperfusion injury: role of myocardial hypoxanthine and xanthine in free radical–mediated reperfusion injury. *Circulation* 1988;78:III-224–III-235.

27. Grum CM, Gallagher KP, Kirsh MM, Shlafer M. Absence of detectable xanthine oxidase in human myocardium. *J Mol Cell Cardiol* 1989;21:263–267.
28. Podzuweit T, Beck H, Muller A, Bader A, Gorlach G, Scheld HH. Absence of xanthine oxido-reductase activity in human myocardium. *Cardiovasc Res* 1991;25:820–830.
29. Werns SW, Lucchesi BR. Leukocytes, oxygen radicals, and myocardial injury due to ischaemia and reperfusion. *Free Rad Biol Med* 1988;4:31–37.
30. Halliwell B, Gutteridge JMC. *Free radicals in biology and medicine.* Oxford: Clarendon Press, 1989;377.
31. Menasche P, Pasquier C, Belluci S, Lorente P, Jaillon P, Piwnica A. Deferoxamine reduces neutrophil-mediated free radical production during cardiopulmonary bypass in man. *J Thorac Cardiovasc Surg* 1988;96:582–589.
32. Lucchesi BR, Werns SW, Fantone JC. The role of the neutrophil and free radicals in ischaemic myocardial injury. *J Mol Cell Cardiol* 1989;1421–1251.
33. Go LO, Murry CE, Richard VJ, Weischedel GR, Jennings RB, Reimer KA. Myocardial neutrophil accumulation during reperfusion after reversible and irreversible ischaemic injury. *Am J Physiol* 1988;235:H1188–H1198.
34. Granger DN. Role of xanthine oxidase and granulocytes in ischaemia–reperfusion injury. *Am J Physiol* 1988;255:H1269–H1275.
35. Nohl H, Koltover V, Stolze K. Ischaemia/reperfusion impairs mitochondrial energy conservation and triggers $O_2^{\cdot -}$ release as a byproduct of respiration. *Free Rad Res Commun* 1993;18:127–137.
36. Jennings RB, Ganote CE. Structural changes in myocardium during acute ischaemia. *Circ Res* 1974;34:III-156–III-172.
37. Subramanian R, Volovsek A, Ho YS. Lack of change in MnSOD during ischaemia/reperfusion of isolated rat heart. *J Mol Cell Cardiol* 1993;25:1179–1186.
38. Manning AS, Hearse DJ. Reperfusion-induced arrhythmias: mechanisms and prevention. *J Mol Cell Cardiol* 1984;16:497–518.
39. Katz AM. *Physiology of the heart.* New York: Raven Press; 1992;124.
40. Fisher DJ. Oxygenation and metabolism in the developing heart. *Sem Perinatol* 1984;8:217–225.
41. Dawes GS, Mott JC, Shelley JH. The importance of cardiac glycogen for the maintenance of life in fetal lambs and newborn animals during anoxia. *J Physiol (Lond)* 1959;146:516–538.
42. Lopaschuk GD, Collins-Nakai RL, Itoi T. Developmental changes in energy substrate use by the heart. *Cardiovasc Res* 1992;26:1172–1180.
43. Nakamura H, del Nido PJ, Jimenez E, Sarin M, Feinberg H, Levitsky S. Age-related differences in cardiac susceptibility to ischaemia/reperfusion injury: response to deferoxamine. *J Thorac Cardiovasc Surg* 1992;104:165–172.
44. Vettenranta K, Raivio KO. Xanthine oxidase during human fetal development. *Pediatr Res* 1990;27:286–288.
45. Achterberg PW, Nieukoop AS, Schoutsen B, De Jong JW. Different ATP-catabolism in reperfused adult and newborn rat hearts. *Am J Physiol* 1988;254:H1091–H1098.
46. Muxfeld M, Schaper W. The activity of xanthine oxidase in hearts of pigs, guinea pigs, rabbits, rats, and humans. *Basic Res Cardiol* 1987;82:486–492.
47. De Jong JW, Achterberg PW. Developmental differences in myocardial ATP metabolism. *Basic Res Cardiol* 1987;82:121–126.
48. Breda MA, Drinkwater DC, Laks H, Bhuta S, Corno AF, Davtyan HG, Chang P. Prevention of reperfusion injury in the neonatal heart with leukocyte-depleted blood. *J Thorac Cardiovasc Surg* 1989;97:654–665.
49. Kelly FJ, Rickett GMW. Temporal development of antioxidants in the newborn rat. *Biochem Soc Trans* 1986;225–226.
50. Das DK, Engelman RM, Flansaas D, Otani OJ, Rousou J, Breyer RH. Developmental profiles of protective mechanisms of heart against peroxidase injury. *Basic Res Cardiol* 1987;82:36–50.
51. Dhaliwal H, Kirschenbaum LA, Randhawa AK, Singal PK. Correlation between antioxidant changes during hypoxia and recovery on reoxygenation. *Am J Physiol* 1991;261:H632–H638.
52. Das DK, Flansaas RM, Engelman JA, Rousou RH, Breyer R, Jones S, Lemeshow A, Otani H. Age-related developmental profiles of the antioxidative defence system and the peroxidation status of the pig heart. *Biol Neonate* 1987;51:156–169.

The Developing Heart,
edited by Bohuslav Ošťádal et al.
Lippincott-Raven Publishers,
Philadelphia

33

Postnatal Development: Metabolic and Functional Determinants of Response to Oxygen Stress

Carin Wittnich, DVM, MSc

Institute of Medical Science, Departments of Physiology and Surgery, University of Toronto and Division of Cardiovascular Surgery, Hospital for Sick Children, Toronto, Ontario M5S 1A8, Canada

ABSTRACT

This chapter explores the effects of maturation on systemic and myocardial responses to a variety of oxygen stresses, including hypoxia, myocardial ischemia, and hyperoxia. It examines the neonatal hemodynamic and metabolic response to graded hypoxia, and identifies oxygen-restricted metabolism as confirmed by the development of lactic acidosis and altered oxygen handling in 3-day-old piglets exposed to 2 hours of graded arterial hypoxia (arterial partial pressure of oxygen = PaO_2), including mild (60 mmHg), moderate (40 mmHg), moderately severe (30 mmHg), or severe (20 mmHg) hypoxia. In mild and moderate hypoxia, lactate and acid–base homeostasis were unaltered because of a significant increase in oxygen extraction that was sufficient to maintain oxygen uptake ($C_{a\text{-}v}O_2$). However, in moderately severe hypoxia, despite an increase in oxygen extraction, oxygen uptake was reduced. Increased arterial lactate, decreased bicarbonate (HCO_3^-), and base excess were evidence of anaerobic metabolism and indicated the onset of oxygen-restricted metabolism. With severe hypoxia increased oxygen extraction was severely limited by availability, resulting in significantly reduced oxygen uptake, anaerobic metabolism, and profound lactic acidosis. The neonatal heart appeared to tolerate up to moderately severe hypoxia with minimal alterations in energy levels. However, severe hypoxia caused an 85% reduction in glycogen, a 10-fold increase in lactate, and a 50% reduction in ATP levels, which impaired the heart's tolerance to ischemia. Although hypothermia provided some protection to neonates, it was only 50% as effective in hearts with depressed ATP levels. High oxygen levels (hyperoxia) in neonates induced a more adultlike metabolic response in the heart, which afforded some metabolic benefit during early ischemia but provoked a higher incidence of ventricular fibrillation. This fibrillation, in hyperoxic neonatal hearts, eliminated any metabolic benefit and resulted in a reduction in ischemic tolerance.

ENERGY METABOLISM

Age-dependent differences in myocardial energy metabolism exist that may be important in understanding cardiac function in the neonatal heart (1). Among these is an increased capacity for aerobic glycolysis in immature hearts (1) and higher glycogen levels in many species, including man (1). There is also immaturity of the enzyme carnitine palmitoyl-CoA-transferase (2), whose timing of maturation may be species dependent (3). These differences impact on the ability of young hearts to utilize free fatty acids (2). We have explored whether these differences contribute

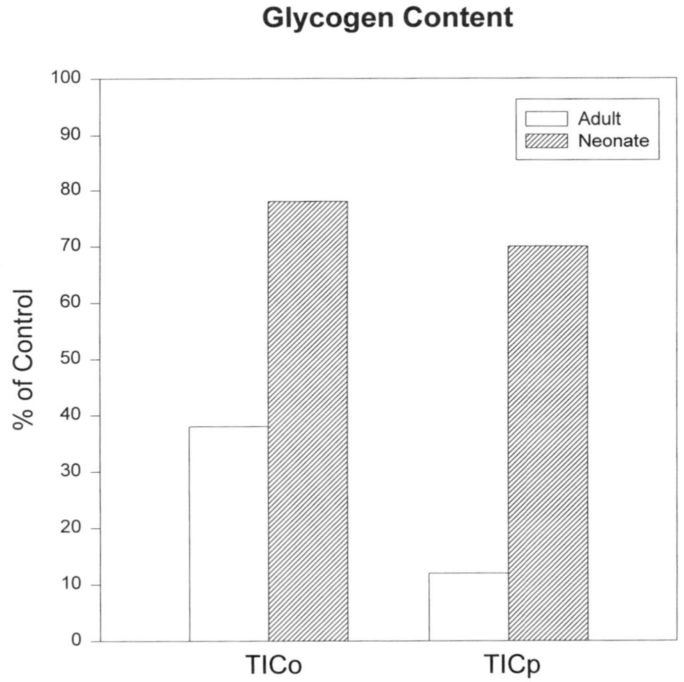

FIG. 33–1. Glycogen content of the myocardium in adult (open bar, $n = 6$) vs neonatal hearts (hatched bar, $n = 6$) in response to global ischemia is expressed as percent of control (pre-ischemia). A significant decrease in glycogen was noted in the adults that continued until near-total depletion by ischemic contracture peak (TICp). In neonates there was a more modest decrease at ischemic contracture onset (TICo), after which time no further decline was noted. Values are group means.

to age-specific metabolic responses to ischemia and found that the rate of ATP decline was significantly less in adult pig hearts (.05 μmol $g^{-1}min^{-1}$) during global ischemia compared to 3-day-old piglet hearts (.095 μmol $g^{-1}min^{-1}$) (4). Interestingly, myocardial glycogen use was incomplete in neonates compared to adults (Fig. 33–1). Since glycogen is the main source of substrate for the ischemic heart, this incomplete glycogen use could have significant implications. The key regulatory enzyme for glycolysis is phosphofructokinase (PKF). This enzyme is sensitive to hydrogen ion, lactate, and ATP/ADP ratios. Inhibition of PFK would result in accumulation of glycolytic intermediates such as glucose-6-phosphate (G6P) and an impaired ability to further utilize glycogen for glycolysis. Our work showed a very rapid and significant accumulation of G6P in piglet hearts during early ischemia, confirming the inhibition of this pathway (4). It has been reported that fetal and newborn hearts of rabbits and guinea pigs have higher glycolytic enzyme activity, particularly PFK, compared to adults of the same species (5). Since lactate accumulates during anaerobic glycolysis, age-related differences in the amount and rate of this accumulation could offer one explanation for this apparent earlier PFK inhibition. More rapid lactate accumulation during global normothermic ischemia was indeed found in piglet hearts (.66 μmol $g^{-1}min^{-1}$) compared to adult hearts (.46 $\mu mol/g^{-1}/min^{-1}$) (4), which could result in earlier inhibition of PFK in the neonate. Additionally, differences in cellular ability to buffer the hydrogen ion produced during a period of global ischemia could impact on hydrogen ion accumulation and thereby contribute to PFK inhibition and the extent of tissue injury (6).

BUFFERING CAPACITY

The net accumulation of hydrogen ion at any one time is determined by the amount produced and its removal. Hydrogen removal involves a number of cellular mechanisms that fall under the general categories of physicochemical buffering, transmembrane fluxes and exchangers of hydrogen ion (7). Although exchangers play a major role in recovery from an acid load, they are rapidly inactivated during ischemia. This occurs because of an accumulation of interstitial hydrogen ion resulting in a loss of the hydrogen ion gradient across the cell membrane (8–10). Because of this, during ischemia intracellular buffers become crucial. We, as well as others, have explored age-related differences in the heart's buffering capacity. Buffering capacity is the ability of tissue to resist changes in pH when an acid or base is added. It was found that when the hearts of adult pigs were compared to those of 3-day-old piglets, the immature heart had at least a 20% lower buffering capacity (6). This would clearly make the immature heart more susceptible to developing acidosis during an ischemic episode compared to its adult counterpart. This was confirmed when we documented a greater accumulation of hydrogen ion in immature hearts compared to adults over the same ischemic interval (6). The lower buffering capacity in young compared to adult hearts has also been reported in sheep (11). Interestingly, some species differences may exist as neonatal rabbit hearts have been reported to maintain higher pH than adults during an ischemic period (3).

CALCIUM HANDLING

It has been reported that influx of calcium during ischemia contributes to ischemic injury (12). Age-related differences in calcium handling could also impact on neonatal myocardial function (12). The heart is said to undergo three phases of development with respect to calcium handling (13). In the fetal heart, calcium for excitation–contraction coupling is derived almost exclusively from extracellular stores. In the newborn heart, although extracellular calcium does continue to be the major contributor to excitation–contraction coupling, it also begins to mediate calcium release from the developing sarcoplasmic reticulum (SR). In the adult heart, extracellular calcium causes induced calcium release from the SR, which then causes myofilament shortening. Many structural and metabolic differences exist between the adult and neonatal heart that contribute to these different phases of development. These include a poorly developed SR in neonates that is incapable of the rate of calcium uptake seen in adults (14). In addition, the SR regulatory protein phospholamban, which controls calcium pump activity, is not mature at birth and is only activated by cAMP-dependent kinase, not calcium-calmodulin or calcium–phospholipid-dependent kinases as seen at maturity (15). Immature hearts have decreased amounts of SR calcium–ATPase and calsequestrin, the SR calcium storage protein, compared to mature hearts. They also have decreased density and activity of sarcolemmal sodium–calcium exchangers and calcium–ATPase pumps, *t*-tubule density and myofibrillar calcium-activated ATPase (16,17).

Clearly, changes in the heart's reliance on extracellular calcium contribute not only to differences in function but, since extracellular calcium entry into the cell during ischemia is known to contribute to ischemic injury (12), may contribute to neonatal susceptibility to ischemic injury. We challenged this experimentally by altering the extracellular calcium concentration in adult and 3-day-old piglet hearts and assessing the time to development of ischemic injury (18). Contrary to adult pig hearts, which did not alter their time to ischemic injury even when exposed to high extracellular calcium levels (4.44 mM), neonatal pig hearts significantly decreased their time to ischemic injury in response to high extracellular calcium. This increased sensitivity to ischemia in neonatal hearts created by high extracellular calcium was eliminated if the hearts were pretreated with the L-calcium channel blocker, verapamil (18). This work confirmed that age-related differences in calcium handling do contribute to susceptibility to ischemic injury and that neonates appear unable to "buffer out" the high extracellular calcium compared to adults.

REPERFUSION

A number of metabolic differences have been identified in the immature heart that appear to impact on its ability to tolerate ischemia. Whether these differences affect recovery from an ischemic episode to the same degree is not clear, for reports conflict (3). We compared the neonatal heart's ability to recover from varying durations of ischemia in a normothermic blood-perfused 3-day-old piglet maintained on cardiopulmonary bypass (19). Hearts were reperfused after development of peak ischemic contracture, which has been reported in adult hearts to mark irreversible ischemic injury (20). In the neonatal heart, a minimal 18–20% recovery of function was seen. It has been felt by some that the immature heart could recover almost completely from this insult; however, this was clearly not the case in this model. Other 3-day-old piglet hearts that were reperfused at the onset of ischemic contracture had a more variable recovery but still averaged only 50–60%, indicating some degree of injury was present (19). Ongoing research should provide further clarification on this issue.

HYPOXIA

Tissue hypoxia challenges the intact whole body system to maintain adequate heart function, despite reduced oxygen availability. Oxygen is the terminal electron acceptor for the mitochondrial electron transport chain. Inadequate cellular oxygen availability impairs mitochondrial oxidative phosphorylation, inducing a shift from aerobic to anaerobic glycolysis and ultimately producing lactic acid. Although hypoxia-induced lactic acidosis has been investigated extensively in adults (21–23), it has not been clearly defined in neonates. Two short-duration (<1 hour) studies found neonatal lambs undergoing severe hypoxia, where the PaO_2 was 19 ± 12 mmHg, had significant acid–base changes (24,25). Previous work in our laboratory elucidated that, in addition to acidosis, significant CO_2 production occurred during 2 hours of severe hypoxia (PaO_2 = 20 mmHg) (26). The etiology of this observation in neonates, the relative role of CO_2 in the observed acid–base disturbances, and the precise PaO_2 identifying the onset of metabolic stress remained unclear. At the threshold for oxygen-restricted metabolism, the switch from aerobic to anaerobic glycolysis generates both lactate and hydrogen ion intracellularly. Excess hydrogen ion is released into the circulation and is ultimately buffered by the blood bicarbonate buffer system (27). We undertook a PaO_2 dose–response study of blood lactate, acid–base balance, and oxygen handling to identify, in neonates, the threshold for oxygen-restricted metabolism (28). This was done since the PaO_2 threshold for the development of hypoxia-induced lactic acidosis, as confirmed by altered blood lactate and oxygen handling, had not been evaluated in neonates. This is crucial since the extent of hypoxia-induced metabolic acidosis could ultimately influence the ability to tolerate varying levels of hypoxia (29). A wide range of hypoxia levels was studied without the confounding variable of respiratory acidosis, to identify the PaO_2 threshold at which impaired oxygen uptake and extraction induces a shift to oxygen-restricted metabolism, ultimately resulting in lactate accumulation and acidosis. Hypoxia was induced by adding 100% nitrogen to the inspired medical air, thus creating an appropriate inspired gas ratio to achieve each level of hypoxia; mild (60 mmHg), moderate (40 mmHg), moder-

TABLE 33–1. *Pao_2, $MSao_2$, Pvo_2 and $MSvo_2$ in the neonatal pig hypoxia model*

Parameter	Normoxia	Moderate hypoxia	Moderately severe hypoxia	Severe hypoxia
Pao_2*	81.13 ± 2.75	40.46 ± 0.71	32.30 ± 0.64	24.47 ± 1.03
$MSao_2$§	97.87 ± 0.57	67.32 ± 1.16	50.67 ± 1.71	34.87 ± 1.57
Pvo_2*	26.26 ± 0.67	19.20 ± 0.53	12.49 ± 0.67	8.31 ± 0.89
$MSvo_2$§	42.09 ± 1.70	22.33 ± 1.12	13.33 ± 1.03	9.41 ± 0.96

Values are mean ± SEM (* = mmHg, § = percent). For each parameter, all groups were significantly different ($p < .05$). (Reprinted with permission from *J Appl Physiol* 1994; 77(5) 2318–2324.)

ately severe (30 mmHg), or severe (20 mmHg) hypoxia. These various levels of hypoxia resulted in significantly altered measured saturations in both the arterial and venous systems (Table 33–1). Oxygen contents, both arterial (Cao_2) and venous (Cvo_2), were used to calculate oxygen uptake and extraction. Oxygen uptake ($C_{a\text{-}v}o_2$) was defined as the arteriovenous oxygen content difference. Oxygen extraction was taken as the ratio of oxygen uptake to arterial oxygen content ($C_{a\text{-}v}o_2/Cao_2$). Only in response to moderately severe and severe hypoxia was there a progressive reduction in $C_{a\text{-}v}o_2$. Two distinct relationships between oxygen uptake and

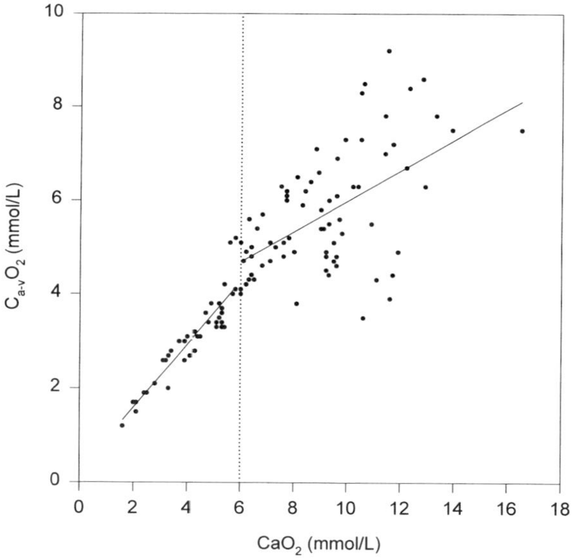

FIG. 33–2. Arterial oxygen content (CaO_2) versus oxygen uptake ($C_{a\text{-}v}O_2$) in all animals during the study period ($mmol/L^{-1}$ = mmol/L). This graph shows the linear regression lines for the oxygen-restricted (<6 mmol/L) and oxygen-unrestricted (>6 mmol/L) portions of the graph. The regression equations and correlation coefficients for the high and low CaO_2 regions are $y = 0.3267x + 2.7222$ ($r = 0.55608$) and $y = 0.6688x + 0.2560$ ($r = 0.92099$), respectively. (Reprinted with permission from *J Appl Physiol,* 1994; 77(5) 2318–2324.)

Cao_2 were identified (Fig. 33–2). In Cao_2 range above 6 mmol/L^{-1}, a very weak correlation coefficient ($r = 0.56$) was seen, while the Cao_2 range below 6 mmol/L^{-1} had a very strong correlation ($r = 0.92$). Thus, in this study, moderately severe hypoxia ($CaO_2 \cong 6$ mmol/L^{-1}) marked the onset of oxygen-restricted metabolism. Below this threshold, oxygen availability limited oxygen uptake, thus confirming oxygen-restricted metabolism.

As previously mentioned, anaerobic glycolysis yields lactic acid, which releases lactate and hydrogen ion intracellularly. When the rate of hydrogen ion production is sufficiently high, excess hydrogen ion enters the circulation and is neutralized by the blood buffer systems (27) in an attempt to maintain pH. The primary blood buffer is the bicarbonate buffer system (27). In the moderately severe hypoxia group at 1 hour, there was a doubling in arterial lactate (Fig. 33–3a), but HCO_3^- was unaltered, suggesting that there was adequate compensation. By 2 hours, however, decreased HCO_3^- indicated excess hydrogen ion production was stressing the buffering system. Although there was only a slight Pao_2 decrease from moderately severe to severe hypoxia, it has profound metabolic significance. In the severe hypoxia group, the decreased HCO_3^- was concomitant with significantly and progressively decreased pH (Fig.33–3b) and base excess. In this group, the rate of lactic acid production overwhelmed the intracellular buffers and rapidly exceeded the blood buffering capacity, inducing profound progressive lactic acidosis (Fig. 33–3b) (30). For each level of hypoxia, the rate of lactic acid production and the buffering capacity were the primary factors that influenced acid–base homeostasis (27,31–34). Unlike our previous study, which was confounded by respiratory acidosis (26), in this normocapnic model, decreased pH confirmed metabolic acidosis. Thus, both acid–base status and oxygen handling identified moderately severe hypoxia as the threshold for oxygen-restricted metabolism.

In summary, anesthetized neonatal pigs maintained adequate cellular oxygen delivery in a Pao_2 range from 80 to 40 mmHg. In the moderate hypoxia group, systemic oxygen extraction increased significantly and was sufficient to maintain oxygen uptake, preventing oxygen-restricted metabolism and acid–base disturbances. When the Pao_2 was further reduced, an inability to increase oxygen extraction resulted in significantly reduced oxygen uptake and ultimately induced a shift from aerobic to anaerobic glycolysis, causing net lactic acid production. In the moderately severe hypoxia group, reduced oxygen uptake and elevated arterial blood lactate indicated the onset of oxygen-restricted metabolism. However, at this level ($Pao_2 = 30$ mmHg), the intact neonate successfully buffered this metabolic acid. In severe hypoxia, with only a slight further Pao_2 reduction, oxygen uptake decreased to 50% of normal, resulting in extensive anaerobic glycolysis. This oxygen-restricted metabolism caused a high rate of H^+ production that rapidly exceeded the buffering capacity, resulting in profound progressive lactic acidosis.

Since sustained heart function is dependent on adequate myocardial energy supply, hypoxia severe enough to impair myocardial metabolism could limit energy supply and impact on performance. Therefore, the effect of graded hypoxia on metabolism of the neonatal heart was studied (35). It was found that the 3-day-old piglet heart could tolerate up to moderately severe hypoxia with minimal alter-

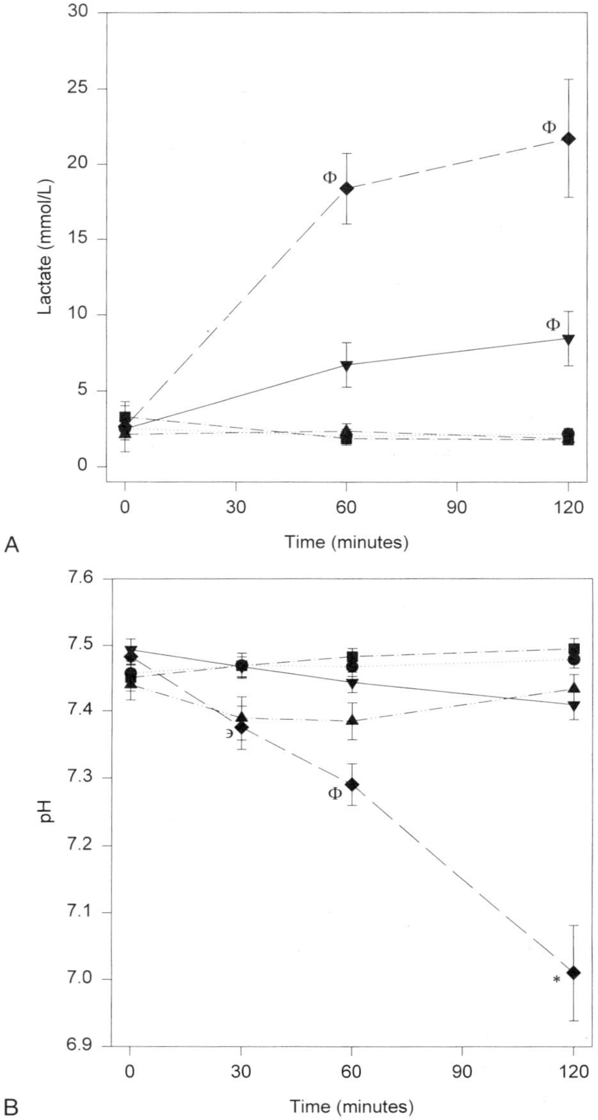

FIG. 33–3. Groups shown are normoxia (●) and mild (■), moderate (▲), moderately severe (▼), and severe (◆) hypoxia. (**A**) Arterial lactate concentration with graded hypoxia in neonatal pigs (mmol/L^{-1}). Control values are 2.5 ± 0.3 mmol/L (mean ± standard error of the mean). Significantly different from control $^{\Phi}$ $p < .0001$. (Reprinted with permission from *J Appl Physiol,* 1994.) (**B**) Arterial pH with varying degrees of hypoxia in neonatal pigs. Control values are 7.46 ± 0.01 (mean ± standard error of the mean). Significantly different from * all other time intervals ($p < .0001$); $^{\Phi}$ control ($p < .0001$), and ϵ control ($p < .001$). (Reprinted with permission from *J Appl Physiol,* 1994; 77(5) 2318–2324.)

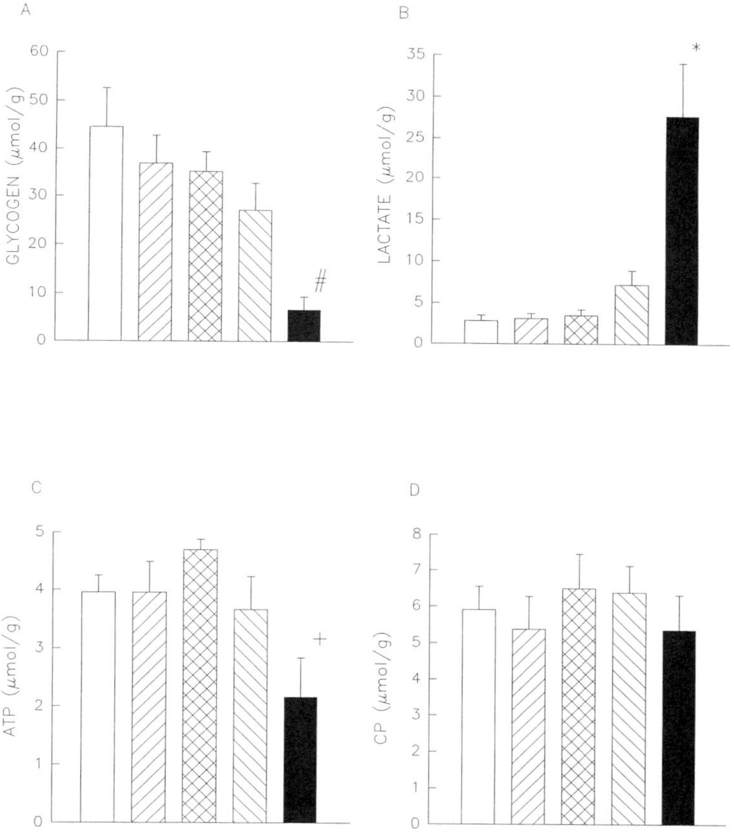

FIG. 33–4. Neonatal myocardial metabolic parameters subsequent to 2 hours of ventilation at varying levels of systemic hypoxia. Values shown are mean ± standard error of the mean (μmol/g^{-1} wet weight). Groups shown are normoxia ( ), mild ( ), moderate ( ), moderately severe ( ), and severe ( ) hypoxia. (**A**) Myocardial glycogen. Significantly different from all except the moderately severe hypoxia group # $p < 0.05$. (**B**) Myocardial lactate. Significantly different from all others at the same time interval * $p < 0.0001$. (**C**) Myocardial ATP. Significantly different from the moderate hypoxic group + $p < 0.05$. (**D**) Myocardial CP. No significant difference (NS) in any of the experimental groups. (Reprinted with permission from *J Mol Cell Cardiol,* 1994; (26) 675–682.)

ations in glycogen, lactate, creatine phosphate (CP), and ATP (Fig. 33–4). However, in the face of severe hypoxia there was an 85% reduction in myocardial glycogen, a 10-fold increase in lactate, and a 50% reduction in ATP. Despite this stress profile, CP stores remained unaltered. In adult hearts, it is known that CP stores are immediately utilized to maintain ATP levels (36). The activity of creatine phosphokinase, the enzyme responsible for CP hydrolysis, has been reported to be depressed in immature hearts and could result in an inability to metabolize endogenous CP stores (37,38). Despite some controversy, particularly in the adult literature, ATP levels have been correlated with tolerance to ischemia (39–41). An impaired ability to utilize CP could put the hypoxic neonatal heart with both reduced ATP levels and glycogen reserves "at risk" of a subsequent ischemic stress. This was confirmed in our hypoxic hearts, where a greater than 50% reduction in tolerance to ischemia was seen (35).

It is also interesting to note that during *hypoxic* stress, where blood flow can remove byproducts of anaerobic metabolism, glycogen use was almost complete in the severely hypoxic neonatal heart. This is in stark contrast to the neonatal hearts' *ischemic* response, where glycogen use was only 30% (Fig. 33–1).

Since survival is ultimately determined, not only by oxygenation and degree of acidosis, but by the acute hemodynamic response over the first few hours as well, the combined systemic and myocardial effects of hypoxia on hemodynamics was also documented. Some controversy exists in the literature on whether arterial pressure is increased (42,43), maintained (29,44), or decreased (24,45) in response to hypoxia in the neonate. This appears to depend partly on the duration and severity of the exposure. Our studies allowed us to clarify this by conducting a Pao_2 dose-dependent evaluation of the hemodynamic responses. Tachycardia was induced at a Pao_2 threshold of moderate hypoxia (40 mmHg). This tachycardia effectively maintained arterial blood pressure (46). Below this threshold there was a heart rate, CNS, and chemoreceptor-mediated pressor response, resulting in an initial Pao_2-dependent hypertension. In response to severe hypoxia there was also an initial increase in pulse pressure (systolic–diastolic). An increase in peripheral vascular resistance at this level of hypoxia most likely contributed to the initial hypertension. As the duration of hypoxia was extended, the hypertension seen initially at more profound hypoxia levels could not be sustained, likely because of subsequent peripheral vasodilation in response to local tissue hypoxia. In severe hypoxia this was exacerbated by depressed myocardial function (46).

HYPOTHERMIA

Systemic hypothermia with or without circulatory arrest continues to be used to protect hearts during pediatric heart surgery. Cooling slows heart rate and metabolism, which in turn, results in decreased oxygen consumption (47). The effectiveness of this method has been evaluated in children using such markers as cardiac index (48) and other clinical parameters such as urine output, amount of inotropes needed, and need for defibrillation (49). Gross measures such as hospital mortality have also been published (48,50). It has been reported that in the neonatal heart, hypothermia permits a "safe" ischemic period for at least 90 minutes and possibility even up to 120 min in some cases (50). Despite this, clinical studies have reported a 10% mortality using deep hypothermia, with 50% of these deaths ascribed to acute cardiac insufficiency (51). It would appear that not all hearts are afforded equal "protection" with hypothermia. We undertook to carefully study the meta-

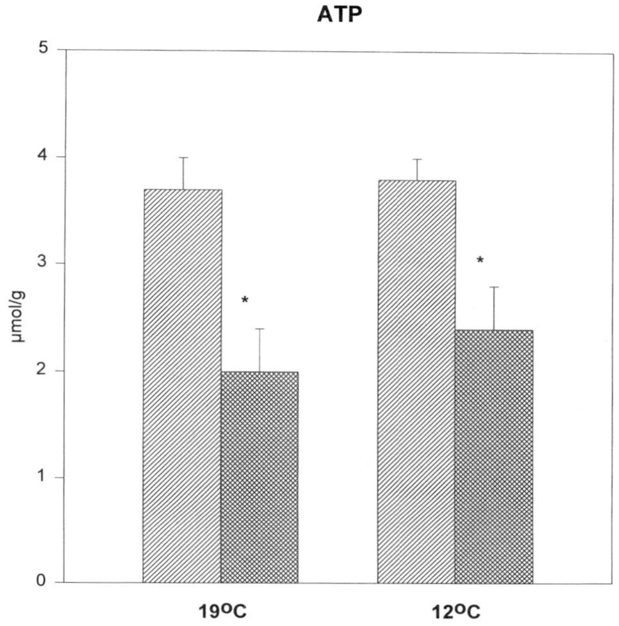

A

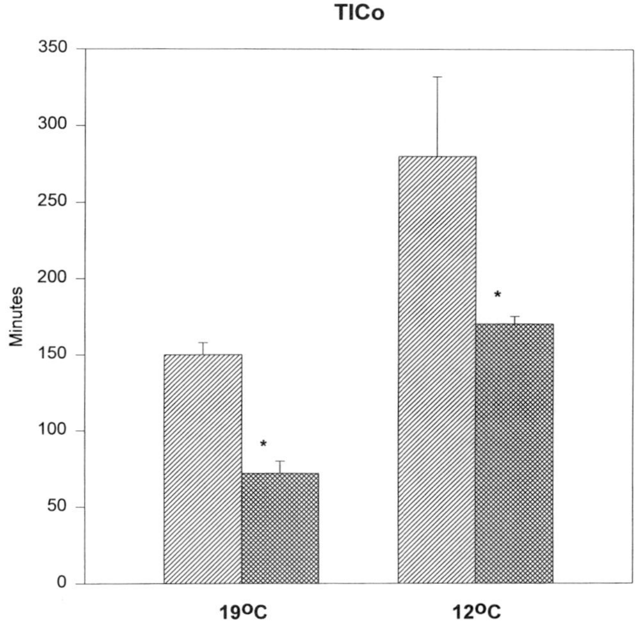

B

FIG. 33–5. (**A**) Adenosine triphosphate values before ischemia were significantly lower in a subgroup of hearts in both 19°C ($n = 5$) and 12°C ($n = 5$) (cross-hatched bars) compared with the group mean at 19°C or 12°C (diagonally hatched bars). Values (μmol/g^{-1} wet weight) shown are mean ± the standard error of the mean (* $p < 0.01$.) (Reprinted [redrawn] with permission from *Ann Thorac Surg,* 1991; (52) 1000–1004.) (**B**) Time to onset of ischemic contracture was significantly less in both "at-risk" groups at 19°C and 12°C (cross-hatched bars) compared with the group mean for 19°C or 12°C (diagonally hatched bars). Note the small variation in the "at-risk" groups. Data shown as the mean ± the standard error of the mean (* $p < 0.01$). (Reprinted [redrawn] with permission from *Ann Thorac Surg,* 1991; (52) 1000–1004.)

bolic effects of various clinically employed levels of hypothermia (25°C, 19°C, 12°C) on 3-day-old piglet hearts (52,53). As expected, each level of hypothermia extended the time before onset of ischemic injury in neonatal hearts. However, it was interesting to note that even with the deepest hypothermia (12°C), ATP depletion by as much as 25% was seen in the first 30 min of ischemia (52). Although this was significantly less than that seen during 30 min of normothermic ischemia (50%), clearly some ATP use was still present. When deep hypothermia was further investigated, a group of "at risk" hearts was identified that even prior to ischemia had 50% less ATP than normal (Fig. 33–5a) (53). The "safe" ischemic time afforded these "at risk" hearts by the use of deep hypothermia was significantly reduced to approximately half that of the group mean (Fig. 33–5b). Clearly, hypothermia does not offer equal protection in all immature hearts, especially those with lower ATP levels, which then have shorter "safe" ischemic times. This could include neonatal hearts exposed to severe hypoxia. Since their ATP levels were depleted to approximately 50% after 2 hours of exposure (Fig. 33–4), hypothermia may not be able to provide the anticipated protection.

HYPEROXIA

Administration of oxygen is used to improve tissue oxygen transport and counteract the leftward shift of the oxygen–hemoglobin dissociation curve occurring with cold temperatures. Despite experimental evidence of detrimental effects of high oxygen (hyperoxia) in adults (54), and more recently in neonates undergoing cardiopulmonary bypass with subsequent myocardial ischemia/reperfusion (55), the excessive levels of oxygen achieved during clinical management of patients have not been traditionally of concern. We chose to study the effects of two clinically relevant levels of hyperoxia (PaO_2=250 mmHg, 500 mmHg) on 3-day-old piglets (56). Interestingly, despite benefits to the heart such as better preservation of ATP during early ischemia and an apparently more adultlike metabolic profile during this stress, there was a significant up to 50% incidence of ventricular fibrillation with hyperoxia. Those hearts that did fibrillate lost any metabolic benefit provided by hyperoxia during early ischemia (56).

SUMMARY

Clearly, there are age-related metabolic differences with the potential to impact on the performance of the heart and its ability to respond to oxygen stress. Adaptations such as enhanced glycolysis in neonates, which allow for some resistance to hypoxia, require that the byproducts such as lactate and hydrogen ion be removed from the cell. These may actually be maladaptations in the face of global ischemia where the byproducts of anaerobic metabolism cannot be removed. This was confirmed by the rapid lactate and hydrogen ion accumulation during global ischemia in immature hearts, in the face of poorer buffering capacity, which put them at risk of earlier damage. Importantly, the time-honored technique of hypothermia, employed to reduce metabolism and protect the heart, was not uniformly effective in neonates. Hearts with reduced energy levels were only offered approximately 50% of the anticipated protection. Other risk factors of concern in immature hearts exposed to low oxygen conditions include the apparent diminished ability to mobilize CP to maintain energy levels as well as restricted capacity to increase oxygen uptake to maintain extraction. Both of these also predispose the neonate to earlier injury. Even the use of high oxygen levels, in neonates, appeared to be a double-edged sword. It provided some metabolic benefit by preserving energy levels during early ischemia and yet resulted in a greater incidence of ventricular fibrillation with the onset of global ischemia. Further research is ongoing in various centers around the world to clarify these issues. Clearly, techniques employed to enhance the neonatal heart's ability to tolerate such oxygen stresses will have to take into account these differences if they are to be successful.

ACKNOWLEDGMENTS

The author wishes to acknowledge the assistance of Mr. Michael P. Belanger and the hard work of all the graduate students that made this work possible; Ms. Cathy E. Carlyle, Dr. Jun Su, Ms Shona M. Torrance, and Mr. W. Jack Wallen. Grant funding was provided by the Heart & Stroke Foundation of Ontario and trainee support by the Heart & Stroke Foundation of Canada and the Ontario Ministry of Health.

REFERENCES

1. Wells RJ, Friedman WF, Sobel BE. Increased oxidative metabolism in the fetal and newborn lamb heart. *Am J Physiol* 1972;222:1488.
2. Fisher DJ. Oxygenation and metabolism in the developing heart. *Semin Perinatol* 1984;8:217.
3. Riva HE, Hearse DJ. *The Developing Myocardium.* Mount Kisco, NY: Futura Publishing, 1991.
4. Wittnich C, Peniston C, Ianuzzo D, Abel JC, Salerno TA. Relative vulnerability of neonatal and adult hearts to ischemic injury. *Circ* 1987;769(suppl V):156–160.
5. Werner JC, Whitman V, Fripp RR, Schuler HG, Morgan HE. Carbohydrate metabolism in isolated working newborn pig heart. *Am J Physiol* 1981;241:E364.
6. Wittnich C, Su J, Porter P, O'Brien P. Age related differences in myocardial hydrogen ion handling. 1996 (submitted).
7. Lowenstein J. *Acid and basics: a guide to understanding acid–base disorders.* Oxford: Oxford University Press, 1993.
8. Williamson JR, Schaffer SW, Ford C, Saffer B. Contribution of tissue acidosis to ischemic injury in the perfused rat heart. *Circ* 1976;53(suppl 1):3–14.
9. de Hamptinne A. Intracellular pH and surface pH in skeletal and cardiac muscle measured with a double-barrelled pH microelectrode. *Pflugers Arch* 1980;386:121–126.
10. Pierce GN, Philipson KD. Na^+/H^+ exchange in cardiac sarcolemmal vesicles. *Biochim Biophys Acta* 1985;818:109–116.
11. Griffiths RI, Baldwin J, Berger PJ. Metabolic development of sheep diaphragm during fetal and newborn life. *Respir Physiol* 1994;95(3):337–347.
12. Ikonomidis JS, Salerno TA, Wittnich C. Calcium and the heart: an essential partnership. *Can J Cardiol* 1990;6(7):305–316.

13. Nakanishi T, Seguchi M, Takao A. Development of the myocardial contractile system. *Experientia* 1988;44:936–944.
14. Boland R, Martonosi A, Tillack TW. Developmental changes in the composition and function of sarcoplasmic reticulum. *J Biol Chem* 1974;249:612–623.
15. Pegg W, Michalak M. Differentiation of sarcoplasmic reticulum during cardiac myogenesis. *Am J Physiol* 1987;252:H22–H31.
16. Legato MJ. *The developing heart.* Boston: Martinus Nijhoff, 1985.
17. Corno AF, Bethencourt DN, Laks H. Myocardial protection in the neonatal heart: a comparison of topical hyperthermia and crystalloid and blood cardioplegic solutions. *J Thorac Cardiovasc Surg* 1987;93:163–172.
18. Wallen WJ, Wittnich C, Ikonomidis JS. Alterations in extracellular calcium affects neonatal not adult tolerance to ischemia. 1997 (submitted).
19. Wittnich C, Torrance SM. Is there functional recovery after ischemic contracture in the immature heart? 1997 (submitted).
20. Hearse DJ, Garlick PB, Humphrey SM. Ischemic contracture of the myocardium: mechanisms and prevention. *Am J Cardiol* 1977;39:986–993.
21. Cain SM. Appearance of excess lactate in anesthetized dogs during anemia and hypoxic hypoxia. *Am J Physiol* 1965;209:604–610.
22. Huckabee WE. Relationships of pyruvate and lactate during anaerobic metabolism. III. Effect of breathing low-oxygen gases. *J Clin Invest* 1958;37(2):264–271.
23. Ruggles TN, Lavietes MH, Miller M, Woodward H, Treister M. Effect of phenformin on the elevated blood lactic acid produced by hypoxia in normal and diabetic rats. *Ann NY Acad Sci* 1968;148:662–670.
24. Moss M, G Moreau G, Lister G. Oxygen transport and metabolism in the conscious lamb: the effects of hypoxemia. *Pediatr Res* 1987;22(2):177–183.
25. Sidi D, Kuipers JRG, Teitel D, Heymann MA, Rudolph AM. Developmental changes in oxygenation and circulatory responses to hypoxemia in lambs. *Am J Physiol* 1983;245:H674–H682.
26. Torrance SM, Wittnich C. The effect of varying arterial oxygen tension on neonatal acid-base balance. *Pediatr Res* 1992;31(2):112–116.
27. Despopoulos A, Silbernagi S, eds. *Color atlas of physiology.* Stuttgart: Thieme, 1986.
28. Torrance SM, Wittnich C. Blood lactate and acid-base balance in graded neonatal hypoxia: evidence for oxygen-restricted metabolism. *J Appl Physiol* 1994;77(5):2318–2324.
29. Hurst JW, Schlant RC, eds. *The Heart,* 7th ed. New York: McGraw-Hill, 1990.
30. Jones NL. A quantitative physicochemical approach to acid-base physiology. *Clin Biochem* 1990;23(3):189–195.
31. Arieff AI, DeFronzo RA. *Fluid, electrolyte, and acid-base disorders,* vol. 1. New York: Churchill Livingstone, 1985.
32. Goldberger E. *A primer of water, electrolyte and acid–base syndromes,* 7th ed. Philadelphia: Lea and Febiger, 1986.
33. Halperin ML, Goldstein MB. *Fluid, electrolyte, and acid-base emergencies,* 2nd edition. Philadelphia: WB Saunders, 1994.
34. Rawn JD. *Biochemistry.* Burlington: Carolina Biological Supply Company, 1988.
35. Wittnich C, Torrance SM. Does the severity of acute hypoxia influence neonatal myocardial metabolism and sensitivity to ischemia? *J Mol Cell Cardiol* 1994;26:675–682.
36. Narins KG, Jones ER, Townsend R, Goodkin DA, Shay RJ. Metabolic acid–base disorders: pathophysiology, classification, and treatment. In: Arieff AI, DeFronzo RA, eds. *Fluid, electrolyte, and acid-base disorders.* New York: Churchill Livingston, 1985; 281–309.
37. Baldwin KH, Cook DA, Cheadle WC. Enzyme alterations in neonatal heart muscle during development. *J Mol Cell Cardiol* 1977;9:651–660.
38. Peneksky ZJ. Perinatal development of cardiac contractile mechanisms. In: Gootman N, Gootman PM, eds. *Perinatal Cardiovascular Function.* New York: Marcel Dekker, 1983; 109–199.
39. Quantz M, Tchervenchov C, Chiu RJ. Unique responses of immature hearts to ischemia: functional recovery versus initiation of contracture. *J Thorac Cardiovasc Surg* 1992;103(5):927–935.
40. Koretsune Y, Marban E. Mechanism of ischemic contracture in ferret hearts: relative roles of $[Ca^{2+}]_i$ elevation and ATP depletion. *Am J Physiol* 1990;258:H9–H16.
41. Jennings RB, Hawkins HK, Lowe JE, Hill ML, Klotman S, Reimer SA. Relation between high energy phosphate and lethal injury in myocardial ischemia in the dog. *Am J Pathol* 1978;92:187–214.
42. Zugaib M, Forsythe AB, Nuwayhid B et al. Mechanisms of beat to beat variability in the heart rate of the neonatal lamb: II effects of hypoxia. *Am J Obstet Gynecol* 1980;138:453–458.

43. Covert RF, Drummond WH, Gimotty PA, Carter RL. Chloralose alters both basal hemodynamics and cardiovascular responses to alveolar hypoxia in chronically instrumented, spontaneously breathing lambs. *Pediatr Res* 1989;25:389–395.
44. Sidi D, Teitel DF, Kuipers JRG, Heymann MA, Rudolph AM. Effect of β-adrenergic receptor blockade on responses to acute hypoxemia in lambs. *Pediatr Res* 1988;23:229–234.
45. Rootwelt T, Loberg EM, Moen A, Oyasaeter S, Suagstad OD. Hypoxemia and reoxygenation with 21% or 100% oxygen in newborn pigs: changes in blood pressure, base deficit, and hypoxanthine and brain morphology. *Pediatr Res* 1992;32:107–113.
46. Torrance SM, Wittnich C. Neonatal hemodynamic responses to extreme ranges of controlled graded hypoxia. *Crit Care Med* 1996; 24(11) 1886–1892.
47. Hearse DJ. Hypothermia. In: Hearse DJ, Braimbridge MV, Jynge P, eds. *Protection of the ischemic myocardium: cardioplegia.* New York: Raven Press, 1981; 167–208.
48. Alexi-Meskhishvili VV, Nikoljuk AP, Churkin VM, Abdurachimov ZZ. Deep hypothermia with reduced flow rates for correction of ventricular septal defects in infants: an alternative approach. *Thorac Cardiovasc Surg* 1985;33:157–161.
49. Yamaguchii M, Imai M, Ohashi H, Hosokawa Y, Tachibana H, Ito H. Enhanced myocardial protection by systemic deep hypothermia in children undergoing total correction of tetralogy of Fallot. *Ann Thorac Surg* 1986;41:639–646.
50. Lamberti JJ Jr, Cohon LH, Laks H, Braunwald NS, Collins JJ Jr, Castaneda AR. Local cardiac hypothermia for myocardial protection during correction of congenital heart disease. *Ann Thorac Surg* 1975;20:446–455.
51. Litasova EE, Lomivorotov VN. Hypothermic protection (26–25°C) without perfusion cooling for surgery of congenital cardiac defects using prolonged occlusion. *Thorax* 1988;43:206–211.
52. Wittnich C, Vicente W, Salerno TA. Comparison of mild and deep hypothermia: do they provide similar protection in all neonatal hearts? *Can J Surg* 1991;34(4):317–321.
53. Wittnich C, Maitland A, Vicente W, Salerno TA. Not all neonatal hearts are equally protected from ischemic damage during hypothermia. *Ann Thorac Surg* 1991;52:1000–1004.
54. Balentine JD. *Pathology of Oxygen Toxicity.* New York: Academic Press, 1982.
55. Buckberg GD. Studies of hypoxemic/reoxygenation injury: I Linkage between cardiac function and oxidant damage. *J Thorac Cardiovasc Surg* 1995;110(4) part 2: 1164–1171.
56. Wittnich C, Carlyle CE. The effects of varying levels of hyperoxia on neonatal myocardial energy status and tolerance to global ischemia. 1997 (submitted).

The Developing Heart,
edited by Bohuslav Ošt'ádal
et al. Lippincott-Raven Publishers,
Philadelphia © 1997.

34

Influence of Taurine Treatment on Sodium Homeostasis in Developing Rats

*Rana M. Temsah and **Jack M. McBroom

**Institute of Cardiovascular Sciences, St. Boniface General Hospital Research Center, Winnipeg, Manitoba, Canada **Department of Physiology, Faculty of Medicine, Kuwait University, Kuwait*

Homeostasis is the ability to maintain a constant or a limited variable internal environment where the body volume and osmolality are kept within narrow ranges. This stability is sustained by the integration of neural, humoral, and local factors that manipulate the most two important factors, sodium (the major determinant of osmolality) and water homeostasis. A group of hormones is well known to be involved in the homeostatic mechanisms—antidiuretic hormone (vasopressin), renin–angiotensin–aldosterone system, and the atrial natriuretic factor (ANF) that was discovered by De Bold et al. (1), who have documented its diuretic and natriuretic effect. Many studies have been carried out to investigate the phenomenon of imbalances in sodium homeostasis in different species fed a variety of dietary sodium content, particularly with reference to atrial natriuretic peptide and the effects of synthetic atriopeptine III (sAP III) (2).

Regulation of osmolality and the extracellular fluid volume (ECFV) is a function of the kidney, with the osmolality of the ECF reflected mainly by the Na^+ concentration. Yet the plasma concentration of Na^+ is usually not affected as much by the Na^+ balance as by the water balance. However, the ECFV is dependent on the Na^+ balance, which is regulated by the kidneys (i.e., urinary Na^+ excretion constitutes more than 95% of the total Na^+ excretion). This interdependent relationship between volume and Na^+ concentration activates the regulatory mechanisms that maintain homeostasis in abnormal conditions (3). Body weight is an excellent indicator of Na^+ and water balance because an increase in Na^+ intake will be accompanied by an increase in water ingestion because of the plasma hyperosmolality. This combined intake will cause an increase in body weight (4).

It is well documented that rapidly growing organisms are always in a state of positive sodium balance and are generally less able to excrete a sodium load than adults (5). This would indicate that a developing kidney is able to conserve Na^+ efficiently. Grunet et al. (6) have reported that the Na^+ requirement of the rat for maximum growth rate is 0.05% (22 μEq/g) of the diet by weight. This requirement remained relatively constant throughout the 6-week growing period and was independent of the K^+ content within the limits of 0.25–1.0% K^+. Brensilver et al. (4) reported that adult rats receiving more sodium than the required amount for growth (247 ± 33 μEq/day) will continue to gain weight and to excrete the excess in urine. Adults receiving lower amounts than the daily requirement gained weight at a slower rate and remained in a positive Na^+ balance state.

Wistar Kayoto normotensive (WKY) rats offered a diet high in Na^+, after ingestion of a low-Na^+ diet, were able to maintain a positive Na^+ balance. No substantial elevation in blood pressure was recorded in this group because of the high salt intake (7). Adult WKY fed a normal Na^+ diet followed by a high-Na^+ diet showed an increase in their water consumption and urine volume. Moreover, their fractional urinary Na^+ excretion increased because of the increased Na^+ intake (8). In spite of the different dietary sodium content introduced to the rats, all were able to maintain positive Na^+ balance values.

It has also been reported (9) that two levels of high-sodium diet (1.44% and 4%) could cause further cardiac enlargement in the genetically hypertensive (SHR) adult rats with moderate increases in mean arterial pressure and total peripheral resistance. These changes were consort with decreased heart rate and organ blood flows to the heart, kidneys, and splanchnic area. On the other hand, the 4% sodium diet caused an increased cardiac mass in normotensive WKY rats without any hemodynamic changes, suggesting that dietary sodium intake plays an important role in the pathogenesis of cardiac hypertrophy.

Similar studies have been carried out on Wistar rats (Table 34–1), and it has been shown that high-sodium diet treatment has no effect on hemodynamic or sympathetic neuronal activity, while it has a trophic effect. Left ventricular mass was significantly increased in young rats, an effect that was not detected in older rats. Furthermore, a moderately high- (2% NaCl) and a high-sodium diet had no effect on blood pressure at any age (10). This study also showed that food sodium can cause significant left ventricular hypertrophy, depending upon the strain and age of the rats independent of cardiac volume or pressure overload.

On the other hand, by studying the effect of intracerebroventricular loading of hypertonic sodium on blood pressure, water and sodium balance in rats, it was

TABLE 34–1. *Effects of dietary sodium on cardiac anatomy, MAP, TPRI, and cardiac index in normotensive Wistar rats of different ages.*[a]

	4–8 wk of age (n = 9)		9–13 wk of age (n = 9)		26–30 wk of age (n = 8)	
Measured parameters	0.6% NaCl	8% NaCl	0.6% NaCl	8% NaCl	0.6% NaCl	8% NaCl
LV dry wt, mg/100 g body wt	51 ± 2	59 ± 2*	45 ± 1	49 ± 1*	43 ± 2	44 ± 1
RV dry wt, mg/100 g body wt	13 ± 0.5	14 ± 0.4	11 ± 0.5	12 ± 0.4	7 ± 0.6	7 ± 0.4
MAP, mmHg	107 ± 3	107 ± 3	102 ± 2	105 ± 3	108 ± 3	109 ± 5
TPRI, mmHg ml^{-1} min^{-1} kg^{-1}	0.31 ± 0.02	0.30 ± 0.01	0.32 ± 0.01	0.34 ± 0.02	–	–
Cardiac index, ml^{-1} min^{-1} kg^{-1}	329 ± 11	357 ± 9	338 ± 8	318 ± 15	–	–

[a]Values are means ± SE; n = no. of rats used in each diet. LV, left ventricular; RV, right ventricular; MAP, mean arterial pressure; TPRI, total peripheral resistance index. *$p < 0.05$ vs 0.6% NaCl (10).

found that blood pressure was elevated accompanied by increased plasma catecholamine with no changes in the vasopressin content. This suggests the role of the sympathetic nervous system in developed hypertension (11). It is also demonstrated that this treatment caused a positive water balance while sodium balance was negative. Therefore, in sodium loading, the central nervous system and the renal response may be critical in developing and maintaining salt-induced hypertension.

In general, developing animals will always try to maintain their internal homeostatic balance as a growth requirement, even if they receive different dietary sodium contents. The regulatory responses will involve the neuronal, hormonal, renal, and cardiac interferences.

TAURINE AND ITS POSSIBLE HOMEOSTATIC ROLE

Taurine, 2-aminoethanesulfonic acid (NH^+_3-CH_2-CH_2-SO_3^-), is the most abundant intracellular free amino acid present in mammalian tissue, especially in the sarcoplasm of heart cells. It can arise by the decarboxylation of cysteic acid and/or the oxidation of hypotaurine (cysteine sulfonic acid) (12). Spaeth and Schneider (13) have studied taurine and its distribution in different tissues of the rat and have recorded the following: 20.4 μmol/g in the heart, 7.1 μmol/g in the kidney, and 5 μmol/g in the brain. Urinary taurine was reported to equal 15.8 ± 2.0 μmol 100 g^{-1} 12 hr^{-1} (14) while plasma taurine level was 29.1 ± 5.9 μmol/L (15). Taurine is metabolized very slowly and is not incorporated into protein synthesis. It is also well known that the total body pools of taurine (as in brain) are controlled by the kidney (16). Therefore, an excess of body taurine will be excreted in urine, while a deficiency in the diet will stimulate the kidney to conserve it by increasing reabsorption (17).

There is a growing body of evidence that taurine has a major role in cellular osmoregulatory in different tissues: brain (15), neurons and glial cells (18). Oral taurine treatment could normalize the blood pressure of SHR (19–21). In addition, it also inhibited renin-induced salt appetite but not water intake. This suggested that an intrinsic brain system activated by renin administration into the preoptic area in the brain is attenuated by oral taurine treatment (20). Fujita and Sato (22) observed this antihypotensive effect of taurine in uninephrectomized DOCA–salt hypertensive rats receiving 1% NaCl solution.

It is well cited in the literature that the uptake of taurine by the heart and kidney is sodium dependent (23). Zelikovic et al. (24) have suggested that sodium–taurine cotransport in the rat kidney is Cl^-/Br^- dependent and that the transport mechanism most probably occurs through a $2Na^+$:1taurine:$1Cl^-$/Br^- carrier complex. Recently, the cDNA encoding of the Na^+- and Cl^--dependent taurine transporter has been isolated (25) from the renal medulla and Madin-Darby canine kidney (MDCK) cells, and the sequence is found to correspond to a protein of 655 amino acids. The mRNA for the transporter was present in renal cortex and medulla, ileal mucosa, brain, liver, and heart, in descending order. Furthermore, the abundance of mRNA for the taurine transporter is increased in cells cultured in hypertonic medium, suggesting that regulation of transport activity by medium hypertonicity occurs at the level of mRNA accumulation.

In the heart, studies have indicated the increased intracellular sodium concentration, or decreased concentration extracellularly, would cause the development of a concentration gradient that would cause the efflux of taurine from the heart cells. Moreover, increased plasma taurine concentration will lead to increased cotransport of both sodium and taurine intracellularly, which in turn will increase both the release of calcium ions from the sarcoplasmic reticulum and the sensitivity of the contractile proteins (26). It was also concluded that the cotransport will be in either direction across the cell membrane of mammalian ventricular myocytes.

Studies have also been made to investigate the effect of taurine on the cardiovascular system, especially on ion movement. It is now known that taurine can play a protective cardiovascular role by regulating intracellular calcium concentration through calcium channel modulation (27) and by altering the potassium rectifying current to induce action potential modulation (28). Furthermore, it is suggested that taurine may also have an inhibitory effect on the sodium current, which would protect the heart muscles by antiarrhythmic action and would decrease the intracellular calcium concentration through the Na^{+}-Ca^{2+} exchanger. In general, taurine would act on the transport system and ion channels in a manner to keep the intracellular calcium concentration level relatively constant and to maintain the cell viability (29).

Frequent reports have been published about the effect of intracellularly raised taurine concentration in the perfusion solution and the culture media used in myocyte isolation or storage of enzymatically isolated myocytes, in affecting their sensitivity to calcium depletion and repletion. These observations were supported recently by isolating 70–90% rod-shaped myocytes from guinea pig hearts perfused with taurine containing Tyrode when compared to the 50–80% obtained in the absence of taurine (30). In the same study an induced rise of taurine in the sarcoplasm, produced either during cell isolation or via diffusion from the solution in a microelectrode, was accompanied by a fall in intracellular sodium activity. These data are consistent with the presence of a Na^{+}:taurine symport, which is activated to cause efflux of both ions when either rises above its physiologic level.

Great interest was given to studying the effect of dietary taurine when included in diets containing different concentrations of salt. Meldrum et al. (21) have reported that low- and high-taurine diet caused an increase in urine volume and fluid intake in SHR with decreased blood pressure, whereas there was no difference in sodium excretion as compared to controls. Calcium has shown an interesting pattern as its urinary excretion increased after the first week of treatment. Moreover, taurine concentration was elevated in the kidney, skeletal muscle, serum, and brain tissue. On the other hand, long-term administration of high-taurine content in a high-salt diet supplied to Dahl-sensitive rats retarded the development of salt-induced hypertension and myocardial hypertrophy. This effect is induced by the inhibitory effect of taurine on the sympathetic system as suggested by the reduced pulse rate. Another mechanism may be involved in this effect: activated renal kallikrein (31). These results point at the protective role of taurine on the renal and cardiovascular system.

In a trial to study the osmoregulatory response of the kidney due to infusion with a hypertonic solution of saline for a 2-day period (32), a concentration gradient of taurine in the renal tissue increasing monotonically from the cortex to the inner medulla has been demonstrated. This suggests that taurine content is highly osmoregulated by hyperosmolality. In these animals, sodium concentration and osmolality in urine and serum were significantly higher in salt-loaded rats when compared to the hydrated ones. This is in accordance with the nature of taurine as a compatible organic osmolyte that is present intracellularly. That is, its accumulation is controlled by uptake from extracellular fluid and dissipation is mediated by rapid efflux of osmolytes from the cells (33).

Dlouha and McBroom (34) studied cardiomyopathic hamsters that were challenged with taurine solution, and showed that they developed moderate hypernatremia. The same result was found in a similar group drinking 0.6% NaCl (S) solution. Assay rats treated with the atrial extracts from hamsters of these two drinking groups showed a natriuretic and diuretic response. Moderate hypernatremia produced by oral intake of 1.8% NaCl in adult rats was reported by Dlouha and Krecek (35). Injection with adult or prepubertal atrial extract was not able to suppress hypernatremia, while the animals responded by increasing the renal excretory activity. The study of Dlouha and Krecek (36) on adult intact rats has shown that the ingestion of 1.8% NaCl or a combined solution of 0.1 M T + 1.8% NaCl caused higher mortality rates and hypernatremia in the T + S treatment group. On the other hand, decreasing the taurine concentration (0.01 M) in the combined drinking solution caused only a moderate rise in plasma Na^+ as compared with the group drinking 0.1 M T + 1.8% NaCl. When animals drinking the combined solution (0.1 M T + 1.8% NaCl) were challenged with atrial extract, a decreased natriuretic and diuretic response in comparison with the controls was seen. This suggested that drinking taurine might interfere with the ANF regulatory action. As the ANP caused diuresis and natriuresis in animals drinking T + S, it is possible that it may be associated with altered Na^+ balance in this treatment.

Al-Kady (37) recorded plasma and blood volume expansion in adult rats receiving 0.3 M S or 0.1 M T + 0.3 M S, but not in weanlings. On the other hand, weanlings drinking either solution had an increase in plasma sodium (2,37). This increase was recorded in adults drinking the combined solution only. Though hypernatremia developed in both age groups receiving T + S, weanling rats were found to suffer a more rapid development of severe hypernatremia and earlier mortality than the adults (2,37). This response occurred faster in weanlings than in adults and was accompanied by an augmented fluid intake and urine output with depressed feeding and an increase in right and left atrial immunoreactive AP III. Those drinking the same concentration of taurine alone or saline alone suffered no serious ill effects (2).

From the preceding information, it is clear that the amino acid, taurine, plays an important role in cellular osmoregulation because it is involved in ion movement in different tissues. It also has a protective role at the renal and cardiovascular levels in regulating the distribution of excess ions (mainly sodium), manipulating currents (calcium and potassium), and affecting the homeostatic mechanisms.

ROLE OF ATRIAL NATRIURETIC PEPTIDE IN SODIUM BALANCE

De Bold et al. (1) first discovered the natriuretic and diuretic effect of the extract of atrial muscle homogenates. Their findings showed a marked increase in urinary sodium concentration and urine volume. These observations paralleled the decrease in blood pressure induced by the associated atrial extracts and an increased haematocrit value. This effect was caused by a polypeptide stored in the secretory granules of atrial myocytes (38) and was found to play an important role in regulating salt and water balance (1,39) in response to volume expansion (40), atrial distension (41), and chronic sodium loading (42).

Different studies have focused on synthetic atriopeptine III (sAP III) and its effects on the imbalances of Na^+ homeostasis in different species. Borenstein et al. (43) studied the renal hemodynamic changes produced by atrial extracts. They found that the atrial extract caused a significant increase in the total and medullary renal blood flow. Many investigations have concentrated on the renal responses to ANF. For example, Cogan (44) was able to show that ANF caused a significant rise in the urine excretion primarily by increasing the glomerular filtration rate (GFR) in the single nephron and in the whole kidney.

The natriuretic response was further confirmed by Sonnenberg et al. (45) when an infusion of AP II was associated with an increase of Na^+ delivery to the medullary collecting ducts and reduced fractional Na^+ reabsorption in the duct. It was found that ANP not only has a direct inhibitory action on Na^+ reabsorption, but also indirectly acts on the inhibition of aldosterone production from the zona glomerulosa (46). Intracerebroventricular administration of ANP in rats was adequate to decrease their sympathetic outflow, heart rate, and arterial pressure (47). These responses were similar to the inhibitory effects evoked by systemic administration of the peptide, but each may have a special mechanism to induce its effect.

The volume homeostatic role of ANP in newborn infants was reported by Bierd et al. (48). It was speculated that plasma ANP concentration is elevated in response to an expanded extracellular volume state in the period of adaptation from intrauterine to extrauterine life. This is accompanied by an increase in the atrial size and total body fluids. The ANP level will decrease after 3 days of age accompanied by isotonic volume contraction reflected by decreasing body weight and atrial size. Furthermore, cGMP, the second messenger and biological marker of ANP activity, will decrease with diminished diuretic response.

Muchant et al. (49) have recorded a significant increase of atrial pro-ANP and ANP content and decreased basal plasma ANP concentration resulting from increased dietary sodium intake in preweaned rat pups, whereas these changes were not detected after similar dietary sodium manipulation in adult rats. Furthermore, increased sodium intake caused no changes in cardiac ANP mRNA levels in both age groups. These results suggest that the changes that occurred in weanlings are due to alterations in storage or release of the peptide rather than to changes in protein transcription. In the same lab (50), it was found that plasma ANP levels were higher in the preweaned rats than in adults postexpansion with saline (1% body weight), regardless of dietary sodium content, although the natriuretic response was more greatly augmented in adults. Furthermore, neonatal compensation to increased sodium intake is incomplete, as plasma sodium continued to elevate during the period of the experiment independently of plasma ANP. The dietary sodium intake had no effect on the hemodynamic factors (Table 34–2) when these factors showed an inclining pattern with age. Therefore, the lack of effect of sodium in diet suggests that the adaptive response is renal maturation dependent.

In mature Wistar rats fed a high-sodium diet, plasma ANF concentration increased from 69 ± 52 pg/ml before starting the treatment to 95 ± 32 pg/ml in the first day of the treatment, which then declined again to a normal level (51). This study suggests that 1 day on a diet high in sodium is considered a sufficient stimulus to increase the release of atrial ANF into circulation. It was also recognized that right and left atrial ANF concentration increases with age and more so in the right atria. High-salt treatment increased the plasma ANF levels in older rats as compared to their controls or younger rats. Also, this treatment decreased the left atrial content of ANF, but not the right atria, and the ANF content was lower in the older rats than their controls.

ANP clearance was also found to be age related (52). Throughout life, two mechanisms are responsible for modulating the plasma ANP level in circulation: one is the C-receptors (in glomerulus and proximal tubules), the other is the neutral endopeptidase (in glomerulus). It was found that the C-receptor activity decreases with age from 18 days to adulthood, contributing in part to decreased systemic clearance of ANP. The endopeptidase pathway was recorded to contribute in the regulation of plasma ANP levels and urinary cGMP (the second messenger) excretion within physiologic concentrations. Furthermore, this study has proven that each pathway compensates for the other in case of blocking. Therefore, limited diuretic and natriuretic response after acute volume expansion in early days of life may be at least in part due to enhanced activity of C-receptors, impaired signal transduction, or altered processing of cGMP.

TABLE 34–2. *Effect of high dietary sodium on hemodynamic factors in Sprague-Dawley rats (preweaned and adults)*[a]

	7 day-old (preweaned)		7–8 wk old (adults)	
Measured parameters	Control	145 mEq Na/L	Control	145 mEq Na/L
MAP (mmHg)	59 ± 2*	56 ± 2*	139 ± 4	140 ± 4
HR (Beat/min)	329 ± 8*	300 ± 13*	381 ± 16	393 ± 13

[a]Values are means ± SE; MAP, mean arterial pressure; HR, heart rate. *$p < 0.05$ vs adult groups, same treatment (50).

Out of the previously mentioned background, we found it important to study the effect of dietary taurine in a hypertonic solution on the body homeostasis. As a second objective, it was also interesting to detect the homeostatic responses of the developing animals in the designed model of our study.

MATERIALS AND METHODS

Animals

Two age groups of Wistar rats of both sexes were used: adults (65–85 days old) weighing 170–390 g and weanlings (28–32 days old) weighing 58–160 g. Animals were housed under automatically controlled conditions of temperature (20–22°C), humidity (50–60%) and a 12-hr light/dark cycle. Each animal was located in a separate metabolic cage as per the specificity of the study.

Diet

All animals were fed, *ad libitum,* powdered rat chow (Pillsbury's LTD, Birmingham, UK) containing 0.51% (w/w) sodium (Na^+) that was checked during the experiment to maximize the accuracy of the balance study.

Experimental Protocol

Animals representing the two age groups were housed in the metabolic cages for 10 days (day −2 to day 8). Tapwater was provided to all the groups for the first 2 days so that the animals could adapt to this new environment (53). From day 0 each age group was divided into four treatment groups, with each group comprising 10 rats, that were given, *ad libitum:* (C) Control, water; (T) 0.1 M taurine (T-Fluka Chemie AG, CH-9470 Buchs); (S) 1.5% sodium chloride (sodium chloride, crystal - 'Baker analyzed' reagent); or (T+S) 0.1 M taurine + 1.5% saline until day 8 (final day in the cage). The treatment solutions were prepared using distilled water, where no appreciable amounts of Na^+ were detected. Daily solution consumption and therefore Na^+ intake in the solution were measured and calculated. The solutions used were chosen according to a study performed in the laboratory (54). Measurements of body weight (Bwt), solution consumption, food consumption, and urine volume were taken daily, whereas blood samples were collected for analysis on alternate days.

Blood Analysis

A volume of blood, collected from the tail, was drawn to fill three microhematocrit tubes (68 μl/tube) to centrifuge and collect the plasma. Plasma Na^+ concentration (P_{Na}) (mmol/L) was measured using a flame photometer with a lithium internal standard (Corning 435/455 Flame Photometer with Diluter, CME). Plasma analysis during the balance study was too small for duplicate measurements. If more samples were taken, the animal may have experienced hemodynamic changes that could interfere with the experimental aims.

Urine Analysis

Urine was collected daily and two analytical determinations were made, in duplicate: urinary sodium concentration (U_{Na}) (mmol/L) measured by a flame photometer, and urine osmolality (U_{Osm}) measured by a cryoscopic osmometer (Advanced Digi Matic Osmometer Model 3D2, Needham Heights, MA 02144, USA). Daily urine output and urinary Na^+ excretion were determined. Preliminary measurements have shown that sodium excreted in feces is negligible when compared to urinary sodium; therefore, the decision was made to consider the urinary Na^+ content only.

Balance Studies

From the measurement of total Na intake (in solution and diet), Na^+ output (in urine), and total solution consumption and urine volume, the following balance studies were performed: Na^+-balance and visible water balance (55). A high degree of accuracy and uniformity in the balance determination was ensured by the feeding technique and collection procedure.

Mortality Study

Mortality rates were monitored for all groups continued on the same treatment solutions for 2 months following the beginning of the regime. During the first month after removal from the metabolic cages, weekly recordings of Bwt and P_{Na} were measured. For this part of the study, the animals were kept in individual conventional cages and were checked for mortality on alternate days for the remaining month (to day 64).

Statistical Analysis

The Biomedical Data Statistical Package (BMDP) was used to perform the univariate and simple effects analysis of variance (4V) with grouping factor for repeated measures designed experiments (56). For more detailed analysis, the Statistical Package for Social Sciences-X (SPSSX) was used. In some of the measured parameters, the Mann-Whitney analysis of variance test was used to detect the differences between each pair of treatment groups on each day of the regime. Moreover, the statistical tests were also performed to detect the effect of age on the animal's response to each treatment solution. Paired comparison between T and S was excluded from the fulfilled analysis, since the difference between the two groups will not serve our aims. If no comparison is mentioned between the C and T groups, it will be considered an indication of similar responses. The threshold for statistical significance was $p < 0.05$, which indicates a confidence limit larger than 95%. Sigmaplot V3.10 program was used for plotting the graphs in which mean values were used with the standard errors (SE).

RESULTS

Sodium Balance Study

In Fig. 34–1A weanling S drinkers showed a higher level of P_{Na} than in the C and T groups ($p < 0.05$); and the T + S group showed an even higher increase than the other three groups ($p < 0.001$). It is clear that in the adult groups (Fig. 34–1B), the only significant difference was the increased pattern in the P_{Na} level in the group receiving T + S solution when compared to the other three treatment groups starting from day 4 of the treatment ($p < 0.001$). S drinkers have shown a transient drop in their P_{Na} on day 4 ($p < 0.05$) when compared to the adults and then leveled back to the normal value. Besides, weanlings receiving S or T + S have shown higher levels as compared to their adult counterparts.

Total sodium intake in the two age and four treatment groups was calculated. As expected (Fig. 34–2 A and B), the S drinkers in both groups were consuming more sodium when compared with the C drinkers ($p < 0.01$ in weanlings; $p < 0.001$ in adults). The T + S group in general was consuming even more Na^+ than the S group. They have shown a significant difference ($p < 0.001$) when compared to the other three treatment groups in weanlings, whereas in adult groups, the increased total intake was remarkable versus C, T ($p < 0.001$) and versus S ($p < 0.05$). T + S solution was the only treatment that caused a difference in the response of the compared groups due to age, as the weanlings were consuming relatively more sodium than their adult counterparts.

Sodium excretion rates are presented in (Fig. 34–3A and B). It is obvious that the S and T + S drinkers show increased rates that are more pronounced in the T + S in both age groups. This increased excretion is highly significant when S drinkers were compared to C ($p < 0.001$) and T + S to the C and T ($p < 0.001$) groups. When comparing T + S versus S, a notable increase in sodium excretion rate was also recorded in weanlings ($p < 0.01$) and adults ($p < 0.05$). Moreover, only the T + S drinkers showed an age-dependent relationship; the weanlings displayed a higher sodium excretion rate than adults.

Sodium balance was calculated after the total sodium intake and output were determined. From Fig. 34–4A and B, it is obvious that the C, T, and S drinkers were keeping a state of positive sodium balance in both age groups that was even significantly higher in S drinkers ($p < 0.05$ versus C). Contrarily, T + S drinkers devel-

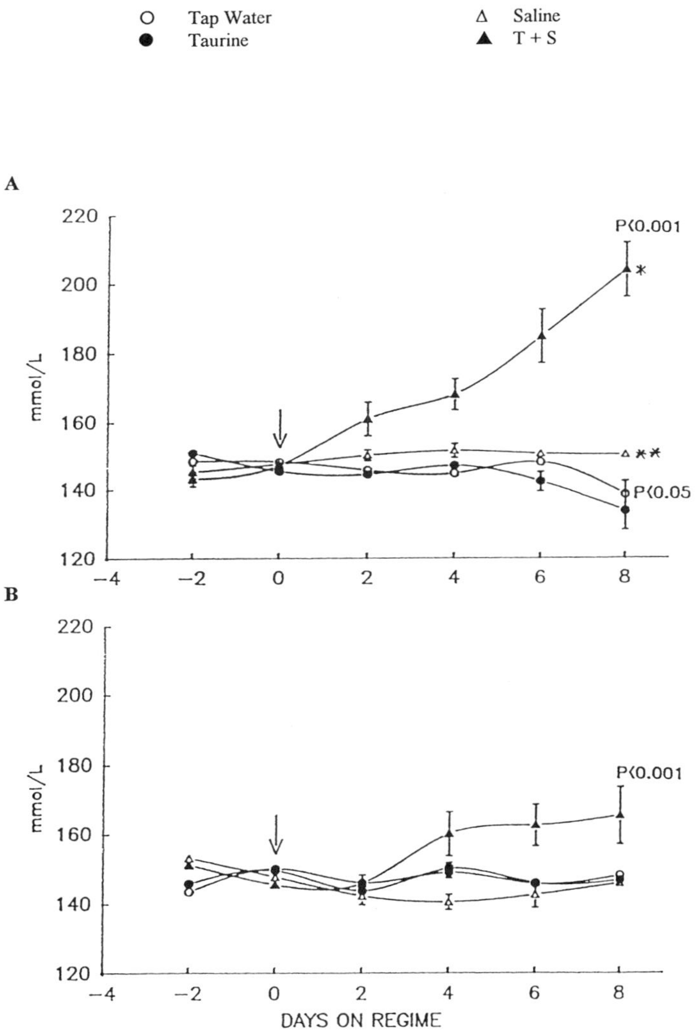

FIG. 34–1. Plasma sodium concentration in (**A**) weanling and (**B**) adult rats receiving the four treatment regimes (mean ± SE). *p* values show the statistical changes during the treatment period in each group. (Groups with no *p* values indicate no significant changes.) Some SE bars are not seen because of their very small values. * $p < 0.05$ and ** $p < 0.001$ vs adults. ↓ = Starting the regime.

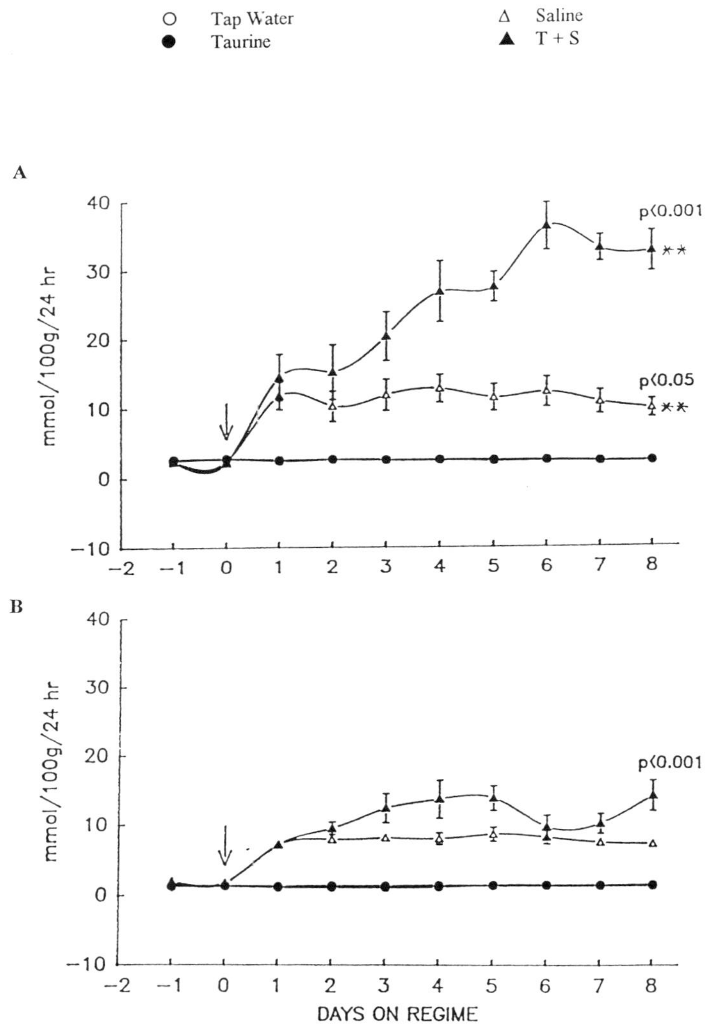

FIG. 34–2. Total sodium consumption in (**A**) weanling and (**B**) adult rats receiving the four treatment regimes (mean ± SE). Water and taurine plots are superimposed. Indications of statistical comparisons are the same as in Fig. 34–1. ↓ = Starting the regime.

oped a state of negative sodium balance. Weanlings had a fluctuating state between negative and positive as the homeostatic mechanism failed at the end to maintain a positive balance. The fluctuation clearly started from the second day of the treatment. The magnified difference was recorded when T + S were compared to the C ($p < 0.001$) where it was also high as compared to C and T ($p < 0.05$). Adults were trying to maintain in the positive range when, as speculated, their homeostatic mechanisms deteriorated starting from the fifth day until the end of the treatment

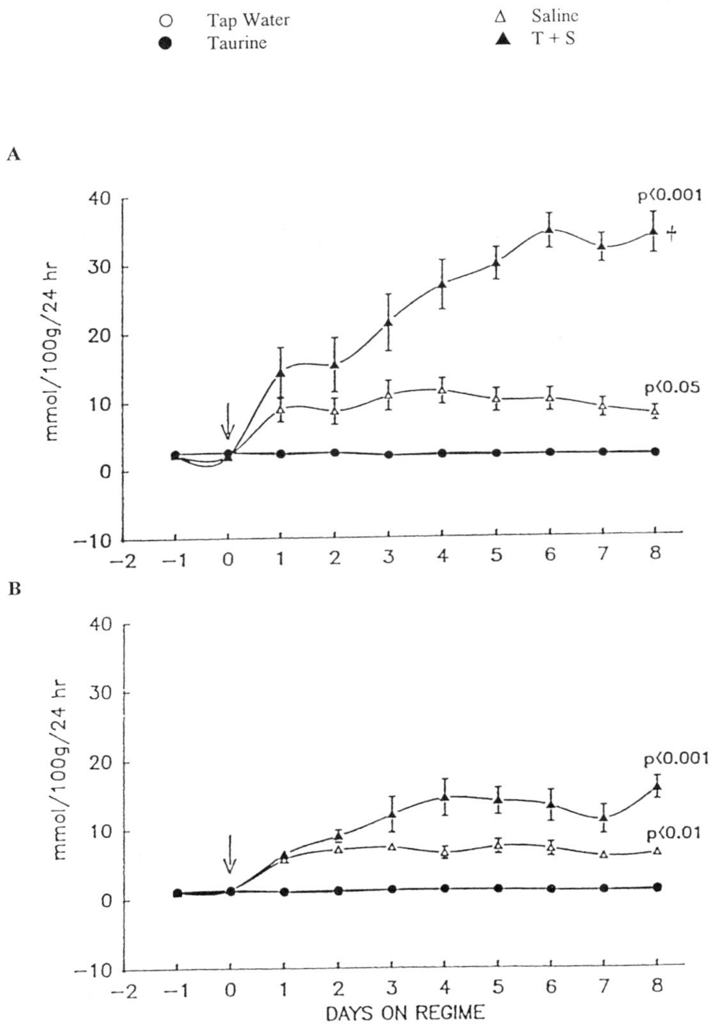

FIG. 34–3. Sodium excretion rate in (**A**) weanling and (**B**) adult rats receiving the four treatment regimes (mean ± SE). Indications of statistical comparisons are the same as in Fig. 34–1. †$p < 0.01$ vs adults. ↓ = Starting the regime.

period. The T + S drinkers have shown the highest drop in their Na^- balance level at day 6 as compared to the other groups ($p < 0.05$). This difference was maintained until the end of the treatment period as compared to the S ($p < 0.05$) but was significant only at days 6 and 8 when compared to C ($p < 0.05$). None of the studied treatment groups showed any age-related differences.

Since water is the second parameter that is vital in maintaining homeostasis, it was crucial to study the visible water balance. Figures 34–5A and B show that all

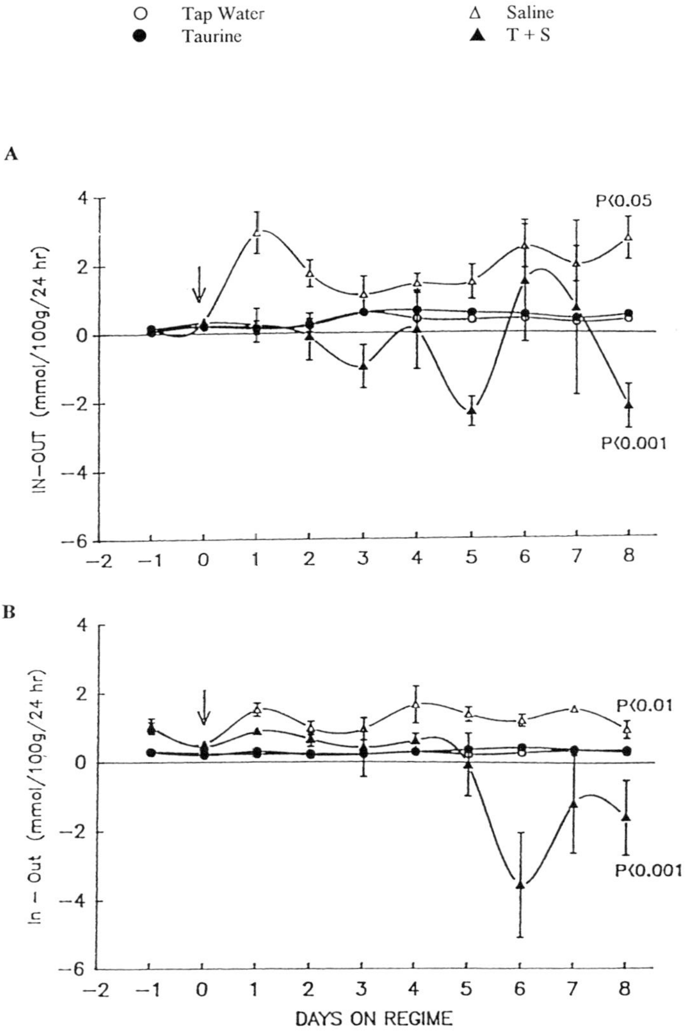

FIG. 34–4. Sodium balance in (**A**) weanling and (**B**) adult rats receiving the four treatment regimes (mean ± SE). Indications of statistical comparisons are the same as in Fig. 34–1. ↓ = Starting the regime.

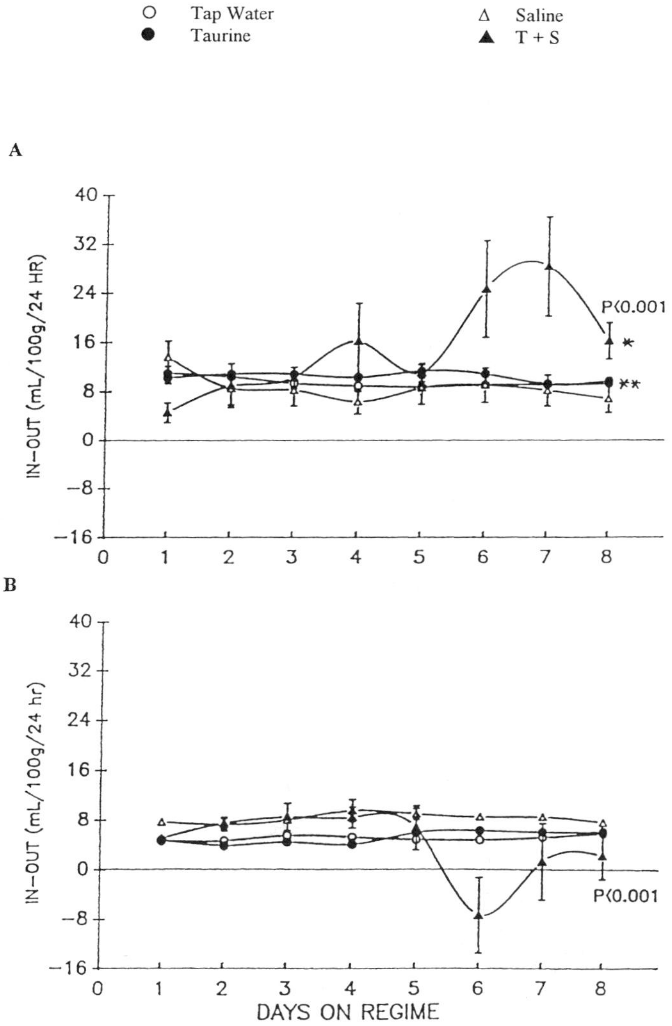

FIG. 34–5. Visible water balance in (**A**) weanling and (**B**) adult rats receiving the four treatment regimes (mean ± SE). Indications of statistical comparisons are the same as in Fig. 34–1. ↓ = Starting the regime.

age and treatment groups were able to maintain their water balance, although the T + S adults showed some variation in their response toward the end of the treatment period. Adult S drinkers showed significantly higher water balance values than did the C group ($p < 0.001$), whereas no differences were reported between the weanlings of these groups. Interestingly, adult T + S drinkers were able to conserve more water during the first period of the treatment. On days 2 and 4, their water balance was significantly higher as compared to C ($p < 0.01$). It was also higher on days 2, 3 ($p < 0.05$), and 4 ($p < 0.01$) as compared to T. For some reason, on day 6 they lost more water when compared to the other three groups ($p < 0.05$), and they then tried again to conserve their water balance till the end of the treatment period. Adults drinking C, T, or T + S displayed lower water balance values as compared to the weanlings.

Mortality Study

For the adult group, the C and S drinkers managed to survive until the end of the second month (day 64). Only one of the T-drinking animals died on day 6 of the sodium balance study. However, animals receiving T + S showed an increase in their mortality rate, starting from day 7 until the end of the next month, with 10% survival. Weanlings drinking C, T, or S have recorded 100% survival rate until day 64, whereas the animals started to die at day 6 in the T + S drinkers and the mortality continued drastically throughout the period of the study.

Growth rate was recorded to be increasing in adults drinking either C, T, or S, whereas the T + S group was losing weight. S adults gained more weight than the C drinkers of the same age ($p < 0.001$). Weanlings, on the other hand, drinking C, T, or S showed an increase in their body weight while the T + S drinkers lost weight. Moreover, S drinkers had lower values when compared to controls ($p < 0.05$). Age was an important factor affecting the change in body weight. Only in the C ($p < 0.001$) and T ($p < 0.01$) drinkers did the weanlings drinking either solution record higher growth rate than the adults.

For the P_{Na} measurement during the mortality period, at day 64 in adults the records were (mmol/L) as follows: 138.7 ± 3.44 (C), 136.0 ± 1.18 (T), 146.2 ± 2.64 (S), and 162 (T + S) as they ended with one animal (no SE). In the weanlings the records were 147.7 ± 1.55 (C), 149.4 ± 3.38 (T), and 147.4 ± 1.11 (S), where none of the T + S survived. In general, only S drinkers ($p < 0.001$ in adults and $p < 0.01$ in weanlings) displayed different patterns of response as compared to the C drinkers. Weanlings drinking T were the only group that showed a difference in their trend of response ($p < 0.01$). Taking age into consideration, no significant differences were recorded in the four treatment groups.

DISCUSSION

Many studies have been done in an attempt to determine the role of taurine in the body as an osmoregulator (15) and as a hypotensive agent (19,20,22). It was reported that a combined drinking solution of taurine plus saline caused hypernatremia in rats (2,35,37) that was much more pronounced in the weanlings (37). The concentrations of the combined solution used was 0.1 M T + 1.8% S. Previous studies performed in our laboratory (54) have shown that lower concentrations of sodium in the combined solution caused fewer adverse effects. It was therefore decided to study the effect of this combined solution of 0.1 M taurine plus 1.5% saline on the sodium balance in both adult and weanling rats.

In this study, 0.1 M taurine-drinking animals appeared healthy and responded in a normal manner, when compared to the control group, as taurine had no effect on either the growth rate or the solution consumption. This similarity in response was found in both age groups, which was consistent with the results reported in other studies (2,17,19) even when high taurine concentration was used for spontaneously hypertensive rats (21).

The adult drinkers that received a hypertonic saline solution developed an increased plasma osmolality. This would activate the first defense mechanisms: first, to shift water from the cells to the extracellular fluid to maintain the osmotic balance; second, to activate the thirst center continuously, which caused a repeated intake of the provided solution (i.e., hypertonic saline); and third, to release vasopressin (57). Therefore, the increased intake caused plasma expansion (37,58) from the first day of the treatment, which would stretch the atria, providing a sufficient stimulus for releasing ANP into the circulation (51). This peptide stimulates the kidneys to respond to diuresis (increased UV) and natriuresis (increased $U_{Na} \times UV$), because of inhibition of vasopressin (59,60) and aldosterone (46), respectively. This combined effect results in a more diluted urine (decreased U_{Osm}).

In the radioimmunoassay study of ANP (iAP III) in adult rats drinking saline (2), it was reported that after 4 days of saline treatment, the serum iAP III concentration was not changed from that of the normal rats. Agreeable results (51) were reported to show that the plasma levels of ANP will start to drop after day 1, even by maintaining the same treatment. The increased diuretic effect recorded in this study caused a further rise in the plasma osmolality, which again stimulated the thirst center and caused the animals to drink more of the solution and to release vasopressin to reabsorb water. As a result, plasma sodium concentration was kept constant and normal.

Because the animals drinking the hypertonic saline solution were ingesting the same amount of food as the controls, and drinking more (2–3X C), the excess amount of solution and salt consumed may be reflected by an increase in their body weight (Data not shown.) The activated mechanisms shifted the body homeostatic level and the animals displayed high water balance values. Moreover, the saline-drinking animals showed a positive and high steady state of sodium balance level, proposing that the regulatory mechanisms responsible for maintaining the stability of the body composition of electrolytes (mainly sodium) were not affected by the treatment. This suggested that the challenge with the saline solution probably would release ANP during a short period of time to adapt to the stress and then the ANP level will return to its normal concentration. During this time course the animals were able to shift to a new level of homeostasis.

The kidneys of the 1.5% saline adult drinkers showed an increased ability to deal with this sodium load efficiently as they were able to excrete the excess Na^+ in their urine (2X C) with a reduced osmolality of 20–30% as compared to controls. Even during the mortality period study, the animals continued to gain weight and survived at the same rate as the controls. The ability of the kidney to deal with a similar excess sodium intake and to display a positive sodium balance was previously reported by Lundin et al. (8).

Weanlings drinking 1.5% saline increased the amount of their solution consumption resulting from increased osmolality of the plasma. This condition may well have caused the stimulation of the thirst center in an attempt to dilute the plasma, which might cause a transient plasma volume expansion. Stretching of the atria would release ANP (50), thus causing diuresis and natriuresis.

It is well documented that the kidneys of young rats reach their functional maturity by the age of 41 days (61,62). Therefore, the kidneys of the weanlings (28–32 days old) have a limited ability to retain water and sodium from the filtrate. This explains the high renal response of their kidneys (increased UV, U_{Na}, and decreased osmolality) to a level that was not different from that of the adults. Different results were reported by Muchant et al. (50) as the animals used in their experiment were preweaned (7 days old); that is, they are less mature and are less efficient dealing with the induced experimental conditions. Strain may be another factor that could rule out the differences reported (10). Since the diuretic response to ANP was higher than the natriuretic response, no water retention could occur and plasma sodium concentration probably increased with no plasma volume expansion. This inability to develop plasma volume expansion was previously reported in weanlings receiving 1.8% saline (37). Developed hypernatremia will overactivate the thirst center so that the animals drink more and dilute the plasma. Since the third mechanism was the main compensatory maneuver, the animals drank as much as their adult counterparts.

In young rats, as the amounts of sodium offered were greater than the sodium requirement for maximum growth rate (4), the animals continued to gain weight. We suppose that consumed sodium could be utilized for growth purposes and that it would attract water into the cells to maintain the osmotic equilibrium. Therefore, salt and water utilized for growth shifted the sodium–water balance values to a high and steady level similar to the level displayed by the adults.

During the mortality period, weanlings receiving saline continued to gain weight. At the end of the sodium-balance study (starting the mortality period), the kidneys of the weanlings are functionally mature. Therefore, they would function more efficiently to maintain the stability of the plasma osmolality. This could be achieved by water reabsorption from the renal tubules that would participate in diluting plasma and therefore return the plasma sodium concentration back to normal. These animals also survived to the end of the mortality study period.

Taurine administered alone in the solution, whether to adults or weanlings, showed no ill effects. Whenever it was combined with salt, it increased the mortality rate. In our study, taurine plus saline caused a dramatic increase in the plasma sodium concentration in the weanlings and earlier deaths than in the adults. This is in accordance with previous studies (2,36,37).

Adults receiving taurine plus saline were able to respond to the stress induced by the solution directly after 24 hours. The ingested solution contained 1.5% saline and raised the plasma osmolality, which activated the regulatory mechanisms responsible for maintaining the osmotic balance. This in turn may well cause plasma volume expansion, which would stretch the atria to release ANP, stimulating the kidney to respond by diuresis and natriuresis to excrete the excess load of salt and water. In spite of the activated regulatory mechanisms, the taurine plus saline drinkers displayed higher positive sodium balance (not significant) and higher positive water balance values than the controls (during the first period of the experiment).

The response of the taurine plus saline group is due to the special handling of the taurine by the body. It is well documented that the taurine transport is mediated by a saturable sodium-dependent system in different organs of the body. This transport mechanism is present across the renal brush-border membrane (24), suggesting the release of sodium out into the interstitium through the Na^+–K^+–ATPase pump. Taurine was also documented to accumulate in the intestinal mucosal membrane (63) stimulated by the presence of Na^+ extracellularly. This high-affinity, Na^+-dependent cotransport system was also reported to be present in the jejunum (64) and the brain capillary endothelial cells (65) as well as cardiac myocytes (26). Therefore, as the sodium is cotransported with taurine across these membranes, it is possible that it was trapped inside other types of cells. Consequently, water would be trapped intracellularly to maintain the cellular osmolality (15). As a result, the animals were able to conserve part of the consumed solution intracellularly and to excrete the excess amounts of sodium and solution in the urine (increased UV and U_{Na}, decreased U_{Osm}). This maintained situation was followed up to day 4, at which time the animals developed hypernatremia. Since the animals showed no change in the amounts of solutions (source of sodium) consumed and a stable balance state, the developed hypernatremia may well be due to sodium release from the cells that trapped Na^+ with taurine by the Na^+–K^+–ATPase pump. Another possibility might be a decrease in the plasma and cellular fluid content. A judgment on the events taking place would be facilitated by measuring water distribution between the intra- and extracellular compartments.

Increased plasma osmolality further stimulates intake of solution (4–7X C) to dilute the plasma. Because of an unknown mechanism, this intake of solution failed to correct the increased sodium concentration in the plasma because the kidneys were still excreting the excess urine. The combined solution of T + S may be responsible for the renal impairment. Furthermore, solution consumption dropped at day 6 of the treatment, which caused a decrease in the water balance (not significant) and in the sodium balance. A possible reason for this is the accumulation of taurine in the brain cells, which would inhibit fluid intake (20).

Although urine output was slightly depressed, the kidneys continued to excrete the excess sodium (1.5X C) in a larger urine volume as in the prehypertonic period (U_{Osm} was 50–60% X C). The large urine volume was higher than the solution consumption, which caused the drop in the water balance to a negative value. A possible meaning for the increased output is that the kidneys were utilizing needed water as a vehicle to excrete the salt load, thus losing water that could serve to dilute the extracellular osmolality. It is possible that the thirst center was then stimulated to overcome the depressed intake of the solution. However, the regulatory mechanisms in the body failed to restore the Na^+–water balance or even to correct the high plasma concentration back to normal. Studying the taurine balance in the body could be integrated into future studies, since it would then be possible to know how the body would deal with taurine in the combined solution. Furthermore, studying the plasma concentration of aldosterone and vasopressin in the taurine plus saline model may be essential.

Weanlings receiving taurine and saline were able to respond after 24 hours, as did their adult counterparts. These animals showed an increasing pattern of positive water balance and a fluctuating Na^--balance when compared to normal rats. These animals developed severe and increasing hypernatremia earlier and greater than their adult counterparts.

As the weanlings were drinking the combined solution, plasma hyperosmolality activated the thirst center, inducing further intake of the solution. We suggest that a transient plasma volume expansion might have occurred, causing the release of ANP and thus diuresis and natriuresis. Since renal maturity is known to be incomplete in rats until the age of 41 days (61,62), the kidneys will not be effectively capable of retaining water or even sodium from the filtrate. This would explain the high urine sodium concentration and urine volumes excreted. Therefore, continuous increase in solution consumption accompanied with a continuous increase in the urine volume, adding to that the limited ability to retain water from the kidneys, would prevent plasma volume expansion. A study performed on weanlings drinking the combined solution of taurine plus saline (1.8%) showed no volume expansion (37).

It is well documented that the young rats have a higher taurine accumulative capacity than the adults (63), since taurine is important for growth as reported in the literature (66). This uptake of taurine would increase the pattern of positive water balance throughout the treatment period in the weanlings, more so than in the adults. Since Na^+ will be released from the cells by the Na^+–K^+–ATPase pump, the osmolality would increase, causing a continuous increase in solution consumption that was higher than that of the adults drinking the combined solution. Also, the Na^+ concentration in urine was similar to that of the adults, and the urine volume output (/100 g Bwt) was 50% higher than that of their adult counterparts. This suggests that the hypernatremia that developed may well be due to the larger loss of relative water in the weanlings than in the adults.

Throughout the experiment, the two age groups drinking the combined solution of taurine and saline displayed a decrease in their feeding pattern that was probably due to the taurine added to the solution. It has been reported that the increase in the hypothalamic concentration of taurine will depress food drives (67). Therefore, these animals lost weight and died earlier than the other adults.

In conclusion, adults receiving the combined solution of taurine plus saline showed maintained Na^+-balance during the first period of the treatment, while it dropped towards the end of the experiment. Weanlings, on the other hand, showed a fluctuation in their Na^+-balance pattern as soon as they started on the regime. This may be due to the interference by taurine, in the combined solution, with the regulatory mechanisms in the body. The water balance study suggested that the combined solution drinking rats (adults and weanlings) were facing a homeostatic dilemma in their attempt to correct Na^+-balance. Since these animals displayed a reduced ability to concentrate urine, their unsuccessful attempt to correct P_{Na} occurred at the expense of water conservation and/or osmolality regulation. Moreover, since taurine introduced in the diet with saline would cause these renal disturbances, they may also be interfering with the distribution of other ions, such as calcium, which is highly related to sodium, in a way that may cause hemodynamic oscillation of catastrophic action on the cardiovascular system. Further studies on the effect of the combined solutions on the cardiac system in both age groups are endorsed. Also, it is difficult to judge the hormonal changes taking place in this model, knowing that the pattern of response of the animals studied will help in studying the changes taking place in the proposed mechanisms.

SUMMARY

It has been shown repeatedly that animals that drink a combined solution of taurine (T) and saline (S) develop hypernatremia within a few days. In the present study, the effect of a combined solution of 0.1 M T + 1.5% S on sodium and water balance for 8 days in two age groups was studied. Experiments were performed on adult (65–85 days old) and weanling (28–32 days old) rats. Each group was subdivided into four treatment regimes: C (tapwater): T (0.1 M T): S (1.5% NaCl) and T + S. In both age groups, Na^+-balance was positive and stable in groups C, T, and S throughout the treatment period. Plasma sodium concentration (P_{Na}) remained normal (i.e., 150 mmol/L or less in the C, T, and S drinkers), except that weanlings drinking S developed moderate hypernatremia (151.5 ± 1.7 mmol/L). In the adult T + S drinkers, the mean P_{Na} had risen from 145 ± 1.2 mmol/L to 160.0 ± 6.4 mmol/L by day 4 and the Na^+-balance became negative toward the end of the experimental period. These changes persisted throughout the treatment period. On the other hand, weanlings drinking T + S developed a dramatic increase in the P_{Na} starting from day 2 (161.0 ± 4.9 mmol/L) and increasing to a level of 204.7 ± 8.2 mmol/L by the end of the experimental period. Na^+-balance fluctuated during the treatment period, following a decreasing trend. Among other parameters, in both adults and weanlings, no appreciable differences were noted between C and T groups. Solution consumption (and thus, Na^+ intake) and urine volume were elevated in both S and T + S, with higher values in T + S. Urine Na^+ concentration was also elevated in both S and T + S, while urine osmolality was reduced, although more so in T + S. In S drinkers, age differences were detected in the elevated P_{Na} (147.6 mmol/L in adults; 151.5 mmol/L in weanlings) and urine volume of weanlings was up to 50% higher as compared to their adult counterparts; whereas no significant differences were found in the other parameters. On the other hand, weanlings drinking T + S displayed significantly higher values for solution consumption, P_{Na}, urine volume, sodium excretion rate, and water balance as compared to the adults receiving the combined solution. Based on the data, the water balance explains the ability of the S drinkers to maintain a normal P_{Na} as they excreted part of the volume consumed to eliminate the Na^+ excess. By contrast, T + S drinkers excreted more than the volume consumed in an unsuccessful attempt to restore P_{Na} to normal. This was much more exaggerated in weanlings than in their adult counterparts, because their P_{Na} continued to increase and was associated with an earlier death. This suggests that rats drinking T + S face a homeostatic dilemma in which attempts at Na^+-balance (given the reduced ability to concentrate urine) occur at the expense of water conservation and/or osmolality regulation.

ACKNOWLEDGMENT

This work was supported by a grant MY019 from Kuwait University, Research Administration department. The author would like to acknowledge the technical assistance of Mrs. M. Mathew.

REFERENCES

1. De Bold AJ, Borenstein HB, Veress AT, and Sonnenberg H. A rapid and potent natriuretic response to intravenous injection of atrial myocardial extract in rats. *Life Sci* 1981;28:89–94.
2. McBroom MJ, Rinaudo MS, Clough DL, Mueller GP, Haddy FJ. Taurine and NaCl: untoward effects and a possible role for the heart. In: Iwata H, Lombardini JB, Segawa T, eds. *Taurine and the heart.* Boston: Kluwer; 1989:99–115.
3. Valtin H. Disorders of Na^+ balance: edema renal dysfunction—mechanisms involved in fluid and solute imbalance. Boston: Little, Brown; 1979:57–65.
4. Brensilver JM, Daniels FH, Lefavour GS, Maseptic RM, Lorch JA, Ponte ML, Cortell S. Effect of variations in dietary sodium intake on sodium excretion in mature rats. *Kidney Int* 1985; 27:497–502.
5. Spitzer JA. The role of the kidney in sodium homeostasis during maturation. *Kidney Int* 1982;21:539–545.
6. Grunet RR, Meyer JH, Phillips PH. The sodium and potassium requirements of the rat for growth. *J Nutr* 1950;42:609–618.
7. Peuler JD, Beyer KH. Sodium balance and blood pressure during high sodium ingestion in spontaneously hypertensive and Wistar Kyoto normotensive rats. *Pharmacology* 1985;30:83–85.
8. Lundin S, Herlitz H, Hallbck-Nordlander M, Ricksten S, Gtheberg G, Berglund G. Sodium balance during development of hypertension in the spontaneously hypertensive rat (SHR). *Acta Physiol Scand* 1982;115:317–323.
9. Frohlich ED, Chien Y, Sesoko S, Pegram BL. Relationship between dietary sodium intake, hemodynamics and cardiac mass in SHR and WKY. *Am J Physiol* 1993;264:R30–R34.
10. Yuan B, Leenen FHH. Dietary intake and left ventricular hypertrophy in normotensive rats. *Am J Physiol* 1991;261:H1397–H1401.
11. Kawano Y, Sudo RT, Ferrario CM. Effects of chronic intraventricular sodium on blood pressure and fluid balance. *Hypertension* 1991;17:28–35.
12. Awapara J. The metabolism of taurine in the animal. In: Huxtable R, Barbeau A, eds. *Taurine.* New York: Raven Press; 1976:1–19.
13. Spaeth DG, Schneider DL. Taurine metabolism: effects of diet and bile salt metabolism. In: Huxtable R, Barbeau A, eds. *Taurine.* New York: Raven Press; 1976:35–44.
14. Iwata H, Baba A, Yoneda Y. Some factors affecting the concentration of tissue or urinary taurine. In: Huxtable R, Barbeau A, eds. *Taurine.* New York: Raven Press; 1976:85–90.
15. Trachtman H, Del Pizzo R, Sturman JA, Huxtable RJ, Finberg L: Taurine and osmoregulation: II. Administration of taurine analogues affords cerebral osmoprotection during chronic hypernatremic dehydration. *Am J Dis Child* 1988;142:1194–1198.

16. Chesney RW, Lippincott S, Gusowski N, Padilla M, Zelikovic I. Studies on renal adaptation to altered dietary amino acid intake: tissue responses in nursing and adult rats. *J Nutr* 1986;116:1965–1976.
17. Sturman JA. Taurine pool sizes in rat: Effects of vitamin B-6 deficiency and high taurine diet. *J Nutr* 1973;103:1566–1580.
18. Walz W, Allen AF. Evaluation of the osmoregulatory function of taurine in brain cells. *Exp Brain Res* 1987;68:290–298.
19. Nara Y, Yamori Y, Lovenberg W. Effect of dietary taurine on blood pressure in spontaneously hypertensive rats. *Biochem Pharmacol* 1978;27:2689–2692.
20. Abe M, Shibata K, Matsuda T, Furukawa T. Inhibition of hypertension and salt intake by oral taurine treatment in hypertensive rats. *Hypertension* 1987;10:383–389.
21. Meldrum MJ, Tu R, Patterson T Jr RD, Petty T. The effect of taurine on blood pressure, and urinary sodium, potassium and calcium excretion. In: Huxtable R and D.V. Michalk eds. *Taurine in health and disease.* D.V. Michalk. New York: Plenum Press; 1994:207–215.
22. Fujita T, Sato Y. Hypotensive effect of taurine: possible involvement of the sympathetic nervous system and endogenous opiates. *J Clin Invest* 1988;993–997.
23. Awapara J, Berg M. Uptake of taurine by slices of rat heart and kidney. In: Huxtable R, Barbeau A, eds. *Taurine.* New York: Raven Press; 1976;82(3):135–143.
24. Zelikovic I, Stejskal-Lorenz E, Lohstroh P, Budreau A, Chesney RW. Anion dependence of taurine transport by rat renal brush-border membrane vesicles. *Am J Physiol* 1989;256:F646–F655.
25. Uchida S, Kwon HM, Yamauchi A, Preston AS, Marumo F, Handler JS. Molecular cloning of the cDNA for an MDCK cell Na^+- and Cl^--dependent taurine transporter that is regulated by hypertonicity. *Proc Natl Acad Sci USA* 1992;89:8230–8234.
26. Chapman RA, Suleiman M-S, Earm YE. Taurine and the heart. *Cardiovasc Res* 1993;27:358–363.
27. Satoh H, Sperelakis N. Effect of taurine on Ca^{2+} currents in young embryonic chick cardiomyocytes. *Gen Pharmacol* 1993;26(3):517–521.
28. Satoh H. Regulation by taurine of the spontaneous activity in young embryonic chick cardiomyocytes. *J Cardiovasc Pharmacol* 1995;25:3–8.
29. Satoh H. Taurine-induced hyperpolarizing shift of the reversal potential of the fast Na^+ current in embryonic chick cardiomyocytes. *Eur J Pharmacol* 1995;231:443–449.
30. Suleiman M-D, Rodrigo GC, Chapman RA. Interdependence of intracellular taurine and sodium in guinea pig heart. *Cardiovasc Res* 1992;26:897–905.
31. Ideishi M, Miura S-I, Sakai T, Sasaguri M, Misumi Y, Arakawa K. Taurine amplifies renal kallikrein and prevents salt-induced hypertension in Dahl rats. *J Hypertension* 1994;12:653–661.
32. Nakanishi T, Uyama O, Sugita M. Osmotically regulated taurine content in rat renal inner medulla. *Am J Physiol* 1991;261:F957–F962.
33. García-Pérez A. Organic osmolytes in the kidney. *Semin Nephrol* 1993;13:182–190.
34. Dlouha H, McBroom MJ. Atrial natriuretic factor in taurine-treated normal and cardiomyopathic hamsters. *Proc Soc Exp Biol Med* 1986;181:411–415.
35. Dlouha H, Krecek J. Age-dependent differences in the effect of atrial natriuretic factor. *Life Sci* 1985;37:2523–2529.
36. Dlouha H, Krecek J. Hypernatremia in taurine and saline drinking rats any link to atrial natriuretic factor (ANF). *Fed Proc* 1986;45:1023.
37. Al-Kady MM. The effect of drinking taurine and NaCl solutions on the volume and composition of blood in young and adult rats. M.Sc. Thesis, Kuwait University College of Graduate Studies, Kuwait, 1986.
38. Jamieson JD, Palade GE. Specific granules in atrial muscle cells. *J Cell Biol* 1964;23:151–172.
39. Needleman P, Greenwald JE. Atriopeptin: a cardiac hormone intimately involved in fluid, electrolyte, and blood pressure homeostasis. *N Engl J Med* 1986;314:828–834.
40. Garcia R, Cantin M, Thibault G, Ong H, Genest J. Relationship of specific granules to the natriuretic and diuretic activity of rat atria. *Experientia* 1982;38:1071–1073.
41. Ledsome JR, Wilson N, Courneya CA, Rankin AJ. Release of atrial natriuretic peptide by atrial distension. *Can J Physiol Pharmacol* 1985;63:739–742.
42. Shenker Y, Sider RS, Ostafin EA, Grekin RJ. Plasma levels of immunoreactive atrial natriuretic factor in health subjects and in patients with edema. *J Clin Invest* 1985;76:1684–1687.
43. Borenstein HB, Cupples WA, Sonnenberg H, Veress AT. The effect of a natriuretic atrial extract on renal haemodynamics and urinary excretion in anaesthetized rats. *J Physiol* 1983;334:133–140.
44. Cogan MG. Atrial natriuretic factor can increase renal solute excretion primarily by raising glomerular filtration. *Am J Physiol* 1986;250:F710–F714.

45. Sonnenberg H, Honrath U, Chong CK, Wilson DR. Atrial natriuretic factor inhibits sodium transport in medullary collecting duct. *Am J Physiol* 1986;250:F963–F966.
46. Atarashi K, Mulrow PJ, Franco-Saenz R. Effect of atrial peptides on aldosterone production. *J Clin Invest* 1985;76:1807–1811.
47. Schultz HD, Steele MK, Gardner DG. Central administration of atrial peptide decreases sympathetic outflow in rats. *Am J Physiol* 1990;258:R1250–R1256.
48. Bierd TM, Kattwinkel J, Chevalier RL, Rheuban KS, Smith DJ, Teague WG, Carey RM, Linden J. Interrelationship of atrial natriuretic peptide, atrial volume, and renal function in premature infants. *J Pediatr* 1990;116:753–759.
49. Muchant DG, Belmonte DC, Garmey MJ, Baertschi AJ, Pence RA, Chevalier RL. Dietary sodium modulates neonatal but not adult cardiac atrial natriuretic peptide in rats. *Pediatr Res* 1995;37: 310–315.
50. Muchant DG, Thornhill BA, Belmonte DC, Felder RA, Baertschi AJ, Chevalier RL. Chronic sodium loading augments natriuretic response to acute volume expansion in the preweaned rat. *Am J Physiol* 1995;269:R15–R22.
51. Korytkowski MT, Ladenson PW. Age-related changes in basal and sodium-stimulated atrial and plasma atrial natriuretic factor (ANF) in the rat. *J Gerentol* 1991;46(3):B107–B110.
52. Chevalier RL, Garmey M, Scarborough RM, Linden J, Gomez RA, Peach MJ, Carey RM. Inhibition of ANP clearance receptors and endopeptidase 24.11 in maturing rats. *Am J Physiol* 1991;260:R1218–R1228.
53. Lachance D, Garcia R. Atrial natriuretic factor release by angiotensin II in the conscious rat. *Hypertension* 1988;11:502–508.
54. Al-Bader M. The effect of a combined taurine and saline intake on rats: role of atrial natriuretic peptide; effect of uninephrectomy. M.Sc. Thesis, Kuwait University College of Graduate Studies, Kuwait, 1992.
55. McCance RA, Widdowson EM. The response of the new-born puppy to water, salt and food. *J Physiol* 1958;141:81–87.
56. Dixon WJ, Brown MB, Engelman L, Jennrich RI. BMDP statistical software manual. Los Angeles: University of California Press; 1990:1170–1176.
57. Ota M, Crofton JT, Liu H, Festavan G, Share L. Increased plasma osmolality stimulates peripheral and central vasopressin release in male and female rats. *Am J Physiol* 1994;267:R923–R928.
58. Schiffrin E. Regulation of receptors for atrial natriuretic peptide in the rat and human. *Cardiovasc Drug Ther* 1988;2:493–500.
59. Nonoguchi H, Sands JM, Knepper MA. Atrial natriuretic factor inhibits vasopressin-stimulated osmotic water permiability in rat inner medullary collecting duct. *J Clin Invest* 1988;282:1383–1390.
60. Nonoguchi H, Sands JM, Knepper MA. ANF inhibits NaCl and fluid absorption in cortical collecting duct of rat kidney. *Am J Physiol* 1989;256:F179–F186.
61. Solomon S. Developmental changes in nephron number, proximal tubular length and superficial nephron glomerular filtration rate of rats. *J Physiol* 1977;272:573–589.
62. Dobrovic-Jenik D, Ozegovic B, Malkovic S. Postnatal development of rat kidney plasma membrane Na-K-ATPase. *Biol Neonate* 1984;46:115–121.
63. Sharfafuddin M, Nassar GM, Nassar CF. Taurine transport across the small intestine of adult and suckling rats. *Comp Biochem Physiol* 1987;91(1):33–36.
64. Barnard JA, Thaxter S, Kikuchi K, Ghisham FK. Taurine transport by rat intestine. *Am J Physiol* 1988;254:G334–G338.
65. Tayarani I, Cloz I, Lefauconnier JM, Bourre JM. Sodium-dependent high-affinity uptake of taurine by isolated rat brain capillaries. *Biochem Biophys Acta* 1989;985:168–172.
66. Sturman JA. Taurine in development. *J Nutr* 1988;118:1169–1176.
67. Thut PD, Hruska RE, Huxtable R, Bressler R. Effect of taurine on eating and drinking behaviour. In: Huxtable R, Barbeau A, eds. *Taurine*. New York: Raven Press; 1976:357–364.

Subject Index

R